Advanced Nanoscience of Biomaterials for Biomedical Applications (Volume II)

Advanced Nanoscience of Biomaterials for Biomedical Applications (Volume II)

Guest Editor

Kwang-Sun Kim

MDPI

Basel • Beijing • Wuhan • Barcelona • Belgrade • Novi Sad • Cluj • Manchester

Guest Editor
Kwang-Sun Kim
Department of Chemistry and
Chemistry Institute for
Functional Materials
Pusan National University
Busan
Republic of Korea

Editorial Office
MDPI AG
Grosspeteranlage 5
4052 Basel, Switzerland

This is a reprint of the Special Issue, published open access by the journal *Pharmaceutics* (ISSN 1999-4923), freely accessible at: https://www.mdpi.com/journal/pharmaceutics/special_issues/1CPL9IHZVW.

For citation purposes, cite each article independently as indicated on the article page online and as indicated below:

Lastname, A.A.; Lastname, B.B. Article Title. *Journal Name* **Year**, *Volume Number*, Page Range.

ISBN 978-3-7258-7302-9 (Hbk)
ISBN 978-3-7258-7303-6 (PDF)
https://doi.org/10.3390/books978-3-7258-7303-6

Contents

About the Editor . . . . **vii**

Atanu Naskar and Kwang-sun Kim
Photo-Stimuli-Responsive CuS Nanomaterials as Cutting-Edge Platform Materials for Antibacterial Applications
Reprinted from: *Pharmaceutics* **2022**, *14*, 2343,
https://doi.org/10.3390/pharmaceutics14112343 . . . . **1**

Atanu Naskar and Kwang-sun Kim
Friends against the Foe: Synergistic Photothermal and Photodynamic Therapy against Bacterial Infections
Reprinted from: *Pharmaceutics* **2023**, *15*, 1116,
https://doi.org/10.3390/pharmaceutics15041116 . . . . **18**

Ugo D'Amora, Sawsan Dacrory, Mohamed Sayed Hasanin, Angela Longo, Alessandra Soriente, Samir Kamel, et al.
Advances in the Physico-Chemical, Antimicrobial and Angiogenic Properties of Graphene-Oxide/Cellulose Nanocomposites for Wound Healing
Reprinted from: *Pharmaceutics* **2023**, *15*, 338,
https://doi.org/10.3390/pharmaceutics15020338 . . . . **40**

Hala N. ElShagea, Rana R. Makar, Alaa H. Salama, Nermeen A. Elkasabgy and Emad B. Basalious
Investigating the Targeting Power to Brain Tissues of Intranasal Rasagiline Mesylate-Loaded Transferosomal In Situ Gel for Efficient Treatment of Parkinson's Disease
Reprinted from: *Pharmaceutics* **2023**, *15*, 533,
https://doi.org/10.3390/pharmaceutics15020533 . . . . **73**

Gabriela Petrișor, Ludmila Motelica, Denisa Ficai, Cornelia-Ioana Ilie, Roxana Doina Trușcă, Vasile-Adrian Surdu, et al.
Increasing Bioavailability of Trans-Ferulic Acid by Encapsulation in Functionalized Mesoporous Silica
Reprinted from: *Pharmaceutics* **2023**, *15*, 660,
https://doi.org/10.3390/pharmaceutics15020660 . . . . **96**

Dina Saeed Ghataty, Reham Ibrahim Amer, Mai A. Amer, Mohamed F. Abdel Rahman and Rehab Nabil Shamma
Green Synthesis of Highly Fluorescent Carbon Dots from Bovine Serum Albumin for Linezolid Drug Delivery as Potential Wound Healing Biomaterial: Bio-Synergistic Approach, Antibacterial Activity, and In Vitro and Ex Vivo Evaluation
Reprinted from: *Pharmaceutics* **2023**, *15*, 234,
https://doi.org/10.3390/pharmaceutics15010234 . . . . **115**

Eun Jo Jang, Rajkumar Patel and Madhumita Patel
Electrospinning Nanofibers as a Dressing to Treat Diabetic Wounds
Reprinted from: *Pharmaceutics* **2023**, *15*, 1144,
https://doi.org/10.3390/pharmaceutics15041144 . . . . **140**

Nikolay Zahariev, Milena Draganova, Plamen Zagorchev and Bissera Pilicheva
Casein-Based Nanoparticles: A Potential Tool for the Delivery of Daunorubicin in Acute Lymphocytic Leukemia
Reprinted from: *Pharmaceutics* **2023**, *15*, 471,
https://doi.org/10.3390/pharmaceutics15020471 . . . . **162**

Atanu Naskar, Hyejin Cho and Kwang-sun Kim
A Nanocomposite with Extracellular Vesicles from *Lactobacillus paracasei* as a Bioinspired Nanoantibiotic Targeting *Staphylococcus aureus*
Reprinted from: *Pharmaceutics* **2022**, *14*, 2273,
https://doi.org/10.3390/pharmaceutics14112273 . . . . **179**

Lucas Prestianni, Eric R. Espinal, Sarah F. Hathcock, Nadine Vollmuth, Pixiang Wang, Robert A. Holler, et al.
Synthesis and Characterization of Quercetin–Iron Complex Nanoparticles for Overcoming Drug Resistance
Reprinted from: *Pharmaceutics* **2023**, *15*, 1041,
https://doi.org/10.3390/pharmaceutics15041041 . . . . **194**

Md. Khalid Anwer, Mohammed Muqtader Ahmed, Mohammed F. Aldawsari, Muzaffar Iqbal, Gamal A. Soliman and Ibrahim A. Aljuffali
Eluxadoline-Loaded Eudragit Nanoparticles for Irritable Bowel Syndrome with Diarrhea: Formulation, Optimization Using Box–Behnken Design, and Anti-Diarrheal Activity
Reprinted from: *Pharmaceutics* **2023**, *15*, 1460,
https://doi.org/10.3390/pharmaceutics15051460 . . . . **211**

Abdullah I. El-Kholy, Maha Fadel, Maha Nasr, Ibrahim El-Sherbiny, Abeer Tawfik, Yasser O. Mosaad, et al.
Gold-Polypyrrole-Loaded Eosin in Photo-Mediated Treatment of Hidradenitis Suppurativa: In Vivo Trans-Epidermal Permeation Study and Clinical Case Report
Reprinted from: *Pharmaceutics* **2022**, *14*, 2197,
https://doi.org/10.3390/pharmaceutics14102197 . . . . **228**

Mihaela Balas, Simona Liliana Iconaru, Anca Dinischiotu, Nicolas Buton and Daniela Predoi
Response of the Endogenous Antioxidant Defense System Induced in RAW 264.7 Macrophages upon Exposure to Dextran-Coated Iron Oxide Nanoparticles
Reprinted from: *Pharmaceutics* **2023**, *15*, 552,
https://doi.org/10.3390/pharmaceutics15020552 . . . . **236**

Michal Kluknavsky, Andrea Micurova, Martin Skratek, Peter Balis, Monika Okuliarova, Jan Manka, et al.
A Single Infusion of Polyethylene Glycol-Coated Superparamagnetic Magnetite Nanoparticles Alters Differently the Expressions of Genes Involved in Iron Metabolism in the Liver and Heart of Rats
Reprinted from: *Pharmaceutics* **2023**, *15*, 1475,
https://doi.org/10.3390/pharmaceutics15051475 . . . . **254**

About the Editor

Kwang-Sun Kim

Kwang-Sun Kim is a Professor of Chemistry at Pusan National University (PNU), Korea. His research focuses on understanding antibiotic resistance and developing innovative antimicrobial platforms, including nanomaterials and extracellular-vesicle-based vaccines and therapeutics. He received his Ph.D. in Biochemistry from KAIST in 2004 and completed postdoctoral training at KAIST and in Stanley N. Cohen's lab at Stanford University. From 2009 to 2015, he served as a Senior Researcher at the Korea Research Institute of Bioscience and Biotechnology (KRIBB). His work integrates biomedical and environmental applications of advanced vaccine and antimicrobial technologies.

pharmaceutics

MDPI

Review

Photo-Stimuli-Responsive CuS Nanomaterials as Cutting-Edge Platform Materials for Antibacterial Applications

Atanu Naskar and Kwang-sun Kim *

Department of Chemistry and Chemistry Institute for Functional Materials, Pusan National University, Busan 46241, Korea

* Correspondence: kwangsun.kim@pusan.ac.kr; Tel.: +82-51-510-2241

Abstract: Photo-stimuli-responsive therapeutic nanomaterials have gained widespread attention as frontline materials for biomedical applications. The photoactivation strategies are classified as single-modality (based on either reactive oxygen species (ROS)-based photodynamic therapy (PDT), hyperthermia-based photothermal therapy (PTT)), or dual-modality (which combines PDT and PTT). Due to its minimal invasiveness, phototherapy has been extensively applied as an efficient therapeutic platform for many diseases, including skin cancers. However, extensive implementation of phototherapy to address the emergence of multidrug-resistant (MDR) bacterial infections remains challenging. This review focuses on copper sulfide (CuS) nanomaterials as efficient and cost-effective PDT and PTT therapeutic nanomaterials with antibacterial activity. The features and merits of CuS nanomaterials as therapeutics are compared to those of other nanomaterials. Control of the dimensions and morphological complexity of CuS nanomaterials through judicious synthesis is then introduced. Both the in vitro antibacterial activity and the in vivo therapeutic effect of CuS nanomaterials and derivative nanocomposites composed of 2D nanomaterials, polymers, metals, metal oxides, and proteins are described in detail. Finally, the perspective of photo-stimuli-responsive CuS nanomaterials for future clinical antibacterial applications is highlighted. This review illustrates that CuS nanomaterials are highly effective, low-toxic, and environmentally friendly antibacterial agents or platform nanomaterials for combatting MDR bacterial infections.

Keywords: photo-stimuli-responsive nanomaterial; CuS; photodynamic therapy; photothermal therapy; antibacterial

1. Introduction

Bacterial infection has become one of the largest healthcare challenges for humans that requires immediate attention. According to World Health Organization (WHO) predictions, by 2050, ten million people will die every year from infectious bacterial diseases [1]. Moreover, the overuse and misuse of antibiotics are serious issues, as bacteria are becoming increasingly resistant to most available antibiotics [2]. Hence, it is easy to understand the urgent need for a solution or alternative to antibiotics. In this regard, researchers are targeting light sources a modern medical or alternative tool for treating bacterial infections [3]. Different wavelengths of light, ranging from ultraviolet (UV) to near-infrared (NIR), have been utilized with photo-stimuli-responsive nanomaterials to eliminate various bacteria [4]. This method is target-specific and, more importantly, the possibility of bacterial resistance can be avoided.

Reactive oxygen species (ROS)-based photodynamic therapy (PDT) and hyperthermia-based photothermal therapy (PTT) are the two modes of this photoactivated antibacterial activity [4]. Despite the wide use of these approaches for enhancing antibacterial activity, each has its own limitations, such as UV light contamination of healthy tissues in PDT and the high temperature/high dosage of the photothermal agent (PTA) required in PTT [5]. Therefore, researchers have proposed a multimodal strategy in which PDT and PTT can be combined in a single nanomaterial or nanocomposite to achieve more effective antibacterial activity [5].

CuS, a p-type semiconductor, is known for its multifunctional properties and is widely used in various biomedical nanomaterials for anticancer, bioimaging, antibacterial, and other applications [6]. The optical properties of CuS are comparable to those of widely used noble metals (Au and Ag), which are extensively utilized for biomedical applications. However, the advantage of CuS over other NIR-absorbing nanomaterials (e.g., Ag and Au) is that the NIR absorption range of CuS is 700–1000 nm. It is also known that the absorption of CuS at >900 nm can be tuned by altering the stoichiometry [6]. Notably, biological tissues have almost no absorption in this NIR region, which in turn enhances the spatial resolution of photoacoustic imaging by reducing background noise and reducing the harm to healthy tissue.

The photodynamic and photothermal properties of CuS also depend on the morphology of the sample [7], and thus can be controlled by morphology modulation. Moreover, the antibacterial activity can be enhanced by the multimodal strategy of combining PDT and PTT through the use of CuS nanomaterials or CuS nanocomposites [7–10]. Furthermore, for clinical application in the NIR region, both PDT and PTT can be combined using a singular nanomaterial.

In this review, we highlight the importance of photo-stimuli-responsive nanomaterials with antibacterial activity and different types of such nanomaterials. The advantages of CuS nanomaterials upon achieving antibacterial action are compared with those of other photo-stimuli-responsive nanomaterials. A detailed description of methods to synthesize dimension-controlled CuS nanomaterials [zero-dimensional (0D), one-dimensional (1D), two-dimensional (2D), and three-dimensional (3D)] is presented, after which the photo-stimuli-responsive antibacterial applications of CuS and its nanocomposites are discussed. Finally, the prospects and challenges of obtaining CuS nanomaterials with antibacterial activity are described.

2. Phototherapy and Antibacterial Activity

2.1. Importance of Photo-Stimuli-Responsive Nanomaterials with Antibacterial Activity

In recent years, phototherapy has received a great deal of attention for its obvious advantages of minimal invasiveness and clinical safety [11,12]. Moreover, light sources with a specific wavelength range can enable confined irradiation of a pre-defined area using advanced instruments [3]. Niels Ryberg Finsen, the founder of modern phototherapy, showed that the skin disease lupus vulgaris can be treated using sunlight and ultraviolet (UV) irradiation, for which he was awarded the Nobel Prize in 1903 [13,14]. From that point onward, phototherapy has continued to gain increasing importance in biomedical applications. After the introduction of phototherapeutic agents, such as photosensitizers and photothermal conversion agents, the use of phototherapy in many biomedical applications, including anticancer and antibacterial treatments, has grown rapidly [7–10,15]. Moreover, the development of various phototherapeutic nano-agents has given more impetus to this already important sector [16].

In terms of antibacterial activity, phototherapy or photo-activated sterilization has shown immense potential in combatting infectious bacterial diseases and is regarded as an apt alternative to antibiotics that does not induce bacterial resistance [4,5]. In general, photoactivated sterilization can be simplified by utilizing suitable wavelengths of light, ranging from ultraviolet (UV) to NIR, to activate photo-stimuli-responsive nanomaterials. These photo-stimuli-responsive nanomaterials absorb the light energy, inhibiting the growth of pathogens in a short time by producing ROS and/or forming hyperthermic environments [4]. Therefore, this technique can be used to avoid bacterial resistance, which occurs with the long-term use of conventional antibiotics. Moreover, this technique is time-controlled and site specific, i.e., it can selectively target infected sites without damaging other healthy organs or cells.

2.2. Different Types of Photo-Stimuli-Responsive Nanomaterials with Antibacterial Activity

Photoactivated sterilization (Figure 1), also known as photoactivated antibacterial activity, can be categorized into two types: (1) ROS-based photodynamic therapy (PDT); and (2) hyperthermia-based photothermal therapy (PTT).

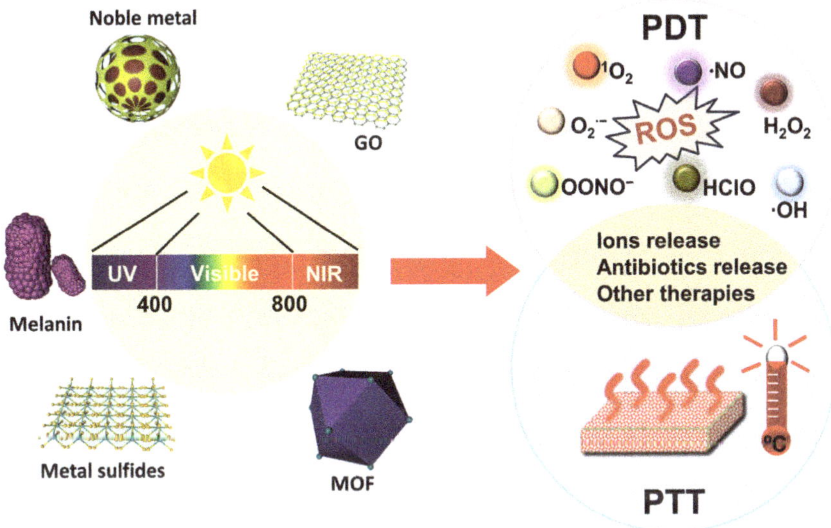

Figure 1. Schematic of photo-stimuli-responsive antibacterial materials and mechanism. Reproduced with permission from Ref. [4]. Copyright 2020 Elsevier.

Generally, light of a given wavelength will excite photosensitizers or photocatalysts to their higher excited state, which will then undergo intersystem crossing and generate free radicals and ROS, such as hydrogen peroxide (H_2O_2), singlet oxygen ($^1O_2$), and hydroxyl radicals (·OH). ROS are commonly believed to be capable of penetrating bacterial membranes and destroying proteins and lipids, thereby killing bacteria. Therapy based on this light-dependent ROS production and the resulting antibacterial activity is called PDT. ROS can also adhere to the bacterial cell membrane and destroy its defense system [17]. Compared with conventional antibiotics, PDT exhibits significant advantages. PDT enables broad-spectrum therapeutic modes, which can simultaneously act on many metabolic pathways and cellular structures of various bacteria, unlike the singular action mode of antibiotics. Moreover, most photosensitizers used for PDT act only after irradiation with light; therefore, the chance of bacterial resistance is remote. However, most photosensitizers for PDT can be activated only in the UV or visible light range and can be harmful to normal tissue [4,17]. Hence, controlling the clinical range of phototherapy, i.e., NIR-light-activated PDT, might well be the future direction for widespread use. Notably, PDT is less effective against Gram-negative bacteria than Gram-positive bacteria due to differences in the membrane structures [18]. These differences in the ROS activity can be attributed to the dense lipopolysaccharide (LPS) structure outside the cell wall (hard to penetrate) of Gram-negative bacteria and multiple layers of loose, porous peptidoglycan (PG) (easy penetration) in Gram-positive bacteria. This is another limitation of PDT that should be overcome in future studies. Photocatalysts, such as TiO_2 [19], ZnO [20], WO_3 [21], and graphitic carbon nitride (g-C_3N_4) [22], as well as photosensitizers, such as porphyrins [23], phthalocyanines [24], phenothiazines [25], and up-conversion luminescence nanomaterials [26], have been effectively used in PDT. Au [27], Ag [28], and CuS [4] can also be used to produce surface plasmon resonance (SPR), which can enhance the effect of PDT, also providing effective antibacterial activity. Similarly, carbon quantum dots [29,30] and organic photosensitizers such as indocyanine green (ICG) [31] can be used synergistically for PDT-based antibacterial activity.

PTT is generally regarded as a safer option compared to PDT in terms of its effectiveness and minimal damage to normal tissues [5]. The basic concept of PTT is that under light stimulation, photothermal agents (PTAs), such as noble-metal nanomaterials (e.g., Ag and Au) [32], metallic sulfides (e.g., CuS) [7–10], carbon-based nanomaterials (e.g., graphene [33] and carbon dots [34]), organic nanomaterials [35], and black phosphorus (BP) [36], can convert solar energy into heat, thereby destroying bacterial cells through hyperthermia. From the earlier days (before the discovery of penicillin), it was recognized that bacteria can be killed at temperatures above 55 °C due to the denaturization of heat-shock proteins [16,37]. Although this approach was previously limited to food preservation, after the invention of PTT, it was regarded as a safe and effective option for killing bacterial cells. NIR light ranging from 700 to 1300 nm is considered as the most non-detrimental light energy for PTT due to its deeper penetration into tissues (more than 3 mm) with minimal damage to healthy tissues, compared to other light sources (e.g., UV and visible), and lower absorption by water and hemoglobin [3]. PTT offers many advantages compared to traditional antibiotic therapy. Firstly, PTT has broad-spectrum antibacterial activity toward various pathogens as the local hyperthermia damages the bacterial structure and disrupts the cell membrane, ultimately inducing bacterial death. Due to this mechanism, the chances of bacteria becoming resistant to PTAs is remote. Furthermore, the treatment time is also short (only a few minutes). Additionally, PTT has the potential to destroy the structure of biofilm by inactivating the inherent bioactive matrix and enabling the penetration of antibacterial agents to kill the protected bacteria [38]. Despite these several advantages of PTT, there are also some limitations that need to be overcome. There is an inevitable chance of damage to normal tissues due to the high power of the excitation light and high dosage of PTAs, which are sometimes needed for hyperthermia treatment [39]. In this regard, the combination of PTT with PDT has recently been considered [7,40]. These multimodal strategies lower the laser density and dosage requirements of PTAs in PTT, and also facilitate cell permeation by ROS generated by the photosensitizers in PDT due to the heat induced by PTT. Therefore, PTT combined with PDT has the ability to not only solve the problems of singular PTT, but also compensate the shortcomings of PDT. Researchers are trying to synthesize nanomaterials that can simultaneously enable PTT and PDT.

2.3. *Photo-Stimuli-Responsive CuS Nanomaterials with Antibacterial Potential*

As discussed earlier (Section 2.2), as isolated strategies, PTT and PDT have intrinsic disadvantages. These include the requirement for high temperatures (PTT), UV-vis irradiation (PDT), and possible damage to healthy biological tissues [5]. Therefore, researchers are trying to design a novel synergistic antibacterial platform, where the advantageous properties of both PDT and PTT are combined and the limitations of each therapy are compensated. CuS is a potentially superior nanomaterial, as it shows both PTT and PDT under irradiation with different wavelengths of light [7–10].

CuS, a semiconducting metal chalcogenide with a narrow bandgap, displays suitable photocatalytic and exceptional photothermal properties [7]. Most importantly, CuS is considered as an excellent PTA due to its excellent potential for antibacterial activity. The light-to-heat conversion characteristics of CuS nanomaterials can be attributed to the d–d energy band transition of Cu^{2+} ions [41]. Due to the excellent NIR absorption and conversion ability of CuS, CuS nanomaterials have the potential to effectively eradicate pathogenic infection. Cu^{2+} is also considered one of the most important trace elements in the human body, playing an essential role in stimulating the wound healing process [42]. The basic advantage of CuS, along with other widely used photoactive nanomaterials, such as Ag and Au, is the ability to absorb NIR light by means of a localized surface plasmonic resonance (LSPR) originating from the collective oscillation of holes in these materials. However, for noble metals, the electrons act as carriers for the same LSPR phenomenon [43]. Unlike noble metals, the LSPR position of CuS can be controlled by modulation of the number of carriers. Hence, relative to other samples, this feature has given CuS-based nanomaterials a significant push toward photoactive applications (e.g., anticancer and antibacterial), especially under NIR irradiation.

Furthermore, CuS exhibits excellent antibacterial properties when doped with metals or non-metals. For example, a CuS/protonated g-C_3N_4 composite showed effective antibacterial activity against Gram-positive and Gram-negative bacteria due to collaborative photodynamic and photothermal bactericidal effects [44]. Similarly, Mutalik et al. [7] demonstrated the potential of CuS with morphology-dependent photodynamic and photothermal antibacterial activity against *E. coli*, facilitated by NIR light. Zhou et al. [45] presented a CuS hybrid hydrogel with the potential to completely eradicate *E. coli* and *S. aureus* via photothermal/photodynamic effects under NIR laser irradiation. A collection of poly(5-(2-ethyl acrylate)-4-methylthiazole-*g*-butyl)/copper sulfide nanoclusters (PATA-C_4@CuS) was also synthesized to effectively kill levofloxacin-resistant Gram-negative and Gram-positive bacteria after NIR laser irradiation [9]. The dual function of PDT and PTT was exploited to achieve effective antibacterial activity. Qiao et al. [46] also demonstrated similar antibacterial potential of CuS nanodots against methicillin-resistant *S. aureus* (MRSA) and extended-spectrum β-lactamase *E. coli* by combining PTT and PDT with NIR laser irradiation. More recently, our group [47] published a BP-based CuS nanoplatform with similar antibacterial activity against *P. aeruginosa* and *S. aureus* in response to NIR light, along with ROS generation.

Despite the numerous advantages of CuS nanomaterials for multimodal PDT and PTT, there are still some limitations to overcome before these materials can be finally utilized for some worthy clinical applications. The toxicity of CuS remains an issue requiring immediate resolution; toxicity is an ever-present issue for nanomaterials for clinical applications. Additionally, the synthesis of CuS is slightly more complex than that of certain other nanomaterials. Therefore, a simple and cost-effective route needs to be established for the synthesis of CuS to facilitate related antibacterial applications. In addition, the required dosage of photo-stimuli-responsive nanomaterials (such as CuS) is still higher than that of antibiotics, which requires more attention when used in clinics. The nondegradable property of photo-stimuli-responsive CuS nanomaterials, along with the phototoxicity of light, are areas that require significant future emphasis.

3. Controllable Synthesis of CuS Nanomaterials

Nanomaterials have attracted great attention for biomedical applications due to their unique physical, chemical, and electronic properties [48,49], which are significantly dependent on the dimensions of the nanomaterials, making them important entities for various applications. We classified the synthesis of CuS nanomaterials in terms of the dimensions (zero-dimensional (0D), one-dimensional (1D), two-dimensional (2D), and three-dimensional (3D)). Various synthesis techniques have been utilized to synthesize CuS nanomaterials with different dimensions, as the morphology of the CuS nanomaterials may vary with the synthesis processes, eventually affecting the final applications. For example, spherical CuS nanomaterials [50] are mainly used in photoacoustic imaging and therapeutics, along with photothermal ablation, whereas hollow nanocubes and nanocages are utilized in drug delivery [51,52]. Furthermore, CuS nanorods and nanowires have been successfully used in biosensing applications to detect food pathogens and immunologically relevant moieties [6]. Therefore, it is easy to agree on the fact that the synthesis technique is a determining factor for CuS nanomaterials and on the corresponding biomedical applications. Therefore, the synthesis of CuS nanomaterials, such as CuS nanoparticles (0D), CuS nanorods, nanowires, nanotubes (1D), CuS nanoplates (2D) and nanospheres, nanocages, and nanoflowers (3D), are discussed according to the dimensionality of the samples.

3.1. *Synthesis of Zero-Dimensional (0D) CuS Nanomaterials*

Despite the availability of various methods of synthesizing 0D materials, only a few 0D CuS nanomaterials have been successfully prepared. Qiao et al. [46] successfully synthesized CuS nanodots by a facile single-step hydrothermal route, where a biocompatible and highly soluble protein, bovine serum albumin (BSA), was utilized to control the particle size and stability of the sample. The CuS nanodots not only eradicated multidrug-resistant bacteria, but also expedited wound healing due to their NIR light-mediated photothermal effect. In another experiment, CuS quantum dots (QDs) were obtained via green synthesis [53]. A transparent solution of starch, which is a natural biodegradable polymer, was used as both a reducing and capping agent for the synthesis of CuS QDs. Moreover, the size of the synthesized CuS QDs was controlled by adjusting the reaction parameters. The CuS QDs selectively sensed Hg^{2+} ions, demonstrating potential toward sustainable nanotechnology. These syntheses demonstrate that 0D CuS nanomaterials can be obtained by simple approaches, and we envision numerous potential biomedical applications of 0D CuS nanomaterials in the future.

3.2. *Synthesis of One-Dimensional (1D) CuS Nanomaterials*

The excellent optical, magnetic, and mechanical properties of 1D nanomaterials are always attractive for researchers [54]. Due to their enhanced catalytic and electrochemical characteristics, 1D CuS nanomaterials are mainly used for biosensor application [6]. However, attempts have been made to use them for other biomedical applications, especially as antibacterial agents [55]. Notably, 1D CuS nanomaterials can vary in diameter from 1 to 100 nm, with nanotube, nanorod, and nanowire morphologies [54].

A wide range of approaches for synthesizing 1D CuS nanomaterials have been explored, varying from hydrothermal to template-assisted, high-pressure autoclave, and other approaches [6]. Along with the synthesis process, the composition, growth conditions, and precursors also play important roles in the formation of 1D CuS nanomaterials, such as CuS nanotubes (30–120 nm) and nanowires (30–80 nm). The basic advantage of CuS nanorods/nanotubes for biomedical applications is their intrinsically high surface area. Bekhit et al. [55], synthesized CuS nanotubes via a green, simple, and effective gamma-radiolysis method without adding any capping or reducing agents. The synthesized CuS nanotubes showed broad-spectrum antimicrobial activity against *Aspergillus niger, Bacillus subtilis, Escherichia coli, Pseudomonas aeruginosa, Staphylococcus aureus*, and yeast. CuS nanotubes have also been utilized in various biomedical applications, including biosensor and anticancer applications [56]. Similarly, CuS nanorods have been synthesized via various methods, such as microwave irradiation and hydrothermal techniques. Manikandan et al. [57] utilized a hydrothermal method to synthesize cellulose acetate (CA)-templated nanorods like CuS fibers using vegetable extract (*Brassica oleracea* var. *italica*). This vegetable extract itself acts as a reducing agent. The synthesized CuS nanorods showed effective antibacterial activity against *E. coli* and *Bacillus cereus*. CuS nanowires are another nanomaterial that has captured research interest due to their basic advantage of a high contact area [58].

3.3. *Synthesis of Two-Dimensional (2D) CuS Nanomaterials*

Although 1D and 3D CuS nanomaterials have been widely synthesized for many applications, including antibacterial agents, 2D CuS nanomaterials are comparatively less explored and limited to nanoplates and thin films [59,60]. Because the biomedical applications of these nanomaterials are not extensively reported, we herein only briefly discuss the structures and related syntheses.

Similar to 1D CuS, hydrothermal and solvothermal approaches are the most explored approaches for synthesizing 2D CuS nanomaterials, where the size of the plates range from 50 to 200 nm. To exploit their antibacterial activity, Mirzaei et al. [59] synthesized CuS nanoplates and anchored them onto g-C_3N_4 nanosheets suspended in a poly(methyl methacrylate) (PMMA) matrix. A hydrothermal method was also used to synthesize CuS nanoplates and the antibacterial activity against *E. coli* and *S. aureus* was assessed, confirming the antibacterial properties of the CuS nanoplates. Nishi et al. [60] successfully synthesized CuS nanoplates for potential localized surface plasmon resonance (LSPR)-

mediated biosensors. Sonochemical [61] and chemical vapor methods were also used to synthesize CuS nanoplates [62].

3.4. Synthesis of Three-Dimensional (3D) CuS Nanomaterials

Researchers have always preferred 3D nanomaterials in comparison with their 0D, 1D, and 2D counterparts for various applications, including biomedical applications. This is due to the unique high surface area and large surface-to-volume ratio, along with the greater structural stability of 3D nanomaterials [54]. Hence, it is easy to understand the extensive use of 3D CuS nanomaterials, such as CuS nanospheres [63], CuS nanocages [64], hierarchical CuS nanomaterials [65], CuS microflowers [66], and hollow CuS [51], for various applications compared to the 0D, 1D, and 2D versions. Several methods, such as the sol–gel, hydrothermal, solvothermal, microwave, and sonochemical approaches, have been used to synthesize 3D CuS nanomaterials [6].

The hydrothermal method seems to be the preferred choice for researchers due to the ready availability of water, low cost, and environment friendly nature. Water can dissolve non-ionic covalent compounds with the use of high temperature and pressure. Water can also be used as both a pressure-transmitting medium and solvent medium, which in-turn lowers the activation energy of the reactions. For example, sodium thiosulfate ($Na_2S_2O_3$) and copper sulfate ($CuSO_4$) aqueous solutions were mixed in deionized water and transferred into Teflon-lined stainless-steel autoclaves for hydrothermal reaction at 180 °C for 12 h to obtain CuS nanospheres [67]. Shu et al. [68] utilized a facile one-pot, template-assisted hydrothermal method to synthesize porous hollow CuS nanospheres. AL-Jawad et al. [69] utilized the hydrothermal process to prepare CuS nanomaterials with strong antibacterial potential against *E. coli*, *P. aeruginosa*, and *S. aureus*.

Microwave irradiation is another simple and widely used approach for synthesizing CuS nanomaterials which is also fast and energy efficient. For example [70], microwave irradiation of a mixture of Cu and S precursors in an aqueous medium yielded CuS nanomaterials in a specific timeframe.

Han et al. [63] utilized a simple template-assisted approach to synthesize 3D hollow CuS nanospheres, which were further used for the controlled delivery of doxorubicin, improving the photothermal-chemotherapeutic effect.

From the above discussion of the synthesis methods, it is clear that various factors, such as the precursor salt, solvent, reaction temperature, applied pressure, and surfactant, govern the synthesis of various CuS nanomaterials, which in turn directs the resulting applications.

4. Photo-Stimuli-Responsive Antibacterial Applications of CuS and Its Nanocomposites

As discussed in Section 2.3, CuS has excellent photoactivated antibacterial properties and shows promising antibacterial activity when irradiated in the so-called biological window (i.e., NIR region) [71]. In this section, we further discuss the photo-stimuli-responsive antibacterial applications of CuS and its nanocomposites (Table 1).

4.1. CuS Nanomaterials

CuS nanomaterials exhibit inherent photoactivated antibacterial potential, especially in the NIR region. For example, Qiao et al. [46], developed ultrasmall copper sulfide (covellite) nanodots (CuS NDs), which showed effectiveness in the treatment of multidrug-resistant bacteria-infected chronic non-healing wounds. The dual functional mode of the CuS nanosystem enabled eradication of extended-spectrum β-lactamase (ESBL) *E. coli* and methicillin-resistant *S. aureus* (MRSA) in both in vitro and in vivo studies, while simultaneously expediting wound healing. The NIR laser (808 nm, 2.5 W·cm^{-2})-mediated photothermal effect and remote control of copper-ion (Cu^{2+}) release were the main origins of the dual-mode activity. Ren et al. [72] utilized CuS nanoparticles (NPs) to prepare a photothermal antibacterial silk fabric. A chitosan quaternary ammonium salt (QCS) was used as a template. The antibacterial efficiency of CuS NP-deposited silk fabric with QCS as a template (SF/QCS/CuS) resulted in 99.99% bacterial death of *S. aureus* and *E. coli* within 5 min of irradiation (400 mW·cm^{-2}). The nanocomposite also showed good UV-resistance and superb light-to-heat conversion efficiency. Even after 10 washes, the antibacterial activity of the nanocomposite remained at a high level, demonstrating excellent bonding between the photothermal nanomaterials. In a similar experiment, CuS NPs were coated onto glass slides, and the antibacterial properties were investigated [43]. The CuS NP–glass samples showed good stability and an admirable photothermal effect when irradiated with NIR light. The samples were also effective for the controlled release of copper in water. Hence, the antibacterial activity of the CuS NP-glass samples against *E. coli* and *S. aureus* was attributed to the dual mechanism of hyperthermia-induced NIR laser irradiation and the slow and sustained copper release. As discussed earlier, CuS has shown morphology-dependent photodynamic and photothermal antibacterial activities [7]. This study also proves that CuS itself can be employed for simultaneous ROS-mediated photodynamic therapy and hyperthermia-mediated photothermal therapy (Figure 2). A hydrothermal process was utilized to synthesize CuS microspheres (MSs), CuS nanosheets (NSs), and CuS nanoparticles (NPs) by using three different solvents (ethanol, glycerol, and water, respectively). In this case, the antibacterial activity against *E. coli* was attributed to ROS production and heat generation after irradiation with simulated solar and NIR light. Thus, all the above reports on CuS demonstrate its immense inherent photoactive antibacterial potential. However, CuS can also be utilized in nanocomposites by combining it with a polymer, 2D nanomaterial, metal, protein, or other material, as discussed in the ensuing sections.

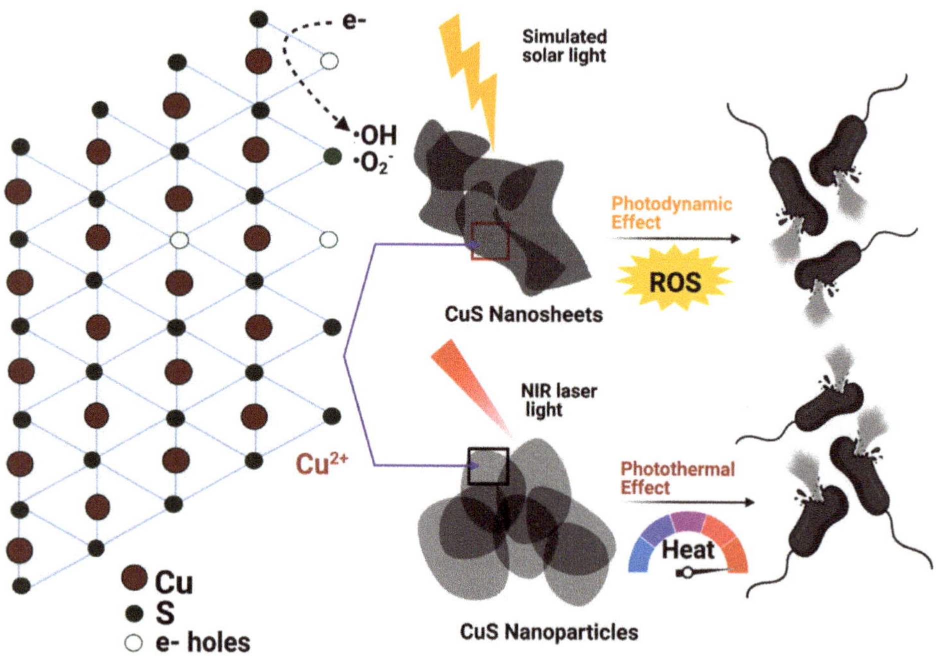

Figure 2. Schematic illustration of CuS NSs and NPs mediated photodynamic and photothermal antibacterial pathways. Reproduced with permission from Ref. [7]. Copyright 2022 Elsevier.

Table 1. Antibacterial activity of phoactivated CuS nanomaterials.

Photoactivated CuS	Antibacterial Mechanism	Light Source	Bacteria	Efficacy	Ref.
CuS NDs	PTT & Cu^{2+} release	NIR (808 nm, 2.5 W·cm^{-2})	ESBL *E. coli*, MRSA	~100%	[46]
CuS NPs	PTT	UV (400 mW·cm^{-2})	*E. coli*, *S. aureus*	99.99%	[72]
CuS NPs	PTT	NIR (800, 900, and 1000 nm, 0.26 W·cm^{-2})	*E. coli*, *S. aureus*	95% (>5 h)	[43]
CuS MSs, NSs, NPs	PDT, PTT	Simulated solar light and NIR (808 nm, 1.5 W·cm^{-2})	*E. coli*	Effective	[7]
CuS/GO	PTT	Visible light (0.2 W·cm^{-2})	*E. coli*, *S. aureus*	99.98%	[73]
PEG-CuS@g-C_3N_4	PTT	NIR (808 nm, 2.5 W)	*E. coli*, *S. aureus*	~99%	[74]
$Ti_3C_2T_x$@CuS	PDT, PTT	NIR (808 nm, 1.5 W)	*E. coli*, *S. aureus*	~99%	[8]
CuS-BP	PDT, PTT	NIR (808 nm, 2.5 W)	*P. aeruginosa*, *S. aureus*	~100%	[47]
PATAC4@CuS	PDT, PTT	NIR (980 nm, 1.5 W·cm^{-2})	*Bacillus amyloliquefaciens*, *E. coli*, *P. aeruginosa*, Levofloxacin-resistant *S. aureus*	Effective	[9]
MUH@CuS NCs	PTT	NIR	*E. coli*	~100%	[75]
BSA-CuS NPs	PTT	NIR (808, 8.0 W·cm^{-2})	*A. baumannii*, *S. aureus*, *S. haemolyticus*	Effective	[76]
Ce6-labeled BSA-CuS NPs	PDT, PTT	NIR (980 nm, 1.59 W·cm^{-2})	*E. coli*, *S. aureus*	97%	[10]
CuS-BSA/lysozyme	PTT	NIR (980 nm, 0.7 W·cm^{-2})	*B. subtilis*, *E. coli*	~100%	[77]
Au@CuS	PTT	NIR	*E. coli*	~100%	[78]

Abbreviations: Near-infrared, NIR; Methicillin-resistant *Staphylococcus aureus*, MRSA; Extended-β-lactamase, ESBL; Polyethylene glycol, PEG; Graphene oxide, GO; Microsphere, MS; Nanosheet, NS; Nanoparticle, NP; Nanodot, ND; poly(5-(2-ethyl acrylate)-4-methylthiazole-g-butyl)/copper sulfide nanoclusters, PATAC4@CuS; thiol-terminated, alkyl-containing short-chain poly(ethylene glycol) (HS-$(CH_2)_{11}$-$(OCH_2CH_2)_6$-OH, MUH.

4.2. CuS with 2D Nanomaterials

In recent times, 2D nanomaterials have revolutionized research due to their unique physiochemical properties, non-toxicity, and excellent utility in various biomedical applications, including antibacterial treatments [79–81]. After the immense success of graphene [82,83], researchers have been exploring different 2D nanomaterials as antibacterial agents, namely graphitic carbon nitride (g-C_3N_4) nanosheets [22,59], titanium carbide (Mxene) [84], boron nitride (BN) [85], transition metal dichalcogenides [e.g., molybdenum disulfide (MoS_2)] [86], BP [36,47,87,88], and others. The basic advantage of using 2D nanomaterials with CuS is the synergetic improvement in the antibacterial activity, with less chance of toxicity, due to the biocompatibility of 2D materials.

In this respect, Lv et al. [73] demonstrated the importance of CuS nanocomposites with graphene oxide (GO) for photothermal antibacterial applications by utilizing visible light. A simple one-pot hydrothermal method was utilized to synthesize flower-like CuS anchored on GO sheets. Due to the morphology-dependent high surface area of CuS and defects in GO, the nanocomposite showed excellent photocatalytic performance. The nanocomposite showed excellent antibacterial activity against *E. coli* and *S. aureus*. This antibacterial activity was attributed to the excellent photocatalytic activity of the nanocomposite, coupled with the visible-light-induced (0.2 $W \cdot cm^{-2}$) photothermal response and release of Cu ions. The nanomaterial was also biocompatible with L929, a murine fibroblast cell line. Another 2D nanomaterial, graphitic carbon nitride (g-C_3N_4) nanosheets [74], were utilized with CuS nanomaterials for the photothermal eradication of bacteria. In that study, a simple hydrothermal process was again utilized to fabricate CuS nanomaterial-decorated graphitic carbon nitride (g-C_3N_4) nanosheets. Thereafter, polyethylene glycol (PEG) was capped with the nanocomposite to make it more biocompatible. The PEG-CuS@g-C_3N_4 nanocomposite was effective as an antibacterial agent, killing up to 99% of both *E. coli.* and *S. aureus* in a 200 $\mu g \cdot mL^{-1}$ suspension within 20 min of NIR irradiation (808 nm, 2.5 W). The biocompatibility of the nanocomposite was also verified using mouse skin fibroblast NIH-3T3 cell lines. $Ti_3C_2T_x$ Mxene was also used with CuS to achieve PDT- and PTT-mediated multimodal activity against *E. coli* and *S. aureus*, with bactericidal rates of 99.6 and 99.1%, respectively [8]. $Ti_3C_2T_x$@CuS composites were synthesized by a simple hydrothermal method, where the CuS NPs were distributed on the surface of $Ti_3C_2T_x$, affording synergistic effects. ROS generation, which eventually facilitated destruction of the bacterial cells, was attributed to the formation of the $Ti_3C_2T_x$@CuS heterojunction, which promoted the separation of electrons and holes, leading to improved electron transport efficiency. Furthermore, the nanocomposite had a stronger photothermal effect than the individual components, confirming its synergistic action. Recently, our group reported a BP-based CuS nanoplatform (CB) with photothermal activity, demonstrating antibacterial activity against environmental bacterial pathogens [47]. In our work, a low-temperature solution synthesis method was utilized to prepare CuS nanomaterials, which were then immobilized on BP nanosheets. The synthesized CB nanocomposites showed excellent antibacterial activity against *P. aeruginosa* and *S. aureus*, and also showed good activity against the MDR strains of these bacteria after irradiation with NIR light (808 nm, 2.5 W). The CB nanocomposite also showed exceptional ROS generation ability under NIR irradiation relative to the non-NIR-irradiated sample. Therefore, the multi-modal action of ROS and hyperthermia was also successfully applied therein under NIR irradiation (Figure 3).

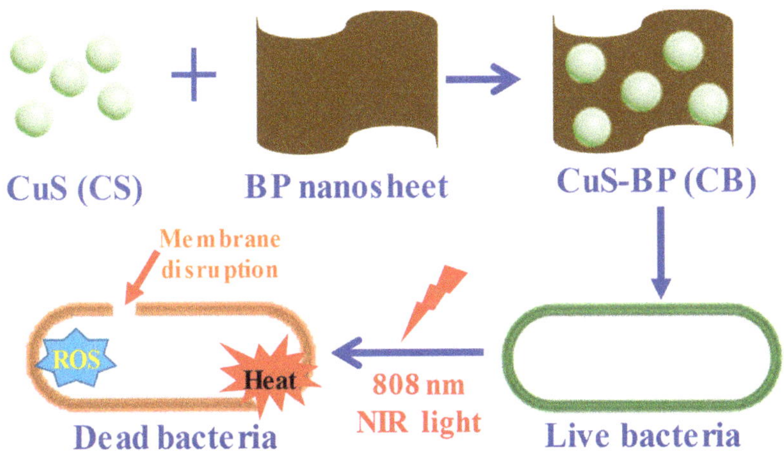

Figure 3. Schematic of CuS-BP synthesis and its PTT- and PDT-dependent antibacterial activity. Reproduced with permission from Ref. [47]. Copyright 2022 Elsevier.

4.3. CuS with Polymers

CuS nanomaterials were also utilized with different polymers to achieve synergistic photoactivated antibacterial activity. Dai et al. [9] synthesized a collection of poly(5-(2-ethyl acrylate)-4-methylthiazole-g-butyl)/copper sulfide nanoclusters (PATAC4@CuS), which were applied to levofloxacin-resistant Gram-negative and Gram-positive bacteria for efficient capture and effective ablation by NIR laser irradiation. The nanoclusters not only showed excellent photothermal activity under NIR irradiation, but also demonstrated admirable photodynamic properties (Figure 4). PATAC4@CuS nanoclusters showed excellent antibacterial activity against *B. amyloliquefaciens*, *E. coli*, *P. aeruginosa*, and levofloxacin-resistant *S. aureus* at 5.5 μg·mL^{-1} under NIR laser irradiation (980 nm, 1.5 W·cm^{-2}, 5 min). The heat and ROS generated from the NIR-irradiated PATAC4@CuS nanoclusters were stated as the reasons for the effective elimination and prevention of regrowth of the bacteria. The nanocluster also showed wound healing potential in bacteria-infected rat wounds without nonspecific harm to normal tissue. In another similar experiment, Wang et al. [75] introduced a thiol-terminated, alkyl-containing short-chain poly(ethylene glycol) (HS-$(CH_2)_{11}$-$(OCH_2CH_2)_6$-OH, abbreviated as MUH, onto CuS nanoclusters (NCs) to achieve photothermal antibacterial activity under NIR irradiation. The MUH-coated CuS NCs exhibited excellent stability in solutions with various pH values and stayed stable in pure water for at least 10 months. The MUH-coated CuS NCs showed strong antibacterial activity toward *E. coli* bacteria at 800 μM (76.8 μg·mL^{-1}) concentration.

4.4. CuS with Protein

Despite numerous advantages of CuS nanomaterials for biomedical applications, toxicity remains an issue that needs to be resolved. To address this issue, researchers have tried to coat CuS with proteins, especially bovine serum albumin (BSA). BSA is selected as a coating for CuS due its various advantageous properties, such as versatility, non-toxicity, stability, and biodegradability. Additionally, its functional groups allow easy binding and capping of nanomaterials, such as CuS.

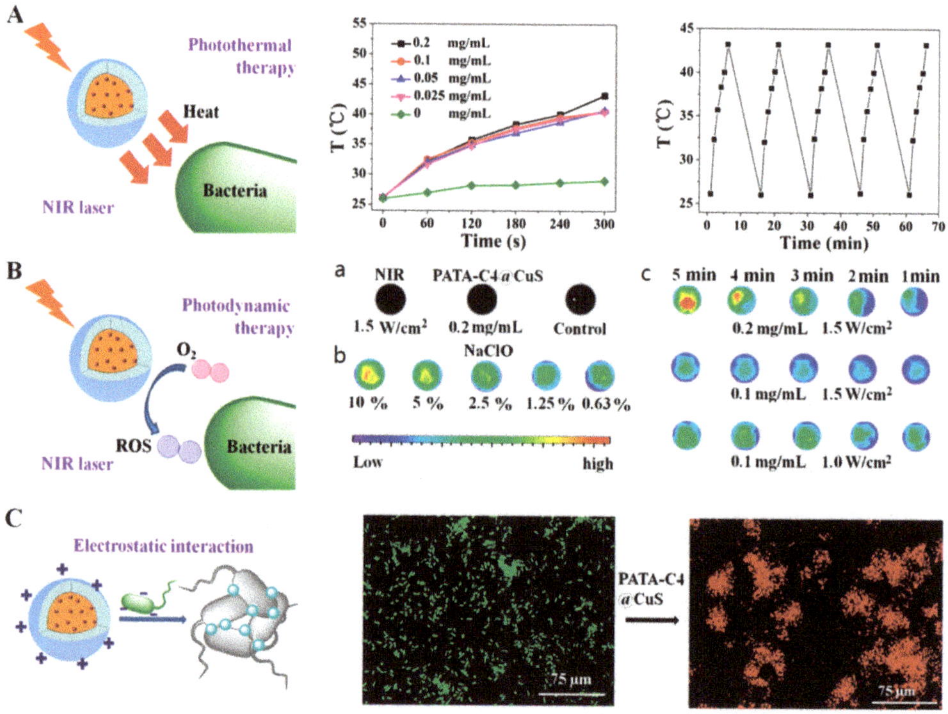

Figure 4. (**A**): Photothermal temperature change of PATA3-C4@CuS at different concentrations under NIR laser irradiation. (**B**) Fluorescence imaging of ROS generation detected by DCFH-DA assay: (**a**) single PBS and PBS containing PATA3-C4@CuS/NIR treated with DCFH-DA (black map indicates no ROS generation), (**b**) NaClO solution at different concentrations treated with DCFH-DA, and (**c**) solution containing PATA3-C4@CuS treated with DCFH-DA under various conditions. (**C**) Fluorescence micrographs of *B. amyloliquefaciens* stained with acridine orange (AO) and ethidium bromide (EB) before and after treatment with PATA3-C4@CuS. Reproduced with permission from Ref. [9]. Copyright 2017 American Chemical Society.

Zhao et al. [76] applied BSA-CuS NPs to the treatment of diabetic wound infection in vivo as a method of photothermal therapy. A facile biomineralization method was used to synthesize BSA-CuS nanomaterials, which were successfully used to destroy *A. baumannii*, *S. aureus*, and *S. haemolyticus* under NIR irradiation (808 nm, 8.0 W·cm^{-2}) for 10 min at 200 mg·L^{-1} concentration. Both in vitro and in vivo experiments were performed in this case. The BSA-CuS NPs showed excellent NIR-mediated photothermal antibacterial activity, with low cytotoxicity, in vivo toxicity, and excellent water solubility. Dual-mode PTT and PDT was applied using Ce6-labeled BSA-CuS NPs, enabling a synergistic effect against *E. coli and S. aureus* both in vitro and in vivo [10]. Most importantly, the same NIR light source was utilized to generate the ROS required for PDT activity and for PTT. The CuS NPs were prepared in the presence of BSA, which prevents aggregation of the CuS NPs. BSA also acts as a linker between the CuS and Ce6 molecules through amide bonds. The Ce6-labeled BSA-CuS NPs showed an overall bacterial killing efficacy of 97% in vitro due to the synergistic effects of combined PTT and PDT. The nanocomposite also successfully eliminated bacterial infection in vivo. BSA was also utilized as a template to synthesize uniform CuS NPs by a biomineralization method, and its NIR-mediated photothermal antibacterial activity against *E. coli* and *S. aureus* was evaluated (Figure 5). The as-prepared BSA-CuS nanocomposites showed good biocompatibility with skin fibroblast cells. Moreover, the nanocomposites showed excellent antibacterial activity under NIR light (980 nm, 1.59 W·cm^{-2}). The biocompatible CuS-BSA/lysozyme nanocomposite was also effective against *B. subtilis* and *E. coli* under NIR irradiation (980 nm, 0.7 W·cm^{-2}) [77].

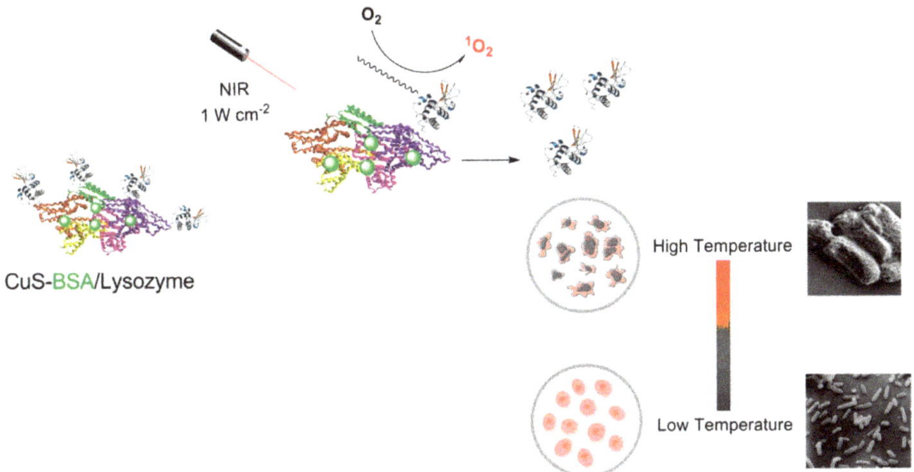

Figure 5. Schematic illustration of PDT and PTT mediated antibacterial activity of BSA-CuS nanocomposite. Reproduced with permission from Ref. [77].

4.5. CuS with Metals

The use of intrinsic antibacterial agents, such as Ag [83,86], Au [36], and ZnO [20,86], in combination with CuS to achieve photothermal antibacterial activity, is still in the infancy stage. Addae et al. [78] demonstrated the strong photothermal antibacterial potential of Au/CuS NPs against *Bacillus anthracis*. The antibacterial effect was dependent on both the NP concentration and treatment time. Similarly, Park et al. [89] showed the photothermal antibacterial potential of Au@CuS against *E. coli*. The Au@CuS yolk-shell nanomaterials on a PDMS film induced excellent photothermal sterilization against *E. coli*, where the photothermal efficiency of the nanocomposite reached 79.8%. Further research in this area is still necessary to completely understand the antibacterial mechanism of the nanocomposites.

5. Conclusions and Future Perspectives

In conclusion, it is certain that research to tackle MDR bacteria and their associated infections has seen remarkable advancements in recent years. The urgent need for alternatives to current antibiotics is well recognized. Consequently, therapeutic agents for PDT and PTT are prospective game-changers for antibacterial therapy. CuS is an especially promising material due to its multiple beneficial properties as an antibacterial agent. As discussed earlier, CuS absorbs NIR light through an LSPR, which originates from the collective oscillation of holes rather than electrons in other widely used photoactive nanomaterials such as Ag and Au. Furthermore, Cu^{2+} is recognized as an important trace element in the human body, stimulating the wound healing process. Therefore, the advantages of CuS over other photoactive nanomaterials are noteworthy. The most important aspect is that the PDT and PTT can be effectively utilized with CuS nanomaterials to achieve excellent antibacterial activity. Furthermore, the odds of bacterial resistance are almost non-existent. The multimodal strategy of combining PDT and PTT is also possible with CuS. Despite these remarkable antibacterial properties and advantages, some challenges still remain to be resolved. First and foremost, all the reported studies on PDT and PTT with CuS were performed under laboratory conditions. Hence, the same significant antibacterial activity remains elusive in clinical trials. There is also the ever-present issue of the toxicity of nanomaterials, such as CuS, which requires attention. The biocompatibility, target specificity, and stability of CuS can be amended with the help of functional nanoconjugates. Nevertheless, the synthesis of CuS nanomaterials is somewhat complicated in comparison with that of other well-known antibacterial agents, along with the relatively high cost of the former. This pricey aspect of CuS synthesis could hinder its application in large-scale clinical settings. Hence, the affordable preparation of CuS by economical and green methods is a future direction for large-scale synthesis. The high dose of CuS nanomaterials required to achieve antibacterial activity also needs to be addressed. Different synthesis methods and various CuS morphologies can prospectively be utilized to diminish the problem of high dosage. In summary, we expect the emergence of more therapeutic strategies involving CuS nanomaterials or nanocomposites to combat bacterial infection in clinical applications in the global research arena.

Author Contributions: A.N.: Conceptualization, writing—original draft. K.-s.K.: Conceptualization, writing—review & editing, and funding acquisition. All authors have read and agreed to the published version of the manuscript.

Funding: This research was funded by a National Research Foundation of Korea (NRF) grant, funded by the Korean Government (MSIT) (grant number NRF-2021R1A2C1007413).

Institutional Review Board Statement: Not applicable.

Informed Consent Statement: Not applicable.

Data Availability Statement: Not applicable.

Acknowledgments: Graphical abstract (GA) of this manuscript has been prepared utilizing BioRender.com (accessed on 10 October 2022).

Conflicts of Interest: The authors declare that they have no conflict of interest.

References

1. Mendelson, M.; Matsoso, M.P. The World Health Organization Global Action Plan for antimicrobial resistance. *S. Afr. Med. J.* **2015**, *105*, 325. [CrossRef] [PubMed]
2. Naskar, A.; Kim, K.-S. Nanomaterials as delivery vehicles and components of new strategies to combat bacterial infections: Advantages and Limitations. *Microorganisms* **2019**, *7*, 356. [CrossRef] [PubMed]
3. Lee, H.P.; Gaharwar, A.K. Light-Responsive Inorganic Biomaterials for Biomedical Applications. *Adv. Sci.* **2020**, *7*, 2000863. [CrossRef] [PubMed]
4. Ren, Y.; Liu, H.; Liu, X.; Zheng, Y.; Li, Z.; Li, C.; Yeung, K.W.K.; Zhu, S.; Liang, Y.; Cui, Z.; et al. Photoresponsive Materials for Antibacterial Applications. *Cell Rep. Phys. Sci.* **2020**, *1*, 100245. [CrossRef]
5. Huo, J.; Jia, Q.; Huang, H.; Zhang, J.; Li, P.; Dong, X.; Huang, W. Emerging photothermal-derived multimodal synergistic therapy in combating bacterial infections. *Chem. Soc. Rev.* **2021**, *50*, 8762–8789. [CrossRef]
6. Ain, N.U.; Abdul Nasir, J.; Khan, Z.; Butler, I.S.; Rehman, Z. Copper sulfide nanostructures: Synthesis and biological applications. *RSC Adv.* **2022**, *12*, 7550–7567. [CrossRef]
7. Mutalik, C.; Okoro, G.; Krisnawati, D.I.; Jazidie, A.; Rahmawati, E.Q.; Rahayu, D.; Hsu, W.T.; Kuo, T.R. Copper sulfide with morphology-dependent photodynamic and photothermal antibacterial activities. *J. Colloid Interface Sci.* **2022**, *607*, 1825–1835. [CrossRef]
8. Li, Q.; Wang, W.; Feng, H.; Cao, L.; Wang, H.; Wang, D.; Chen, S. NIR-triggered photocatalytic and photothermal performance for sterilization based on copper sulfide nanoparticles anchored on $Ti_3C_2T_x$ MXene. *J. Colloid Interface Sci.* **2021**, *604*, 810–822. [CrossRef]
9. Dai, X.; Zhao, Y.; Yu, Y.; Chen, X.; Wei, X.; Zhang, X.; Li, C. Single Continuous Near-Infrared Laser-Triggered Photodynamic and Photothermal Ablation of Antibiotic-Resistant Bacteria Using Effective Targeted Copper Sulfide Nanoclusters. *ACS Appl. Mater. Interfaces.* **2017**, *9*, 30470–30479. [CrossRef]
10. Gao, D.Y.; Ji, X.; Wang, J.L.; Wang, Y.T.; Li, D.L.; Liu, Y.B.; Chang, K.W.; Qu, J.L.; Zheng, J.; Yuan, Z. Engineering a protein-based nanoplatform as an antibacterial agent for light activated dual-modal photothermal and photodynamic therapy of infection in both the NIR I and II windows. *J. Mater. Chem. B* **2018**, *6*, 732–739. [CrossRef]
11. Yang, X.; Liu, G.; Shi, Y.; Huang, W.; Shao, J.; Dong, X. Nano-black phosphorus for combined cancer phototherapy: Recent advances and prospects. *Nanotechnology* **2018**, *29*, 222001. [CrossRef] [PubMed]
12. Zhang, B.; Wang, Y.; Liu, J.; Zhai, G. Recent Developments of Phototherapy Based on Graphene Family Nanomaterials. *Curr. Med. Chem.* **2017**, *24*, 268–291. [CrossRef] [PubMed]

13. Gøtzsche, P.C. Niels Finsen's treatment for lupus vulgaris. *J. R. Soc. Med.* **2011**, *104*, 41–42. [CrossRef] [PubMed]
14. Moller, K.I.; Kongshoj, B.; Philipsen, P.A.; Thomsen, V.O.; Wulf, H.C. How Finsen's light cured lupus vulgaris. *Photodermatol. Photoimmunol. Photomed.* **2005**, *21*, 118–124. [CrossRef] [PubMed]
15. Zhang, X.; Wang, S.; Cheng, G.; Yu, P.; Chang, J. Light-Responsive Nanomaterials for Cancer Therapy. *Engineering* **2022**, *13*, 18–30. [CrossRef]
16. Xu, J.W.; Yao, K.; Xu, Z.K. Nanomaterials with a photothermal effect for antibacterial activities: An overview. *Nanoscale* **2019**, *11*, 8680–8691. [CrossRef]
17. Memar, M.Y.; Ghotaslou, R.; Samiei, M.; Adibkia, K. Antimicrobial use of reactive oxygen therapy: Current insights. *Infect. Drug. Resist.* **2018**, *11*, 567–576. [CrossRef]
18. Sun, Y.D.; Zhu, Y.X.; Zhang, X.; Jia, H.R.; Xia, Y.; Wu, F.G. Role of Cholesterol Conjugation in the Antibacterial Photodynamic Therapy of Branched Polyethylenimine-Containing Nanoagents. *Langmuir* **2019**, *35*, 14324–14331. [CrossRef]
19. Yang, M.; Qiu, S.; Coy, E.; Li, S.; Załęski, K.; Zhang, Y.; Pan, H.; Wang, G. NIR-Responsive TiO_2 Biometasurfaces: Toward In Situ Photodynamic Antibacterial Therapy for Biomedical Implants. *Adv. Mater.* **2022**, *34*, e2106314. [CrossRef]
20. Gupta, J.; Mohapatra, J.; Bahadur, D. Visible light driven mesoporous Ag-embedded ZnO nanocomposites: Reactive oxygen species enhanced photocatalysis, bacterial inhibition and photodynamic therapy. *Dalton Trans.* **2017**, *46*, 685–696. [CrossRef]
21. Duan, G.; Chen, L.; Jing, Z.; De Luna, P.; Wen, L.; Zhang, L.; Zhao, L.; Xu, J.; Li, Z.; Yang, Z.; et al. Robust Antibacterial Activity of Tungsten Oxide (WO_{3-x}) Nanodots. *Chem. Res. Toxicol.* **2019**, *32*, 1357–1366. [CrossRef] [PubMed]
22. Huang, J.; Ho, W.; Wang, X. Metal-free disinfection effects induced by graphitic carbon nitride polymers under visible light illumination. *Chem. Commun.* **2014**, *50*, 4338–4340. [CrossRef] [PubMed]
23. Amos-Tautua, B.M.; Songca, S.P.; Oluwafemi, O.S. Application of Porphyrins in Antibacterial Photodynamic Therapy. *Molecules* **2019**, *24*, 2456. [CrossRef]
24. Xu, Z.; Mei, L.; Shi, Y.; Yun, M.; Luan, Y.; Miao, Z.; Liu, Z.; Li, X.M.; Jiao, M. Multivalent Phthalocyanine-Based Cationic Polymers with Enhanced Photodynamic Activity for the Bacterial Capture and Bacteria-Infected Wound Healing. *Biomacromolecules* **2022**, *23*, 2778–2784. [CrossRef] [PubMed]
25. Vara, J.; Gualdesi, M.S.; Aiassa, V.; Ortiz, C.S. Evaluation of physicochemical properties and bacterial photoinactivation of phenothiazine photosensitizers. *Photochem. Photobiol. Sci.* **2019**, *18*, 1576–1586. [CrossRef]
26. Liang, G.; Wang, H.; Shi, H.; Wang, H.; Zhu, M.; Jing, A.; Li, J.; Li, G. Recent progress in the development of upconversion nanomaterials in bioimaging and disease treatment. *J. Nanobiotechnol.* **2020**, *18*, 154. [CrossRef]
27. Mohamed, M.M.; Fouad, S.A.; Elshoky, H.A.; Mohammed, G.M.; Salaheldin, T.A. Antibacterial effect of gold nanoparticles against *Corynebacterium pseudotuberculosis*. *Int. J. Vet. Sci. Med.* **2017**, *5*, 23–29. [CrossRef]
28. Sun, P.; Ye, L.; Tan, X.; Peng, J.; Zhao, L.; Zhou, Y. Silver Nanoparticle-Assisted Photodynamic Therapy for Biofilm Eradication. *ACS Appl. Nano Mater.* **2022**, *5*, 8251–8259. [CrossRef]
29. Han, D.; Ma, M.; Han, Y.; Cui, Z.; Liang, Y.; Liu, X.; Li, Z.; Zhu, S.; Wu, S. Eco-friendly Hybrids of Carbon Quantum Dots Modified MoS_2 for Rapid Microbial Inactivation by Strengthened Photocatalysis. *ACS Sustain. Chem. Eng.* **2020**, *8*, 534–542. [CrossRef]
30. Nie, X.; Jiang, C.; Wu, S.; Chen, W.; Lv, P.; Wang, Q.; Liu, J.; Narh, C.; Cao, X.; Ghiladi, R.A.; et al. Carbon quantum dots: A bright future as photosensitizers for in vitro antibacterial photodynamic inactivation. *J. Photochem. Photobiol. B* **2020**, *206*, 111864. [CrossRef]
31. Garin, C.; Alejo, T.; Perez-Laguna, V.; Prieto, M.; Mendoza, G.; Arruebo, M.; Sebastian, V.; Rezusta, A. Chalcogenide nanoparticles and organic photosensitizers for synergetic antimicrobial photodynamic therapy. *J. Mater. Chem. B* **2021**, *9*, 6246–6259. [CrossRef] [PubMed]
32. Ye, L.; Cao, Z.; Liu, X.; Cui, Z.; Li, Z.; Liang, Y.; Zhu, S.; Wu, S. Noble metal-based nanomaterials as antibacterial agents. *J. Alloys Compd.* **2022**, *904*, 164091. [CrossRef]
33. Lv, Y.K.; Mei, L.; Zhang, L.X.; Yang, D.H.; Yin, Z.Y. Multifunctional graphene-based nanocomposites for simultaneous enhanced photocatalytic degradation and photothermal antibacterial activity by visible light. *Environ. Sci. Pollut. Res. Int.* **2021**, *28*, 49880–49888. [CrossRef] [PubMed]
34. Qie, X.; Zan, M.; Gui, P.; Chen, H.; Wang, J.; Lin, K.; Mei, Q.; Ge, M.; Zhang, Z.; Tang, Y.; et al. Design, Synthesis, and Application of Carbon Dots With Synergistic Antibacterial Activity. *Front Bioeng. Biotechnol.* **2022**, *10*, 894100. [CrossRef] [PubMed]
35. Zhu, K.; Qian, S.; Guo, H.; Wang, Q.; Chu, X.; Wang, X.; Lu, S.; Peng, Y.; Guo, Y.; Zhu, Z.; et al. pH-Activatable Organic Nanoparticles for Efficient Low-Temperature Photothermal Therapy of Ocular Bacterial Infection. *ACS Nano* **2022**, *16*, 11136–11151. [CrossRef]
36. Naskar, A.; Lee, S.; Kim, K.-s. Au-ZnO Conjugated Black Phosphorus as a Near-Infrared Light-Triggering and Recurrence-Suppressing Nanoantibiotic Platform against *Staphylococcus aureus*. *Pharmaceutics* **2021**, *13*, 52. [CrossRef]
37. Pan, W.Y.; Huang, C.C.; Lin, T.T.; Hu, H.Y.; Lin, W.C.; Li, M.J.; Sung, H.W. Synergistic antibacterial effects of localized heat and oxidative stress caused by hydroxyl radicals mediated by graphene/iron oxide-based nanocomposites. *Nanomedicine* **2016**, *12*, 431–438. [CrossRef]
38. Nguyen, T.K.; Duong, H.T.; Selvanayagam, R.; Boyer, C.; Barraud, N. Iron oxide nanoparticle-mediated hyperthermia stimulates dispersal in bacterial biofilms and enhances antibiotic efficacy. *Sci. Rep.* **2015**, *5*, 18385. [CrossRef]
39. Wang, Y.; Jin, Y.; Chen, W.; Wang, J.; Chen, H.; Sun, L.; Li, X.; Ji, J.; Yu, Q.; Shen, L.; et al. Construction of nanomaterials with targeting phototherapy properties to inhibit resistant bacteria and biofilm infections. *Chem. Eng. J.* **2019**, *358*, 74–90. [CrossRef]

40. Meeker, D.G.; Jenkins, S.V.; Miller, E.K.; Beenken, K.E.; Loughran, A.J.; Powless, A.; Muldoon, T.J.; Galanzha, E.I.; Zharov, V.P.; Smeltzer, M.S.; et al. Synergistic Photothermal and Antibiotic Killing of Biofilm-Associated *Staphylococcus aureus* Using Targeted Antibiotic-Loaded Gold Nanoconstructs. *ACS Infect Dis.* **2016**, *2*, 241–250. [CrossRef]
41. Huang, J.; Zhou, J.; Zhuang, J.; Gao, H.; Huang, D.; Wang, L.; Wu, W.; Li, Q.; Yang, D.P.; Han, M.Y. Strong Near-Infrared Absorbing and Biocompatible CuS Nanoparticles for Rapid and Efficient Photothermal Ablation of Gram-Positive and -Negative Bacteria. *ACS Appl Mater. Interfaces* **2017**, *9*, 36606–36614. [CrossRef] [PubMed]
42. Wang, P.; Yuan, Y.; Xu, K.; Zhong, H.; Yang, Y.; Jin, S.; Yang, K.; Qi, X. Biological applications of copper-containing materials. *Bioact. Mater.* **2020**, *6*, 916–927. [CrossRef] [PubMed]
43. Gargioni, C.; Borzenkov, M.; D'Alfonso, L.; Sperandeo, P.; Polissi, A.; Cucca, L.; Dacarro, G.; Grisoli, P.; Pallavicini, P.; D'Agostino, A.; et al. Self-Assembled Monolayers of Copper Sulfide Nanoparticles on Glass as Antibacterial Coatings. *Nanomaterials* **2020**, *10*, 352. [CrossRef] [PubMed]
44. Ding, H.; Han, D.; Han, Y.; Liang, Y.; Liu, X.; Li, Z.; Zhu, S.; Wu, S. Visible light responsive CuS/ protonated g-C_3N_4 heterostructure for rapid sterilization. *J. Hazard. Mater.* **2020**, *393*, 122423. [CrossRef] [PubMed]
45. Zhou, L.; Chen, F.; Hou, Z.; Chen, Y.; Luo, X. Injectable self-healing CuS nanoparticle complex hydrogels with antibacterial, anti-cancer, and wound healing properties. *Chem. Eng. J.* **2021**, *409*, 128224. [CrossRef]
46. Qiao, Y.; Ping, Y.; Zhang, H.; Zhou, B.; Liu, F.; Yu, Y.; Xie, T.; Li, W.; Zhong, D.; Zhang, Y.; et al. Laser-Activatable CuS Nanodots to Treat Multidrug-Resistant Bacteria and Release Copper Ion to Accelerate Healing of Infected Chronic Nonhealing Wounds. *ACS Appl. Mater. Interfaces* **2019**, *11*, 3809–3822. [CrossRef]
47. Naskar, A.; Cho, H.; Kim, K.S. Black phosphorus-based CuS nanoplatform: Near-infrared-responsive and reactive oxygen species-generating agent against environmental bacterial pathogens. *J. Environ. Chem. Eng.* **2022**, *10*, 108226. [CrossRef]
48. Naskar, A.; Cho, H.; Lee, S.; Kim, K.-s. Biomimetic Nanoparticles Coated with Bacterial Outer Membrane Vesicles as a New-Generation Platform for Biomedical Applications. *Pharmaceutics* **2021**, *13*, 1887. [CrossRef]
49. Naskar, A.; Kim, K.S. Recent Advances in Nanomaterial-Based Wound-Healing Therapeutics. *Pharmaceutics* **2020**, *12*, 499. [CrossRef]
50. Li, Y.; Lu, W.; Huang, Q.; Huang, M.; Li, C.; Chen, W. Copper sulfide nanoparticles for photothermal ablation of tumor cells. *Nanomedicine* **2010**, *5*, 1161–1171. [CrossRef]
51. Li, M.; Wang, Y.; Lin, H.; Qu, F. Hollow CuS nanocube as nanocarrier for synergetic chemo/photothermal/photodynamic therapy. *Mater. Sci. Eng. C Mater. Biol. Appl.* **2019**, *96*, 591–598. [CrossRef] [PubMed]
52. Wang, Y.; Xiao, Y.; Zhou, H.; Chen, W.; Tang, R. Ultra-high payload of doxorubicin and pH-responsive drug release in CuS nanocages for a combination of chemotherapy and photothermal therapy. *RSC Adv.* **2013**, *3*, 23133–23138. [CrossRef]
53. Raj, S.I.; Jaiswal, A.; Uddin, I. Ultrasmall aqueous starch-capped CuS quantum dots with tunable localized surface plasmon resonance and composition for the selective and sensitive detection of mercury(ii) ions. *RSC Adv.* **2020**, *10*, 14050–14059. [CrossRef] [PubMed]
54. Kalimuldina, G.; Nurpeissova, A.; Adylkhanova, A.; Adair, D.; Taniguchi, I.; Bakenov, Z. Morphology and Dimension Variations of Copper Sulfide for High-Performance Electrode in Rechargeable Batteries: A Review. *ACS Appl. Energy Mater.* **2020**, *3*, 11480–11499. [CrossRef]
55. Bekhit, M.; Abo El Naga, A.O.; El Saied, M.; Abdel Maksoud, M.I.A. Radiation-induced synthesis of copper sulfide nanotubes with improved catalytic and antibacterial activities. *Environ. Sci. Pollut. Res. Int.* **2021**, *28*, 44467–44478. [CrossRef] [PubMed]
56. Zhang, X.; Wang, G.; Gu, A.; Wei, Y.; Fang, B. CuS nanotubes for ultrasensitive nonenzymatic glucose sensors. *Chem. Commun.* **2008**, *45*, 5945–5947. [CrossRef] [PubMed]
57. Manikandan, T.; Padmalaya, G.; Mahalakshmi, S.; Nivethitha, A.S.; Pavithran, V.; Perumal, S.; Sreeja, B.S.; Senthil Kumar, P. Facile hydrothermal bio-synthesis of cellulose acetate templated CuS nanorods like fibres: Antibacterial, cytotoxicity effects and DNA cleavage properties against A549 lung cancer cells. *IET Nanobiotechnol.* **2020**, *14*, 47–52. [CrossRef]
58. Kwon, Y.T.; Ryu, S.H.; Shin, J.W.; Yeo, W.H.; Choa, Y.H. Electrospun CuS/PVP Nanowires and Superior Near-Infrared Filtration Efficiency for Thermal Shielding Applications. *ACS Appl. Mater. Interfaces* **2019**, *11*, 6575–6580. [CrossRef] [PubMed]
59. Mirzaei, A.; Peymanfar, R.; Javanshir, S.; Fallahi, R.; Karimi, J. Antibacterial Characteristics of CuS Nanoplates Anchored onto g-C_3N_4 Nanosheets, Suspended in PMMA Matrix. *Int. J. Nanosci. Nanotechnol.* **2021**, *17*, 249–260.
60. Nishi, H.; Asami, K.; Tatsuma, T. CuS nanoplates for LSPR sensing in the second biological optical window. *Opt. Mater. Express* **2016**, *6*, 1043–1048. [CrossRef]
61. Palanisamy, S.; Velmurugan, S.; Yang, T.C.K. One-pot sonochemical synthesis of CuS nanoplates decorated partially reduced graphene oxide for biosensing of dopamine neurotransmitter. *Ultrason. Sonochem.* **2020**, *64*, 105043. [CrossRef] [PubMed]
62. Wang, K.-J.; Li, G.-D.; Li, J.-X.; Wang, Q.; Chen, J.-S. Formation of Single-Crystalline CuS Nanoplates Vertically Standing on Flat Substrate. *Cryst Growth Des.* **2007**, *7*, 2265–2267. [CrossRef]
63. Han, L.; Hao, Y.N.; Wei, X.; Chen, X.W.; Shu, Y.; Wang, J.H. Hollow Copper Sulfide Nanosphere-Doxorubicin/Graphene Oxide Core-Shell Nanocomposite for Photothermo-chemotherapy. *ACS Biomater. Sci. Eng.* **2017**, *3*, 3230–3235. [CrossRef] [PubMed]
64. Wu, S.; Zhang, P.; Jiang, Z.; Zhang, W.; Gong, X.; Wang, Y. Enhanced Peroxidase-like Activity of CuS Hollow Nanocages by Plasmon-Induced Hot Carriers and Photothermal Effect for the Dual-Mode Detection of Tannic Acid. *ACS Appl. Mater. Interfaces* **2022**, *14*, 40191–40199. [CrossRef] [PubMed]

65. Cui, Y.; Li, J.; Liu, M.; Tong, H.; Liu, Z.; Hu, J.; Qian, D. Convenient synthesis of three-dimensional hierarchical CuS@Pd core-shell cauliflowers decorated on nitrogen-doped reduced graphene oxide for non-enzymatic electrochemical sensing of xanthine. *Mikrochim. Acta* **2020**, *187*, 589. [CrossRef]
66. Deng, X.; Wang, C.; Yang, H.; Shao, M.; Zhang, S.; Wang, X.; Ding, M.; Huang, J.; Xu, X. One-pot hydrothermal synthesis of CdS decorated CuS microflower-like structures for enhanced photocatalytic properties. *Sci. Rep.* **2017**, *7*, 3877. [CrossRef]
67. Fang, J.; Zhang, P.; Chang, H.; Wang, X. Hydrothermal synthesis of nanostructured CuS for broadband efficient optical absorption and high-performance photo-thermal conversion. *Sol. Energy Mater. Sol. Cells* **2018**, *185*, 456–463. [CrossRef]
68. Shu, Q.W.; Li, C.M.; Gao, P.F.; Gao, M.X.; Huang, C.Z. Porous hollow CuS nanospheres with prominent peroxidase-like activity prepared in large scale by a one-pot controllable hydrothermal step. *RSC Adv.* **2015**, *5*, 17458–17465. [CrossRef]
69. AL-Jawad, S.M.H.; Taha, A.A.; Redha, A.M. Studying the structural, morphological, and optical properties of CuS:Ni nanostructure prepared by a hydrothermal method for biological activity. *J. Sol.-Gel. Sci. Technol.* **2019**, *91*, 310–323. [CrossRef]
70. Thongtem, T.; Phuruangrat, A.; Thongtem, S. Characterization of copper sulfide nanostructured spheres and nanotubes synthesized by microwave-assisted solvothermal method. *Mater. Lett.* **2010**, *64*, 136–139. [CrossRef]
71. Krajnik, B.; Golacki, L.W.; Fiedorczyk, E.; Bański, M.; Noculak, A.; Hołodnik, K.M.; Podhorodecki, A. Quantitative comparison of luminescence probes for biomedical applications. *Methods Appl. Fluoresc.* **2021**, *9*, 045001. [CrossRef] [PubMed]
72. Ren, Y.; Yan, B.; Wang, P.; Yu, Y.; Cui, L.; Zhou, M.; Wang, Q. Construction of a Rapid Photothermal Antibacterial Silk Fabric via QCS-Guided In Situ Deposition of CuSNPs. *ACS Sustain. Chem. Eng.* **2022**, *10*, 2192–2203. [CrossRef]
73. Lv, R.; Liang, Y.-Q.; Li, Z.-Y.; Zhu, S.-L.; Cui, Z.-D.; Wu, S.-L. Flower-like CuS/graphene oxide with photothermal and enhanced photocatalytic effect for rapid bacteria-killing using visible light. *Rare Met.* **2022**, *41*, 639–649. [CrossRef]
74. Liu, X.; Li, X.; Shan, Y.; Yin, Y.; Liu, C.; Lin, Z.; Kumar, S.S. CuS nanoparticles anchored to g-C3N4 nanosheets for photothermal ablation of bacteria. *RSC Adv.* **2020**, *10*, 12183–12191. [CrossRef]
75. Wang, H.Y.; Hua, X.W.; Wu, F.G.; Li, B.; Liu, P.; Gu, N.; Wang, Z.; Chen, Z. Synthesis of ultrastable copper sulfide nanoclusters via trapping the reaction intermediate: Potential anticancer and antibacterial applications. *ACS Appl. Mater. Interfaces* **2015**, *7*, 7082–7092. [CrossRef]
76. Zhao, Y.; Cai, Q.; Qi, W.; Jia, Y.; Xiong, T.; Fan, Z.; Liu, S.; Yang, J.; Li, N.; Chang, B. BSA-CuS Nanoparticles for Photothermal Therapy of Diabetic Wound Infection *In Vivo*. *ChemistrySelect* **2018**, *3*, 9510–9516. [CrossRef]
77. Swaidan, A.; Ghayyem, S.; Barras, A.; Addad, A.; Szunerits, S.; Boukherroub, R. Enhanced Antibacterial Activity of CuS-BSA/Lysozyme under Near Infrared Light Irradiation. *Nanomaterials* **2021**, *11*, 2156. [CrossRef]
78. Addae, E.; Dong, X.; McCoy, E.; Yang, C.; Chen, W.; Yang, L. Investigation of antimicrobial activity of photothermal therapeutic gold/copper sulfide core/shell nanoparticles to bacterial spores and cells. *J. Biol. Eng.* **2014**, *8*, 11. [CrossRef]
79. Derakhshi, M.; Daemi, S.; Shahini, P.; Habibzadeh, A.; Mostafavi, E.; Ashkarran, A.A. Two-Dimensional Nanomaterials beyond Graphene for Biomedical Applications. *J. Funct. Biomater.* **2022**, *13*, 27. [CrossRef]
80. Naskar, A.; Kim, S.; Kim, K.-s. A nontoxic biocompatible nanocomposite comprising black phosphorus with Au-γ-Fe_2O_3 nanoparticles. *RSC Adv.* **2020**, *10*, 16162–16167. [CrossRef]
81. Naskar, A.; Lee, S.; Ko, D.; Kim, S.; Kim, K.-s. Bovine Serum Albumin-Immobilized Black Phosphorus-Based γ-Fe_2O_3 Nanocomposites: A Promising Biocompatible Nanoplatform. *Biomedicines* **2021**, *9*, 858. [CrossRef] [PubMed]
82. Ansari, M.O.; Gauthaman, K.; Essa, A.; Bencherif, S.A.; Memic, A. Graphene and Graphene-Based Materials in Biomedical Applications. *Curr. Med. Chem.* **2019**, *26*, 6834–6850. [CrossRef] [PubMed]
83. Naskar, A.; Khan, H.; Sarkar, R.; Kumar, S.; Halder, D.; Jana, S. Anti-biofilm activity and food packaging application of room temperature solution process based polyethylene glycol capped Ag-ZnO-graphene nanocomposite. *Mater. Sci. Eng. C Mater. Biol. Appl.* **2018**, *91*, 743–753. [CrossRef] [PubMed]
84. Zheng, K.; Li, S.; Jing, L.; Chen, P.Y.; Xie, J. Synergistic Antimicrobial Titanium Carbide (MXene) Conjugated with Gold Nanoclusters. *Adv. Healthc. Mater.* **2020**, *9*, e2001007. [CrossRef] [PubMed]
85. Li, M.; Wang, S.; Li, R.; Wang, Y.; Fan, X.; Gong, W.; Ma, Y. The Mechanical and Antibacterial Properties of Boron Nitride/Silver Nanocomposite Enhanced Polymethyl Methacrylate Resin for Application in Oral Denture Bases. *Biomimetics* **2022**, *7*, 138. [CrossRef] [PubMed]
86. Naskar, A.; Shin, J.; Kim, K.-s. A MoS_2 based silver-doped ZnO nanocomposite and its antibacterial activity against β-lactamase expressing *Escherichia coli*. *RSC Adv.* **2022**, *12*, 7268–7275. [CrossRef] [PubMed]
87. Naskar, A.; Kim, K.-s. Black phosphorus nanomaterials as multi-potent and emerging platforms against bacterial infections. *Microb. Pathog.* **2019**, *137*, 103800. [CrossRef]
88. Cho, H.; Naskar, A.; Lee, S.; Kim, S.; Kim, K.-s. A New Surface Charge Neutralizing Nano-Adjuvant to Potentiate Polymyxins in Killing Mcr-1 Mediated Drug-Resistant *Escherichia coli*. *Pharmaceutics* **2021**, *13*, 250. [CrossRef]
89. Park, E.; Selvaraj, R.; Kim, Y. High-efficiency photothermal sterilization on PDMS film with Au@CuS yolk-shell nanoparticles. *J. Ind. Eng. Chem.* **2022**, *113*, 522–529. [CrossRef]

pharmaceutics

MDPI

Review

Friends against the Foe: Synergistic Photothermal and Photodynamic Therapy against Bacterial Infections

Atanu Naskar and Kwang-sun Kim *

Department of Chemistry and Chemistry Institute for Functional Materials, Pusan National University, Busan 46241, Republic of Korea; atanunaskar@pusan.ac.kr
* Correspondence: kwangsun.kim@pusan.ac.kr; Tel.: +82-51-510-2241

Abstract: Multidrug-resistant (MDR) bacteria are rapidly emerging, coupled with the failure of current antibiotic therapy; thus, new alternatives for effectively treating infections caused by MDR bacteria are required. Hyperthermia-mediated photothermal therapy (PTT) and reactive oxygen species (ROS)-mediated photodynamic therapy (PDT) have attracted extensive attention as antibacterial therapies owing to advantages such as low invasiveness, low toxicity, and low likelihood of causing bacterial resistance. However, both strategies have notable drawbacks, including the high temperature requirements of PTT and the weak ability of PDT-derived ROS to penetrate target cells. To overcome these limitations, a combination of PTT and PDT has been used against MDR bacteria. In this review, we discuss the unique benefits and limitations of PTT and PDT against MDR bacteria. The mechanisms underlying the synergistic effects of the PTT–PDT combination are also discussed. Furthermore, we introduced advancements in antibacterial methods using nano-based PTT and PDT agents to treat infections caused by MDR bacteria. Finally, we highlight the existing challenges and future perspectives of synergistic PTT–PDT combination therapy against infections caused by MDR bacteria. We believe that this review will encourage synergistic PTT- and PDT-based antibacterial research and can be referenced for future clinical applications.

Keywords: photodynamic therapy; photothermal therapy; synergistic effect; antibacterial; multidrug-resistant bacteria

1. Introduction

The prevalence of multidrug-resistant (MDR) bacteria and their infections in humans has frightened the global health system. Identifying them is a critical issue that must be addressed to ensure that people live in safe and healthy environments [1]. The overall number of deaths from bacterial infections is expected to increase to 10 million per year by 2050, illustrating the severity of MDR bacterial infections [2]. Currently, it is feasible that a bacterial infection might not respond to current antibiotic therapies. The overuse or misuse of conventional antibiotics is to blame for this unbelievable situation [3]. Notably, bacteria develop resistance to antibiotics at a considerably higher rate than that at which new antibiotics are discovered.

Bacteria have evolved various protection mechanisms against antibiotics over time [4,5]. These include the development of the drug efflux pump in bacteria for allowing drugs to be expelled outside of cells, evolved abilities to break down antibiotics using enzymes produced by bacteria, modifications of bacterial metabolic pathways to protect them from antibiotics, formations of biofilms, and structured colonization of bacterial cells with a self-produced extracellular polymeric substance matrix. Antibiotics cannot function through this protective biofilm matrix and are captured in the matrix [6]. Furthermore, bacteria enclosed in the biofilm matrix can efficiently communicate and transfer antibiotic-resistance genes among all bacteria, making it more difficult to kill using antibiotics from outside the biofilms. Unsurprisingly, approximately 80% of chronic and recurrent infections in the human body are associated with the formation of dense bacterial biofilms [6]. Therefore, an urgent need exists for thorough and methodical research on techniques for preventing MDR bacteria from rapidly multiplying after infecting humans, in addition to techniques for eliminating bacteria.

Research has explored various alternatives to conventional antibiotics to manage this constantly hazardous and demanding scenario with varying degrees of effectiveness. However, these alternatives are not perfect solutions for overcoming the limitations of antibiotic therapies. For instance, naturally occurring antimicrobial compounds have been investigated; however, they are expensive to use [7]. Antimicrobial peptides (AMPs) have been characterized and suggested as promising alternatives owing to their potent antibacterial activity and species selectivity; however, they are unstable and very vulnerable to proteolysis, limiting their potential for use [8]. To overcome these limitations, molecules designed to mimic the properties of antimicrobial peptides have resulted in synthetic mimics of antimicrobial peptides [9]. These are polymeric mimics of AMPs, peptidomimetic oligomers, or small molecules. Most are prepared with the aim of overcoming the issues of protease lability, toxicity, and high costs in manufacturing AMPs. However, optimizing these materials to achieve controlled bioactivity remains challenging. Quaternary ammonium compounds have been used because of their antibacterial activity; however, their bacterial resistance after long-term use needs to be resolved [10]. Metal-based nanoparticles have recently been extensively developed in view of their well-received antibacterial activity, but their toxicity to mammalian cells is yet to be fully resolved [11].

Following the above trends, phototherapy has emerged as a promising strategy against bacteria owing to its excellent antibacterial activity, non-invasive nature, and fewer chances of bacteria generating bacterial resistance [12]. Hyperthermia-mediated photothermal therapy (PTT) and reactive oxygen species (ROS)-mediated photodynamic therapy (PDT) are the two most widely utilized phototherapies against bacterial infections. The basic mechanism of PTT depends on the light-to-heat conversion ability of photothermal agents (PTAs) after irradiation with desirable light sources. PTAs damage and kill bacteria through various processes (for example, membrane disruption and intracellular component disintegration of bacteria) [13]. Owing to their non-invasive nature, the chances of bacteria becoming resistant to this process are very unlikely relative to those with antibiotic therapies. Moreover, the usual light source utilized in this strategy is near-infrared (NIR) light between 700 and 1100 nm, which shows good tissue penetration ability owing to its longer wavelength. Accordingly, it can influence deep tissues for photothermal antibacterial treatment [14]. Additionally, a biofilm structure can be damaged by hyperthermia, facilitating the penetration of antibacterial agents through the biofilm matrix and efficiently killing bacteria [15]. This localized hyperthermia-mediated strategy for broad-spectrum antibacterial activity has potential clinical applications. However, it also has certain limitations, such as requiring high temperatures ($\geq$60 °C), long-term laser exposures, and a high PTA dosage, which may cause inevitable thermal damage to normal tissues [16].

PDT is another non-invasive therapy. It utilizes a light source to activate photoresponsive materials to generate ROS. The ROS inflict oxidative damage on intracellular components of bacteria and eventually kill them [17]. Similar to PTT, the chance of bacteria becoming resistant to PDT is very unlikely, owing to its light source mechanism. Over the years, the biocompatibilities of the photoresponsive materials for PDT have been optimized with various types of functionalization for more productive and effective antibacterial activity, thereby providing greater potential for clinical applications [12]. However, limitations such as the weak penetration ability of the short-wavelength light for PDT [18] and the lifetime of ROS [19] need to be addressed before the strategy can be fully utilized in clinics.

In this regard, a combination of PTT and PDT seems promising, as both strategies can complement each other's limitations [20]. The PTT and PDT synergistic therapy combination not only maintains the beneficial properties of each strategy but also compensates for the deficiencies of each strategy. The high-temperature requirement of PTT and the weak penetration ability of PDT can be easily overcome if PTT and PDT are synergistically utilized. Therefore, in this review, we briefly describe the advantages and limitations of using PTT and PDT individually, along with their antibacterial mechanisms. Following this, the importance of synergistic PTT and PDT and why they complement each other is discussed. Various advances in antibacterial therapy based on synergistic PTT and PDT are extensively discussed. Finally, future perspectives on the synergistic potential are discussed.

2. Photothermal Therapy (PTT) and Photodynamic Therapy (PDT)

2.1. Photothermal Therapy (PTT)

PTT is a therapeutic method in which light energy is converted into heat energy after PTAs are irradiated by external light sources, such as NIR [20]. This converted heat energy can effectively kill bacteria through a variety of thermal effects, such as cell membrane rupture, cell fluid evaporation, protein/enzyme degeneration, and cell hollowing. Previously, anti-cancer applications were the most used fields for PTT [21]. However, researchers have also utilized PTT in various ways for antibacterial activity and wound healing [13,20]. PTT is a non-invasive technique with low side effects and high specificity. Owing to these beneficial attributes, PTT has emerged as a promising strategy for combatting MDR pathogenic infections.

2.1.1. Mechanism of PTT

The working mechanism of PTT involves the conversion of light energy into heat energy for use in the surrounding environment by photothermal materials. Owing to the distinct photophysical characteristics of various materials, it is evident that photothermal conversion mechanisms are different for different materials. In this section, the photothermal conversion mechanisms (Figure 1) of all the photothermal materials are broadly described.

PTTs using noble metal (for example, Ag and Au)-based nanomaterials are well-known [22], and their excellent photothermal properties can be attributed to the localized surface plasmon resonance (LSPR) effect of the nanomaterials [23]. Free electrons from the noble metallic nanoparticle surface are excited after the nanoparticles absorb the energy of photons at the appropriate wavelengths. The conduction band electrons then start to vibrate collectively at the same frequency. The LSPR effect is the term applied to this phenomenon [24]. LSPR can decay both radiatively and non-radiatively. The plasmonic enhancement of the electric field in the near-field regime is mainly governed by the radiative decay process, whereas the formation of hot electrons is directed by the non-radiative decay process via intra- or inter-band transitions. As light absorption (for example, NIR light) can be increased by modifying a particle size or structure, the LSPR effect is significantly correlated with several characteristics, including particle morphology, size, and composition [25]. The plasma coupling effect is another approach for enhancing the LSPR effect. Although noble metal (Ag and Au)-based nanomaterials are mostly used for the plasmonic effect, some materials, such as Al, Cu, Co, Ni, and CuS, have also been investigated for the same purpose [23].

Another photothermal conversion mechanism comprises the generation and relaxation of electron (e^-)–hole (h^+) pairs (Figure 1); these often occur in semiconductors [26]. In this process, the semiconductor absorbs photons to produce active e^-–h^+ pairs after being irradiated with light energy (the energy should be equal to or greater than the band gap energy of the semiconductor). After light irradiation, electrons are generated in the conduction band (CB), followed by electronic vacancies or holes in the valence band (VB). At this point, either the radiative (photons) or non-radiative (phonons) process is used for the subsequent relaxation from the higher excited states to the lower-energy states. This non-radiative process releases heat, resulting in a thermal (vibrational) energy increment of the lattice, which can be measured as an increase in their temperature.

Lattice vibrations are another photothermal conversion mechanism by which carbon and polymer-based materials exhibit excellent photothermal properties [26]. In this mechanism, less tightly held electrons in Π bonds from the Π orbital can be easily excited to the Π* orbital with lower energy input. Notably, the light-irradiated excitation of electrons (Π→Π*) induces a strong absorption in the NIR region. The excited electrons released the absorbed energy as heat during their return to the ground state, resulting in an increase in the temperature (Figure 1).

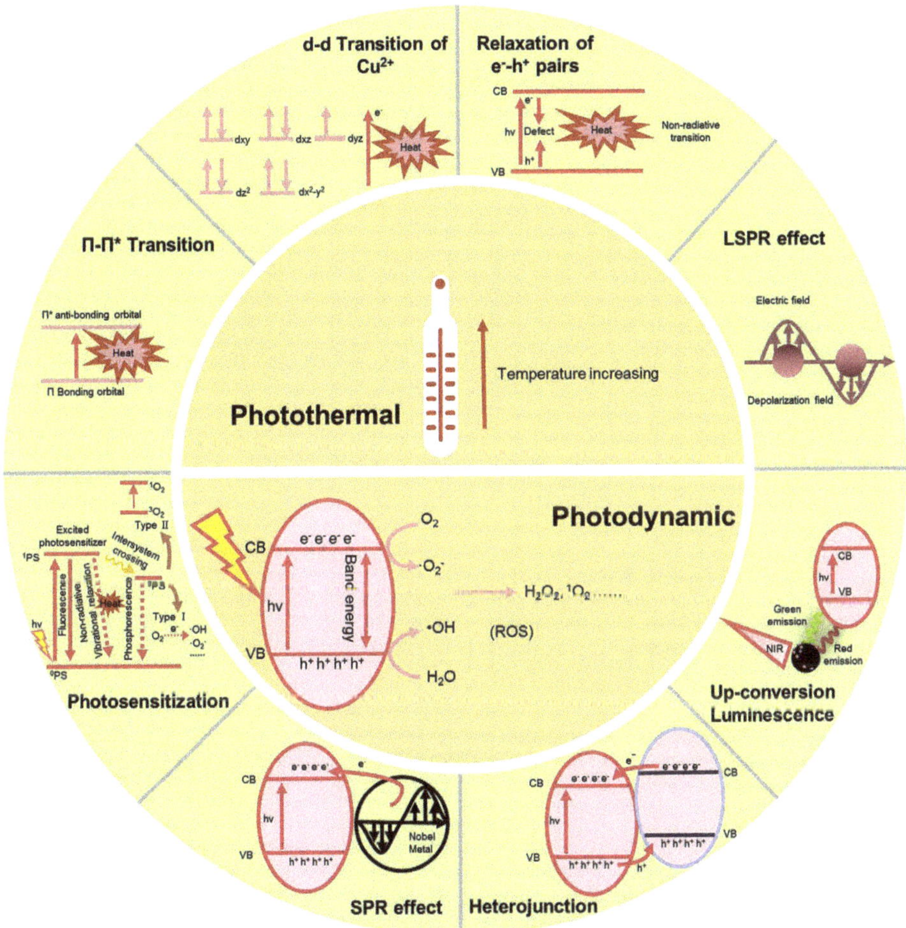

Figure 1. Mechanisms of photothermal therapy (PTT) and photodynamic therapy (PDT). Reproduced with permission from Ref. [12]. Copyright 2020 Elsevier. LSPR: localized surface plasmon resonance, SPR: surface plasmon resonance, CB: conduction band, VB: valence band.

2.1.2. Advantages of PTT

PTT has emerged as a potential solution for treating MDR pathogens and a viable alternative to antibiotics [13,20,27] owing to the following advantages: (1) broad-spectrum antibacterial effects for both Gram-negative (G−) bacteria and Gram-positive (G+) bacteria irrespective of the membrane structure, owing to the penetration ability of the light sources (for example NIR) utilized in PTT; (2) a good tissue penetration ability without causing tissue damage based on the commonly utilized NIR light source (700–1400 nm), which enhances the chances for successful bacterial treatments (even in deep tissues); (3) localized hyperthermia for the antibacterial activity to reduce the risk of damaging normal cells; (4) facilitation of antibacterial agent penetration inside the biofilm via hyperthermia;

and (5) a non-invasive and non-contact mechanism which minimizes the opportunity for bacteria to obtain resistance against the therapy. From the above features, it is easy to understand why PTT-mediated therapy for combatting MDR pathogens is gathering significant attention.

2.1.3. Limitations of PTT

Despite the considerable interest in PTT, significant obstacles remain before PTT can be fully employed for practical applications. First, PTT usually requires high temperatures (≥60 °C) to kill bacteria [20]. Such prolonged hyperthermia kills bacterial cells and thermally harms the normal tissues around bacterial infection sites [16]. Therefore, a more strategic design is necessary to optimize the conditions, for example, with shorter treatment times at lower temperatures (~50 °C). Additionally, normal tissues may be critically affected by the necessity for a high excitation light power and high PTA dosage; these aspects require quick attention to ensure safer and more efficient PTT.

2.2. Photodynamic Therapy (PDT)

PDT combines photoresponsive materials such as photocatalysts and photosensitizers (PSs) and a light source to kill bacterial cells [17]. Currently, PDT has mainly been applied to cancers as a clinical therapeutic approach to treating non-invasive tumors. It is regarded as a major step in anti-cancer applications, including surgery, chemotherapy, and radiotherapy [28]. Additionally, PDT has been applied to other hard-to-treat diseases such as rheumatoid arthritis, actinic keratosis, and bacterial infections. Researchers have used PDT for antibacterial activity owing to its low toxicity, the negligible chance of drug resistance with mild adverse reactions, and excellent antibacterial potential.

2.2.1. Mechanism of PDT

The primary mechanism of PDT relies on the generation of ROS, including hydroxyl radicals (·OH), singlet oxygens ($^1O_2$), or superoxide radicals ($\cdot O^{2-}$) after photoresponsive materials are exposed to laser irradiation [29]. It is widely acknowledged that "toxic" cellular waste (i.e., ROS) can permanently damage macromolecules such as nucleic acids, lipids, and proteins after entering bacterial cells. The ROS generated by the PDT can directly or indirectly interfere with the physiological activities of the cells, ultimately leading to cell death [30]. In a different procedure, ROS can attach to bacterial cell walls and membranes, leading to cell death. As illustrated in Figure 1, photocatalysts, photosensitization, surface plasmon resonance (SPR), heterojunctions, and up-conversion luminescence routes can be utilized under light irradiation for PDT-mediated antibacterial activity.

The basic antibacterial mechanism of photocatalysts, such as ZnO [31] and TiO_2 [32], depends on the nature of the ROS produced during the photoexcitation process. As illustrated in Figure 1, after photoirradiation, the excited electrons (e^-) on the CB reduce O_2 into $\cdot O^{2-}$. Similarly, the photoinduced holes (h^+) on the VB oxidize H_2O to ·OH. These ROS can be further converted to other types of ROS for antibacterial activity [17]. Another effective approach for ROS generation is to form heterojunctions with two or more semiconductors. This can promote charge separations and transfers in single semiconductors instead of the rapid recombination of electron–hole pairs [33], eventually stimulating ROS production and antibacterial activity.

The ROS generation mechanism for PSs differs from that for photocatalysts [34]. There are two main molecular-level mechanisms in the photosensitization route [35] for controlling PDT-mediated antibacterial activity (Figure 1). One of the mechanisms normally occurs in bacterial cell membranes. In this mechanism, molecules from the PS temporarily migrate from the ground state to the singlet state (^{1}PS) and subsequently reach the time-extended triplet state (^{3}PS) by inter-system scurrying. In this scenario, the ^{3}PS produces ROS, such as ·OH and $\cdot O^{2-}$, through electron transfer after reacting with biomolecules in the surrounding environment. Subsequently, the ROS disrupt the bacterial cell membranes and increases their ion permeability for killing bacteria. In the second mechanism, the ^{3}PS can directly react with oxygen molecules to undergo an energy transfer for the formation of $^1O_2$ with a very short lifetime (and only able to react within a micrometer range of its generation site). This singlet oxygen can cause oxidative damage to intracellular bacterial compounds and eventually kill them. The PS molecules return to their ground states for the next cycle of reactions after the reactions are complete.

SPR also has the potential to enhance PDT-mediated antibacterial activity [36]. Photoinduced noble metals (Ag and Au) and metallic compounds (CuS) can produce SPR, which activates electrons that can be transferred to the CBs of the photocatalysts (Figure 1). As a second mechanism, the irradiation near the plasmon resonance frequency of noble metals can substantially enhance the local electric field, accelerating the separation of e^--h^+ pairs. In this regard, PSs and noble metals can be applied together for better antibacterial activity [37].

Up-conversion nanoparticles (UCNPs) represent another approach to resolving the poor penetration ability of PDT. UCNPs can convert the excitation of long-wavelength light into short-wavelength light for PDT based on visible light-responsive photocatalysts [38].

2.2.2. Advantages of PDT

Researchers are eager to seek alternatives to antibiotics owing to the ever-increasing number of MDR pathogens. In this regard, PDT has emerged as a viable option for treating MDR pathogens, owing to the following advantages: (1) broad-spectrum activity with ROS production, which disrupts many metabolic pathways of bacteria and their cellular structures rather than focusing on a single process or structure; (2) light-irradiation-induced antibacterial activity with photoresponsive ROS-generating materials; correspondingly, the chances of bacteria becoming resistant to the photoresponsive materials are very minimal; (3) preferential control of the binding to bacteria at the infected site of the body, light time, and location [39]; (4) low cytotoxicity to normal cells when treating bacterial infections in living organisms; (5) combinations with other therapies, such as radiotherapy, chemotherapy, and PTT; and (6) remote chances of any self-adaptability transferring to the next generation of bacterial cells in a very short time. Hence, the chances of bacteria becoming resistant are greatly reduced.

2.2.3. Limitations of PDT

Despite the above-mentioned advantages of PDT, certain limitations must be addressed before it can be fully utilized to treat bacterial infections in living organisms. ROS-mediated PDT depends on photoresponsive materials and a light source for the irradiation of biological tissues. However, owing to the thickness of human tissue, the poor penetration ability or shallow depth of short-wavelength light or both has hindered the application of PDT to human tissues for antibacterial infections [40]. A longer-wavelength light source could provide greater tissue penetration. However, the ROS production for PDT is directly correlated with the energy of the light; therefore, light sources with longer wavelengths and low energies limit the production of ROS. Thus, UV light with a short wavelength and high energy can produce more ROS and is highly effective in killing microorganisms [41]. However, UV irradiation can also damage normal cells and tissues. Hence, the selection of an appropriate light source must be addressed to improve PDT applications.

Additionally, the development of PDT for clinical use is constrained by the limited release distance and lifespan of the ROS, as well as the low stability, toxicity, and ineffective bacterial targeting of certain photoresponsive materials [17]. Notably, PDT is less effective for G− bacteria than for G+ bacteria owing to the different membrane structures and limited penetration ability of ROS; this also requires further research. Therefore, the limitations of PDT need to be fully addressed before it can be further applied in practical applications.

3. Promising Aspects of Synergistic Action of PTT and PDT Combination

From the information on PTT and PDT discussed above, individual PTT and PDT for antibacterial activity have certain limitations hindering their potential growth for broad-scale and/or clinical application. To overcome this, researchers have attempted to improve the functionality of the individual strategies to resolve the limitations of PTT (for example, higher temperature requirements) and PDT (for example, limited tissue penetration) for excellent antibacterial activity. Notably, however, a synergistic combination of PTT and PDT has recently emerged with excellent potential to overcome the individual disadvantages of PTT and PDT [12,17,20]. The synergistic strategy is quite simple, as the combination enhances the antibacterial potential and retains the potential advantages of each process and compensates for the deficiencies of each strategy [42].

To understand the synergistic mechanisms of PTT and PTT, we must first understand the individual mechanisms of PTT and PDT, as discussed above. In PDT, photoresponsive materials are irradiated by light energy, generating ROS, and quickly killing bacteria. However, a single photodynamic agent requires large amounts of ROS to fulfill the requirements of PDT and kill bacteria. The main drawback, in this case, is that a large amount of ROS also causes problems for normal cells, such as inflammation and fibrosis [43]. To counter this problem, PTT can be employed together for better efficiency for both processes. The heat generated by the PTT can reduce the cell activity of the bacteria and make them more sensitive to ROS, correspondingly reducing the amount of ROS required. Similarly, the higher temperature requirement of PTT to kill bacteria if utilized alone can be reduced if used with PDT, as the ROS generated from the PDT process damages the bacteria and reduces the singular burden of the high-temperature generation by the PTT. Following a similar strategy and synergistic mechanisms, the higher dosage requirements for PTAs could be reduced.

Similarly, the weak penetration ability of ROS can be improved using PTT. As discussed above, the ROS production for PDT directly depends on the energy of the light source, where a higher-energy light source can produce more ROS but reduces the chances of tissue penetration owing to the shorter wavelength [40]. UV light has mostly been used to produce more ROS and kill microorganisms owing to its short wavelength and high energy. However, it also runs the risk of damaging normal healthy tissues because of the negative effect of UV light on mammalian cells [44]. In this scenario, PTT and PDT can be conducted together to achieve synergistic activity. The synergistic mechanism of this process can be realized by the fact that the PTT with the longer-wavelength light source and low energy can penetrate easily to the infection site and induce heat to improve the permeability of the pathogenic cell membrane, which in turn enables easier cellular permeation of the ROS into the membrane and compensates for the lower ROS permeability for PDT [45]. Simultaneously, the ROS can also reduce the heat resistance of the bacteria, thereby reducing the higher temperature requirements for PTT efficacy.

Various researchers have utilized several nanomaterials to achieve synergistic PTT- and PDT-based antibacterial applications (Table 1). Carbon-based materials have shown excellent potential for antibacterial activity as photoresponsive materials [46]. For example, in one study, carbon-based materials were utilized for dual-modal PTT and PDT owing to their potential for hyperthermia and ROS generation through light activation [47]. Zhang et al. [48] utilized cationic carbon dots (CCDs) on black phosphorus (BP) nanosheets, which could bind to the anionic sites of bacteria via electrostatic attraction. BP@CCD produced BP-derived photothermal effects and CCD-originating photodynamic effects in response to mixed laser radiation (660 and 808 nm) for synergistic antibacterial activity. Similarly, graphene quantum dots (GQDs) have been synergistically utilized with germicidal chitosan oligosaccharide (COS) for the simultaneous production of ROS and hyperthermia after 450 nm visible light irradiation, providing highly efficient removal of bacterial infections both in vitro and in vivo [49].

PSs have also been used with PTAs for synergistic PDT with PTT. For example, graphene nanoribbons (GNRs) as PTA have been applied with polycationic porphyrin

(Pp4N) as the PS for hyperthermia generation along with the electrostatic interactions between the cationic Pp4N and negatively charged bacterial cells for wide-spectrum drug-resistant antibacterial activity [50]. In a similar experiment, novel polyfluoroalkyl-substituted silicon phthalocyanine and single-walled carbon nanotubes (SWNTs) were utilized together for heat generation and ROS production after light irradiation and showed synergistic antibacterial activity [51]. Similarly, indocyanine green (ICG) loaded 3-aminopropylsilane coated superparamagnetic iron oxide nanoparticles (APTMS@SPIONs) were evaluated on planktonic cells and biofilms of G- (*Esherichia coli*, *Klebsiella pneumoniae*, *Pseudomonas aeruginosa*) and G+ (*Staphylococcus epidermis*) bacteria for synergistic PTT- and PDT-based antibacterial activity [52]. Cai et al. [53] also encapsulated ICG and manganese pentacarbonyl bromide ($MnBr(CO)_5$) into a 2,2′-bipyridine-4-carboxylic (BPY)-modified peptide dendrimer-based nanogel (G3KBPY) for ICG&CO@G3KBPY nanocomposite which was experimented to treat biofilm infection by synergistic PTT and PDT.

Nanomaterial-based dual-modal PTT and PDT approaches have also been explored for synergistic antibacterial activity. In various studies, gold nanoparticles and polydopamine (PDA)-loaded hydroxyapatite [54], a poly(5-(2-ethylacrylate)-4-methylthiazole-g-butyl)/copper sulfide (CuS) cluster [55], Ce6 combined with ultrasmall protein-modified CuS nanoparticles [56], and CuS-BP nanocomposites [57] have shown PTT and PDT effects under NIR laser irradiation for effective antibacterial activity. Polyethylene glycol-functionalized poly(N-phenylglycine) nanoparticles (PNPG-PEG NPs) also showed an excellent synergistic PTT and PDT potential for antibacterial activity against *E. coli* and *Staphylococcus aureus* [58]. Different small organic molecules were also explored for synergistic PTT- and PDT-based anti-cancer activity [59–61], but not much for antibacterial activity.

The approach to PTT and PDT combination therapy should be synergistic and not only a one-plus-one combination method. Hence, proper experimental procedures and functionalization must be performed to achieve the final synergistic goal of "1 + 1 > 2".

Table 1. Photothermal therapy (PTT)- and photodynamic therapy (PDT)-based synergistic antibacterial applications.

Material	Light Source	Microorganisms	Ref.
BP@CCD	660 and 808 nm	*E. coli*, *S. aureus*	[48]
GQDs-COS	450 nm	*E. coli*, *S. aureus*	[49]
Pp4N/GNR	660 and 808 nm	*A. baumannii*, MRSA	[50]
SiPc-F-SWNTs	680 nm	*E. coli*	[51]
ICG loaded APTMS@SPIONs	808 nm	*E. coli*, *K. pneumoniae*, *P. aeruginosa*, *S. epidermidis*	[52]
PDA@Au-HAp	808 nm	*E. coli*, *S. aureus*	[54]
PATA-C_4@CuS	980 nm	Levofloxacin-resistant *S. aureus*, *E. coli*, *P. aeruginosa*, *B. amyloliquefaciens*	[55]
Ce6-BSA-CuS NPs	660 and 1064 nm	*E. coli*, *S. aureus*	[56]
PNPG-PEG NPs	810 nm	*E. coli*, *S. aureus*	[58]
CuS nanostructures	808 nm, Simulated solar light	*E. coli*	[62]
CuS nanoparticle complex hydrogels	808 nm	*E. coli*, *S. aureus*	[63]
CuS nanodots	808 nm	β-lactamase *E. coli*, MRSA	[64]
PDA-Cur	405 and 808 nm	*E. coli*, *S. aureus*	[65]
Fe_3O_4–Au–PDA	808 nm	*E. coli*	[66]
BC/MoS_2-CS	≥420 nm, xenon lamp	*E. coli*, *S. aureus*	[67]
MoS_2@Au nanorods	808 nm, xenon lamp	*E. coli*	[68]
UCNPs@TiO_2@GO-PVDF	980 nm	*E. coli*, *S. aureus*	[69]
GO-tobramycin@CuS	980 nm	Antibiotic-resistant *P. aeruginosa*, *S. aureus*	[70]
GO/nGO	630 nm	*E. coli*, *S. aureus*	[71]
ICG-GO	808 nm	MRSA	[72]
VCL/PEGDA-MNPs-MWCNTs-ZnMintPc	630 nm	*E. coli*, *S. aureus*, *C. albicans*	[73]
nGO-BSA-AIEgen	795 nm	AMO-resistant *E. coli*, *S. aureus*	[45]

Table 1. *Cont.*

Material	Light Source	Microorganisms	Ref.
BP@Te doped CDs	808 nm	*E. coli, S. aureus*	[74]
N doped CDs@Cur	405 and 808 nm	*E. coli, S. aureus*	[75]
Cu-CDs-C35	808 nm	*E. coli, S. aureus*	[76]
GQD–AgNP	450 nm	*E. coli, S. aureus*	[77]
DMCPNs	808 nm, White light	Ampicillin-resistant *E. coli*	[78]
PEDOT:ICG@PEG-GTA	808 and 1064 nm	*E. coli, S. aureus*	[79]
Ti-RP/PCP/RSNO	808 nm	MRSA	[80]
Ti-PDA/ICG/RGD	808 nm	*S. aureus*	[81]
AuNRs@Cur	405 and 808 nm	*E. coli, S. aureus*	[82]
Au@Bi_2S_3	808 nm	*E. coli, S. aureus*	[83]

Abbreviations: *A. baumannii, Acinetobacter baumannii; B. amyloliquefaciens, Bacillus amyloliquefaciens;* BP, Black Phosphorus; *C. albicans, Candida albicans;* CCD, cationic carbon dots; GQDs, graphene quantum dots; COS, chitosan oligosaccharide; Pp4N, polycationic porphyrin; GNR, graphene nanoribbon; MRSA, Methicillin-resistant *S. aureus;* SiPc-F, polyfluoroalkyl substituted silicon phthalocyanine; SWNTs, single wall carbon nanotubes; ICG, indocyanine green; APTMS, 3-aminopropylsilane; PDA, polydopamine; Hap, hydroxyapatite; PATA,C_4-poly(5-(2-ethyl acrylate)-4-methylthiazole-*g*-butyl); PNPG, poly(*N*-phenylglycine); Cur, Curcumin; BC, bacterial cellulose; CS, chitosan; GO, graphene oxide; UCNP, up-conversion nanoparticle; PVDF, poly(vinylidene) fluoride; VCL/PEGDA, poly (N-vinylcaprolactam-co-poly(ethylene glycol diacrylate)) poly (VCL-co-PEGDA) polymer; MNPs, iron magnetic nanoparticles; MWCNTs, multiwall carbon nanotubes; ZnMintPc, menthol-Zinc phthalocyanine; AIE, aggregation-induced emission fluorogen; AMO, amoxicillin; CDs, carbon quantum dots; C35, cocoamidopropyl betaine; DMCPNs, dual-mode conjugated polymer nanoparticles; PEDOT, poly(3,4-ethylenedioxythiophene) nanoparticle; GTA, glutaraldehyde; Ti-RP, red phosphorus modified Ti implants; PCP, PVA/CS/PDA hydrogel; RSNO; S-nitrosuccinic acid.

Synergistic PTT and PDT Agents

To overcome the individual limitations of PTT and PDT, researchers have utilized dual-mode synergistic PTT- and PDT-based antibacterial therapies. In this respect, research works based on synergistic PTT- and PDT-based antibacterial activity have mostly combined PTT and PDT agents [50,55,56]. The purpose of this conceptual approach to research was to exploit the advantageous properties and overcome the limitations of each process for synergistic antibacterial activity. In one study, owing to the absorption mismatch between the photoresponsive agents for individual PTT and PDT, two different wavelengths of light sources were applied in a nanocomposite to excite PSs and PTAs, respectively [50,56]. Despite obtaining impressive outcomes after exploiting this concept, certain limitations must be resolved. (1) Utilizing both agents together and irradiation with different wavelengths of light is economically costly. (2) The synthesis process for the combination of PTT and PDT is more complex than the individual processes. (3) Proper functionalization is needed for nanocomposite formation with PTT and PDT agents because the various physiochemical characteristics (for example, surface potential, solubility, stability, toxicity, and biodegradability) can interfere with nanocomposite formation and eventually hinder the outcome.

Hence, combining a single nanomaterial or nanocomposite with NIR light irradiation can represent a potential solution to the aforementioned problems, where the heat generation for PTT and ROS production for PDT can be achieved using a single photoresponsive nanomaterial or nanocomposite with a single NIR light source. Notably, the penetration ability of NIR light is far greater than that of UV or visible light [84] and can be utilized by photoresponsive materials to generate ROS and increase temperatures for antibacterial or anti-cancer activity [63,64]. Moreover, NIR light has clinical potential considering its anti-cancer or antibacterial activity [21,28]. Hence, it is easy to understand the extensive use of NIR light not only for antibacterial activity but also for other biomedical applications. Therefore, the aim of researchers in recent years has been to synthesize nanomaterials with the ability of NIR light-mediated photothermal conversion as well as the capacity for singlet oxygen generation [63,64]. Although research in this direction is scarce, there are some materials, such as CuS, PDA, and molybdenum disulfide (MoS_2), which show potential for use in further research regarding NIR light-mediated synergistic PTT- and PDT-based antibacterial activity.

CuS, a semiconducting metal chalcogenide with a narrow bandgap, is widely known as a photothermal nanomaterial with anti-cancer and antibacterial activities owing to its excellent NIR light absorption properties [85]. As discussed above, CuS can absorb NIR light using the LSPR originating from the collective oscillation of holes instead of the electron-mediated LSPR for noble metals [85]. Therefore, unlike noble metals, the LSPR position of CuS (and, accordingly, its photothermal properties) can be controlled by modulating the number of carriers. Moreover, CuS shows the ability to generate ROS after irradiation with NIR light. Thus, it can be functionalized for use as a PTT- and PDT-based synergistic antibacterial agent without the need for individual materials. For example, Mutalik et al. [62] demonstrated the morphology-dependent photodynamic and photothermal antibacterial activity of NIR light-irradiated CuS against *E. coli*. Similarly, Zhou et al. [63] demonstrated an injectable self-healing hydrogel system consisting of a CuS-based complex with the potential to completely eradicate *E. coli* and *S. aureus* via synergistic PTT and PDT under NIR laser irradiation. Qiao et al. [64] demonstrated a similar NIR laser-irradiated PTT- and PDT-based antibacterial potential of CuS nanodots against methicillin-resistant *S. aureus* (MRSA) and extended-spectrum β-lactamase *E. coli*.

PDA is another material with excellent PTT- and PDT-based synergistic potential for NIR light-mediated antibacterial activity [86]. Several advantageous properties of PDA, such as its simple preparation process, easy functionalization, excellent photothermal and photoacoustic properties, biocompatibility, and biodegradability, have led to several PDA-based biomedical research studies. Regarding antibacterial activity, PDA is regarded as an excellent PTA with a good ROS generation ability after laser irradiation. Hence, a single nanomaterial or nanocomposite can be used for synergistic PTT and PDT after NIR light irradiation using PDA. Su et al. [65] demonstrated the excellent PTT- and PDT-based synergistic antibacterial activity of PDA-based nanocomposites. PDA–curcumin (PDA–Cur) nanocomposites) were prepared via self-polymerization. The PDA–Cur nanocomposites showed good antibacterial activity against *S. aureus* and *E. coli* with good biocompatibility. In another experiment, magnetic Fe_3O_4–Au–PDA hybrid microcapsules were developed for NIR laser-irradiated synergistic PTT- and PDT-based antibacterial activity against *E. coli* [66].

MoS_2 is another nanomaterial that has shown significant potential in this category. Similar to PDA, MoS_2 is an excellent PTA material with remarkable photothermal antibacterial properties and has the potential to generate ROS after laser irradiation. Hence, synergistic PTT- and PDT-based antibacterial activity is possible with MoS_2-based nanocomposites. Shen et al. [67] developed in situ-grown bacterial cellulose/MoS_2–chitosan nanocomposite materials for PTT- and PDT-based antibacterial activities. The nanocomposite showed excellent antibacterial efficacy against *E. coli* (99.998%) and *S. aureus* (99.988%) after visible-light irradiation. Yougbaré et al. [68] also demonstrated antibacterial activity against *E. coli* like that of MoS_2@Au nanorods with NIR laser irradiation.

4. Synergistic Antibacterial Applications of PTT and PDT

Synergistic combination therapies of PTT and PDT have been designed based on multi-target bactericidal activity, where the deficiencies of a single treatment therapy are overcome via the synergistic combination. Researchers have tested various materials for synergistic antibacterial activity. In this review, we summarized (1) carbon-, (2) polymer-, and (3) metal-based materials for synergistic antibacterial PTT and PDT combinations.

4.1. Carbon-Based Combination of PTT and PDT

Carbon-based materials have been considered ideal for various biomedical applications owing to their negligible cytotoxicity and environmentally benign nature [87,88]. Additionally, their tunable parameters (such as size, shape, and layer number) can generate excellent physiochemical properties and have proven excellent assets for antibacterial activity [49,50,70–72,87]. Typically, graphene, carbon dots, and carbon nanotubes (CNTs) have been explored for synergistic PTT and PDT therapies owing to their NIR light absorption properties and photothermal conversion abilities.

The immense success of graphene in biomedical applications is well-known, with numerous studies on graphene as a core material [70–72,87,88]. The unique optical properties of graphene and its derivatives \[graphene oxide (GO) and reduced GO (RGO)], that is, their ability to absorb light energy and release it as heat energy, have encouraged researchers to utilize it for PTT applications [70–72]. Furthermore, graphene can produce ROS after irradiation with NIR light. It is also believed that 2D graphene can utilize its sharp edges to destroy the cellular membranes of bacteria, ultimately killing them [89]. The broad-spectrum antibacterial activities of GO and RGO have also been exploited by researchers [70–72,87].

Another advantage of graphene is that it can be functionalized into a single nanocomposite for synergistic photothermal and photodynamic antibacterial activity using a single NIR light source. For example, Sun et al. [69] reported the utilization of up-conversion nanoparticles (UCNPs) consisting of $NaYF_4$:Yb:Tm nanorods with a hierarchical core-shell structure (UCNPs@TiO_2) (Figure 2). Subsequently, photothermal GO was incorporated into the UCNPs@TiO_2 for a UCNPs@TiO_2@GO (UTG) nanocomposite. Finally, the mixture was electrospun in a poly(vinylidene) fluoride (PVDF) membrane to prepare a UTG–PVDF nanocomposite. A single NIR light (980 nm) source was used to irradiate the UTG–PVDF nanocomposites for 5 min. Simultaneously, ROS were generated, and the temperature increased, providing synergistic antibacterial effects against both G- and G+ bacteria. This antibacterial activity is difficult to achieve using individual photodynamic or photothermal nanocomposite membranes. Furthermore, the graphene-based nanocomposite membrane accelerated wound healing, further enhancing its potential for infectious wound healing studies.

The NIR light absorption of graphene has been frequently used for heat energy generation and ROS production [49,50,70–72]. However, the fast recombination rate of the electrons and holes in GO hinders its application in synergistic PTT and PDT. Dai et al. [70] found a solution to this problem by introducing CuS and the aminoglycoside antibiotic tobramycin (Tob) to form a GO–Tob@CuS hybrid nanoplatform. CuS was added to solve the problem of fast recombination of the electrons and holes. Additionally, the broad-spectrum antibiotic Tob was selected to modify the surface charge potential of the GO because the surface charge of GO is usually negative and is not ideal for interactions with electronegative bacterial surface charges. The GO–Tob@CuS nanocomposite showed excellent PTT and PDT effects after NIR laser (980 nm, 1.5 $W \cdot cm^{-2}$) irradiation for 5 min, with a temperature increment of up to 65 °C at a concentration of 100 $\mu g \cdot mL^{-1}$. ROS were also produced after the NIR irradiation. Moreover, the GO–Tob@CuS nanocomposite showed irreversible damage to antibiotic-resistant *P. aeruginosa* and *S. aureus* species after NIR laser irradiation by utilizing the nano-knife effect along with the PTT and PDT properties of the nanocomposite.

In another experiment, Romero et al. [71] demonstrated the broad-spectrum and selective antibacterial activity of GO and nanographene oxide (nGO) against *E. coli* and *S. aureus* species by utilizing the synergistic PTT and PDT effects. The GO and nGO showed the ability to form ROS with an increase in temperature from 55 to 60 °C when irradiated with an LED red light at 630 nm (65 $mW \cdot cm^{-2}$), effectively killing the targeted bacterial cells using the synergistic PTT and PDT effects. In another direct synergistic procedure, the PS indocyanine green (ICG), usually used for PDT, was loaded onto photothermal GO nanosheets for NIR-irradiated anti-MRSA activity [72]. The NIR (808 nm, 1 $W \cdot cm^{-2}$)-irradiated ICG–GO showed a photothermal temperature increment of 43.1 °C and the highest ROS generation (increments of 316.51% and 157.11% compared with ICG and GO alone, respectively), representing a potent material for inhibiting the growth of MRSA. In a similar study, the PS menthol-zinc phthalocyanine was encapsulated in magnetic nanocomposites with GO and multiwall CNTs to prepare a biocompatible hydrogel [73].

Subsequently, its broad-spectrum antibacterial activity was evaluated based on its synergistic PTT and PDT effects. The magnetic nanocomposite was irradiated with a red light of 630 nm/65.5 mW·cm^{-2}. The nanocomposite was able to eliminate three types of microbial colonies (*C. albicans*, *E. coli*, and *S. aureus*) using the synergistic PTT and PDT effect and could be considered a broad-spectrum photoresponsive antibacterial agent. GNRs [50] and SWNTs [51] have also been utilized for synergistic antibacterial activities. Zhang et al. [45] entrapped hydrophobic aggregation-induced emission fluorogens (AIEgens) in amphiphilic nGO and bovine serum albumin (BSA) nanocomposites. The biocompatibility of the nanoparticles was enhanced by conjugation with the BSA. Moreover, the nanocomposite formed a dual-mode (PTT and PDT) antibacterial application using the heat produced by the nGO- and AIEgen-produced ROS for collaborative antibacterial results under light irradiation.

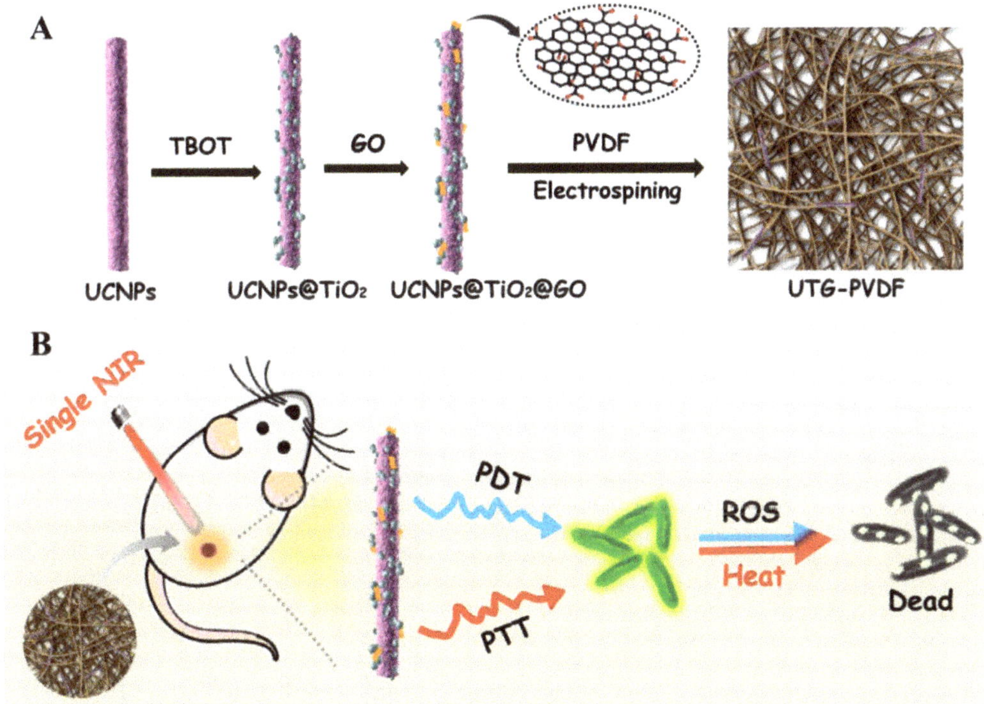

Figure 2. (**A**) Schematic diagram of up-conversion nanoparticles@TiO_2@graphene oxide (UTG)-poly(vinylidene) fluoride (PVDF) nanocomposite membrane synthesis, (**B**) Near-infrared (NIR) light-mediated PTT- and PDT-based synergistic antibacterial activities of UTG-PVDF membrane. Reproduced with permission from Ref. [69]. Copyright 2019, American Chemical Society.

Despite the immense success of graphene in biomedical applications (including those based on antibacterial activity), many hurdles remain before it can be fully applied in clinical applications. For example, the complex interactions of graphene with biological membranes can lead to endotoxin contamination during synthesis, mitochondria-mediated apoptosis, and septic shock [90]. In this regard, researchers have developed carbon quantum dots (CDs), a new carbon-based nanomaterial for biomedical applications [74–76]. CDs are well-known for their biocompatibility, excellent water solubility, and stability. However, the NIR absorption properties of CDs are not satisfactory for phototherapy. Therefore, more functionalized CDs for CD-based nanocomposites are required for the synergistic PTT and PDT effect to achieve antibacterial activity.

Liu et al. [74] constructed a 2D antibacterial nanoplatform by combining liquid-phase exfoliated BP and hydrothermally prepared tellurium-doped CDs, thereby combining the favorable biomedical properties of CDs with the photothermal properties of BP. A single 808 nm NIR laser irradiation process was used to induce the photothermal conversion of BP with ROS generation from the CDs. The BP@CDs showed PTT- and PDT-mediated excellent synergistic antibacterial activity against *E. coli* and *S. aureus* (as high as 98.4 and 92.7%, respectively), coupled with a faster wound closure ratio than other infected wounds. The BP@CD nanoplatform also showed good hemocompatibility, cytocompatibility, and biocompatibility; thus, it could be utilized clinically. Zhang et al. [48] performed a similar experiment using BP and CCDs.

In another study, nitrogen-doped CDs were compounded with Cur to prepare a synergistic nanocomposite showing dual-mode PTT and PDT antibacterial activity [75]. In this synergistic nanocomposite, the biocompatibility and rich amphiphilic functional group-mediated solubility of the CDs perfectly complemented the Cur, a natural PS with powerful antibacterial properties but with insolubility in water. Blue (405 nm) and near-infrared (808 nm) light sources were utilized for generating ROS and hyperthermia, respectively. The CD-based Cur nanocomposite showed synergistic PTT- and PDT-based antibacterial activity against *E. coli* and *S. aureus* under the dual light source (405 + 808 nm) irradiation, along with low toxicity and good hemocompatibility. A similar approach was reported by Mei et al. [49], in which COS-functionalized GQDs were utilized to kill *E. coli* and *S. aureus* after short-term exposure to 450 nm visible light (Figure 3). The nanocomposite also showed good hemocompatibility and low cytotoxicity for infected wound healing.

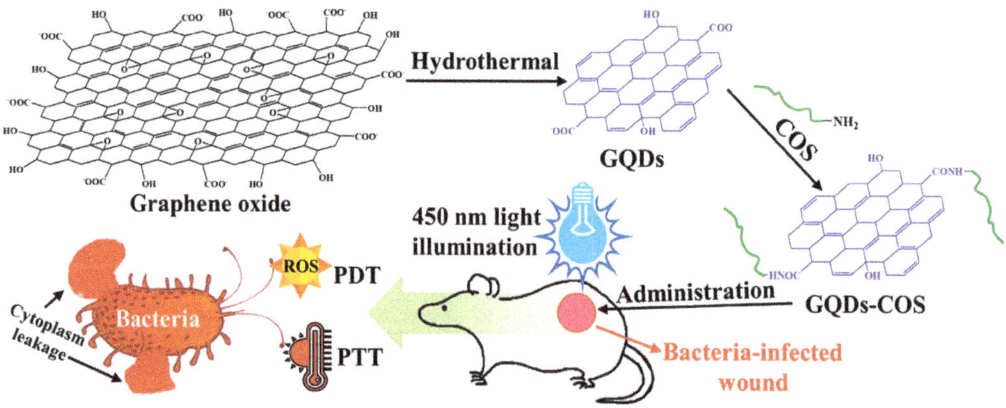

Figure 3. Schematic illustration of graphene quantum dots (GQDs)-chitosan oligosaccharide (COS) synthesis and its PTT- and PDT-based synergistic antibacterial wound healing. Reproduced with permission from Ref. [49]. Copyright 2020 American Chemical Society.

Metal-based nanoparticles also have antibacterial and excellent NIR absorption properties, with numerous reports supporting these claims [91–93]. However, their toxicity hinders their further growth. A combination of metal nanoparticles with CDs reduces the risk of toxicity owing to the CDs and increases the chances of obtaining photothermal properties owing to metal-based nanoparticles. For example, Chu et al. [76] proposed a combination of copper ions with CDs and quaternary amino compounds for synergistic photothermal and photodynamic-based antibacterial activity against *E. coli* and *S. aureus*. with 808 nm NIR light irradiation, leading to a temperature increment of up to 57.3 °C and efficient ROS production. Thus, a synergistic PTT and PDT approach was established. In another similar experiment [77], Ag-conjugated GQDs were utilized as blue light-enhanced nanotherapeutics for antimicrobial therapy. The nanocomposite showed improved production of ROS combined with a significant increase in temperature for synergistic PTT- and PDT-mediated antibacterial activity.

4.2. Polymer-Based PTT and PDT

Conjugated polymers (CPs) have shown excellent potential for biomedical applications owing to their unique conjugated backbone structures and exceptional photophysical properties [78,79]. One of the major advantages of CPs is that they can generate ROS and heat based on light energy irradiation after synthesis by regulating the backbone structures. Additionally, CPs are biocompatible and photostable, and the cost of their synthesis is low. Unsurprisingly, CPs have emerged as potential candidates for PSs (PDT) and PTAs (PTT). Moreover, water-insoluble CPs can be developed into nanoparticles with good dispersibility and biocompatibility for use in aqueous media without complicated water-soluble modifications [94]. These water-insoluble CPs can also be utilized for the photothermal releases of drugs. Researchers are constantly trying to exploit the beneficial properties of PTT and PDT while limiting the deficiencies of each process. CPs may represent a valid force for synergistic PTT- and PDT-mediated antibacterial activity.

Cui et al. [95] developed a water-insoluble conjugated polymer (PDPP)-mediated antibacterial hydrogel with synergistic PTT and PDT antibacterial capabilities. A nano-precipitation method was used to convert the PDPP into water-insoluble nanoparticles. Subsequently, the cell-penetrating peptide "TAT" was grafted onto the PDPP surface. Finally, a polyisocyanide (PIC) hydrogel was added. The PIC hybrid intelligently regulated its antibacterial ability when sequentially irradiated with white light and NIR light and showed stronger antibacterial ability than PDT or PTT alone.

In another study, Zhang et al. [78] utilized dual-mode antibacterial conjugated polymer nanoparticles (DMCPNs) for PTT and PDT for the efficient killing of ampicillin-resistant *E. coli* (Figure 4). A co-precipitation method was employed for the self-assembly of DM-CPNs using poly(diketopyrrolopyrrole-thienothiophene) as the PTA and poly [2-methoxy-5-((2-ethylhexyl)oxy)-p-phenylenevinylene] as a PS. Poly(styrene-co-maleic anhydride) has also been used for nanoparticle dispersion in water via hydrophobic interactions. The DM-CPNs produced a 93% inhibition rate of ampicillin-resistant *E. coli.* after dual irradiation with near-infrared light (550 mW$\cdot$cm^{-2}, 5 min) and white light (65 mW$\cdot$cm^{-2}, 5 min). This antibacterial activity was attributed to the ability of DMCPNs to generate photothermal effects and ROS after exposure to oxygen in the surroundings after light irradiation.

Despite the excellent potential of CPs for PTT- and PDT-mediated antibacterial activity, more CP nanoparticles absorbed NIR light in the first biological window (NIR-I, 700 and 950 nm) than in the second NIR window (NIR-II, 1000 and 1250 nm) [96]. The NIR-II window has advantages regarding the spatial scattering effect and penetration depth. Following this principle, Li et al. [79] synthesized a poly(3,4-ethylenedioxythiophene) nanoparticle (PEDOT)-based nanocomposite for dual-mode (PTT + PDT) antibacterial activity owing to the broad absorbance of PEDOT in the NIR region (700 and 1250 nm). In this work, ICG dye was conjugated with PEDOT using an environmentally friendly hydrothermal method utilizing the electrostatic attraction between them. The PEDOT nanoparticles were initially modified with glutaraldehyde (GTA) for bacterial targeting. The functionalized and stable PEDOT:ICG@PEG-GTA nanocomposite exhibited excellent synergistic antibacterial potential against pathogenic bacteria in the presence of NIR irradiation (808 nm for PDT and 1064 nm for PTT) in both the NIR-I and -II windows and was considerably more effective than PTT or PDT alone.

An MRSA infection through biofilm was also managed using a hydrophilic and viscous hydrogel consisting of PVA modified with chitosan, PDA, and an NO release donor formed on a red phosphorus nanofilm deposited on a titanium (Ti) implant. The MRSA biofilm was synergistically destroyed by ROS and hyperthermia under NIR irradiation [80]. Yuan et al. [81] exploited NIR light-triggered PTT and PDT to eradicate biofilms on Ti implants. Mesoporous PDA (MPDA) nanoparticles were immobilized onto an amino-modified Ti surface. An ICG PS was then integrated into the MPDA by π–π stacking. Finally, to eliminate the NIR-triggered *S. aureus* biofilm in vivo through the synergistic PDT and PTT effects, the system was functionalized with an RGD peptide for the final sample (Ti-M/I/RGD).

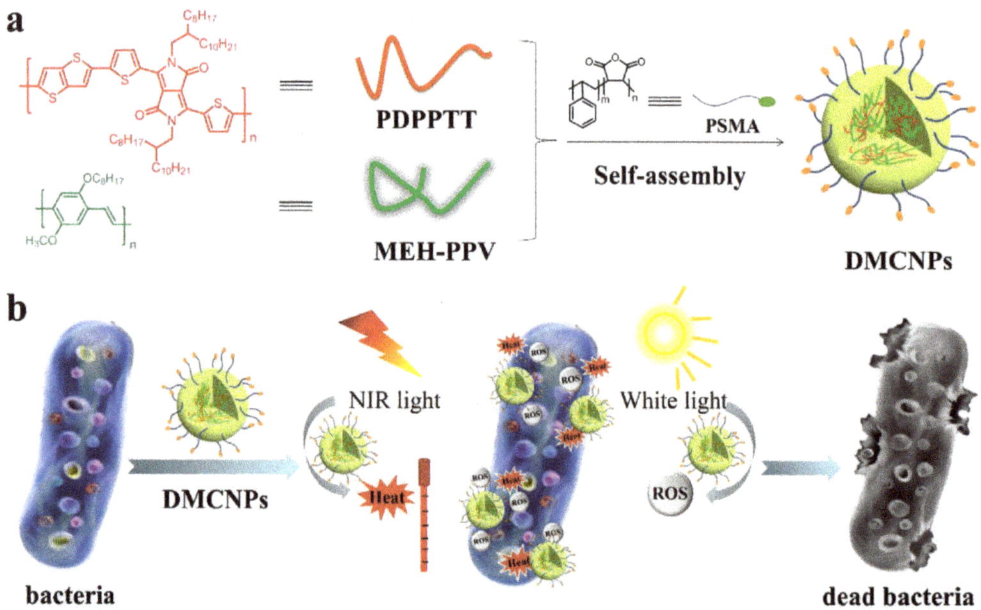

Figure 4. (**a**) Schematic illustration for the synthesis of utilized dual-mode antibacterial conjugated polymer nanoparticles (DMCPNs), (**b**) PTT- and PDT-based synergistic antibacterial activity of DMCPNs. Reproduced with permission from Ref. [78]. Copyright 2019 Wiley.

4.3. Metal-Based Combination of PTT and PDT

Metal-based nanoparticles are well-known for their inherent antibacterial properties. Au, Ag, Pd, ZnO, CuO, and CuS have been reported to exhibit antibacterial activities owing to their favorable physicochemical properties [1,97]. Moreover, some of them are considered photoresponsive materials due to their ability to absorb light sources and convert them into heat energy or to produce ROS after light irradiation [85,98]. However, their poor photostability, low targeting efficiency, and cytotoxicity in mammalian cells have hindered their broad application for clinical antibacterial activity. Hence, researchers are constantly trying to exploit the advantageous properties of metal-based nanoparticles for PDT- and PTT-based antibacterial activity in combination with efforts to limit their deficiencies.

Zhang et al. [82] synthesized core-shell gold nanorod (Au NR)@mesoporous-silica/Cur nanocomplexes for dual-mode PTT and PDT antibacterial activity (Figure 5). Each material in the nanocomposite had a specific role, with the overall goal being synergistic PTT- and PDT-mediated antibacterial activity. Au NRs have been intentionally exploited in gold nanocrystals owing to having the highest photothermal ability. In one study, cationic surfactant cetyltrimethylammonium bromide (CTAB) was used to prepare Au NRs and was essential to improving their stability. However, CTAB also has low compatibility and high toxicity in molecular biofilms. Hence, biocompatible mesoporous silica (SiO_2) was employed to coat the Au NRs to remove the CTAB toxicity. Subsequently, Cur with antibacterial photodynamic potential was constructed onto the mesoporous silica modified Au NRs. The nanocomposite showed excellent dual-mode (PTT and PDT) antibacterial potential after double-wavelength (405 + 808 nm) laser irradiation. The biocompatibility of the nanocomposite was also appropriate for its potential in vivo application.

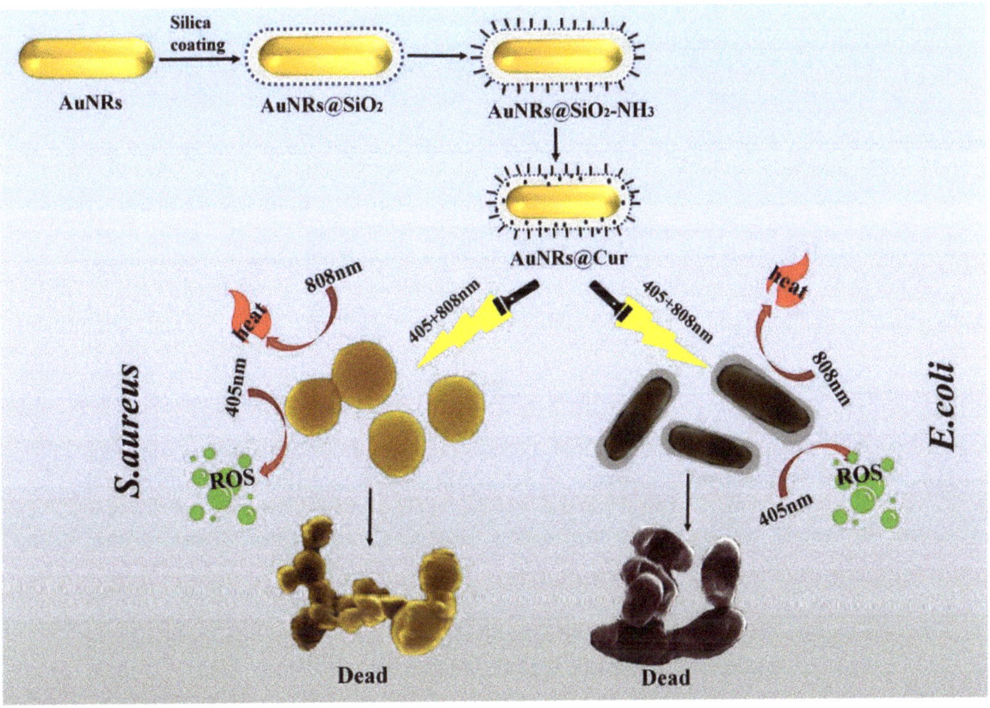

Figure 5. Schematic illustration of preparation and synergistic antibacterial activity of gold nanorods (Au NRs)@curcumin (Cur). Reproduced with permission from Ref. [82]. Copyright 2022 Elsevier.

Similarly, another study successfully exploited sea urchin-like Au@Bi_2S_3 core-shell structures for the synergetic photothermal and photodynamic inactivation of *E. coli* and *S. aureus* after NIR light irradiation [83]. Fang et al. [66] synthesized a magnetic Fe_3O_4–Au–PDA hybrid microcapsule with both photothermal and photodynamic antibacterial potential. Later, tetracarboxyzinc phthalocyanine (ZnPc) was loaded into Fe_3O_4–Au–PDA hybrid microcapsules. The Au–PDA hybrid shell exhibited a photothermal nature and the photodynamic potential was served by the ZnPc PS. The final Fe_3O_4–Au–PDA/ZnPc hybrid microcapsule showed excellent synergistic (PTT and PDT) antibacterial activity against *E. coli* after irradiation with an 808 nm NIR laser.

Metal sulfides have recently emerged as exciting photothermal materials owing to their stability and NIR light-absorption properties [85]. Moreover, Cu-based nanomaterials have gained significant attention for their NIR-mediated antibacterial activity owing to their essential trace element status in the human body. Under these circumstances, CuS has emerged as an excellent NIR light-absorbing nanomaterial with PTT- and PDT-mediated antibacterial activity. For example, Dai et al. [55] prepared poly (5-(2-ethyl acrylate)-4-methylthiazole-g-butyl)/CuS nanoclusters to efficiently capture and eliminate levofloxacin-resistant G- and G+ bacteria using NIR light-mediated synergistic PTT and PDT. A thiazole derivative was applied to this nanocomposite as a membrane-targeting cationic ligand for the bacteria. Under NIR laser irradiation, these conjugated nanoclusters (980 nm, 1.5 $W{\cdot}cm^{-2}$, 5 min) significantly inhibited *B. amyloliquefaciens*, *E. coli*, levofloxacin-resistant *S. aureus*, and *P. aeruginosa* at 5.5 $\mu g{\cdot}mL^{-1}$. The generation of the heat and ROS after NIR light irradiation was attributed to the antibacterial activity, suggesting a synergistic PTT- and PDT-mediated antibacterial activity.

Wang et al. [99] reported that implant-related bacterial infections in orthopedic clinics could be overcome using dual-mode PTT and PDT. In one study, PEG-modified Cu_9S_8

nanoparticles with good biocompatibility were synthesized using a facile one-step wet chemical method. The PEG-modified Cu_9S_8 nanoparticles showed synergistic PTT- and PDT-mediated antibacterial activity with excellent antibiofilm activity against clinically collected pathogenic *S. aureus* growing on Ti surfaces under NIR irradiation (808 nm, 1 W·cm^{-2}).

5. Conclusions and Future Perspectives

Notable developments have been made in killing bacteria and inhibiting their ever-increasing antibiotic resistance. However, it can also be unanimously agreed that a more precise and functionalized strategy is required to tackle MDR bacteria. Following this principle, synergistic PTT and PDT have the potential to be combined with antibiotics to offer a unique opportunity to effectively tackle infections caused by MDR bacteria. Additionally, the chances of bacteria becoming resistant to combination therapy are very remote owing to their non-invasive nature. A multimodal PDT and PTT combination strategy is also possible while using a single nanomaterial instead of using two materials for each individual property.

It is worthwhile to mention that thermal damage to normal tissues owing to the high temperature need of PTT may be managed by employing it with PDT therapy as it lowers the dependency on single-mode PTT use. Furthermore, the targeting ability of photoresponsive materials can be used to solve this problem. This targeting ability, however, necessitates additional research into the precise positioning of synergistic photoresponsive materials that can easily target the intended bacteria or infection site. In this respect, surface modification can be useful, as it is well-known that the surface of photoresponsive materials plays an important role in their antibacterial activity. Because most bacteria have a negative surface potential due to a peptidoglycan coating, electrostatic interactions may play a key role in this scenario. As a result, non-toxic positive charge molecules such as chitosan derivatives have been exploited for specifically targeting bacteria. However, further research is still required with respect to surface functionalization. Moreover, a more tailored synergistic antibacterial activity is required for the precision and accuracy of the antibacterial activity.

Additional PTT and PDT combinations may be relevant in future application-oriented research, such as drug administration and immunotherapy. Similarly, the limited penetration capacity of typical ROS light sources is easily overcome by high-penetration light sources of PTT when they are utilized synergistically. Furthermore, the ability of photoresponsive materials to penetrate the extracellular matrix of biofilm requires more research because bacteria can easily protect themselves within the extracellular matrix of biofilm due to limited options, as high concentrations of antibacterial agents induce cytotoxicity in normal cells. Some structural alteration, such as needle-like nanomaterials as synergistic PTT and PDT agents, is required in this respect. Instead of using nanocomposites, where different PTT and PDT agents are combined for synergistic antibacterial activity, more emphasis should be placed on finding single antibacterial agents, such as CuS, where the PTT- and PDT- based synergistic antibacterial activity can be experienced through a single nanomaterial.

Despite its remarkable potential, issues remain to be resolved. Certain clinical trials regarding the synergistic potential of PTT and PDT need to be established for practical applications. The photosensitive materials utilized for both PTT and PDT have not yet fully proven their non-toxicity. Greater research efforts are still required for photoirradiated synergistic PTT- and PDT-based antibacterial activity and can be further explored in clinical trials. In summary, we sincerely hope that the emergence of synergistic PTT and PDT will fulfill its potential and emerge as a serious force for clinically managing infections caused by MDR bacteria.

Author Contributions: Conceptualization, A.N. and K.-s.K.; writing and review, A.N. and K.-s.K.; funding acquisition, K.-s.K. All authors have read and agreed to the published version of the manuscript.

Funding: This research was funded by a National Research Foundation of Korea (NRF) grant from the Korean Government (MSIT) (grant number NRF-2021R1A2C1007413].

Institutional Review Board Statement: Not applicable.

Informed Consent Statement: Not applicable.

Data Availability Statement: Not applicable.

Conflicts of Interest: The authors declare that there are no conflict of interest.

References

1. Naskar, A.; Kim, K.-S. Nanomaterials as Delivery Vehicles and Components of New Strategies to Combat Bacterial Infections: Advantages and Limitations. *Microorganisms* **2019**, *7*, 356. [CrossRef]
2. Uddin, T.M.; Chakraborty, A.J.; Khusro, A.; Zidan, B.R.M.; Mitra, S.; Emran, T.B.; Dhama, K.; Ripon, M.K.H.; Gajdács, M.; Sahibzada, M.U.K.; et al. Antibiotic resistance in microbes: History, mechanisms, therapeutic strategies and future prospects. *J. Infect. Public Health* **2021**, *14*, 1750–1766. [CrossRef] [PubMed]
3. Kolář, M. Bacterial Infections, Antimicrobial Resistance and Antibiotic Therapy. *Life* **2022**, *12*, 468. [CrossRef] [PubMed]
4. Zhang, F.; Cheng, W. The Mechanism of Bacterial Resistance and Potential Bacteriostatic Strategies. *Antibiotics* **2022**, *11*, 1215. [CrossRef] [PubMed]
5. Reygaert, W.C. An overview of the antimicrobial resistance mechanisms of bacteria. *AIMS Microbiol.* **2018**, *4*, 482–501. [CrossRef]
6. Sharma, D.; Misba, L.; Khan, A.U. Antibiotics versus biofilm: An emerging battleground in microbial communities. *Antimicrob. Resist. Infect. Control* **2019**, *8*, 76. [CrossRef]
7. Kang, S.J.; Nam, S.H.; Lee, B.J. Engineering Approaches for the Development of Antimicrobial Peptide-Based Antibiotics. *Antibiotics* **2022**, *11*, 1338. [CrossRef]
8. Starr, C.G.; Wimley, W.C. Antimicrobial peptides are degraded by the cytosolic proteases of human erythrocytes. *Biochim. Biophys. Acta* **2017**, *1859*, 2319–2326. [CrossRef]
9. Gong, C.; Sun, J.; Xiao, Y.; Qu, X.; Lang, M. Synthetic Mimics of Antimicrobial Peptides for the Targeted Therapy of Multidrug-Resistant Bacterial Infection. *Adv. Healthc. Mater.* **2021**, *10*, 2101244. [CrossRef]
10. Mohapatra, S.; Yutao, L.; Goh, S.G.; Ng, C.; Luhua, Y.; Tran, N.H.; Gin, K.Y. Quaternary ammonium compounds of emerging concern: Classification, occurrence, fate, toxicity and antimicrobial resistance. *J. Hazard Mater.* **2023**, *445*, 130393. [CrossRef]
11. Zhang, N.; Xiong, G.; Liu, Z. Toxicity of metal-based nanoparticles: Challenges in the nano era. *Front. Bioeng. Biotechnol.* **2022**, *10*, 1001572. [CrossRef] [PubMed]
12. Ren, Y.; Liu, H.; Liu, X.; Zheng, Y.; Li, Z.; Li, C.; Yeung, K.W.K.; Zhu, S.; Liang, Y.; Cui, Z.; et al. Photoresponsive Materials for Antibacterial Applications. *Cell Rep. Phys. Sci.* **2020**, *1*, 100245. [CrossRef]
13. Bai, X.; Yang, Y.; Zheng, W.; Huang, Y.; Xu, F.; Bao, Z. Synergistic photothermal antibacterial therapy enabled by multifunctional nanomaterials: Progress and perspectives. *Mater. Chem. Front.* **2023**, *7*, 355–380. [CrossRef]
14. Qu, Y.; Lu, K.; Zheng, Y.; Huang, C.; Wang, G.; Zhang, Y.; Yu, Q. Photothermal scaffolds/surfaces for regulation of cell behaviors. *Bioact. Mater.* **2021**, *8*, 449–477. [CrossRef]
15. Alumutairi, L.; Yu, B.; Filka, M.; Nayfach, J.; Kim, M.H. Mild magnetic nanoparticle hyperthermia enhances the susceptibility of *Staphylococcus aureus* biofilm to antibiotics. *Int. J. Hyperth.* **2020**, *37*, 66–75. [CrossRef]
16. Zhu, X.; Feng, W.; Chang, J.; Tan, Y.W.; Li, J.; Chen, M.; Sun, Y.; Li, F. Temperature-feedback upconversion nanocomposite for accurate photothermal therapy at facile temperature. *Nat. Commun.* **2016**, *7*, 10437. [CrossRef]
17. Hu, X.; Zhang, H.; Wang, Y.; Shiu, B.-C.; Lin, J.-H.; Zhang, S.; Lou, C.-W.; Li, T.-T. Synergistic antibacterial strategy based on photodynamic therapy: Progress and perspectives. *Chem. Eng. J.* **2022**, *450*, 138129. [CrossRef]
18. Fan, W.; Bu, W.; Shi, J. On The Latest Three-Stage Development of Nanomedicines based on Upconversion Nanoparticles. *Adv. Mater.* **2016**, *28*, 3987–4011. [CrossRef]
19. Ming, L.; Cheng, K.; Chen, Y.; Yang, R.; Chen, D. Enhancement of tumor lethality of ROS in photodynamic therapy. *Cancer Med.* **2021**, *10*, 257–268. [CrossRef]
20. Huo, J.; Jia, Q.; Huang, H.; Zhang, J.; Li, P.; Dong, X.; Huang, W. Emerging photothermal-derived multimodal synergistic therapy in combating bacterial infections. *Chem. Soc. Rev.* **2021**, *50*, 8762–8789. [CrossRef]
21. Han, H.S.; Choi, K.Y. Advances in Nanomaterial-Mediated Photothermal Cancer Therapies: Toward Clinical Applications. *Biomedicines* **2021**, *9*, 305. [CrossRef]
22. Lv, Z.; He, S.; Wang, Y.; Zhu, X. Noble Metal Nanomaterials for NIR-Triggered Photothermal Therapy in Cancer. *Adv. Healthc. Mater.* **2021**, *10*, e2001806. [CrossRef] [PubMed]
23. Kim, M.; Lee, J.H.; Nam, J.M. Plasmonic Photothermal Nanoparticles for Biomedical Applications. *Adv. Sci.* **2019**, *6*, 1900471. [CrossRef] [PubMed]

24. Li, J.; Zhang, W.; Ji, W.; Wang, J.; Wang, N.; Wu, W.; Wu, Q.; Hou, X.; Hu, W.; Li, L. Near infrared photothermal conversion materials: Mechanism, preparation, and photothermal cancer therapy applications. *J. Mater. Chem. B* **2021**, *9*, 7909–7926. [CrossRef]
25. Shibu, E.S.; Hamada, M.; Murase, N.; Biju, V. Nanomaterials formulations for photothermal and photodynamic therapy of cancer. *J. Photochem. Photobiol. C* **2013**, *15*, 53–72. [CrossRef]
26. Gao, M.; Zhu, L.; Peh, C.K.; Ho, G.W. Solar absorber material and system designs for photothermal water vaporization towards clean water and energy production. *Energy Environ. Sci.* **2019**, *12*, 841–864. [CrossRef]
27. Chen, Y.; Gao, Y.; Chen, Y.; Liu, L.; Mo, A.; Peng, Q. Nanomaterials-based photothermal therapy and its potentials in antibacterial treatment. *J. Control Release* **2020**, *328*, 251–262. [CrossRef] [PubMed]
28. Gunaydin, G.; Gedik, M.E.; Ayan, S. Photodynamic Therapy for the Treatment and Diagnosis of *Cancer*-A Review of the Current Clinical Status. *Front. Chem.* **2021**, *9*, 686303. [CrossRef]
29. Correia, J.H.; Rodrigues, J.A.; Pimenta, S.; Dong, T.; Yang, Z. Photodynamic Therapy Review: Principles, Photosensitizers, Applications, and Future Directions. *Pharmaceutics* **2021**, *13*, 1332. [CrossRef]
30. Kong, C.; Chen, X. Combined Photodynamic and Photothermal Therapy and Immunotherapy for Cancer Treatment: A Review. *Int. J. Nanomed.* **2022**, *17*, 6427–6446. [CrossRef]
31. Bera, S.; Naskar, A.; Pal, M.; Jana, S. ZnO–graphene–polyaniline nanoflowers: Solution synthesis, formation mechanism and electrochemical activity. *RSC Adv.* **2016**, *6*, 40854–40857. [CrossRef]
32. Wang, J.; Guo, R.T.; Bi, Z.X.; Chen, X.; Hu, X.; Pan, W.G. A review on TiO_{2-x}-based materials for photocatalytic CO_2 reduction. *Nanoscale* **2022**, *14*, 11512–11528. [CrossRef] [PubMed]
33. Pan, C.; Mao, Z.; Yuan, X.; Zhang, H.; Mei, L.; Ji, X. Heterojunction Nanomedicine. *Adv. Sci.* **2022**, *9*, e2105747. [CrossRef] [PubMed]
34. Zhang, L.; Zhu, C.; Huang, R.; Ding, Y.; Ruan, C.; Shen, X.C. Mechanisms of Reactive Oxygen Species Generated by Inorganic Nanomaterials for Cancer Therapeutics. *Front. Chem.* **2021**, *9*, 630969. [CrossRef]
35. Ghorbani, J.; Rahban, D.; Aghamiri, S.; Teymouri, A.; Bahador, A. Photosensitizers in antibacterial photodynamic therapy: An overview. *Laser Ther.* **2018**, *27*, 293–302. [CrossRef] [PubMed]
36. Yeshchenko, O.A.; Kutsevol, N.V.; Tomchuk, A.V.; Khort, P.S.; Virych, P.A.; Chumachenko, V.A.; Kuziv, Y.I.; Naumenko, A.P.; Marinin, A.I. Plasmonic enhancement of the antibacterial photodynamic efficiency of a zinc tetraphenylporphyrin photosensitizer/dextran *graft* polyacrylamide anionic copolymer/Au nanoparticles hybrid nanosystem. *RSC Adv.* **2021**, *12*, 11–23. [CrossRef] [PubMed]
37. Sun, P.; Ye, L.; Tan, X.; Peng, J.; Zhao, L.; Zhou, Y. Silver Nanoparticle-Assisted Photodynamic Therapy for Biofilm Eradication. *ACS Appl. Nano Mater.* **2022**, *5*, 8251–8259. [CrossRef]
38. Lv, H.; Liu, J.; Wang, Y.; Xia, X.; Li, Y.; Hou, W.; Li, F.; Guo, L.; Li, X. Upconversion nanoparticles and its based photodynamic therapy for antibacterial applications: A state-of-the-art review. *Front. Chem.* **2022**, *10*, 996264. [CrossRef]
39. Sun, J.; Fan, Y.; Ye, W.; Tian, L.M.; Niu, S.C.; Ming, W.H.; Zhao, J.; Ren, L.Q. Nearinfrared light triggered photodynamic and nitric oxide synergistic antibacterial nanocomposite membrane. *Chem. Eng. J.* **2021**, *417*, 128049. [CrossRef]
40. Gao, J.; Chen, Z.; Li, X.; Yang, M.; Lv, J.; Li, H.; Yuan, Z. Chemiluminescence in Combination with Organic Photosensitizers: Beyond the Light Penetration Depth Limit of Photodynamic Therapy. *Int. J. Mol. Sci.* **2022**, *23*, 12556. [CrossRef]
41. Wang, Q.; de Oliveira, E.F.; Alborzi, S.; Bastarrachea, L.J.; Tikekar, R.V. On mechanism behind UV-A light enhanced antibacterial activity of gallic acid and propyl gallate against Escherichia coli O157:H7. *Sci. Rep.* **2017**, *7*, 8325. [CrossRef] [PubMed]
42. Youf, R.; Müller, M.; Balasini, A.; Thétiot, F.; Müller, M.; Hascoët, A.; Jonas, U.; Schönherr, H.; Lemercier, G.; Montier, T.; et al. Antimicrobial Photodynamic Therapy: Latest Developments with a Focus on Combinatory Strategies. *Pharmaceutics* **2021**, *13*, 1995. [CrossRef] [PubMed]
43. Zhu, Y.; Matsumura, Y.; Velayutham, M.; Foley, L.M.; Hitchens, T.K.; Wagner, W.R. Reactive oxygen species scavenging with a biodegradable, thermally responsive hydrogel compatible with soft tissue injection. *Biomaterials* **2018**, *177*, 98–112. [CrossRef]
44. McMillan, T.J.; Leatherman, E.; Ridley, A.; Shorrocks, J.; Tobi, S.E.; Whiteside, J.R. Cellular effects of long wavelength UV light (UVA) in mammalian cells. *J. Pharm. Pharmacol.* **2008**, *60*, 969–976. [CrossRef] [PubMed]
45. Zhang, Y.; Fu, H.; Liu, D.E.; An, J.; Gao, H. Construction of biocompatible bovine serum albumin nanoparticles composed of nano graphene oxide and AIEgen for dual-mode phototherapy bacteriostatic and bacterial tracking. *J. Nanobiotechnol.* **2019**, *17*, 104. [CrossRef] [PubMed]
46. Giancarlo, G.V.D.; Janneri, L.Á.K.; Paulina, R.O.M. Antibacterial Strategies: Photodynamic and Photothermal Treatments Based on Carbon-Based Materials. In *Biotechnology—Biosensors, Biomaterials and Tissue Engineering—Annual Volume 2023 [Working Title]*; Intechopen: London, UK, 2022.
47. Lagos, K.J.; Buzzá, H.H.; Bagnato, V.S.; Romero, M.P. Carbon-Based Materials in Photodynamic and Photothermal Therapies Applied to Tumor Destruction. *Int. J. Mol. Sci.* **2021**, *23*, 22. [CrossRef]
48. Zhang, P.; Sun, B.; Wu, F.; Zhang, Q.; Chu, X.; Ge, M.; Zhou, N.; Shen, J. Wound healing acceleration by antibacterial biodegradable black phosphorus nanosheets loaded with cationic carbon dots. *J. Mater. Sci.* **2021**, *56*, 6411–6426. [CrossRef]
49. Mei, L.; Gao, X.; Shi, Y.; Cheng, C.; Shi, Z.; Jiao, M.; Cao, F.; Xu, Z.; Li, X.; Zhang, J. Augmented Graphene Quantum Dot-Light Irradiation Therapy for Bacteria-Infected Wounds. *ACS Appl. Mater. Interfaces* **2020**, *12*, 40153–40162. [CrossRef]

50. Yu, Z.H.; Li, X.; Xu, F.; Hu, X.L.; Yan, J.; Kwon, N.; Chen, G.R.; Tang, T.; Dong, X.; Mai, Y.; et al. A Supramolecular-Based Dual-Wavelength Phototherapeutic Agent with Broad-Spectrum Antimicrobial Activity Against Drug-Resistant Bacteria. *Angew. Chem. Int. Ed.* **2020**, *59*, 3658–3664. [CrossRef]
51. Chen, X.; Wu, S.; Ma, D.; Chen, J.; Guo, Q.; Han, X.; Chen, K.; Yang, H.; Huang, Y.; Peng, Y. A polyfluoroalkyl substituted phthalocyanine based supramolecular light switch for photothermal and photodynamic antibacterial activity against Escherichia coli. *Chem. Commun.* **2018**, *54*, 13279–13282. [CrossRef]
52. Bilici, K.; Atac, N.; Muti, A.; Baylam, I.; Dogan, O.; Sennaroglu, A.; Can, F.; Yagci Acar, H. Broad spectrum antibacterial photodynamic and photothermal therapy achieved with indocyanine green loaded SPIONs under near infrared irradiation. *Biomater. Sci.* **2020**, *8*, 4616–4625. [CrossRef] [PubMed]
53. Ma, W.; Chen, X.; Fu, L.; Zhu, J.; Fan, M.; Chen, J.; Yang, C.; Yang, G.; Wu, L.; Mao, G.; et al. Ultra-efficient Antibacterial System Based on Photodynamic Therapy and CO Gas Therapy for Synergistic Antibacterial and Ablation Biofilms. *ACS Appl. Mater. Interfaces* **2020**, *12*, 22479–22491. [CrossRef]
54. Xu, X.; Liu, X.; Tan, L.; Cui, Z.; Yang, X.; Zhu, S.; Li, Z.; Yuan, X.; Zheng, Y.; Yeung, K.W.K.; et al. Controlled-temperature photothermal and oxidative bacteria killing and acceleration of wound healing by polydopamine-assisted Au-hydroxyapatite nanorods. *Acta Biomater.* **2018**, *77*, 352–364. [CrossRef] [PubMed]
55. Dai, X.; Zhao, Y.; Yu, Y.; Chen, X.; Wei, X.; Zhang, X.; Li, C. Single Continuous Near-Infrared Laser-Triggered Photodynamic and Photothermal Ablation of Antibiotic-Resistant Bacteria Using Effective Targeted Copper Sulfide Nanoclusters. *ACS Appl. Mater. Interfaces* **2017**, *9*, 30470–30479. [CrossRef]
56. Gao, D.Y.; Ji, X.; Wang, J.L.; Wang, Y.T.; Li, D.L.; Liu, Y.B.; Chang, K.W.; Qu, J.L.; Zheng, J.; Yuan, Z. Engineering a protein-based nanoplatform as an antibacterial agent for light activated dual-modal photothermal and photodynamic therapy of infection in both the NIR I and II windows. *J. Mater. Chem. B* **2018**, *6*, 732–739. [CrossRef]
57. Naskar, A.; Cho, H.; Kim, K.-S. Black phosphorus-based CuS nanoplatform: Near-infrared-responsive and reactive oxygen species-generating agent against environmental bacterial pathogens. *J. Environ. Chem. Eng.* **2022**, *10*, 108226. [CrossRef]
58. Ghayyem, S.; Barras, A.; Faridbod, F.; Szunerits, S.; Boukherroub, R. Effective PDT/PTT dual-modal phototherapeutic killing of bacteria by using poly(N-phenylglycine) nanoparticles. *Mikrochim. Acta.* **2022**, *189*, 150. [CrossRef]
59. Kwon, N.; Kim, H.; Li, X.; Yoon, J. Supramolecular agents for combination of photodynamic therapy and other treatments. *Chem. Sci.* **2021**, *12*, 7248–7268. [CrossRef]
60. Shao, W.; Yang, C.; Li, F.; Wu, J.; Wang, N.; Ding, Q.; Gao, J.; Ling, D. Molecular Design of Conjugated Small Molecule Nanoparticles for Synergistically Enhanced PTT/PDT. *Nanomicro Lett.* **2020**, *12*, 147. [CrossRef]
61. Sun, L.; Wang, J.; Yang, B.; Wang, X.; Yang, G.; Wang, X.; Jiang, Y.; Wang, T.; Jiang, J. Assembled small organic molecules for photodynamic therapy and photothermal therapy. *RSC Adv.* **2021**, *11*, 10061–10074. [CrossRef]
62. Mutalik, C.; Okoro, G.; Krisnawati, D.I.; Jazidie, A.; Rahmawati, E.Q.; Rahayu, D.; Hsu, W.T.; Kuo, T.R. Copper sulfide with morphology-dependent photodynamic and photothermal antibacterial activities. *J. Colloid Interface Sci.* **2022**, *607 Pt 2*, 1825–1835. [CrossRef] [PubMed]
63. Zhou, L.; Chen, F.; Hou, Z.; Chen, Y.; Luo, X. Injectable self-healing CuS nanoparticle complex hydrogels with antibacterial, anti-cancer, and wound healing properties. *Chem. Eng. J.* **2021**, *409*, 128224. [CrossRef]
64. Qiao, Y.; Ping, Y.; Zhang, H.; Zhou, B.; Liu, F.; Yu, Y.; Xie, T.; Li, W.; Zhong, D.; Zhang, Y.; et al. Laser-Activatable CuS Nanodots to Treat Multidrug-Resistant Bacteria and Release Copper Ion to Accelerate Healing of Infected Chronic Nonhealing Wounds. *ACS Appl. Mater. Interfaces* **2019**, *11*, 3809–3822. [CrossRef]
65. Su, R.; Yan, H.; Li, P.; Zhang, B.; Zhang, Y.; Su, W. Photo-enhanced antibacterial activity of polydopamine-curcumin nanocomposites with excellent photodynamic and photothermal abilities. *Photodiagn. Photodyn. Ther.* **2021**, *35*, 102417. [CrossRef] [PubMed]
66. Fang, Q.; Xu, K.; Xiong, Q.; Xu, Y.; Hui, A.; Xuan, S. Fe_3O_4–Au–polydopamine hybrid microcapsules with photothermal–photodynamic synergistic anti-bacterial performance. *CrystEngComm* **2021**, *23*, 6610–6619. [CrossRef]
67. Shen, H.; Jiang, C.; Li, W.; Wei, Q.; Ghiladi, R.A.; Wang, Q. Synergistic Photodynamic and Photothermal Antibacterial Activity of In Situ Grown Bacterial Cellulose/MoS_2-Chitosan Nanocomposite Materials with Visible Light Illumination. *ACS Appl. Mater. Interfaces* **2021**, *13*, 31193–31205. [CrossRef]
68. Yougbaré, S.; Mutalik, C.; Chung, P.F.; Krisnawati, D.I.; Rinawati, F.; Irawan, H.; Kristanto, H.; Kuo, T.R. Gold Nanorod-Decorated Metallic MoS_2 Nanosheets for Synergistic Photothermal and Photodynamic Antibacterial Therapy. *Nanomaterials* **2021**, *11*, 3064. [CrossRef]
69. Sun, J.; Song, L.; Fan, Y.; Tian, L.; Luan, S.; Niu, S.; Ren, L.; Ming, W.; Zhao, J. Synergistic Photodynamic and Photothermal Antibacterial Nanocomposite Membrane Triggered by Single NIR Light Source. *ACS Appl. Mater. Interfaces* **2019**, *11*, 26581–26589. [CrossRef]
70. Dai, X.; Zhao, Y.; Yu, Y.; Chen, X.; Wei, X.; Zhang, X.; Li, C. All-in-one NIR-activated nanoplatforms for enhanced bacterial biofilm eradication. *Nanoscale* **2018**, *10*, 18520–18530. [CrossRef]
71. Romero, M.P.; Marangoni, V.S.; de Faria, C.G.; Leite, I.S.; Silva, C.C.C.E.; Maroneze, C.M.; Pereira-da-Silva, M.A.; Bagnato, V.S.; Inada, N.M. Graphene Oxide Mediated Broad-Spectrum Antibacterial Based on Bimodal Action of Photodynamic and Photothermal Effects. *Front. Microbiol.* **2020**, *10*, 2995. [CrossRef]

72. Chen, Y.; Huang, W.; Dong, Y.; Yu, X.; Mo, A.; Peng, Q. Enhanced Antibacterial Activity of Indocyanine Green-Loaded Graphene Oxide via Synergistic Contact Killing, Photothermal and Photodynamic Therapy. *J. Biomed. Nanotechnol.* **2022**, *18*, 185–192. [CrossRef] [PubMed]
73. Cuadrado, C.F.; Díaz-Barrios, A.; Campaña, K.O.; Romani, E.C.; Quiroz, F.; Nardecchia, S.; Debut, A.; Vizuete, K.; Niebieskikwiat, D.; Ávila, C.E.; et al. Broad-Spectrum Antimicrobial ZnMintPc Encapsulated in Magnetic-Nanocomposites with Graphene Oxide/MWCNTs Based on Bimodal Action of Photodynamic and Photothermal Effects. *Pharmaceutics* **2022**, *14*, 705. [CrossRef] [PubMed]
74. Liu, B.; Su, Y.; Wu, S.; Shen, J. Local photothermal/photodynamic synergistic antibacterial therapy based on two-dimensional BP@CQDs triggered by single NIR light source. *Photodiag. Photodyn. Ther.* **2022**, *39*, 102905. [CrossRef]
75. Wen, F.; Li, P.; Meng, H.; Yan, H.; Huang, X.; Cui, H.; Su, W. Nitrogen-doped carbon dots/curcumin nanocomposite for combined Photodynamic/photothermal dual-mode antibacterial therapy. *Photodiagn. Photodyn Ther.* **2022**, *39*, 103033. [CrossRef]
76. Chu, X.; Zhang, P.; Wang, Y.; Sun, B.; Liu, Y.; Zhang, Q.; Feng, W.; Li, Z.; Li, K.; Zhou, N.; et al. Near-infrared carbon dot-based platform for bioimaging and photothermal/photodynamic/quaternary ammonium triple synergistic sterilization triggered by single NIR light source. *Carbon* **2021**, *176*, 126–138. [CrossRef]
77. Yu, Y.; Mei, L.; Shi, Y.; Zhang, X.; Cheng, K.; Cao, F.; Zhang, L.; Xu, J.; Li, X.; Xu, Z. Ag-Conjugated graphene quantum dots with blue light-enhanced singlet oxygen generation for ternary-mode highly-efficient antimicrobial therapy. *J. Mater. Chem. B* **2020**, *8*, 1371–1382. [CrossRef] [PubMed]
78. Zhang, H.; Liang, Y.; Zhao, H.; Qi, R.; Chen, Z.; Yuan, H.; Liang, H.; Wang, L. Dual-Mode Antibacterial Conjugated Polymer Nanoparticles for Photothermal and Photodynamic Therapy. *Macromol. Biosci.* **2020**, *20*, e1900301. [CrossRef] [PubMed]
79. Li, L.; Liu, Y.; Hao, P.; Wang, Z.; Fu, L.; Ma, Z.; Zhou, J. PEDOT nanocomposites mediated dual-modal photodynamic and photothermal targeted sterilization in both NIR I and II window. *Biomaterials* **2015**, *41*, 132–140. [CrossRef]
80. Li, Y.; Liu, X.; Li, B.; Zheng, Y.; Han, Y.; Chen, D.F.; Yeung, K.W.K.; Cui, Z.; Liang, Y.; Li, Z.; et al. Near-Infrared Light Triggered Phototherapy and Immunotherapy for Elimination of Methicillin-Resistant Staphylococcus aureus Biofilm Infection on Bone Implant. *ACS Nano* **2020**, *14*, 8157–8170. [CrossRef]
81. Yuan, Z.; Tao, B.; He, Y.; Mu, C.; Liu, G.; Zhang, J.; Liao, Q.; Liu, P.; Cai, K. Remote eradication of biofilm on titanium implant via near-infrared light triggered photothermal/photodynamic therapy strategy. *Biomaterials* **2019**, *223*, 119479. [CrossRef]
82. Zhang, Y.; Yan, H.; Tang, J.; Li, P.; Su, R.; Zhong, H.; Su, W. Dual-mode antibacterial core-shell gold nanorod@mesoporous-silica/curcumin nanocomplexes for efficient photothermal and photodynamic therapy. *J. Photochem. Photobiol. A* **2022**, *425*, 113722. [CrossRef]
83. Wang, W.-N.; Pei, P.; Chu, Z.-Y.; Chen, B.-J.; Qian, H.-S.; Zha, Z.-B.; Zhou, W.; Liu, T.; Shao, M.; Wang, H. Bi_2S_3 coated Au nanorods for enhanced photodynamic and photothermal antibacterial activities under NIR light. *Chem. Eng. J.* **2020**, *397*, 125488. [CrossRef]
84. Chen, G.; Cao, Y.; Tang, Y.; Yang, X.; Liu, Y.; Huang, D.; Zhang, Y.; Li, C.; Wang, Q. Advanced Near-Infrared Light for Monitoring and Modulating the Spatiotemporal Dynamics of Cell Functions in Living Systems. *Adv. Sci.* **2020**, *7*, 1903783. [CrossRef]
85. Naskar, A.; Kim, K.-s. Photo-Stimuli-Responsive CuS Nanomaterials as Cutting-Edge Platform Materials for Antibacterial Applications. *Pharmaceutics* **2022**, *14*, 2343. [CrossRef] [PubMed]
86. Fan, S.; Lin, W.; Huang, Y.; Xia, J.; Xu, J.F.; Zhang, J.; Pi, J. Advances and Potentials of Polydopamine Nanosystem in Photothermal-Based Antibacterial Infection Therapies. *Front. Pharmacol.* **2022**, *13*, 829712. [CrossRef] [PubMed]
87. Naskar, A.; Bera, S.; Bhattacharya, R.; Saha, P.; Roy, S.S.; Sen, T.; Jana, S. Synthesis, characterization and antibacterial activity of Ag incorporated ZnO–graphene nanocomposites. *RSC Adv.* **2016**, *6*, 88751–88761. [CrossRef]
88. Naskar, A.; Bera, S.; Bhattacharya, R.; Roy, S.S.; Jana, S. Effect of bovine serum albumin immobilized Au–ZnO–graphene nanocomposite on human ovarian cancer cell. *J. Alloys Compd.* **2018**, *734*, 66–74. [CrossRef]
89. Aunkor, M.T.H.; Raihan, T.; Prodhan, S.H.; Metselaar, H.S.C.; Malik, S.U.F.; Azad, A.K. Antibacterial activity of graphene oxide nanosheet against multidrug resistant superbugs isolated from infected patients. *R. Soc. Open Sci.* **2020**, *7*, 200640. [CrossRef] [PubMed]
90. Syama, S.; Mohanan, P.V. Comprehensive Application of Graphene: Emphasis on Biomedical Concerns. *Nanomicro Lett.* **2019**, *11*, 6. [CrossRef]
91. Naskar, A.; Lee, S.; Kim, K.-s. Au-ZnO Conjugated Black Phosphorus as a Near-Infrared Light-Triggering and Recurrence-Suppressing Nanoantibiotic Platform against Staphylococcus aureus. *Pharmaceutics* **2021**, *13*, 52. [CrossRef]
92. Naskar, A.; Cho, H.; Kim, K.-s. A Nanocomposite with Extracellular Vesicles from Lactobacillus paracasei as a Bioinspired Nanoantibiotic Targeting Staphylococcus aureus. *Pharmaceutics* **2022**, *14*, 2273. [CrossRef] [PubMed]
93. Cho, H.; Naskar, A.; Lee, S.; Kim, S.; Kim, K.-S. A New Surface Charge Neutralizing Nano-Adjuvant to Potentiate Polymyxins in Killing Mcr-1 Mediated Drug-Resistant Escherichia coli. *Pharmaceutics* **2021**, *13*, 250. [CrossRef] [PubMed]
94. Sun, H.; Schanze, K.S. Functionalization of Water-Soluble Conjugated Polymers for Bioapplications. *ACS Appl. Mater. Interfaces* **2022**, *14*, 20506–20519. [CrossRef]
95. Cui, Q.; Yuan, H.; Bao, X.; Ma, G.; Wu, M.; Xing, C. Synergistic Photodynamic and Photothermal Antibacterial Therapy Based on a Conjugated Polymer Nanoparticle-Doped Hydrogel. *ACS Appl. Bio Mater.* **2020**, *3*, 4436–4443. [CrossRef] [PubMed]
96. Cheng, L.; Yang, K.; Chen, Q.; Liu, Z. Organic stealth nanoparticles for highly effective in vivo near-infrared photothermal therapy of cancer. *ACS Nano* **2012**, *6*, 5605–5613. [CrossRef] [PubMed]

97. Naskar, A.; Kim, K.-S. Recent Advances in Nanomaterial-Based Wound-Healing Therapeutics. *Pharmaceutics* **2020**, *12*, 499. [CrossRef]
98. Naskar, A.; Kim, K.-S. Black phosphorus nanomaterials as multi-potent and emerging platforms against bacterial infections. *Microb. Pathog.* **2019**, *137*, 103800. [CrossRef]
99. Wang, W.; Cheng, X.; Liao, J.; Lin, Z.; Chen, L.; Liu, D.; Zhang, T.; Li, L.; Lu, Y.; Xia, H. Synergistic Photothermal and Photodynamic Therapy for Effective Implant-Related Bacterial Infection Elimination and Biofilm Disruption Using Cu9S8 Nanoparticles. *ACS Biomater. Sci. Eng.* **2019**, *5*, 6243–6253. [CrossRef]

pharmaceutics

MDPI

Review

Advances in the Physico-Chemical, Antimicrobial and Angiogenic Properties of Graphene-Oxide/Cellulose Nanocomposites for Wound Healing

Ugo D'Amora [1,*,†], Sawsan Dacrory [2,†], Mohamed Sayed Hasanin [2], Angela Longo [1], Alessandra Soriente [1], Samir Kamel [2], Maria Grazia Raucci [1], Luigi Ambrosio [1] and Stefania Scialla [1,*]

1 Institute of Polymers, Composites and Biomaterials, National Research Council (IPCB-CNR), 80125 Naples, Italy
2 Cellulose and Paper Department, National Research Centre, 33 El Bohouth St., Cairo 12622, Egypt
* Correspondence: ugo.damora@cnr.it (U.D.); stefania.scialla@cnr.it (S.S.)
† These authors equally contributed to this work.

Abstract: Graphene oxide (GO) and its reduced form (rGO) have recently attracted a fascinating interest due to their physico-chemical properties, which have opened up new and interesting opportunities in a wide range of biomedical applications, such as wound healing. It is worth noting that GO and rGO may offer a convenient access to its ready dispersion within various polymeric matrices (such as cellulose and its derivative forms), owing to their large surface area, based on a carbon skeleton with many functional groups (i.e., hydroxyl, carboxyl, epoxy bridge, and carbonyl moieties). This results in new synergic properties due to the presence of both components (GO or rGO and polymers), acting at different length-scales. Furthermore, they have shown efficient antimicrobial and angiogenic properties, mostly related to the intracellular formation of reactive oxygen species (ROS), which are advantageous in wound care management. For this reason, GO or rGO integration in cellulose-based matrixes have allowed for designing highly advanced multifunctional hybrid nanocomposites with tailored properties. The current review aims to discuss a potential relationship between structural and physico-chemical properties (i.e., size, edge density, surface chemistry, hydrophilicity) of the nanocomposites with antimicrobials and angiogenic mechanisms that synergically influence the wound healing phenomenon, by paying particular attention to recent findings of GO or rGO/cellulose nanocomposites. Accordingly, after providing a general overview of cellulose and its derivatives, the production methods used for GO and rGO synthesis, the mechanisms that guide antimicrobial and angiogenic processes of tissue repair, as well as the most recent and remarkable outcomes on GO/cellulose scaffolds in wound healing applications, will be presented.

Keywords: cellulose; graphene oxide; antimicrobial; angiogenesis; wound healing

1. Introduction

Surgery, trauma, infection, diabetes and other diseases are among the most common causes of a wound genesis. In particular, skin wound healing is a complex phenomenon upregulated by different cell types and based on a fine orchestration of biological and molecular events, such as cell migration, proliferation, and extracellular matrix (ECM) remodelling [1]. In chronic wounds, sustained inflammation, continuous infections, antibiotic-resistant biofilms development, as well as the incapability of resident cells to reply to reparative stimuli may compromise the overall process.

In this scenario, over the past years, chronic wounds have become a life-threatening issue. Nowadays, worldwide, approximately 10 million people experience chronic wound (i.e., burning), leading to death if not properly handled [2]. For this reason, in the management of those injuries, selecting a suitable wound dressing is crucial. By this point of view, material choice is of paramount importance to ensure an appropriate mechanical stability to support skin injuries, a suitable water retention to absorb exudates, promising antibacterial properties to prevent biofilm formation, and tear resistance. Importantly, the material should be able to promote the healing by guaranteeing a long-term drug and growth factors (GFs) delivery with a controlled biodegradation, as well triggering the angiogenesis [3]. Ointments in the form of cream or natural oils, gels, gauzes, and bandages are among the wound dressings currently available, due to their unique combination of high water content, softness, flexibility, and biocompatibility [4–8]. They generally consist of natural (e.g., chitosan, cellulose, keratin, casein, collagen, hyaluronic acid, alginate, and silk fibroin) and/or synthetic (e.g., polyvinyl alcohol, polyethylene glycol, poly[lactic-co-glycolic acid], polycaprolactone, polylactic acid) polymers, and also bioactive compounds (e.g., chemical drugs, metallic nanoparticles, GFs, stem cells, and plant extracts) [9]. Furthermore, the advent of smart wound dressings by using 3D printing has revolutionized wound care management [5,10,11].

Among the natural polymers, cellulose is emerging as a suitable candidate for wound healing applications, where flexibility and toughness are of paramount importance together with biocompatibility and antibacterial properties. Furthermore, it has excellent properties, including tunable mechanical strength, high purity, good water retention, high specific surface area, biodegradability, and low toxicity [12–14]. The three hydroxyl (-OH) groups in the monomer units, which repeat along the cellulose backbone, are involved in the formation of hydrogen bonds, directing the crystalline regions and controlling the physico-chemical properties. These -OH groups also provide a high reactivity to cellulose towards chemical modification processes, such as carboxymethylation, acetylation, oxidation and silylation [15], to obtain cellulose derivatives useful for medical applications and metals or other inorganic precursors absorption.

However, cellulose naturally lacks antimicrobial properties. Among the antibacterial agents, graphene oxide (GO) and its reduced form (rGO) have recently gained enormous interest in biomedical applications. Studies on antibacterial properties of GO-like materials are contradictory and have raised confusion. Several groups of researchers reported GO and rGO to possess bactericidal properties against both Gram-positive (Gram$^+$) and Gram-negative (Gram$^-$) bacteria. Some works suggested that GO has no effect on bacteria, or in opposition, other papers highlighted GO and rGO as enhancers of microbial growth for *Escherichia coli*. However, it is stated that cell growth has been prevented for Gram$^+$ bacteria, whereas, on Gram$^-$ bacteria, GO-like materials have no effect [16]. These inconsistent results have led to the scope of the present detailed overview, whether GO or rGO-based cellulose biomaterials for wound healing applications, have been analysed in order to find a possible explanation of their action in the destruction of bacteria cells. Indeed, the presence of the polymer matrix can dramatically alter the possible antibacterial potential of GO or rGO. At the point of the present state of art, it is rather complex to give a comprehensive review of all the literature concerning GO or rGO/cellulose nanocomposites for wound healing applications.

In this review, the aim of the present work was to critically discuss the potential relationship between structural and physico-chemical properties of GO or rGO/cellulose nanocomposites on the antimicrobials and angiogenic mechanisms, which synergically regulate the wound healing. This review will then give an overview of: (i) the cellulose-derivatives and related production processes, with a special focus on the agricultural wastes, in view of a more circular and green economy, (ii) GO and rGO synthesis, and (iii) the antimicrobial and angiogenic pathways involved in the wound repair. (iv) To finish, the most recent and remarkable findings of the last 3 years on the multifunctional GO or rGO/cellulose biomaterials, in the form of scaffolds and injectable hydrogel formulations, intended for wound healing, will be presented.

2. Cellulose and Cellulose Derivatives

Among the biomaterials, cellulose is the most abundant, cheap, sustainable, chemical reactive and modifiable natural macromolecular compound on the Earth. It is a carbohydrate homopolymer, which is composed of repeating long linear chains of β-anhydro-D-glucopyranose units, linked together by an ether bond between -OH group of C4, and the C1 carbon atom, via a β-1,4-glycosidic bond, as represented in Figure 1 [17].

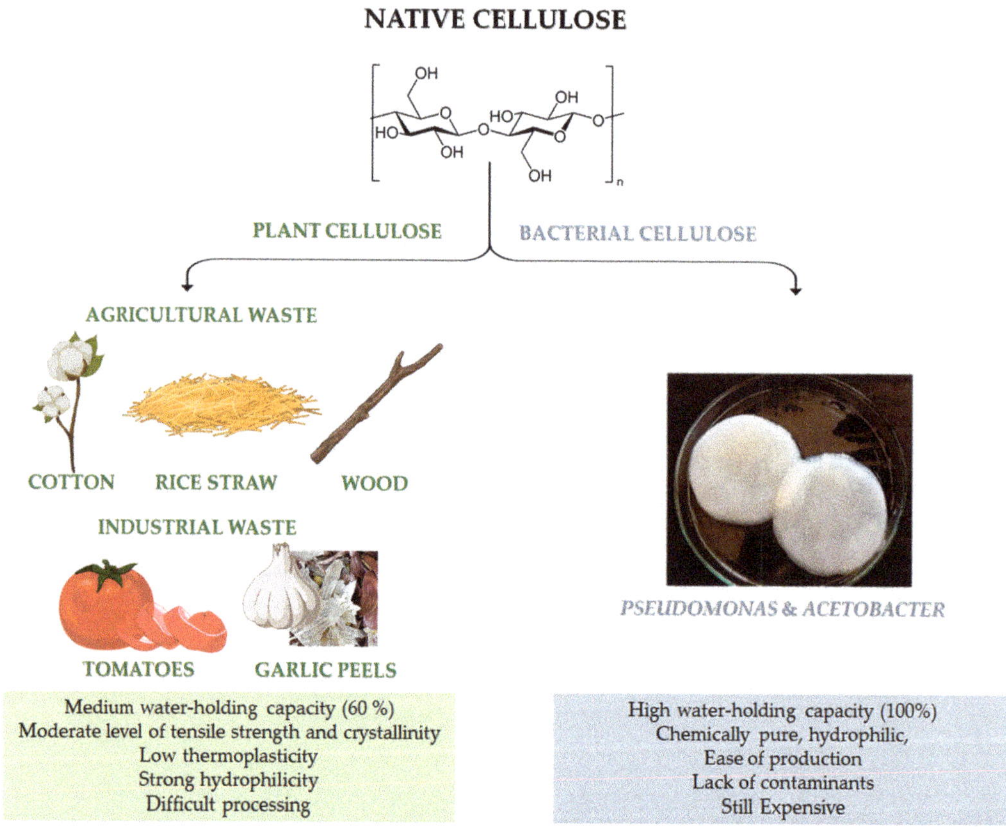

Figure 1. Chemical structure of cellulose and different sources of: native cellulose (from agricultural and industrial wastes) and bacterial cellulose (BC). Advantages and disadvantages of both kinds of cellulose. The image of BC is adapted from [18]. Copyright 2022 by the authors. License MDPI, Basel, Switzerland.

Native cellulose can be mainly classified into plant-derived and bacterial-derived cellulose (BC) [19]. It is worth noting that cellulose can be also obtained by animal sources [20]. In particular, some marine animals, called tunicate, represent the only animal source of cellulose [20]. However, it is still limited and not available for large-scale applications. Naturally-derived cellulose is a versatile, structural polysaccharide polymer, which mainly provides robust mechanical properties to plant cells, thanks to the hierarchical organisation of its natural fibres [21]. However, the structural backbone skeleton of plants represents a non-pure formulation that is usually based on lignocellulose, consisting of lignin, cellulose, hemicellulose, silica and some other impurities with different ratios, according to the plant type, as reported in Table 1. Indeed, plant cellulose widely exists in cotton, wood, and other flora species, such as phloem fibre, seed fibre, and wood fibre, which is the most abundant organic substance in nature [22]. Native cellulose also has the benefit of being able to be derived from agricultural wastes, such as cotton, bamboo, bagasse, and rice straw, which are affordable, readily available, and sustainable material sources [23]. Moreover, food processing is another possible source for cellulose recovery, even though it has highlighted many restrictions related to the solid waste collectability and the status of these wastes after gathering, which are usually contaminated with microorganisms and other impurities. Lately, industrial wastes (i.e., tomato, garlic peels) are also emerging as a promising source of cellulose.

Table 1. Cellulose content within different biomasses from agricultural waste.

Agriculture	Cellulose (%)
Wood	35–50
Wheat straw	33–40
Switchgrass	30–50
Bagasse	44
Olive husk	24
Sunflowers	26
Rice straw	33
Rice husk	49
Cotton	80–95
Nutshells	25–30
Banana fibers	60–65
Corn cob	42–45
Oat straw	33–35
Hazelnut shell	29

Recently, bacterial cellulose has gained particular interest [24]. BC can be produced by strictly aerobic, non-photosynthetic Gram$^-$ bacteria [24,25]. For their growth, these bacteria need carbon sources, which can be found in different raw materials (such as fruit, vegetable or lignocellulosic wastes) and other nutrients (such as nitrogen, iron, zinc and vitamins) [24,26]. *Pseudomonas*, *Gluconacetobacter* and *Acetobacter* are among the most important bacteria for the BC synthesis (Figure 1). Numerous studies have been carried out on the potential benefits of BC and plant-derived cellulose as biomaterials. In particular, the macromolecular characteristics of bacterial- and plant-derived cellulose differ. In addition, 60% of plant-derived cellulose can hold a medium amount of water, and it has a medium level of tensile strength and crystallinity. Conversely, BC is chemically pure, due to its hydrophilic nature, 100% water-holding capacity and lack of lignin, hemicellulose, and other impurities [22]. Furthermore, compared to plant-derived cellulose, BC has high crystallinity [22]. However, BC is still a high cost cellulose if compared to other conventional cellulose [27]. The versatility of BC's biomedical uses is supported by its simple, contaminant-free manufacture and flexibility to modify the material's properties during synthesis, such as crystallinity index, aspect ratio, and morphology, to precisely meet the needs of the intended application [22].

Native cellulose has multiple shortcomings, such as poor solubility in water and most organic solvents, due to intra- and intermolecular hydrogen bonds, low thermoplasticity, strong hydrophilicity, and difficulty in processing, which limit its development and application in the biomedical and pharmaceutical fields [22]. The intra- and intermolecular hydrogen bonds, between the -OH groups of the chain, provide cellulose with a crystalline and stiff structure. For this reason, it is insoluble in water but can be dissolved in strong acidic or alkaline conditions [28] (Figure 2). In particular, cellulose cannot dissolve in common solutions, except for two kinds of solvents: non-derivatizing solvents (i.e., sodium hydroxide, melts of inorganic salts, hydrates of inorganic salts, N, N-dimethylacetamide/lithium chlorideandmineral acids) and derivatizing solvents (i.e., trifluoroacetic acid, formic acid, dimethyl sulfoxide/para-formaldehyde, N, N-dimethyl formamide/dinitrogen tetroxide) [29]. Fortunately, insolubility can be overcome by obtaining cellulose derivatives, also known as cellulosics, through various physical and chemical modification procedures, such as esterification, etherification, or oxidation [30]. By this point of view, cellulose is the most known polysaccharide that can be easily converted to many cellulose derivatives. Among them, there are cellulose derivatives, which can be non-soluble, soluble in organic solvents and water-soluble, with a high safety profile towards biological systems [31].

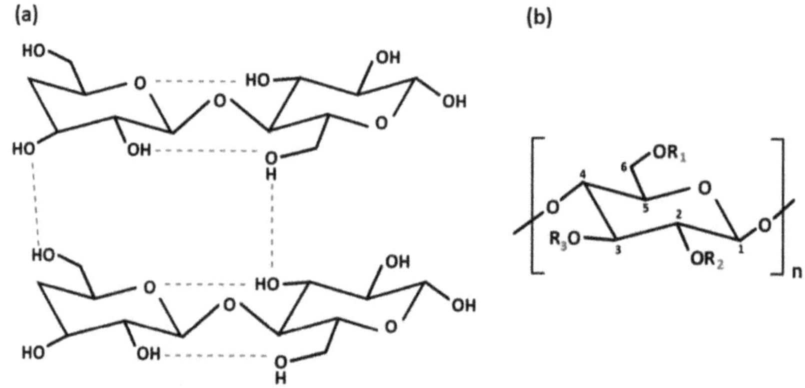

Figure 2. (**a**) Intra- and inter-molecular hydrogen bonds in cellulose; (**b**) repeating unit of cellulose derivatives. "Created with BioRender.com".

2.1. Cellulose Physical Modifications

By altering the structure and surface properties of cellulose, physical modification is mostly used to create new qualities and functions. Briefly, the physical alteration largely entails mechanical swelling, recombining, surface adsorption, and grinding without changing the chemical composition of cellulose. Physically-modified cellulose forms are regenerated cellulose, membrane cellulose, microcrystalline cellulose (MCC), spherical cellulose, and nanocellulose (NC) in its two categories: cellulose nanocrystals (CNC) and cellulose nanofibers (CNF) [21]. NC is attracting a wide research attention for its physico-chemical properties: high specific surface area, easy modification, biodegradability, non-toxicity, biocompatibility, and antimicrobial properties, which are making it a suitable biomaterial for biomedical applications (i.e., wound healing).

2.2. Cellulose Chemical Modifications

With regard to the chemical modification, two different types of reactions are involved: -OH groups derivatisation and cellulose degradation. Acid/base, oxidative, biological, and mechanical processing are all examples of degradation reactions [22]. On the other hand, derivatisation may provide the synthesis of useful chemical products. At a macromolecular level, cellulose is characterised by both crystalline and amorphous regions. The crystalline region is distinguished by densely and firmly packed -OH groups that become unavailable. For this reason, this region is less reactive in comparison with the other one. The amorphous region is more available with high reactivity toward chemical species. Indeed, the majority of the chemical modifications involve the amorphous region [32]. Moreover, cellulose chains are linear, and their aggregation occurs via both intra- and inter-molecular hydrogen bonds as presented in Figure 2a, affecting its degree of crystallinity. This aspect is of paramount importance as the physico-chemical properties of cellulose are fine-tuned by the degree of crystallinity, as well as the hydrogen bonding [33]. Additionally, the reaction behaviour of cellulose and accessibility depend on cellulose morphology, degree of polymerization, crystallinity degree, purity and particle size. It is worth noting that cellulose units have three active -OH groups C6 > C2 > C3, with the C6–OH group, which can react ten times faster than the other two groups C2 and C3 (Figure 2b).

Modification via carboxymethylation, oxidation and Micheal addition reaction can introduce new functional groups in the cellulose backbone including -OH, carboxyl (-COOH), cyano (-C=N), aldehyde (-CH=O) and tetrazole groups, leading to derivatives, such as carboxymethyl cellulose (CMC), methylcellulose (MC), dialdehyde cellulose (DAC) and hydroxyethyl cellulose (HEC), as summarised in Table 2. Over the past years, because of the increasing demand for environmentally eco-friendly and biocompatible products, the possibility to chemically modify the cellulose has boosted great advances in material science and engineering, leading to the use of cellulose derivatives in promising fields of applications, such as pharmaceutical and biomedical [34], but also electronic [35,36], as well as a water treatment one [37,38].

Table 2. Common cellulose derivatives.

Derivative	R_1	R_2	R_3
Carboxymethyl cellulose (CMC)	COONa	COONa	COONa
Methylcellulose (MC)	CH_3	CH_3	CH_3
Dialdehyde cellulose (DAC)	H	C=O	C=O
Hydroxyethyl cellulose (HEC)	CH_2CH_2OH	CH_2CH_2OH	CH_2CH_2OH

Cellulose derivatives are semi-synthetic highly water-soluble biopolymers, having high biocompatibility, biodegradability, non-toxicity, non-immunogenicity properties [39], and also a thermo-gelling behaviour [40]. In addition, cellulose derivatives can absorb and retain a large amount of wound exudates within the interstitial sites of the matrixes, maintaining an optimal local moisture at the lesion site, to avoid skin tissue water loss and tissue necrosis [39,40]. Therefore, they represent a good alternative to water-insoluble cellulose. However, mechanical strength and toughness continue to be the most difficult problems, which scientists have attempted to solve in a variety of ways: (i) by the use of non-covalent (i.e., citric acid, polyphenols) or covalent (i.e., epichlorohydrin, aldehyde-based reagents, urea derivatives, carbodiimides and multifunctional carboxylic acids) crosslinking agents [41], (ii) by designing blends with other synthetic (i.e., polyurethane, poly (vinyl alcohol), polyvinylpyrrolidone) [42] or natural (i.e., collagen, gelatin, chitosan, k-carrageenan, alginate) biopolymers [43]; (iii) by employing gelling agents [44]; (iv) by using nanomaterials as fillers (i.e., graphene oxide derivatives, titanium oxide, silver nanoparticles, zinc oxide, ceramics) [45–47].

2.3. *Cellulose from Agricultural Waste: Extraction Methods and Properties*

Nowadays, taking into consideration the environmental problems arising from a rapidly growing industry, the demand of products obtained starting from renewable and sustainable non-petroleum-based resources is increasing. For this reason, exploring naturally-derived biomaterials, such native cellulose extracted from agricultural wastes, is attracting outstanding attention in the scientific community. Extraction of cellulose can be carried out using different approaches that are mainly based on chemical, biological and physical methodologies [48]. In this context, the chemical method is considered as the best approach, in terms of productivity and low-time consumption. However, low sustainability is among the main drawbacks [49,50]. Additionally, the biological method deals with microbial enzymes, such as ligninolytic enzymes, lignin peroxidases and laccases enzymes, which are able to extract cellulose [51,52]. This approach is highly eco-friendly but has many limitations, such as having low productivity, specificity, high-cost facilities and being time-consuming. The physical method specifically employs a mechanical treatment for lignocellulosic materials to produce high lignin content pulp that is used in specific applications not as pure cellulose [53]. However, each extraction method can build up a unique cellulose in terms of properties and reactivity. The chemical method of cellulose extraction usually produces cellulose contaminated with trace elements that can be found in a cellulose molecular structure during the pulping and the bleaching process, such as sulphur, chlorine, sodium and iodine. On the other hand, this method produces cellulose with good chemical properties with different shapes, including MCC, cellulose fibres and cellulose nanoforms [54]. The biological method overcomes the drawback of the chemical method, obtaining highly pure products. Finally, the physically extracted cellulose enables the production of a material with a high lignin content pulp, which is mainly used in packaging and high mechanical stress applications [55].

3. The Graphene Oxide and Reduced Graphene Oxide

Graphene oxide (GO) is an exceptional 2D material consisting of a single layer of carbon atoms with oxygen-containing functional groups (=O, -OH, -O-, -COOH). Nowadays, it represents a great precursor for preparing reduced-graphene oxide (rGO) [56,57]. Therefore, GO, obtained from the almost complete removal of the oxygen functional groups [56], has mechanical, electrical, and optical properties quite similar to graphene, thus resulting in a convenient 2D material useful for many technological applications [58–63]. Due to its hydrophilic nature, GO can be stably and homogeneously dispersed in aqueous or polar organic solvents, in the form of colloidal suspensions, allowing an easy cast process of new devices, such as transparent conductive films and sensors [64–66]. With a high lateral dimension-to-thickness ratio, an amphiphilic nature due to its many surface functional groups, chemical inertness, and remarkable mechanical qualities, GO combines a number of beneficial properties [64]. In addition, GO is characterised by a large surface area, high thermal conductivity, high drug loading efficiency, bioactivity [47], biocompatibility, and biodegradability [67,68]. Therefore, it has been studied for tissue regeneration [69], gene therapy [70], photothermal treatment [71], and biotechnology techniques such as proteomics [72] and adsorption [73], as an antimicrobial platform [71]. Unfortunately, it is difficult to explain the precise chemical structure of GO and therefore of rGO, due to the irregular density of the carbon-skeleton defects and the different oxygen-containing groups present on the skeleton. The most acceptable structural model proposed for GO is due to Lerf-Klinowski [74], in which the basal planes of carbon atoms are decorated by -OH and epoxide (R−O−R′) groups, whereas the edges are mainly occupied by -COOH and carbonyl (–C=O) groups in a random manner [75–78]. By contrast, rGO can be described as a random distribution of residual oxidized regions, combined with non-oxidized ones [75]. It is well known that the reduction of GO has the effect not only of removing the oxygen-containing groups, but also on repairing some defects, while restoring the conjugated graphitic network [75]. Furthermore, due to the structure deformation and the presence of covalently bonded oxygen-containing groups, the GO layer is atomically rougher than the rGO layer, which appears as a more rigid structure in the basal plane [64,79]. However, GO and rGO sheets show a graphene-like honeycomb lattice, characterised by disorder and deformation [80]. The presence of the oxygen functionality affects the wettability of the GO, and hence the interaction with biological moieties. Several recent theoretical studies demonstrated that highly functionalized GO interacted most favourably with the biomolecules via hydrogen bonding, whereas the GO with low oxygen functional group densities prevalently interacted through $\pi-\pi$ stacking [81–87]. Furthermore, the oxidation and reduction grade of GO sheet are strictly related to the oxidation and reduction method, respectively, whilst the number and the type of the oxygen-containing groups are strictly connected to the graphite precursor. Therefore, GO and rGO properties can be tailored by varying the graphite precursor with different size and number of defects.

3.1. Conventional Synthesis of Graphene Oxide

GO is produced from graphite by means of a two-step approach. Firstly, the graphite crystals are oxidized with strong oxidizing agents (i.e., H_2SO_4, $KMnO_4$), introducing oxygen-containing functional groups. Secondly, the obtained "graphite oxide" adopts oxygen-containing groups, which facilitate the water-dispersion through sonication, thus increasing interlayer distance. Finally, graphite oxide can be exfoliated into either single or multilayers of oxygen-functionalized GO. Brodie was one of the first scientists who described a method to produce GO, where fuming HNO_3 and $KClO_3$ were used as intercalation and oxidative agent of natural graphite, respectively [88]. Later, the Staudenmaier method improved Brodie's one by creating GO with a better C/O ratio by usingH_2SO_4

and HNO_3 solutions [89]. These two techniques, however, rely on a drawn-out oxidation process that can take up to a week. One more method to produce GO was developed by Hummer, in which H_2SO_4 and $NaNO_3/KMnO_4$ were used by completing the oxidation reaction within 2 h [90]. In the last few years, many studies have been focused on improving the methods for GO synthesis by using eco-friendly conditions in order to maximise GO yields.

3.2. Synthesis of Graphene Oxide by Waste

In view of the last sustainable development trends, based on the new paradigm "reduce, re-use, and retain", the valorisation of wastes may constitute an interesting platform in the circular bio-economy for the development of high added-value compounds, such as bioactive compounds and nanomaterials, with remarkable financial and environmental advantages, especially dealing with the problems associated with local and global pollutions. In this section, a summary of the most recent literature advances, focused on graphite extraction from agricultural or industrial waste-biomass, is reported and listed in Table 3. Different natural wastes, such as wood, leaf, sugarcane bagasse [91], tea waste biomass [92] and coconut shell [93], have been employed by a carbonization process for charcoal precursors preparation, to synthesize GO. Somanathan et al. produced GO via single-step reforming of sugarcane bagasse agricultural waste by oxidation under muffled atmosphere conditions [91]. In particular, sugarcane bagasse fine powder was mixed with ferrocene and thermal treated into a muffle furnace at 300 °C for 10 min under atmospheric conditions, outlined in Figure 3a. The successful conversion of solid sugarcane bagasse waste into GO nanosheets was confirmed by morphological and structural investigations (Figure 3b,c).

Table 3. List of GO preparation approaches from agricultural and industrial wastes.

Year	Waste	Physico-Chemical Process and Reagents	References
		Agricultural Wastes	
2015	Sugarcane bagasse	Muffle furnace (T = 300 °C, t = 10 min) Ferrocene	[91]
2020	Coconut shell	Carbonization (T = 600 °C, t = 3 h) + Modified Hummers method ($NaNO_3$, H_2SO_4, $KMnO_4$)	[93]
2020	Tea	Carbonization (T = 750 °C, t = 3 h, argon) + Modified Hummers method ($NaNO_3$, H_2SO_4, $KMnO_4$)	[92]
		Industrial Wastes	
2018	Carbon Tyre	Crushing + Modified Hummers method ($NaNO_3$, H_2SO_4, $KMnO_4$)	[94]
2019	Toner Powder	Modified Hummers method ($NaNO_3$, H_2SO_4, $KMnO_4$)	[95]
2020	Generic	Leaching (6 M HCl, T = 70 °C, t = 210 min) + Modified Hummers method ($NaNO_3$, H_2SO_4, $KMnO_4$)	[96]

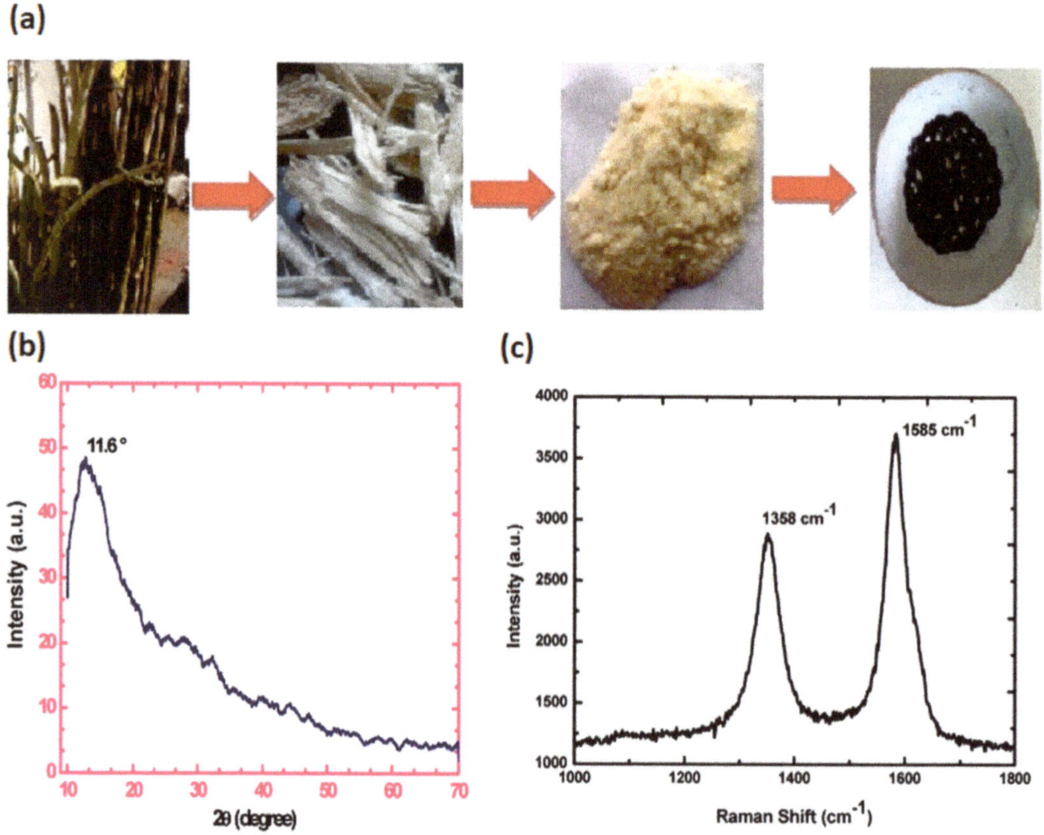

Figure 3. (**a**) Graphic scheme of sugarcane bagasse wastes conversion to GO; (**b**) X-ray diffraction (XRD) pattern; and (**c**) Raman spectrum of bagasse waste-derived GO, adapted from [91]. Copyright © 2015 by the authors; licensee MDPI, Basel, Switzerland.

Recently, Faiz et al. produced GO by conversion of tea waste biomass via carbonization process at high temperature [92]. The following oxidation and exfoliation of graphitized carbon was performed by using an adapted Hummer's method [90]. The oxidation of the graphitized tea waste was confirmed by the presence of oxygen-containing functional groups (i.e., OH, C=O and C–O). Meanwhile, coconut shell wastes were also employed by Sujiono and co-workers to synthesize GO through a modified Hammer's method [90]. Physico-chemical analysis confirmed the GO formation due to the presence of various oxygen-containing functional groups within the structure, while the XRD pattern showed that 71.53% of graphite 2H observed with GO sample tended to form a rGO phase [93]. Lately, industrial wastes have gained growing interest as alternative raw materials for carbonaceous precursors production, through the removal of hazardous metal impurities. The possibility to re-use carbon tyre waste as a precursor to synthesize the GO by Hummer's method was analysed by Bonnaia et al. [94]. Raman spectra characterized by two peaks that can be referred to as D band and G band, located at 1361 cm^{-1} and 1596 cm^{-1} with the intensity ratio of the D band relative to the G band (I_D/I_G) being 0.88, confirmed the obtained GO. Similarly, Tian et al. used toner powder waste as a precursor of GO (Figure 4a) through a one-pot adapted Hummer's method [95]. A 3D porous GO with excellent morphology and microstructure was obtained. In particular, several GO sheets well-assembled and interconnected to form a "cotton-like" 3D structure with wrinkling and "waviness" were observed through scanning electron microscopy (SEM) and transmission electron microscopy (TEM) (Figure 4b,c). The XRD pattern exhibited the characteristic diffraction peak of GO at 2θ = 10.06° (Figure 4d), which was consistent with a lamellar distance of ~8.78 Å. The interlayer spacing of the GO was larger than graphite (3.35 Å), arising from an intercalation of oxygen-containing groups between the GO sheets. Meanwhile, the characteristic D peak (~1345 cm^{-1}) and G peak (~1593 cm^{-1}) of GO were further observed via Raman analysis (Figure 4e). Siaw et al. produced the GO, with a purity of 92.28%, through a leaching process to remove most of the impurities by industrial waste. Subsequently, GO was synthesised via a modified Hummers method with a combination of concentrated H_2SO_4 and $KMnO_4$ [96].

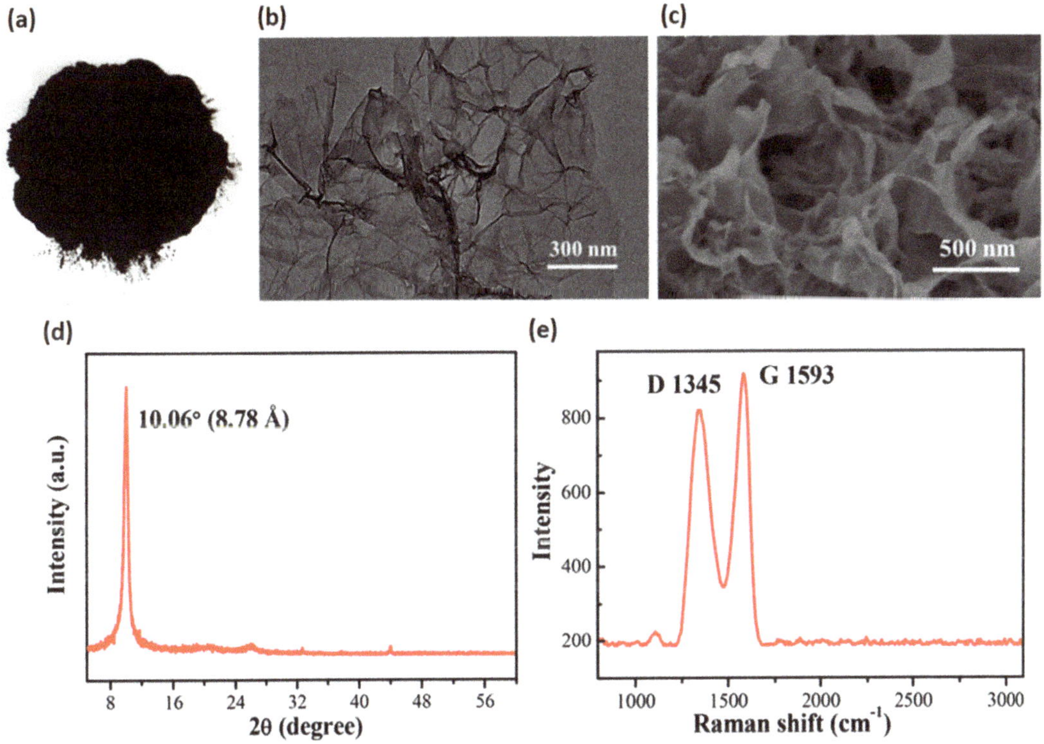

Figure 4. (**a**) Optical photograph; (**b**,**c**) SEM images of 3D porous GO with different magnifications; (right) TEM images with different magnifications; (**d**) XRD and (**e**) Raman spectrum. Reprinted with permission from [95]. Copyright 2022 American Chemical Society.

4. Short Overview of GO-Derivatives' Role in Antimicrobial Activities and Angiogenic Mechanisms

4.1. Antimicrobial Mechanisms Involving GO-Derivatives

The pristine graphene, GO and rGO differently interact with bacteria because of their structural and physico-chemical differences. Graphene-bacteria membrane interaction is strongly influenced by surface charge, which is neutral in the pristine graphene, while negatively charged in GO and rGO. However, several aspects need to be considered when assessing the graphene's antimicrobial action: the physico-chemical properties (i.e., size, number of layers, shape, surface modifications, agglomeration and dispersion), as well as the microorganism category ($Gram^+$/$Gram^-$), shape (rod/spherical), type (aerobic/anaerobic) and stage of maturity. Moreover, differences in graphene inherent properties may arise from the synthesis processes or the (un-)controlled functionalization mechanisms, leading to disputable cytotoxic findings [97]. Similarly, the bacterial cell envelope's complexity also plays a decisive role. Gram$^+$ bacteria own a thicker (20–80 nm) layer of peptidoglycan, surrounding the phospholipid bilayer and acting as barrier towards osmotic pressure changes and harmful molecules; while Gram$^-$ bacteria hold a thinner (2–8 nm) layer of peptidoglycan [98,99]. Therefore, *Staphilococcus aureus* (Gram$^+$ bacteria) is more susceptible to graphene than *Pseudomonas aeruginaosa* (Gram$^-$ bacteria) [100,101]. In addition, Gram$^+$ bacteria interact with graphene through hydrogen bonding, π-π stacking and electrostatic adsorption with the main components of the peptidoglycan [102,103], causing morphological deformation in the membrane [100,101]. Conversely, graphene interacts with Gram$^-$ bacteria via direct contact, leading to membrane disruption [100,101].

To date, a clear knowledge of the mechanisms underlying graphene-based nanosheets antimicrobial activity is still controversial. Several updated reviews have deeply outlined the proposed mechanisms at the cellular level, highlighting the role of the physico-chemical and structural properties of graphene as key factors influencing the interactions with selected bacteria [102,104,105]. Graphene-mediated antimicrobial activities may involve both physical and chemical mechanisms. Graphene may physically damage the bacterial membrane through direct contact with its sharp edge, causing a mechanical stress or a wrapping/trapping effect. Meanwhile, oxidative stress generated by a reactive oxygen species production (ROS-dependent) or electron transfer (ROS-independent) is the antimicrobial chemical mode of action [102,104,105] (Figure 5a). The graphene-induced bacterial cell death can be physically caused by (i) the insertion of blade-like graphene nanosheets within the phospholipid bilayer, (ii) the extraction of lipid molecules from the bilayer with consequent integrity loss, and (iii) the bacteria wrapping or trapping effect. GO interacts with bacterial cell envelopes through direct contact of its sharp edges, lining up in a parallel manner or orthogonally with respect to the membrane. GO tails are trapped within the phospholipid bilayer owing to strong van der Waals and hydrophobic bonds, leading to a spontaneous and rapid insertion of GO within bacteria envelope. GO penetration can cause a cut or deformation in the bacteria membrane, resulting in the leakage of cytoplasmic content (i.e., nucleic acids and proteins) and cell death [102,104,106,107]. This sharp edge effect mostly depends on the lateral size [108], thickness [109] and edge density [110] of GO nanosheets. Micrometer-sized graphene aligns orthogonally to the bacterial membrane, with respect to nanometer-sized graphene, which instead aligns in a parallel manner [108]. Wang et al. observed that a thicker graphene has a higher penetrating ability into bacterial lipid layer than a thinner one [109]. Conversely, Pham and co-workers proved that graphene edges' density significantly affect the antimicrobial behaviour of the graphene nanosheets, causing the formation of pores in the bacterial cell wall, with a subsequent osmotic imbalance and eventually cell death [110]. The bacteria wrapping or trapping effect is another physical damage mechanism mediated by thin and flexible graphene nanosheets [102,104,105]. These last ones may encase bacterial cells, isolating them from the surrounding environment, preventing nutrients from passing through the cell membrane and leading to growth inhibition. Larger GO nanosheets' bactericidal activity towards *Escherichia coli* was stronger than smaller ones, due to an easier and full covering of bacterial cells, inhibiting the proliferation [111]. Chen et al. proved that GO intertwined bacterial (*Pseudomonas syringae* and *Xanthomonas campestris*) and fungal (*Fusarium graminearum* and *Fusarium oxysporum*) pathogens have a wide range of aggregated nanosheets, resulting in a local perturbation of the phospholipid bilayer, decreasing the bacterial membrane potential and the leakage of electrolytes of fungal spores [112].

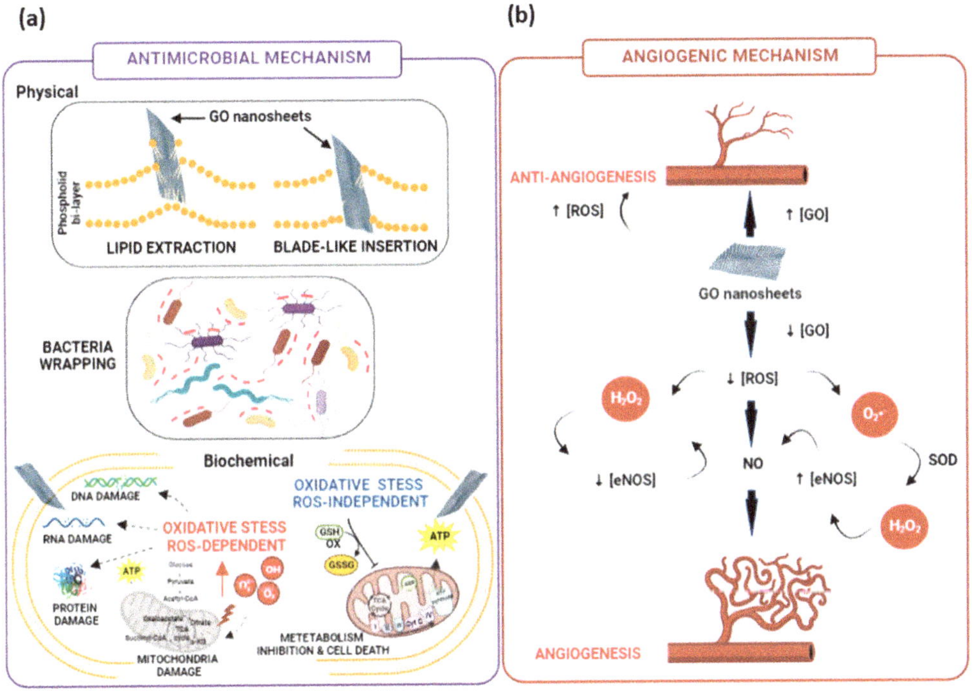

Figure 5. (**a**) Antimicrobial physical and biochemical mechanisms and (**b**) pro- and anti-angiogenic pathways involving GO-derivatives. Created with BioRender.com.

However, oxidative stress is deemed the most widely demonstrated chemical mechanism of graphene's antimicrobial properties [102,104,105]. Oxidative stress interferes with bacterial metabolism by disrupting vital cellular functions and leading to cell death. It may take place through an *ROS-dependent* or an *ROS-independent* pathway. The former occurs as a consequence of an unreasonable accumulation of intracellular ROS species, such as hydroxyl radical ($OH^{\bullet}$), hydrogen peroxide (H_2O_2), singlet molecular oxygen ($^1O_2$) and superoxide anions ($O_2^{\bullet-}$), which trigger protein deactivation, lipid peroxidation, mitochondrial dysfunction and bacterial cell membrane disintegration, leading to cell death. The latter arises from the charge transfer from a bacterial cell membrane to graphene disturbing, oxidizing or depleting vital cellular components and, thereby, killing the cells. Bacterial metabolism relies on several proton–electron transfer reactions, in which the simultaneous reduction of molecular O_2 to water and adenosine triphosphate (ATP) synthesis is fundamental for bacterial cell survival. In the presence of graphene adsorbed on the surface or embedded within the phospholipid bilayer, O_2 can be adsorbed on graphene's edges, or its defective sites undergo reduction reactions catalysed by several reducing enzymes, interrupting the water molecule formation and producing ROS traces in the cell's mitochondria. The expression of epoxy, hydroxyl, and carbon radical moieties on graphene surface, together with -COOH groups on the edges, strongly contributes to bactericidal effects. A graphene-dependent ROS levels increase was observed in *Xanthomonas oryzae pv Oryzae* by Chen et al. [113]; meanwhile, a different increase in ROS level depending on the nature of bacterial cell envelope was also proved: for instance, ROS levels in GO and rGO-treated *P. aeruginosa* cells were 3.8- and 2.7-fold higher than no-treated cells [114]; in addition, $O_2^{\bullet-}$ levels in GO and rGO-treated *E. coli* were 2- and 1-fold higher than no-treated cells [115]. Bacterial cell membrane damage may also be mediated by lipid peroxidation, which depends on the oxidative nature of GO. Krishnamoorthy et al. observed a graphene-concentration dependence of lipid peroxidation levels enhancement in *E. coli, Salmonella typhimurium, Bacillus subtilis* and *Enterococcus faecalis* [116]. Meanwhile, GO-induced lipid peroxidation dependent on the density of defects in the carbon structure, allowing for more oxygen to be absorbed on the surface, was proved by Perreault et al. [117]. Therefore, the manipulation of the oxidative moieties on GO surface may allow for tailoring proper radical expression and the bactericidal potential.

By exploiting the high conductivity properties of graphene, an ROS-independent oxidative stress mechanism has also been proposed. This mechanism relies on the ability of bacteria to exchange electrons from their respiratory chain on the membrane with the surrounding environment, in order to exert the bactericidal effect. Considering this, it was supposed that rGO holds a stronger oxidative capacity than GO, due to its higher conductivity [113]. However, relatively very few reports provided indirect evidence of the oxidative stress mediated by electron transfer between graphene and bacteria, revealing that graphene could oxidize glutathione or other antioxidant compounds without producing high ROS levels [106]. Later, Li and co-workers gave a more direct proof of the electron transfer mechanism by investigating the antibacterial actions of large-area monolayer graphene film on copper (Cu) conductor, Germanium (Ge) semiconductor and silicon dioxide (SiO_2) insulator toward *S. aureus* and *E. coli* [118]. They showed that bacterial growth was significantly inhibited in the case of graphene-Cu and graphene-Ge, but not with graphene-SiO_2. These differences could be explained assuming that an electrical circuit based on electron transfer between bacteria membrane and a conductive substrate (i.e., Cu and Ge) with the graphene takes place.

4.2. Angiogenic Mechanisms Involving GO-Derivatives

Angiogenesis is a complex process, also known as the process of new blood vessels formation, in which many signalling pathways are involved [119]. It includes many important steps, namely: (i) proliferation of endothelial cells by GFs, (ii) migration, and (iii) capillary tube formation. Several studies have emphasized the role of angiogenesis in different diseases, such as cancer, atherosclerosis and cardiovascular disorders. Furthermore, the process regulates embryogenesis, the menstrual cycle, and finally, the wound healing and the formation of granulation tissue, which is the topic of the present review [120]. Particularly, pro- and anti-angiogenic factors, which are naturally occurring in the body, can be used to initiate the process, following an injury. Thrombin, fibrinogen fragments, thymosin- $\beta4$, and GFs are pro-angiogenic mediators. Angiogenic GFs are sequestered inside the ECM and are stored in platelets and inflammatory cells that go through the circulation. Genes like hypoxia-inducible factors (HIF) and cyclooxygenase-2 (COX-2), which are expressed in response to inflammation and hypoxia, control the production of these substances. Indeed, wound angiogenesis is significantly influenced by hypoxia. Vascular endothelial GF (VEGF), which is found in both wound tissue and exudate, is produced as a result of the HIF-1α gene, due to the hypoxic gradient between wounded and healthy tissue. Nitric oxide (NO) generation by endothelial cells is also influenced by hypoxia. Over the past several decades, NO has emerged as a molecule of interest involved in the angiogenesis process. NO has been suggested to modulate different biological events, including vasodilation and angiogenesis, to improve local blood flow.

By contrast, angiogenesis inhibitor factors suppress blood vessel growth. While some inhibitors are stored in the ECM surrounding blood vessels, others circulate in the bloodstream at physiologically low levels. When the physiological equilibrium between angiogenesis stimulators and inhibitors is maintained, vascular growth is inhibited. However, immediately after some damage, angiogenic stimuli are delivered into the wound bed, and a variation in the vascular regulators' levels takes place. [121]. It has been also demonstrated that wound healing response is related to a balance between ROS amount and oxidative stress species production [122]. In fact, H_2O_2 and O_2 act as important redox signalling molecules in the angiogenesis process, with advantages for wound healing treatment. Furthermore, low level of ROS may activate pro-angiogenic response, whereas a high level of ROS may be anti-angiogenic [123]. In particular, ROS appears to be crucial in coordinating lymphoid cell recruitment to the wound site and efficient tissue repair because they act as secondary messengers to various immunocytes and non-lymphoid cells that are engaged in the repair process. Indeed, ROS acts in the host's defense through phagocytes that cause a ROS burst onto the pathogens present in wounds, leading to their destruction. Excess ROS leaking into the environment during this time may have a further bacteriostatic effect [122]. Over the past several years, there is a considerable attention in understanding the GO role in the angiogenesis process. It is well known that GO is a bi-dimensional product of the oxidation and exfoliation of pristine graphene, which exhibits high biocompatibility and angiogenic properties, related to the intracellular formation of ROS. Several studies have shown that GO is able to influence immune response and angiogenic differentiation of endothelial cells, such as human vein umbilical endothelial cells (HUVECs). Moreover, GO possesses intrinsic biological properties, including antimicrobial activity, and it can control immune cell function and modulate the angiogenesis process. Particularly, it is reported that GO nanosheets have pro-angiogenic properties at low doses (1–50 ng/mL) ascribable to controlled intracellular ROS production induced by this material. Meanwhile, the material shows anti-angiogenic activity at high doses (>100 ng/mL), due to the high intracellular ROS levels generated [124]. According to Figure 5, the activity of GO may be primarily attributed to the intracellular production of ROS and reactive nitrogen species as well as the activation of phosphor-eNOS and phosphor-Akt. The understanding of these mechanisms may be important for the potential development of alternative angiogenic treatment approaches for wound care managing. In particular, GO may influence the process by modulating NO production, which plays a critical role in physiological and pathological angiogenesis. In fact, the generation of NO could be useful as pro-angiogenic therapeutic strategy, by controlling the blood pressure, the blood vessel tone and the vascular health. It is generally known that L-citrulline and NO are byproducts of NO synthesis from L-arginine by the enzyme NO synthase (NOS). Endothelial nitric oxide synthase (eNOS), among the NOS isoforms, plays a major role in endothelial cell activity. Additionally, it is widely known that H_2O_2 activates eNOS, which increases intracellular NO levels production [125]. H_2O_2 and NO thus have a direct relationship. For instance, a number of studies revealed that Akt and eNOS signalling is crucial for both angiogenesis and the proliferation of endothelial cells. Other studies have shown that eNOS is phosphorylated in an Akt-dependent manner [125]. However, even though the influence of GO (rGO) on the angiogenesis mechanism is, in part, clear, the possible interaction within the polymer matrix will be analyzed in the next paragraphs.

5. GO-Functionalised Cellulose-Based Nanocomposites for Wound Healing

5.1. GO or rGO/Cellulose Nanocomposites

Nanomaterials, like GO and its derivatives, have been successfully incorporated within cellulose-based matrixes, in the form of hydrogels or scaffolds, to simultaneously stabilise the structure of the nanocomposites and improve the bulk mechanical properties [126]. Among the works published, over the past several years, the majority of them have employed cellulose derivatives as polymer matrix; meanwhile, only one paper was focused on pure cellulose [127] (Table 4). Indeed, Wei and colleagues proposed a multi-modulus components-based strategy for preparing a double cross-linked cellulose/GO composite hydrogel (DCC), with a remarkably high strength and toughness, while retaining a high water content [127]. The authors started from pure cellulose, extracted from cotton linter pulp, dissolved in a 4.6 wt% lithium hydroxide/15 wt% urea solution. The strength and toughness of DCC hydrogel increased because of reversible non-covalent interactions (i.e., hydrogen bonding, hydrophobic and CH-π stacking) established between GO nanosheets and cellulose chains, and irreversible covalent bonds, due to the presence of epichlorohydrin (ECH). GO addition (0–8 wt%) also resulted in a higher storage and viscous moduli compared to cellulose, as reported in Table 4 and shown in Figure 6a,b). Meanwhile, ECH addition (0–3.44 mol_{ECH}:mol_{DCC} ratio) allowed for speeding up the gelation time of the

DCC in 2.5 h, resulting in a storage modulus several orders of magnitude higher than cellulose and DCC (Table 4). Finally, Wei et al. demonstrated that GO nanosheet content, molar ratio between GO and anhydro-glucose units of cellulose, and cross-linker agent concentration were among the critical parameters that allowed for perfectly modulating the mechanical properties of DCC hydrogels, reaching the highest stress and work of fracture in the compressive and tensile mode, as reported in Table 4 and shown in Figure 6c,d. Moreover, the authors showed that the composite hydrogels had broad-spectrum antibacterial properties versus *E. coli* (96.5%, Figure 6e) and *S. aureus* (100%, Figure 6f), upon near-infrared light (NIR) irradiation with a power density of 2 W/cm at 808 nm for 240 s, owing to GO photothermal features. Morphological studies performed via SEM revealed that the bacteria incubated with DCC hydrogels and irradiated with NIR light exhibited a fully collapsed membrane (Figure 6h,j), compared to non-irradiated *E. coli* and *S. aureus* that retained their typical rod and spherical shapes, respectively (Figure 6g,i).

Table 4. List of the papers focused on pure cellulose and derivatives based composites functionalised with GO(rGO) for wound healing application.

Year	Material	Cellulose Biosource	GO Processes	Crosslinker/ Gelling Agents	Inorganic/Organic Compounds Embedded	Physico-Chemical and Mechanical Properties	In Vitro Outcomes	In Vivo Outcomes	Ref.
Pure cellulose									
2022	GO/DCC	Cotton linter pulp	Hummers method	ECH:DCC	-	σ_{comp} = 0.05–13.6 Mpa; w_{comp} = 0.05–1.47 MJ/m^3); σ_{tens} = 0.02–2.8 Mpa; w_{tens} = 0.01–1.49 MJ/m^3 G′ = 0.4–1.5 Pa (GO effect) G″ = 5.8–12.8 Pa (GO effect) G′ = 2037 Pa at 1 rad/s (ECH effect)	*E. coli* death 96.6% *S. aureus* death 100% (8% wt GO, NIR irradiation 2 W/cm, 808 nm, 240 s)	-	[127]
Cellulose-derivatives without bioactive compounds									
2019	rGO/CMC	chemically modified	rGO oxidation by NaOH				HDF cells viability (>90%) *S. aureus* biofilm reduction 81–84%. *P. aeruginosa* biofilm reduction 51–62% *S. aureus* biofilm thickness reduction 47%, *P. aeruginosa* biofilm thickness reduction 40%	Higher biofilm inhibition in *C. elegants* infected with *S. aureus* than *P. aeruginosa*.	[128]
2021	GO/CMC	chemically modified	Hummers method				EA.hy926 migration promotion and increasing of the wound closure rate	Increase of newly formed blood vessels in number and in size. Highly densely packed collagen deposition.	[129]

Table 4. *Cont.*

Year	Material	Cellulose Biosource	GO Processes	Crosslinker/ Gelling Agents	Inorganic/Organic Compounds Embedded	Physico-Chemical and Mechanical Properties	In Vitro Outcomes	In Vivo Outcomes	Ref.
Cellulose-derivatives with bioactive compounds									
2019	AGO/HPC	chemically modified	Hummers method		Ag/ZnO	σ_{tens} = 19.4–28.8 Mpa	*E. coli* inhibition zone 11.25–12.32 mm; *S. aureus* inhibition zone 12.18–13.76 mm	Reduction of wound size after 8 days. Newborn blood vessels filled with red blood cells after 12 days	[130]
2021	GO/TiO_2/Cur/ CA	chemically modified	GO/TiO_2 nanocomposite by hydrothermal method		TiO_2 Cur	σ_{tens} = 35.45 Mpa; swelling ≈ 50–55%	*E. coli* inhibition zone 19 ± 0.2 mm; *S. aureus* inhibition zone 17 ± 0.1 mm; *P. aeruginosa* inhibition zone 16.4 ± 0.2; *E. faecalis* inhibition zone 14 ± 0.2 mm. Wound closure 77 ± 4.18% (12 h)–96 ± 3.26% (24 h)		[131]
2022	O/NA/CA	chemically modified	GO pyrolyzation of cellulose		NA (98%)	σ = 2.46 ± 0.022–4.94 ± 0.027 ($\cdot 10^{-5}$ Mpa); ε = 53.95 ± 0.52–19.05 ± 0.24 %; E = 4.56–25.93 (10^{-7} Mpa).	HeLa cells viability (>80%) *S. aureus* inhibitory zone 9.15 mm		[132]
2022	GO/Cys/DAC GO/Meth/DAC GO/Cys/Meth/ DAC	chemically modified			Cys and Meth		*B. subtilis* inhibition zones (23 ± 0.53 mm and 17 ± 1.27 mm), *S. aureus* inhibition zones (21 ± 0.58 mm and 11 ± 0.69 mm), *E. coli* inhibition zones (12 ± 0.51 mm and 19 ± 1.01 mm), *P. aeruginosa* inhibition zones (24 ± 0.50 mm and 27 ± 0.95 mm), *C. albicans* inhibition zones (12 ± 0.53 mm and 23 ± 0.87 mm) and *C. neoformans* inhibition zones (22 ± 0.52 mm and 32 ± 0.93 mm) for DAC/GO/Cys and DAC/GO/Meth, respectively.		[133]

Table 4. *Cont.*

Year	Material	Cellulose Biosource	GO Processes	Crosslinker/ Gelling Agents	Inorganic/Organic Compounds Embedded	Physico-Chemical and Mechanical Properties	In Vitro Outcomes	In Vivo Outcomes	Ref.
Cellulose with polymeric blend									
2018	rGO/PVA/CMC	chemically modified	rGO reduction under sunlight via convex lens	PVA			EA.hy926 proliferation improved up to 72 h	Number of blood vessels increase 25–62% Blood vessels thickness increase 18.4–44.5%	[134]
2020	rGO/Ag/PU/ Cur/CA	chemically modified	Hummers method	PU	rGO/Ag Cur	σ_{yield} = 0.7 Mpa, σ_{max} = 3.75 Mpa, and E = 0.41 (rGO effect) σ_{yield} = 0.4 Mpa, σ_{max} = 3.4 Mpa, and E = 0.29 (curcumin effect)	*P. aeruginosa* death 100%, and *S. aureus* death 95%.	Wound healing ratio 100%. Collagen fibers deposition after 15 days	[135]
2020	Ag-ZnO@GO/k-car/KG/CMC	chemically modified	Hummers method	k-car	Ag-ZnO KG	$\sigma_{comp} \approx$ 200 kPa; E $\approx$ 150 Mpa	L929 viability 100 % after 7 days. *S. aureus* death 96% and *E. coli* death 98%.	Faster ri-epithelialization process	[136]

Abbreviations: GO, graphene oxide; DCC, double crosslinked cellulose; ECH, epichlorohydine; σ_{comp}, stress at fracture; w_{comp} fracture strain; σ_{tens}, tensile strength; w_{tens} work of fracture; G′, storage modulus; G″, viscous modulus; NIR, near-infrared radiation; MC, methylcellulose; EA.hy926, human vascular endothelial-derived cell line; rGO, reduced graphene oxide; CMC, carboxymethyl cellulose; HDF, human dermal fibroblasts; CA, cellulose acetate; NA, naproxen; σ, stress; ε, strain; E, Young's modulus; HeLa, human tumoral epithelial cell; DAC, dialdehyde cellulose; Cys, cysteine; Meth, methionine; TiO_2, titanium dioxide; Cur, curcumin; HPC, hydroxypropyl cellulose; AGO, GO-grafted silver coated zinc oxide; Ag, silver; ZnO, zinc oxide; PVA, polyvinyl alcohol; PU, polyurethane; σ_{yield}, ultimate strength; k-car, k-carrageenan; KG, Konjac Glucomannan; L929, murine dermal fibroblasts.

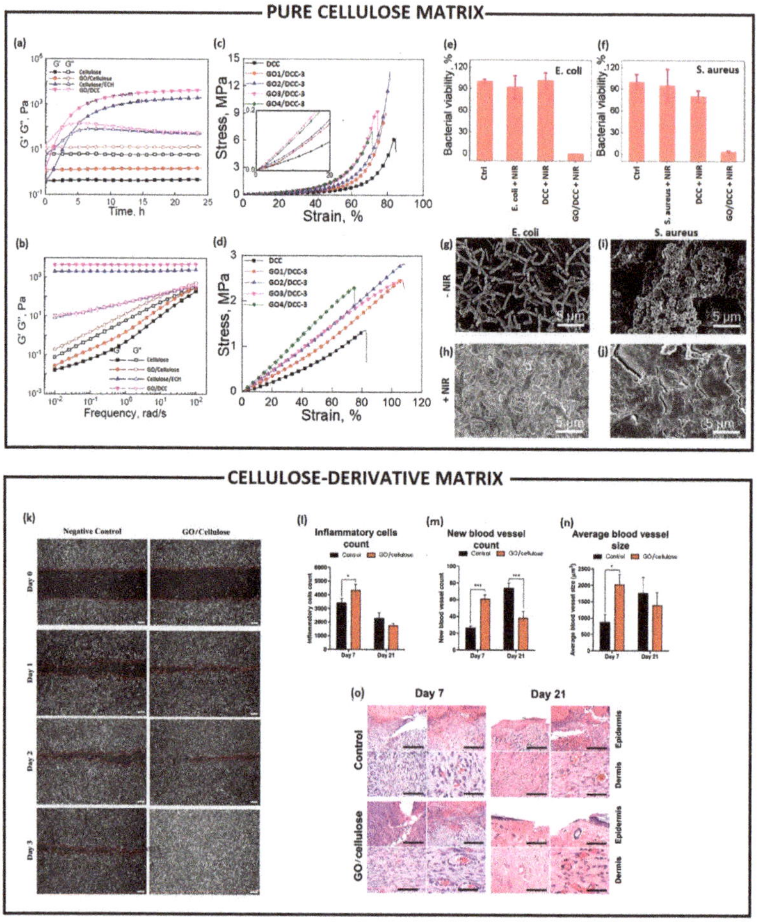

Figure 6. Pure cellulose matrix (top): rheological characterizations: (**a**) time- and (**b**) frequency-dependence of the storage modulus (G′) and loss modulus (G″) of a cellulose, cellulose/GO (2 wt%), cellulose/ECH (ECH:DCC molar ratio = 0.86), and cellulose/GO (2 wt%)/ECH (ECH:AGU molar ratio = 0.86). Mechanical characterizations: (**c**) compression strain–stress curves and (**d**) tensile strain–stress curves of cellulose/GO/ECH composite hydrogels with different GO contents. The insets show magnified plots of the responses in the low-strain range. Antimicrobial studies: relative percentage survival of (**e**) *E. coli* and (**f**) *S. aureus* after incubation with composite hydrogels with and without GO under NIR laser irradiation (power density of 2 W/cm^2 under 808 nm). SEM micrographs of *E. coli* (**g**,**h**) and *S. aureu* (**i**,**j**) on DCC4-3 before (**g**,**i**) and after (**h**,**j**) NIR irradiation. Adapted from [127]. Copyright (2022), with permission from Elsevier. Cellulose-derivatives matrix (bottom): (**k**) evaluation of GO-cellulose nanocomposite effect on in vitro wound healing through scratch assay performed by using a human endothelial cell line (EA.hy926) after 0, 1, 2 and 3 days post wound induction. Red-dotted lines indicate the wound edge (scale bar = 200 μm); (**l**) inflammatory cells counts, (**m**) new blood vessels counts, and (**n**) average blood vessels size measured through ImageJ from a histological section of skin wound in rats treated with or without GO-cellulose nanocomposite for 7 and 21 days. Differences were evaluated using *one-way* ANOVA (* $p < 0.05$; *** $p < 0.0001$); (**o**) haematoxylin and eosin staining of a histological section of skin wound in rats non-treated (control) and treated with GO-cellulose for 7 and 21 days post-wound induction (scale bar = 50 μm). Reprinted from [129]. Copyright (2022), with permission from Elsevier.

Differently from Wei et al., Ali et al. and Soliman et al. developed a GO/cellulose nanocomposite, by using water-soluble MCC [128,129]. Ali and co-workers employed rGO (50, 100, 250, 500 μg/mL), as filler into a water-soluble sodium CMC (NaCMC) hydrogel formulation as functional antibiofilm wound dressing [128]. The rGO/CMC hydrogels exhibited a synergistic antibiofilm effect, inhibiting biofilm formation in *S. aureus* (81–84%) and *P. aeruginosa* (51–62%), respectively. By contrast, the authors reported that GO/CMC hydrogels induced a significant increase in the biofilm formation by *S. aureus* (270%) and *P. aeruginosa* (63%), due to the high level of oxygenated functional groups, which might favour bacteria adhesion. rGO/CMC hydrogel could act in preventing bacteria adhesion in the early adsorption stage because they could be trapped and stacked within rGO agglomerated structures dispersed into the CMC hydrogel matrix. Additional qualitative analysis by using confocal laser scanning microscopy showed that the biofilm thickness was reduced by up to 47% in *S. aureus* and 40% in *P. aeruginosa*, appearing as disintegrated and poorly defined microcolonies. Similarly, GO nanosheets were intercalated within cellulose chains, in a weight ratio 1:1, through non-covalent bonds (i.e., van der Waals, electrostatic and hydrogen bonds) by Soliman and co-workers [129]. GO/MCC nanocomposite retained the viability of human EA.hy926 endothelial cells over time, and enhanced their migration capability in wound scratch assay within 1–3 days (Figure 6k). In addition, GO/MCC significantly promoted the wound healing process in the in vivo rat skin wounds, over the treatment time. Within a short time (day 7), a significant influx of inflammatory cells (Figure 6l) was observed in the dermal region, with a significantly higher number of newly formed vessels (Figure 6m) followed by a significant increase in the size of the blood vessels (Figure 6n) in wounds. Meanwhile, within a longer time (day 21), a mature/remodelled dermis presenting skin appendages (such as hair follicles and sebaceous glands) was observed, with a higher amount of densely arranged collagen fibres (Figure 6o). The authors hypothesized that GO/MCC nanocomposites triggered the in vivo repairing of wounds through GO's capability of scavenging ROS in the wound area, regulating the inflammation and thus driving the healing.

With the aim of improving the inherent potential of the GO and rGO/cellulose nanocomposite as delivery systems, several attempts were investigated by incorporating bioactive compounds (i.e., drugs, amino acids, extracts, nanoparticles, etc.). In this regard, Wang et al. proposed multifunctional composite films consisting of hydroxypropyl cellulose (HPC) matrix and GO-grafted silver-coated zinc oxide nanofillers (AGO) by solution blending [130]. GO was covalently grafted onto the surface with Ag/ZnO by using isophorone diisocyanate, as a coupling agent, which involved the -OH and the -COOH groups on the GO surface and the -OH groups on the Ag/ZnO surface. The AGO intercalation within the HPC matrix contributed to enhancing inter-molecular interactions, resulting in an AGO concentration-dependence increase of the tensile strength (see Table 4). In addition, AGO/HPC films significantly inhibited *E. coli* and *S. aureus* growth with a AGO concentration-dependence (Figure 7a,b). The authors showed that the antimicrobial activity observed in the AGO/HPC films was due to: (i) the generation of OH• and HO_2• radicals, by ZnO nanoparticles upon high energy irradiation, which could destroy the microbial cells' structure [137], followed by (ii) Zn ions penetration through the bacteria cells wall and the reaction with the intracellular active protease [138,139]; (iii) Ag^+ ions interaction with bacteria cell wall, altering its permeability and entering into the cytoplasm promoting the oxidative stress and killing the cells [140]. An in vivo BALB/C mice skinny wound model confirmed a synergistic antibacterial effect and accelerated wound-healing of the AGO/HPC films after 12 days (Figure 7c). Histological images showed many white blood cells and neutrophils recruited in a wound site when bacterial infection occurred in vivo. Over time, new blood vessels filled with red blood cells appeared as highlighted by a red rectangle in Figure 7d. A reliable alternative approach by integrating curcumin (Cur) and GO-grafted titanium dioxide (TiO_2) nanocomposite into CA nanofibers was proposed by Prakash and colleagues. The authors processed the biomaterial by electrospinning, for eradicating the drug-resistant bacteria [131]. GO/TiO_2 nanocomposite incorporation decreased the viscosity of the CA solution, while increasing the conductivity, hence resulting in nanofibers' diameter decrease (≈180 nm). As expected, the integrated GO/TiO_2/Cur/CA nanofibers showed a lower swelling capacity (50–55%) than CA (75–85%) after 7 days, due to strong hydrogen bonding between Cur, GO and CA. However, GO and GO/TiO_2 nanocomposites incorporation in CA matrix created polymeric interactions that hindered the incision sites for triggering the degradation process. Meanwhile, the Cur addition allowed for increasing the degradation. Furthermore, GO/TiO_2/VA nanofibers exhibited a higher tensile strength compared to GO/CA, due to -COOH and -OH functional groups which resulted in intermolecular hydrogel bonding with the CA matrix, whereas Cur addition worked as a nanofiller (discontinuous phase) within a continuous matrix (nanofiber), increasing the density and the mechanical strength. Finally, the GO/TiO_2/CA nanofibers proved the simultaneous antibacterial activity against wounds pathogens and potential wound healing capability. GO/TiO_2/Cur/CA nanofibers showed the highest zone of inhibition. The antimicrobial activity took place through the combined capability of TiO_2 and GO of increasing the ROS-mediated oxidative stress and leading to cell death [141] on one hand; and the possible interference of Cur with the FtsZ protein functions, involved in bacterial cytokinesis, on the other hand, resulting in the bacterial growth inhibition [142,143]. Finally, the GO/TiO_2/CA nanofibers not only proved to be biocompatible, but above all they demonstrated to promote the NIH3T3 fibroblasts proliferation and migration, helping in the closure of wounds of 77% already at 12 h. On the other hand, Purnamasari et al. investigated the potential improvements achieved by simultaneous incorporation of GO and a commercial drug, such as Naproxen (NA), in CA-based hydrogel formulation processed in the form of nanofibers by electrospinning [132]. GO fillers enhanced the mechanical strength of the fibres, driving the production of fibres with a lower diameter (≈447 nm), higher conductivity (1.5 μS/cm) and keeping the NA onto the nanofiber. As the GO increased (0, 0.1, 0.5, 1 g), a corresponding increment in the stress and a reduction in the fibre's strain ability were recorded, thus resulting in Young's modulus increase (Table 4). Even though GO was strictly embedded into the nanocomposite matrix due to a purely physical interaction, it showed the ability to strengthen the nanofibers. GO/CA composite nanofibers were able to sustain the viability of HeLa cells above 80% over 7 h. By contrast, the addition of NA increased HeLa cells' death already after 1 h with a CC_{50} (concentration that reduced the cells proliferation by 50%) of 29.33 μg/mL. However, it showed a strong antibacterial activity against *S. aureus*, with an inhibition zone of 9.15 mm. Concurrently, Hashem et al. developed a potential antimicrobial, antiviral and biocompatible nanocomposite based on DAC, GO and sulphur-containing aminoacids, such as cysteine (Cys) and methionine (Meth) [133]. Both GO/Cys/DAC and GO/Meth/DAC proved a higher and promising antimicrobial activity against $Gram^+$ (*B. subtilis, S. aureus*), $Gram^-$ (*E. coli, P. aeruginosa*) and unicellular fungi (*Candida albicans, Cryptococcus neoformans*). The antimicrobial activity of GO/DAC nanocomposite was improved by the presence and availability of protonated aminoacid residues, which could interact with the bacteria membrane and induce the death.

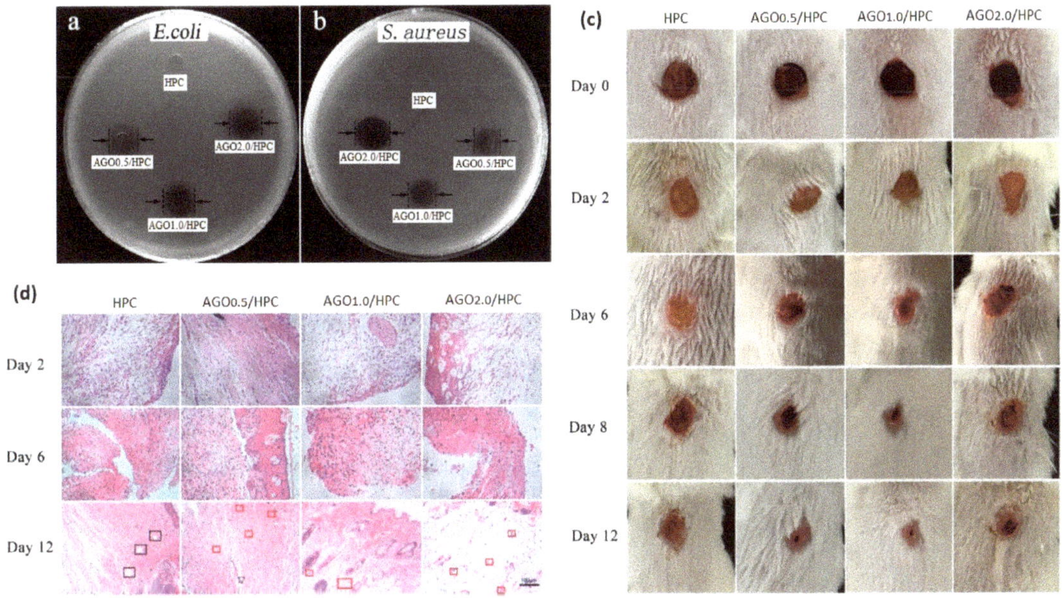

Figure 7. Inhibition zone on plates with solid-state nutrient agar against (**a**) *E. coli* and (**b**) *S. aureus* showing the corresponding diameters of the inhibition zone induced by HPC, $AGO_{0.5}$/HPC, $AGO_{1.0}$/HPC and $AGO_{2.0}$/HPC; (**c**) in vivo BALB/C mouse wound healing model with a 6 mm-diameter of wound on the back, infected with *S. aureus* ($1.0 \cdot 10^7$ CFU/mL) and treated with HPC, $AGO_{0.5}$/HPC, $AGO_{1.0}$/HPC and $AGO_{2.0}$/HPC for 0, 2, 6, 8 and 12 days; (**d**) haematoxylin and eosin staining of histological section of skin wound in mice treated with HPC, $AGO_{0.5}$/HPC, $AGO_{1.0}$/HPC and $AGO_{2.0}$/HPC for 2, 6 and 12 days post-wound induction (scale bar = 100 μm). Adapted from [130] Copyright © 2019 American Chemical Society.

Another possible approach to improve the mechanical strength and toughness of GO/cellulose nanocomposites may involve the use of synthetic or natural polymers as blends [134–136]. Chakraborty et al. synthesised a porous scaffold by freeze-drying, starting from a polymeric blend of polyvinyl alcohol (PVA) and CMC with different amounts of rGO (0, 0.0025, 0.0005, 0.0075 and 0.01% *w*/*v*) [134]. The role of rGO was explored in terms of angiogenesis enhancement. The authors observed that rGO interacted via non-covalent bonding with the polymeric blend, without altering any physico-chemical property of PVA/CMC matrix. NIH3T3 and EA.hy926 cells' good adhesion and proliferation confirmed the biocompatibility of rGO/PVA/CMC scaffolds. Notably, rGO/PVA/CMC with 0.0005 and 0.0075% of rGO successfully increased the EA.hy926 cells proliferation at 72 h, probably due to the slow release of rGO from the scaffold into the culture medium. The pro-angiogenic features of rGO/PVA/CMC were validated in vivo by using the chick chorioallantoic membrane (CAM) model. Two days after scaffolds implanting on the CAM of a developing chick embryo, angiogenesis was remarkably increased (Figure 8a): rGO/PVA/CMC with 0.0005, 0.0075 and 0.01 % rGO induced a significant increase in the number of blood vessels (Figure 8b), along with an absolute increase in blood vessel thickness up to 51.7 % in correspondence with rGO/PVA/CMC with 0.005% rGO. This latter is an evident sign of the newborn blood vessels' maturation, due to a phenomenon called arteriogenesis [144]. The authors ascribed this pro-angiogenic effect to the rGO ability of increasing the intracellular ROS levels [145], triggering the biochemical pathways involved both in the angiogenesis and in the arteriogenesis [145].

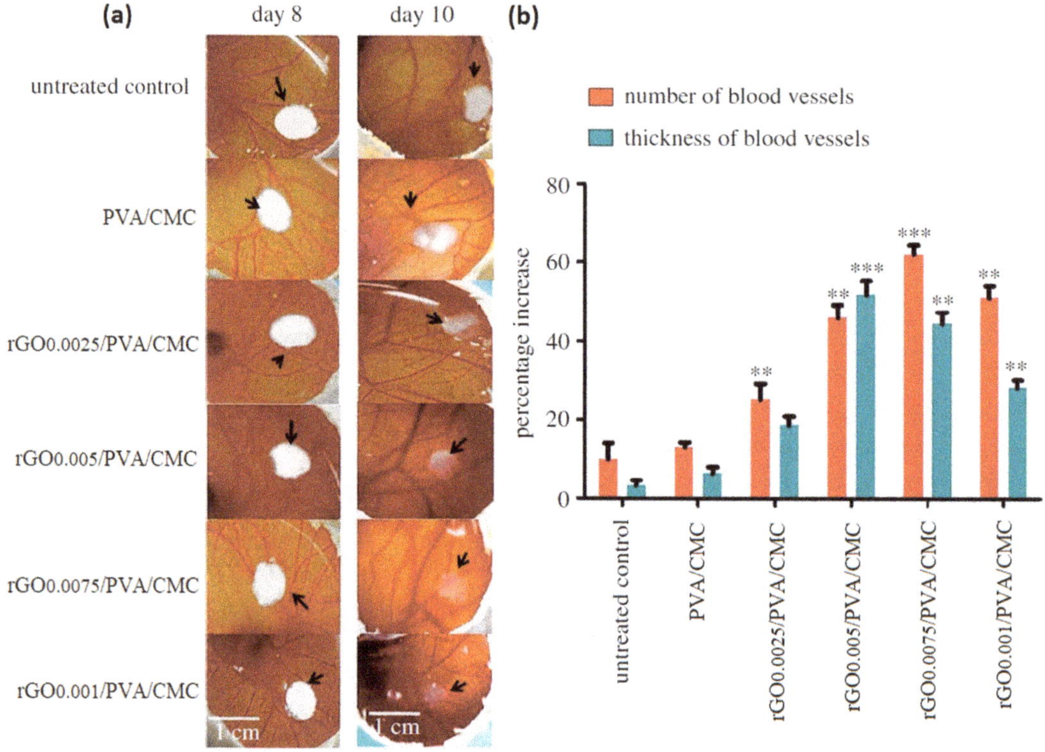

Figure 8. (**a**) Digital photos of chick chorioallantoic membrane (CAM) model untreated and treated with PVA/CMC and PVA/CMC with 0.0025, 0.005, 0.0075 and 0.01% *w*/*v* rGO; (**b**) percentage increase in the number (red bars) and (green bars) blood vessels after 10 days of CAM model (the value are normalised to untreated control at 8 days, ** $p < 0.01$, *** $p < 0.001$ vs. control). Adapted from [134]. Copyright © 2018 by the Royal Society under the terms of the Creative Commons Attribution License.

Later, Esmaeili et al. and Li et al. adopted the same approach by a co-encapsulation of GO/metal oxide nanoparticles, along with a bioactive agent, within a polymeric blend of cellulose derivatives for improving both the mechanical properties and wound healing performances [135,136]. Particularly, Esameili et al. designed a polyurethane (PU)/CA electrospun nanofiber mat, embedding Cur and rGO/Ag [135]. The co-embedding of rGO/Ag and Cur in the PU/CA nanofiber matrix reduced the fibre diameter up to 222 ± 44 nm. Meanwhile, rGO/Ag and Cur showed an opposite effect on the mechanical properties: rGO/Ag enhanced the tensile strength, acting as a nanofiller, while Cur decreased it (Table 4). In addition, the nanocomposite mat with and without Cur exhibited significant antibacterial activity, leading to an inactivation rate of 100% in *P. aeruginosa* and 95% in *S. aureus*, owing to the simultaneous release of Ag ions, which may destroy the bacteria membrane, and the Cur, which can inhibit the shikimate pathway for aromatic amino acid synthesis [142] or the pathway for the protofilament developing [143]. Finally, in vivo histopathological imaging of rat wound skin proved that nanofiber mats significantly stimulated the wound healing process: high level of adnexal growth, mature collagen fibres precipitation and neovascularization were observed after 15 days. Similarly, Li et al. prepared an Ag-ZnO loaded CMC/k-carrageenen/GO/konjac glucomannan hydrogel to validate its efficacy in the antimicrobial and regenerative processes involved in the wound healing [136]. The hydrogel showed a great swelling capability ($\approx$200%), even if the Ag-ZnO nanoparticles addition reduced the swelling compared to the matrix without nanofiller, but mostly high mechanical properties due to a uniform distribution of the Ag-ZnO nanoparticles within the matrix establishing a solid interfacial connection mediated by strong hydrogen bonds. The hydrogel exhibited a strong antibacterial activity, by reducing the viability of *S. aureus* by 96% and *E. coli* by 98%, while it sustained the viability of L929 murine fibroblasts, stimulating their proliferation up to 7 days. Finally, the hydrogel demonstrated promising efficacy in healing an in vivo diabetic ulcer mouse model, promoting a more rapid re-epithelialization process as early as 8 days.

5.2. GO or rGO/Bacterial Cellulose Nanocomposites

Over the past years, BC has been also employed as polymer matrix in combination with GO (rGO) for wound healing applications and the last 3-years advances are summarized in Table 5. A mussel mimetic transdermal patch based on BC was prepared by Khamrai et al. [12]. In particular, BC was modified via an amidation reaction between the carboxylated BC and dopamine (DOPA), a catechol-containing compound. Furthermore, the free -OH group of the DOPA moiety was used to prepare rGO/Ag-NPs/DOPA/BC. rGO is able to confer excellent thermal, electrical and mechanical features. In particular, an increase in the tensile strength was achieved by incorporating 0.2 g of rGO and 2 g of DOPA/BC into 20 mL solution. The antimicrobial action of the prepared film was determined against both Gram$^+$ (*S. aureus* and *Lysinibacillus fusiformis*) and Gram$^-$ (*E. coli* and *P. aeruginosa*) bacteria. Results showed that rGO/Ag-NPs/DOPA/BC exerted a clear bactericidal activity, mainly due to the presence of Ag-NPs. The authors found that the cell surface of *E. coli* and *S. aureus* was drastically altered, and the cell wall was squeezed in the presence of rGO/Ag-NPs/DOPA/BC, indicating its significant antimicrobial activity. The cell compatibility of the composite film over the NIH 3T3 fibroblast cell line was assessed through an MTT assay. The in vitro wound-healing assays over the NIH 3T3 cell line and A549 human lung epithelial cell line revealed that the presence of rGO and Ag-NPs in the composite film accelerated the wound healing process [12]. GO-copper oxide (CuO)/BC nanocomposites were prepared by Xie et al. [146] by mixing GO-CuO solution at different concentrations with BC slurries (1% dry weight). Particularly, GO-CuO (2.5, 5 and 7.5 mg/mL) was introduced to endow antibacterial properties. The proportion of GO-CuO in GO-CuO/BC composites ranged from 5% to 15% (*w*/*w*%). In this case, the presence of CO provided nucleation sites for in situ CuO nanosheets growth. Results from microbiological tests showed that the CuO/BC nanocomposites displayed better antimicrobial properties with higher activity against Gram$^+$ than Gram$^-$ bacteria, underlying the synergic contribution of GO and CuO into the polymer matrix [146]. The authors also tried to elucidate the mechanisms of antimicrobial activity of the nanocomposites, which could be due to (i) a direct contact and interaction of GO sharp nanosheets and CuO nanorods with the cell membrane and lipid membrane, resulting in alteration of membrane permeability, (ii) the disruption of the integrity of the bacterial membrane, accompanied by cellular deformation, surface collapse, surface perforation and roughness, and (iii) an increased production of ROS leading to cell death. Moreover, the GO/CuO nanohybrid-decorated cellulose nanocomposite showed good cell compatibility in vitro towards mice fibroblast cells [146]. Zhang et al. prepared a GO/BC composite film modified with DOPA and immersed in a silver solution [147]. The material was conductive and produced a weak current, generating heat when a voltage was applied. This allowed it to accelerate wound cell migration and promote wound healing. In addition, Ag-NPs immobilized on the surface released Ag$^+$, which generated many oxidizing free radicals that killed bacteria. The in vitro cytotoxicity tests showed that the composite film had excellent biocompatibility, giving it good application prospects for wound dressings [147].

Table 5. List of the papers focused on bacterial cellulose based composites functionalised with GO(rGO) for wound healing application.

Year	Material	Cellulose Biosource	GO Processes	Crosslinker/ Gelling Agents	Inorganic/Organic Compounds Embedded	Physico-Chemical and Mechanical Properties	In Vitro Outcomes	In Vivo Out-comes	Ref.
2019	rGO/Ag/ DOPA/BC	*Gluconacetobacter xylus* (MTCC7795)	Hummers method	–	$AgNO_3$	σ_{tens} = 1–5.52 ± 0.07 MPa σ_{tens} = 5.21 ± 0.03 MPa (Ag NPs effect) Average resistance of 84 kΩ	*E. coli* inhibition zone diameter 15 ± 1 mm; *P. aeruginosa* inhibition zone diameter 11 ± 0.5 mm, *S. aureus* inhibition zone diameter 13 ± 0.5 mm, *L. fusiformis* inhibition zone diameter 14 ± 0.75 mm. High stimulation of NIH3T3 proliferation favouring the wound closure (18 h).	-	[12]
2019	GO-CuO/BC	*Gluconacetobacter xylinus* (traditional Chinese drink)			CuO		*S. aureus* inhibition zone diameter 16.3–18.3 mm; *E. coli* inhibition zone diameter 12.7–15.2 mm, *B. subtilis* inhibition zone diameter 27.8–28.5 mm, *P. aeruginosa* inhibition zone diameter 0–15.2 mm. NIH3T3 viability > 100%	-	[146]
2021	rGO/Ag-pDA/BC	*Gluconacetobacter xylinus*	Hummers method		$AgNO_3$		*E. coli* inhibition zone 6.3 mm ($AgNO_3$ effect)	-	[147]
2022	GQDs/BC	*Komagataeibacter oboediens* (IMBG180)			-		Bacterial inhibition against *S. aureus*, *MRSA*, *E. coli*, *P. aeruginosa* and *S. agalactiae*. Bactericidal effect against *MRSA*, *E. coli* and *P. aeruginosa*. Angiogenesis stimulation validated by up-regulation of eNOS, VEGFA, MMP-9 and vimentin		[148]
2022	GO/PVA/BC	-		TEOS PVA	Cur	Increase of the compressive stress and hydrophilicity by increasing the GO content	*E. coli* inhibition zone 5–15 mm; *S. aureus* inhibition zone 7.5–16 mm; *P. aeruginosa* inhibition zone 7–17 mm		[3]

Abbreviations: BC, bacterial cellulose; DOPA, dopamine; $AgNO_3$, silver nitrate; NIH3T3, mouse embryonic fibroblast cell line; CuO, copper oxide; pDA, polydopamine; GQDs, graphene oxide quantum dots; MRSA, Methicillin-Resistant Staphylococcus Aureus; TEOS, Tetraethyl orthosilicate.

For possible application in the treatment of wounds, BC was impregnated with GO quantum dots (GQDs) by Zmejkoski et al. [148]. Successful loading of approximately 11.7 weight percent of GQDs into the BC was achieved. The GQDs/BC composites demonstrated excellent water and wound fluid absorption, which is in line with good dressing qualities. The biomaterials significantly inhibited *S. aureus* and *S. agalactiae* and had bactericidal effects on *E. coli* and *P. aeruginosa* that were resistant to methicillin. The capacity of the GQDs to interact with bacterial membrane or cell wall, which results in destabilization of its integrity, is associated with the bactericidal effect [148]. The in vitro healing research revealed a significant migration of human fibroblasts following the application of GQDs/BC hydrogels. Furthermore, eNOS, VEGF A, matrix metallopeptidase 9, and vimentin gene expression in fibroblasts were noticeably elevated after 72 h of exposure to GQDs/BC, supporting angiogenesis [148]. Finally, Al-Arjan et al. reported a systematic study by using GO functionalized BC, which was obtained by hydrothermal treatment [3] (Figure 9a). Different concentrations of GO (0.01, 0.02, 0.03 and 0.04 mg) were employed. The presence of GO increased the surface roughness. This aspect is of paramount importance in wound healing, as the surface roughness helps wounds by providing them with important hydration. However, there was a threshold limit behind which a GO amount can cause cracking on drying. Furthermore, wettability as well as the swelling increased by increasing GO concentrations. It is worth noting that the increase of GO concentration allowed for improving mechanical properties (Figure 9b) and decreasing the biodegradation as the GO acted as a crosslinker and as a reinforcement of the polymer matrix [3]. The antibacterial capabilities were tested against microorganisms that cause Gram$^+$ and Gram$^-$ severe infections. By increasing GO concentration, a maximum antibacterial effect was observed (Figure 9c). It can be because the sharp edges of the maximal GO quantity tear the bacterial membrane. In order to prevent bacterial development, the polymeric component of the hydrogel may interact with the bacterial membrane by surrounding and penetrating a number of accessible functional groups [3]. By increasing the quantity of GO, these composite hydrogels demonstrated promising anticancer effects against the U87 cell line. In addition, the biggest anti-cancer effect was observed in the Cur loaded-BC that had the highest GO concentration. This might be as a result of the composite hydrogel's interaction with the cellular membrane, which enabled Cur to carry out anticancer actions. The research findings allowed for concluding that these composite hydrogels have controlled medication release, physico-mechanical, and intrinsic antimicrobial qualities, which make them an appropriate biomaterial for skin wound healing [3].

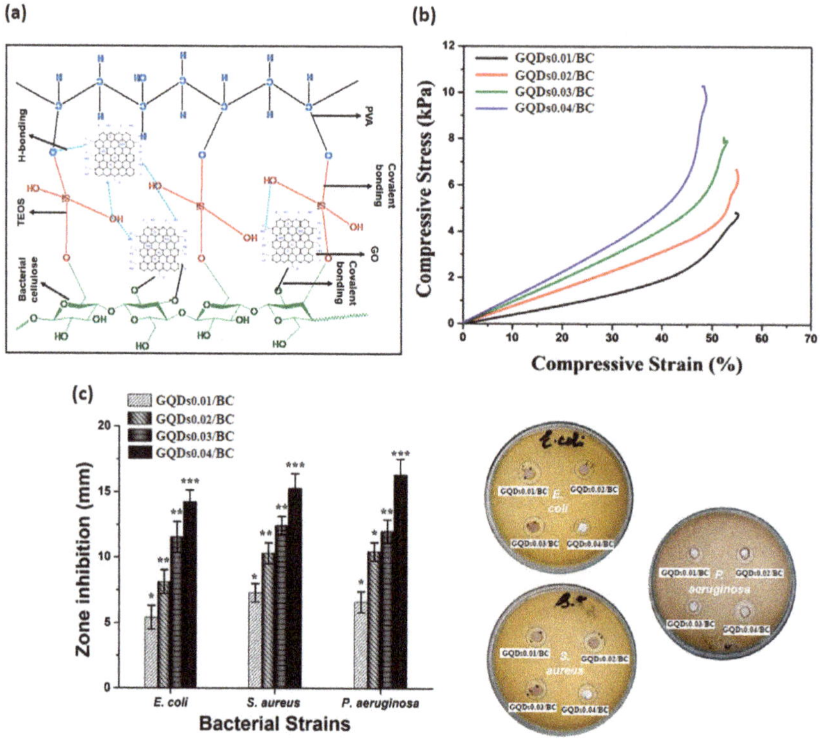

Figure 9. (**a**) The proposed chemical interaction of the bacterial cellulose, polyvinyl alcohol, GO, and crosslinked via TEO; (**b**) stress–strain curve of hydrogels; (**c**) the antibacterial activities of composite hydrogels against different severe skin infections causing Gram$^+$ and Gram$^-$ pathogens. * $p < 0.05$, ** $p < 0.01$ and *** $p < 0.00$. ($GQDs_{0.01}$/BC, $GQDs_{0.02}$/BC, $GQDs_{0.03}$/BC, and $GQDs_{0.04}$/BC) were assigned to these composite hydrogels after a different GO amount (0.01, 0.02, 0.03, and 0.04 mg). Adapted from [3].

6. Conclusions and Future Perspectives

In the last several decades, several research groups have focused on the development of multifunctional GO or rGO/cellulose nanocomposites, in the form of injectable hydrogels or scaffolds for wound healing applications. In particular, several optimized dressings have been specifically designed exploiting the interesting structural and physico-chemical properties of cellulose (i.e., water retention, flexibility, toughness), and the potential antimicrobial and angiogenic effect of GO and rGO. However, despite the encouraging results achieved, there are still several questions that have to be answered and different limitations to overcome. In particular, even though the role of GO or rGO in triggering the bactericidal and pro-/anti-angiogenic properties is well-known when used alone, further investigations are required to understand its role when it is embedded within 3D cellulose-derived matrixes. Indeed, among the studies herein reported, only a few have tried to hypothesise the mechanism of action and also validate their efficacy through suitable in vivo models. However, deeper studies of the main molecular pathways, along with biodegradation and bioaccumulation of the organic and inorganic components in vivo, could be helpful. Furthermore, the presented literature lacks nanocomposites fully based on GO or rGO and cellulose obtained from agricultural or industrial wastes. Indeed, considering the increasing interest in the use of sustainable raw materials, the creation of such nanocomposite biomaterials might represent a promising starting point in the development of innovative smart dressings for wound healing applications.

Author Contributions: Conceptualization, U.D. and S.S.; investigation, U.D., S.D., M.S.H., A.S., A.L. and S.S.; writing—original draft preparation, U.D., S.D., M.S.H., A.S., A.L. and S.S.; writing—review and editing, U.D., S.D., M.S.H., A.S., A.L., S.K., M.G.R., L.A. and S.S.; visualization, U.D. and S.S.; supervision, U.D. and S.S.; funding acquisition, S.D. and S.S. All authors have read and agreed to the published version of the manuscript.

Funding: S.S. and S.D. acknowledged the National Research Council (CNR) of Italy and the Egyptian Academy of Scientific Research and Technology (ASRT) for their financial support through the Joint Bilateral Agreement (Biennial Programme 2022–2023) project "Biowaste-derived Injectable Bionanomaterials Platform for Regenerative Medicine" (CUP B65F22000050005 for CNR and Grant No. 9596 for ASRT).

Institutional Review Board Statement: Not applicable.

Informed Consent Statement: Not applicable.

Data Availability Statement: Not applicable.

Acknowledgments: Figures 2 and 5 were created with BioRender (https://biorender.com/ [accessed on 1 March 2021]).

Conflicts of Interest: The authors declare no conflict of interest.

References

1. Falanga, V. Wound Healing and Its Impairment in the Diabetic Foot. *Lancet* **2005**, *366*, 1736–1743. [CrossRef] [PubMed]
2. Yao, Z.; Niu, J.; Cheng, B. Prevalence of Chronic Skin Wounds and Their Risk Factors in an Inpatient Hospital Setting in Northern China. *Adv. Ski. Wound Care* **2020**, *33*, 1–10. [CrossRef] [PubMed]
3. Al-Arjan, W.S.; Khan, M.U.A.; Almutairi, H.H.; Alharbi, S.M.; Razak, S.I.A. PH-Responsive PVA/BC-f-GO Dressing Materials for Burn and Chronic Wound Healing with Curcumin Release Kinetics. *Polymers* **2022**, *14*, 1949. [CrossRef]
4. Francesko, A.; Petkova, P.; Tzanov, T. Hydrogel Dressings for Advanced Wound Management. *Curr. Med. Chem.* **2018**, *25*, 5782–5797. [CrossRef] [PubMed]
5. Di Mola, A.; Landi, M.R.; Massa, A.; D'Amora, U.; Guarino, V. Hyaluronic Acid in Biomedical Fields: New Trends from Chemistry to Biomaterial Applications. *Int. J. Mol. Sci.* **2022**, *23*, 14372. [CrossRef] [PubMed]
6. Zhang, L.; D'Amora, U.; Ronca, A.; Li, Y.; Mo, X.; Zhou, F.; Yuan, M.; Ambrosio, L.; Wu, J.; Raucci, M.G. In Vitro and in Vivo Biocompatibility and Inflammation Response of Methacrylated and Maleated Hyaluronic Acid for Wound Healing. *RSC Adv.* **2020**, *10*, 32183–32192. [CrossRef] [PubMed]
7. Prelipcean, A.-M.; Iosageanu, A.; Gaspar-Pintiliescu, A.; Moldovan, L.; Craciunescu, O.; Negreanu-Pirjol, T.; Negreanu-Pirjol, B.; Mitran, R.-A.; Marin, M.; D'Amora, U. Marine and Agro-Industrial By-Products Valorization Intended for Topical Formulations in Wound Healing Applications. *Materials* **2022**, *15*, 3507. [CrossRef]
8. Zhu, J.; Li, Z.; Zou, Y.; Lu, G.; Ronca, A.; D'Amora, U.; Liang, J.; Fan, Y.; Zhang, X.; Sun, Y. Advanced Application of Collagen-Based Biomaterials in Tissue Repair and Restoration. *J. Leather Sci. Eng.* **2022**, *4*, 1–19. [CrossRef]
9. Deng, X.; Gould, M.; Ali, M.A. A Review of Current Advancements for Wound Healing: Biomaterial Applications and Medical Devices. *J. Biomed. Mater. Res. Part B Appl. Biomater.* **2022**, *110*, 2542–2573. [CrossRef] [PubMed]
10. Ferroni, L.; Gardin, C.; D'Amora, U.; Calzà, L.; Ronca, A.; Tremoli, E.; Ambrosio, L.; Zavan, B. Exosomes of Mesenchymal Stem Cells Delivered from Methacrylated Hyaluronic Acid Patch Improve the Regenerative Properties of Endothelial and Dermal Cells. *Biomater. Adv.* **2022**, *139*, 213000. [CrossRef]
11. D'Amora, U.; Ronca, A.; Raucci, M.G.; Dozio, S.M.; Lin, H.; Fan, Y.; Zhang, X.; Ambrosio, L. In Situ Sol-Gel Synthesis of Hyaluronan Derivatives Bio-Nanocomposite Hydrogels. *Regen. Biomater.* **2019**, *6*, 249–258. [CrossRef] [PubMed]
12. Khamrai, M.; Banerjee, S.L.; Paul, S.; Ghosh, A.K.; Sarkar, P.; Kundu, P.P. A Mussel Mimetic, Bioadhesive, Antimicrobial Patch Based on Dopamine-Modified Bacterial Cellulose/RGO/Ag NPs: A Green Approach toward Wound-Healing Applications. *ACS Sustain. Chem. Eng.* **2019**, *7*, 12083–12097. [CrossRef]
13. Madaghiele, M.; Demitri, C.; Sannino, A.; Ambrosio, L. Polymeric Hydrogels for Burn Wound Care: Advanced Skin Wound Dressings and Regenerative Templates. *Burn. Trauma* **2014**, *2*, 2321–3868. [CrossRef] [PubMed]
14. Demitri, C.; Raucci, M.G.; Giuri, A.; De Benedictis, V.M.; Giugliano, D.; Calcagnile, P.; Sannino, A.; Ambrosio, L. Cellulose-Based Porous Scaffold for Bone Tissue Engineering Applications: Assessment of h MSC Proliferation and Differentiation. *J. Biomed. Mater. Res. Part A* **2016**, *104*, 726–733. [CrossRef] [PubMed]
15. Oprea, M.; Voicu, S.I. Recent Advances in Composites Based on Cellulose Derivatives for Biomedical Applications. *Carbohydr. Polym.* **2020**, *247*, 116683. [CrossRef] [PubMed]

16. Sengupta, I.; Bhattacharya, P.; Talukdar, M.; Neogi, S.; Pal, S.K.; Chakraborty, S. Bactericidal Effect of Graphene Oxide and Reduced Graphene Oxide: Influence of Shape of Bacteria. *Colloid Interface Sci. Commun.* **2019**, *28*, 60–68. [CrossRef]
17. Hasanin, M.S. Cellulose-Based Biomaterials: Chemistry and Biomedical Applications. *Starch Stärke* **2022**, *74*, 2200060. [CrossRef]
18. Choi, S.M.; Rao, K.M.; Zo, S.M.; Shin, E.J.; Han, S.S. Bacterial Cellulose and Its Applications. *Polymers* **2022**, *14*, 1080. [CrossRef]
19. Naomi, R.; Bt Hj Idrus, R.; Fauzi, M.B. Plant-vs. Bacterial-Derived Cellulose for Wound Healing: A Review. *Int. J. Environ. Res. Public Health* **2020**, *17*, 6803. [CrossRef]
20. Dunlop, M.J.; Clemons, C.; Reiner, R.; Sabo, R.; Agarwal, U.P.; Bissessur, R.; Sojoudiasli, H.; Carreau, P.J.; Acharya, B. Towards the Scalable Isolation of Cellulose Nanocrystals from Tunicates. *Sci. Rep.* **2020**, *10*, 19090. [CrossRef]
21. Szychlinska, M.A.; Bucchieri, F.; Fucarino, A.; Ronca, A.; D'Amora, U. Three-Dimensional Bioprinting for Cartilage Tissue Engineering: Insights into Naturally-Derived Bioinks from Land and Marine Sources. *J. Funct. Biomater.* **2022**, *13*, 118. [CrossRef] [PubMed]
22. Zou, P.; Yao, J.; Cui, Y.-N.; Zhao, T.; Che, J.; Yang, M.; Li, Z.; Gao, C. Advances in Cellulose-Based Hydrogels for Biomedical Engineering: A Review Summary. *Gels* **2022**, *8*, 364. [CrossRef] [PubMed]
23. Malladi, R.; Nagalakshmaiah, M.; Robert, M.; Elkoun, S. Importance of Agriculture and Industrial Waste in the Field of Nano Cellulose and Its Recent Industrial Developments: A Review. *ACS Sustain. Chem. Eng.* **2018**, *6*, 2807–2828.
24. Wang, J.; Tavakoli, J.; Tang, Y. Bacterial Cellulose Production, Properties and Applications with Different Culture Methods—A Review. *Carbohydr. Polym.* **2019**, *219*, 63–76. [CrossRef]
25. Castro, C.; Zuluaga, R.; Álvarez, C.; Putaux, J.-L.; Caro, G.; Rojas, O.J.; Mondragon, I.; Gañán, P. Bacterial Cellulose Produced by a New Acid-Resistant Strain of Gluconacetobacter Genus. *Carbohydr. Polym.* **2012**, *89*, 1033–1037. [CrossRef] [PubMed]
26. Hussain, Z.; Sajjad, W.; Khan, T.; Wahid, F. Production of Bacterial Cellulose from Industrial Wastes: A Review. *Cellulose* **2019**, *26*, 2895–2911. [CrossRef]
27. Abdelraof, M.; Hasanin, M.S.; El-Saied, H. Ecofriendly Green Conversion of Potato Peel Wastes to High Productivity Bacterial Cellulose. *Carbohydr. Polym.* **2019**, *211*, 75–83. [CrossRef]
28. Alves, L.; Medronho, B.; Antunes, F.E.; Topgaard, D.; Lindman, B. Dissolution State of Cellulose in Aqueous Systems. 1. Alkaline Solvents. *Cellulose* **2016**, *23*, 247–258. [CrossRef]
29. Abou-Yousef, H.; Dacrory, S.; Hasanin, M.; Saber, E.; Kamel, S. Biocompatible Hydrogel Based on Aldehyde-Functionalized Cellulose and Chitosan for Potential Control Drug Release. *Sustain. Chem. Pharm.* **2021**, *21*, 100419. [CrossRef]
30. Aziz, T.; Farid, A.; Haq, F.; Kiran, M.; Ullah, A.; Zhang, K.; Li, C.; Ghazanfar, S.; Sun, H.; Ullah, R.; et al. A Review on the Modification of Cellulose and Its Applications. *Polymers* **2022**, *14*, 3206. [CrossRef]
31. Xing, L.; Hu, C.; Zhang, W.; Guan, L.; Gu, J. Biodegradable Cellulose I (II) Nanofibrils/Poly (Vinyl Alcohol) Composite Films with High Mechanical Properties, Improved Thermal Stability and Excellent Transparency. *Int. J. Biol. Macromol.* **2020**, *164*, 1766–1775. [CrossRef] [PubMed]
32. Zaman, A.; Huang, F.; Jiang, M.; Wei, W.; Zhou, Z. Preparation, Properties, and Applications of Natural Cellulosic Aerogels: A Review. *Energy Built Environ.* **2020**, *1*, 60–76. [CrossRef]
33. Wei, Z.; Cai, C.; Huang, Y.; Wang, P.; Song, J.; Deng, L.; Fu, Y. Strong Biodegradable Cellulose Materials with Improved Crystallinity via Hydrogen Bonding Tailoring Strategy for UV Blocking and Antioxidant Activity. *Int. J. Biol. Macromol.* **2020**, *164*, 27–36. [CrossRef] [PubMed]
34. Dacrory, S.; Hashem, A.H.; Kamel, S. Antimicrobial and Antiviral Activities with Molecular Docking Study of Chitosan/Carrageenan@ Clove Oil Beads. *Biotechnol. J.* **2022**, *17*, 2100298. [CrossRef]
35. Dacrory, S.; Kamel, S.; Turky, G. Development of Dielectric Film Based on Cellulose Loaded Nano-Silver and Carbon for Potential Energy Storage. *ECS J. Solid State Sci. Technol.* **2021**, *10*, 123004. [CrossRef]
36. Dacrory, S.; Abou Hammad, A.B.; El Nahrawy, A.M.; Abou-Yousef, H.; Kamel, S. Cyanoethyl Cellulose/BaTiO3/GO Flexible Films with Electroconductive Properties. *ECS J. Solid State Sci. Technol.* **2021**, *10*, 83004. [CrossRef]
37. Al-Shemy, M.T.; Al-Sayed, A.; Dacrory, S. Fabrication of Sodium Alginate/Graphene Oxide/Nanocrystalline Cellulose Scaffold for Methylene Blue Adsorption: Kinetics and Thermodynamics Study. *Sep. Purif. Technol.* **2022**, *290*, 120825. [CrossRef]
38. Dacrory, S. Development of Mesoporous Foam Based on Dicarboxylic Cellulose and Graphene Oxide for Potential Oil/Water Separation. *Polym. Bull.* **2022**, *79*, 9563–9574. [CrossRef]
39. Seddiqi, H.; Oliaei, E.; Honarkar, H.; Jin, J.; Geonzon, L.C.; Bacabac, R.G.; Klein-Nulend, J. Cellulose and Its Derivatives: Towards Biomedical Applications. *Cellulose* **2021**, *28*, 1893–1931. [CrossRef]
40. Tudoroiu, E.-E.; Ghica, M.-V.; Albu-Kaya, G.M.; Dinu-Pirvu, C.-E.; Popa, L.; Anuta, V.; Velescu, B.S.; Kaya, D.A.; Marin, M.M.; Prisada, R.M. Rheological Characterization of Some Cellulose Derivatives-Based Hydrogels. In Proceedings of the 9th International Conference on Advanced Materials and Systems, Online, 26–28 October 2022. [CrossRef]
41. Nasution, H.; Harahap, H.; Dalimunthe, N.F.; Ginting, M.H.S.; Jaafar, M.; Tan, O.O.H.; Aruan, H.K.; Herfananda, A.L. Hydrogel and Effects of Crosslinking Agent on Cellulose-Based Hydrogels: A Review. *Gels* **2022**, *8*, 568. [CrossRef]
42. Manna, S.; Dhanalakshmi, D.; Bhowmik, M.; Jana, S.; Jana, S. Cellulose Derivative-Based Bioadhesive Blend Patch for Transdermal Drug Delivery. *Front. Mater.* **2022**, *9*, 835507. [CrossRef]
43. Douglass, E.F.; Avci, H.; Boy, R.; Rojas, O.J.; Kotek, R. A Review of Cellulose and Cellulose Blends for Preparation of Bio-Derived and Conventional Membranes, Nanostructured Thin Films, and Composites. *Polym. Rev.* **2018**, *58*, 102–163. [CrossRef]
44. Imeson, A. *Food Stabilisers, Thickeners and Gelling Agents*; John Wiley & Sons: Hoboken, NJ, USA, 2011.

45. Oprea, M.; Panaitescu, D.M. Nanocellulose Hybrids with Metal Oxides Nanoparticles for Biomedical Applications. *Molecules* **2020**, *25*, 4045. [CrossRef] [PubMed]
46. Yan, N.; Capezzuto, F.; Lavorgna, M.; Buonocore, G.G.; Tescione, F.; Xia, H.; Ambrosio, L. Borate Cross-Linked Graphene Oxide–Chitosan as Robust and High Gas Barrier Films. *Nanoscale* **2016**, *8*, 10783–10791. [CrossRef]
47. Raucci, M.G.; Giugliano, D.; Longo, A.; Zeppetelli, S.; Carotenuto, G.; Ambrosio, L. Comparative Facile Methods for Preparing Graphene Oxide–Hydroxyapatite for Bone Tissue Engineering. *J. Tissue Eng. Regen. Med.* **2017**, *11*, 2204–2216. [CrossRef]
48. Seo, Y.-R.; Kim, J.-W.; Hoon, S.; Kim, J.; Chung, J.H.; Lim, K.-T. Cellulose-Based Nanocrystals: Sources and Applications via Agricultural Byproducts. *J. Biosyst. Eng.* **2018**, *43*, 59–71.
49. Devi, A.; Singh, A.; Bajar, S.; Pant, D.; Din, Z.U. Ethanol from Lignocellulosic Biomass: An in-Depth Analysis of Pre-Treatment Methods, Fermentation Approaches and Detoxification Processes. *J. Environ. Chem. Eng.* **2021**, *9*, 105798. [CrossRef]
50. Hasanin, M.S.; Kassem, N.; Hassan, M.L. Preparation and Characterization of Microcrystalline Cellulose from Olive Stones. *Biomass Convers. Biorefinery* **2021**, 1–8. [CrossRef]
51. Suryadi, H.; Judono, J.J.; Putri, M.R.; Eclessia, A.D.; Ulhaq, J.M.; Agustina, D.N.; Sumiati, T. Biodelignification of Lignocellulose Using Ligninolytic Enzymes from White-Rot Fungi. *Heliyon* **2022**, *8*, e08865. [CrossRef]
52. Hasanin, M.S.; Darwesh, O.M.; Matter, I.A.; El-Saied, H. Isolation and Characterization of Non-Cellulolytic Aspergillus Flavus EGYPTA5 Exhibiting Selective Ligninolytic Potential. *Biocatal. Agric. Biotechnol.* **2019**, *17*, 160–167. [CrossRef]
53. Liu, K.; Du, H.; Zheng, T.; Liu, W.; Zhang, M.; Liu, H.; Zhang, X.; Si, C. Lignin-Containing Cellulose Nanomaterials: Preparation and Applications. *Green Chem.* **2021**, *23*, 9723–9746. [CrossRef]
54. Nagarajan, K.J.; Ramanujam, N.R.; Sanjay, M.R.; Siengchin, S.; Surya Rajan, B.; Sathick Basha, K.; Madhu, P.; Raghav, G.R. A Comprehensive Review on Cellulose Nanocrystals and Cellulose Nanofibers: Pretreatment, Preparation, and Characterization. *Polym. Compos.* **2021**, *42*, 1588–1630. [CrossRef]
55. Kumar, A.; Gupta, V.; Singh, S.; Saini, S.; Gaikwad, K.K. Pine Needles Lignocellulosic Ethylene Scavenging Paper Impregnated with Nanozeolite for Active Packaging Applications. *Ind. Crops Prod.* **2021**, *170*, 113752. [CrossRef]
56. Bianco, A.; Cheng, H.-M.; Enoki, T.; Gogotsi, Y.; Hurt, R.H.; Koratkar, N.; Kyotani, T.; Monthioux, M.; Park, C.R.; Tascon, J.M.D.; et al. All in the Graphene Family–A Recommended Nomenclature for Two-Dimensional Carbon Materials. *Carbon* **2013**, *65*, 1–6. [CrossRef]
57. Yan, Y.; Nashath, F.Z.; Chen, S.; Manickam, S.; Lim, S.S.; Zhao, H.; Lester, E.; Wu, T.; Pang, C.H. Synthesis of Graphene: Potential Carbon Precursors and Approaches. *Nanotechnol. Rev.* **2020**, *9*, 1284–1314. [CrossRef]
58. Smith, A.T.; LaChance, A.M.; Zeng, S.; Liu, B.; Sun, L. Synthesis, Properties, and Applications of Graphene Oxide/Reduced Graphene Oxide and Their Nanocomposites. *Nano Mater. Sci.* **2019**, *1*, 31–47. [CrossRef]
59. Rowley-Neale, S.J.; Randviir, E.P.; Dena, A.S.A.; Banks, C.E. An Overview of Recent Applications of Reduced Graphene Oxide as a Basis of Electroanalytical Sensing Platforms. *Appl. Mater. Today* **2018**, *10*, 218–226. [CrossRef]
60. Ray, S. *Applications of Graphene and Graphene-Oxide Based Nanomaterials*; William Andrew: Norwich, NY, USA, 2015.
61. Zhu, Y.; Murali, S.; Cai, W.; Li, X.; Suk, J.W.; Potts, J.R.; Ruoff, R.S. Graphene and Graphene Oxide: Synthesis, Properties, and Applications. *Adv. Mater.* **2010**, *22*, 3906–3924. [CrossRef]
62. Chen, D.; Feng, H.; Li, J. Graphene Oxide: Preparation, Functionalization, and Electrochemical Applications. *Chem. Rev.* **2012**, *112*, 6027–6053. [CrossRef]
63. Wan, X.; Huang, Y.; Chen, Y. Focusing on Energy and Optoelectronic Applications: A Journey for Graphene and Graphene Oxide at Large Scale. *Acc. Chem. Res.* **2012**, *45*, 598–607. [CrossRef]
64. Dreyer, D.R.; Park, S.; Bielawski, C.W.; Ruoff, R.S. The Chemistry of Graphene Oxide. *Chem. Soc. Rev.* **2010**, *39*, 228–240. [CrossRef] [PubMed]
65. Rollo, G.; Ronca, A.; Cerruti, P.; Gan, X.P.; Fei, G.; Xia, H.; Gorokhov, G.; Bychanok, D.; Kuzhir, P.; Lavorgna, M.; et al. On the Synergistic Effect of Multi-Walled Carbon Nanotubes and Graphene Nanoplatelets to Enhance the Functional Properties of SLS 3D-Printed Elastomeric Structures. *Polymers* **2020**, *12*, 1841. [CrossRef] [PubMed]
66. Ronca, A.; Rollo, G.; Cerruti, P.; Fei, G.; Gan, X.; Buonocore, G.G.; Lavorgna, M.; Xia, H.; Silvestre, C.; Ambrosio, L. Selective Laser Sintering Fabricated Thermoplastic Polyurethane/Graphene Cellular Structures with Tailorable Properties and High Strain Sensitivity. *Appl. Sci.* **2019**, *9*, 864. [CrossRef]
67. Abdelhamid, H.N.; Hussein, K.H. Graphene Oxide as a Carrier for Drug Delivery of Methotrexate. *Biointerface Res. Appl. Chem.* **2021**, *11*, 14726–14735.
68. Muazim, K.; Hussain, Z. Graphene Oxide—A Platform towards Theranostics. *Mater. Sci. Eng. C* **2017**, *76*, 1274–1288. [CrossRef]
69. Hussein, K.H.; Abdelhamid, H.N.; Zou, X.; Woo, H.-M. Ultrasonicated Graphene Oxide Enhances Bone and Skin Wound Regeneration. *Mater. Sci. Eng. C* **2019**, *94*, 484–492. [CrossRef]
70. Dowaidar, M.; Abdelhamid, H.N.; Hällbrink, M.; Zou, X.; Langel, Ü. Graphene Oxide Nanosheets in Complex with Cell Penetrating Peptides for Oligonucleotides Delivery. *Biochim. Biophys. Acta (BBA) Gen. Subj.* **2017**, *1861*, 2334–2341. [CrossRef]
71. Abdelhamid, H.N.; Khan, M.S.; Wu, H.-F. Graphene Oxide as a Nanocarrier for Gramicidin (GOGD) for High Antibacterial Performance. *RSC Adv.* **2014**, *4*, 50035–50046. [CrossRef]
72. Abdelhamid, H.N.; Wu, H.-F. Synthesis of a Highly Dispersive Sinapinic Acid@ Graphene Oxide (SA@ GO) and Its Applications as a Novel Surface Assisted Laser Desorption/Ionization Mass Spectrometry for Proteomics and Pathogenic Bacteria Biosensing. *Analyst* **2015**, *140*, 1555–1565. [CrossRef]

73. Ashour, R.M.; Abdelhamid, H.N.; Abdel-Magied, A.F.; Abdel-Khalek, A.A.; Ali, M.M.; Uheida, A.; Muhammed, M.; Zou, X.; Dutta, J. Rare Earth Ions Adsorption onto Graphene Oxide Nanosheets. *Solvent Extr. Ion Exch.* **2017**, *35*, 91–103. [CrossRef]
74. Lerf, A.; He, H.; Riedl, T.; Forster, M.; Klinowski, J. 13C and 1H MAS NMR Studies of Graphite Oxide and Its Chemically Modified Derivatives. *Solid State Ionics* **1997**, *101*, 857–862. [CrossRef]
75. Pei, S.; Cheng, H.-M. The Reduction of Graphene Oxide. *Carbon* **2012**, *50*, 3210–3228. [CrossRef]
76. Lerf, A.; He, H.; Forster, M.; Klinowski, J. Structure of Graphite Oxide Revisited. *J. Phys. Chem. B* **1998**, *102*, 4477–4482. [CrossRef]
77. He, H.; Klinowski, J.; Forster, M.; Lerf, A. A New Structural Model for Graphite Oxide. *Chem. Phys. Lett.* **1998**, *287*, 53–56. [CrossRef]
78. Schniepp, H.C.; Li, J.-L.; McAllister, M.J.; Sai, H.; Herrera-Alonso, M.; Adamson, D.H.; Prud'homme, R.K.; Car, R.; Saville, D.A.; Aksay, I.A. Functionalized Single Graphene Sheets Derived from Splitting Graphite Oxide. *J. Phys. Chem. B* **2006**, *110*, 8535–8539. [CrossRef]
79. Mkhoyan, K.A.; Contryman, A.W.; Silcox, J.; Stewart, D.A.; Eda, G.; Mattevi, C.; Miller, S.; Chhowalla, M. Atomic and Electronic Structure of Graphene-Oxide. *Nano Lett.* **2009**, *9*, 1058–1063. [CrossRef] [PubMed]
80. Pandey, D.; Reifenberger, R.; Piner, R. Scanning Probe Microscopy Study of Exfoliated Oxidized Graphene Sheets. *Surf. Sci.* **2008**, *602*, 1607–1613. [CrossRef]
81. Tang, H.; Liu, D.; Zhao, Y.; Yang, X.; Lu, J.; Cui, F. Molecular Dynamics Study of the Aggregation Process of Graphene Oxide in Water. *J. Phys. Chem. C* **2015**, *119*, 26712–26718. [CrossRef]
82. Chen, J.; Chen, L.; Wang, Y.; Chen, S. Molecular Dynamics Simulations of the Adsorption of DNA Segments onto Graphene Oxide. *J. Phys. D Appl. Phys.* **2014**, *47*, 505401. [CrossRef]
83. Baweja, L.; Balamurugan, K.; Subramanian, V.; Dhawan, A. Hydration Patterns of Graphene-Based Nanomaterials (GBNMs) Play a Major Role in the Stability of a Helical Protein: A Molecular Dynamics Simulation Study. *Langmuir* **2013**, *29*, 14230–14238. [CrossRef]
84. Sun, X.; Feng, Z.; Hou, T.; Li, Y. Mechanism of Graphene Oxide as an Enzyme Inhibitor from Molecular Dynamics Simulations. *ACS Appl. Mater. Interfaces* **2014**, *6*, 7153–7163. [CrossRef]
85. Chen, J.; Zhou, G.; Chen, L.; Wang, Y.; Wang, X.; Zeng, S. Interaction of Graphene and Its Oxide with Lipid Membrane: A Molecular Dynamics Simulation Study. *J. Phys. Chem. C* **2016**, *120*, 6225–6231. [CrossRef]
86. Shih, C.-J.; Lin, S.; Sharma, R.; Strano, M.S.; Blankschtein, D. Understanding the PH-Dependent Behavior of Graphene Oxide Aqueous Solutions: A Comparative Experimental and Molecular Dynamics Simulation Study. *Langmuir* **2012**, *28*, 235–241. [CrossRef]
87. Borthakur, P.; Boruah, P.K.; Hussain, N.; Sharma, B.; Das, M.R.; Matić, S.; Reha, D.; Minofar, B. Experimental and Molecular Dynamics Simulation Study of Specific Ion Effect on the Graphene Oxide Surface and Investigation of the Influence on Reactive Extraction of Model Dye Molecule at Water–Organic Interface. *J. Phys. Chem. C* **2016**, *120*, 14088–14100. [CrossRef]
88. Brodie, B.C. XIII. On the Atomic Weight of Graphite. *Philos. Trans. R. Soc. London* **1859**, *149*, 249–259.
89. Staudenmaier, L. Verfahren Zur Darstellung Der Graphitsäure. *Berichte der Dtsch. Chem. Gesellschaft* **1898**, *31*, 1481–1487. [CrossRef]
90. Hummers Jr, W.S.; Offeman, R.E. Preparation of Graphitic Oxide. *J. Am. Chem. Soc.* **1958**, *80*, 1339. [CrossRef]
91. Somanathan, T.; Prasad, K.; Ostrikov, K.; Saravanan, A.; Mohana Krishna, V. Graphene Oxide Synthesis from Agro Waste. *Nanomaterials* **2015**, *5*, 826–834. [CrossRef]
92. Faiz, M.S.A.; Azurahanim, C.A.C.; Yazid, Y.; Suriani, A.B.; Ain, M.J.S.N. Preparation and Characterization of Graphene Oxide from Tea Waste and It's Photocatalytic Application of TiO2/Graphene Nanocomposite. *Mater. Res. Express* **2020**, *7*, 15613. [CrossRef]
93. Sujiono, E.H.; Zabrian, D.; Dahlan, M.Y.; Amin, B.D.; Agus, J. Graphene Oxide Based Coconut Shell Waste: Synthesis by Modified Hummers Method and Characterization. *Heliyon* **2020**, *6*, e04568. [CrossRef]
94. Bonnia, N.N.; Zanuri, A.Z.; Asli, N.A.; Masdar, N.A.; Ratim, S.; Yahaya, S.M.; Mahat, M.M.; Ramli, R. Synthesis of Graphene Oxide from Waste Carbon Tyre Using Modified Hummer's Method. *Int. J. Eng. Technol* **2018**, *7*, 352–355. [CrossRef]
95. Tian, Z.; Cao, K.; Bai, S.; He, G.; Li, J. One-Pot Transformation of Waste Toner Powder into 3D Graphene Oxide Hydrogel. *ACS Sustain. Chem. Eng.* **2018**, *7*, 496–501. [CrossRef]
96. Siaw, W.C.; Tsuji, T.; Manaf, N.A.; Patah, M.F.A.; Jan, B.M. Synthesis of Graphene Oxide from Industrial Waste. *IOP Conf. Ser. Mater. Sci. Eng.* **2020**, *778*, 12050. [CrossRef]
97. Ghosal, K.; Sarkar, K. Biomedical Applications of Graphene Nanomaterials and Beyond. *ACS Biomater. Sci. Eng.* **2018**, *4*, 2653–2703. [CrossRef] [PubMed]
98. Silhavy, T.J.; Kahne, D.; Walker, S. The Bacterial Cell Envelope. *Cold Spring Harb. Perspect. Biol.* **2010**, *2*, a000414. [CrossRef] [PubMed]
99. Yaragalla, S.; Bhavitha, K.B.; Athanassiou, A. A Review on Graphene Based Materials and Their Antimicrobial Properties. *Coatings* **2021**, *11*, 1197. [CrossRef]
100. Pulingam, T.; Thong, K.L.; Ali, M.E.; Appaturi, J.N.; Dinshaw, I.J.; Ong, Z.Y.; Leo, B.F. Graphene Oxide Exhibits Differential Mechanistic Action towards Gram-Positive and Gram-Negative Bacteria. *Colloids Surf. B Biointerfaces* **2019**, *181*, 6–15. [CrossRef]
101. Deokar, A.R.; Lin, L.Y.; Chang, C.C.; Ling, Y.C. Single-Walled Carbon Nanotube Coated Antibacterial Paper: Preparation and Mechanistic Study. *J. Mater. Chem. B* **2013**, *1*, 2639–2646. [CrossRef]

102. Zou, X.; Zhang, L.; Wang, Z.; Luo, Y. Mechanisms of the Antimicrobial Activities of Graphene Materials. *J. Am. Chem. Soc.* **2016**, *138*, 2064–2077. [CrossRef]
103. Romero-Vargas Castrillón, S.; Perreault, F.; De Faria, A.F.; Elimelech, M. Interaction of Graphene Oxide with Bacterial Cell Membranes: Insights from Force Spectroscopy. *Environ. Sci. Technol. Lett.* **2015**, *2*, 112–117. [CrossRef]
104. Mohammed, H.; Kumar, A.; Bekyarova, E.; Al-Hadeethi, Y.; Zhang, X.; Chen, M.; Ansari, M.S.; Cochis, A.; Rimondini, L. Antimicrobial Mechanisms and Effectiveness of Graphene and Graphene-Functionalized Biomaterials. A Scope Review. *Front. Bioeng. Biotechnol.* **2020**, *8*, 465. [CrossRef] [PubMed]
105. Chen, Y.; Pandit, S.; Rahimi, S.; Mijakovic, I. Interactions Between Graphene-Based Materials and Biological Surfaces: A Review of Underlying Molecular Mechanisms. *Adv. Mater. Interfaces* **2021**, *8*, 2101132. [CrossRef]
106. Liu, S.; Zeng, T.H.; Hofmann, M.; Burcombe, E.; Wei, J.; Jiang, R.; Kong, J.; Chen, Y. Antibacterial Activity of Graphite, Graphite Oxide, Graphene Oxide, and Reduced Graphene Oxide: Membrane and Oxidative Stress. *ACS Nano* **2011**, *5*, 6971–6980. [CrossRef]
107. Thakur, V.; Kutty, R.V. Recent Advances in Nanotheranostics for Triple Negative Breast Cancer Treatment. *J. Exp. Clin. Cancer Res.* **2019**, *38*, 430. [CrossRef]
108. Yi, X.; Gao, H. Cell Interaction with Graphene Microsheets Near-Orthogonal Cutting versus Parallel Attachment. *Nanoscale* **2015**, *7*, 5457–5467. [CrossRef]
109. Wang, J.; Wei, Y.; Shi, X.; Gao, H. Cellular Entry of Graphene Nanosheets: The Role of Thickness, Oxidation and Surface Adsorption. *RSC Adv.* **2013**, *3*, 15776–15782. [CrossRef]
110. Pham, V.T.H.; Truong, V.K.; Quinn, M.D.J.; Notley, S.M.; Guo, Y.; Baulin, V.A.; Al Kobaisi, M.; Crawford, R.J.; Ivanova, E.P. Graphene Induces Formation of Pores That Kill Spherical and Rod-Shaped Bacteria. *ACS Nano* **2015**, *9*, 8458–8467. [CrossRef]
111. Liu, S.; Hu, M.; Zeng, T.H.; Wu, R.; Jiang, R.; Wei, J.; Wang, L.; Kong, J.; Chen, Y. Lateral Dimension-Dependent Antibacterial Activity of Graphene Oxide Sheets. *Langmuir* **2012**, *28*, 12364–12372. [CrossRef]
112. Chen, J.; Peng, H.; Wang, X.; Shao, F.; Yuan, Z.; Han, H. Graphene Oxide Exhibits Broad-Spectrum Antimicrobial Activity against Bacterial Phytopathogens and Fungal Conidia by Intertwining and Membrane Perturbation. *Nanoscale* **2014**, *6*, 1879–1889. [CrossRef]
113. Chen, J.; Wang, X.; Han, H. A New Function of Graphene Oxide Emerges: Inactivating Phytopathogenic Bacterium Xanthomonas Oryzae Pv. Oryzae. *J. Nanoparticle Res.* **2013**, *15*, 1658. [CrossRef]
114. Gurunathan, S.; Han, J.W.; Abdal Dayem, A.; Eppakayala, V.; Kim, J.H. Oxidative Stress-Mediated Antibacterial Activity of Graphene Oxide and Reduced Graphene Oxide in Pseudomonas Aeruginosa. *Int. J. Nanomed.* **2012**, *7*, 5901. [CrossRef]
115. Gurunathan, S.; Han, J.W.; Dayem, A.A.; Eppakayala, V.; Park, M.R.; Kwon, D.N.; Kim, J.H. Antibacterial Activity of Dithiothreitol Reduced Graphene Oxide. *J. Ind. Eng. Chem.* **2013**, *19*, 1280–1288. [CrossRef]
116. Krishnamoorthy, K.; Veerapandian, M.; Zhang, L.H.; Yun, K.; Kim, S.J. Antibacterial Efficiency of Graphene Nanosheets against Pathogenic Bacteria via Lipid Peroxidation. *J. Phys. Chem. C* **2012**, *116*, 17280–17287. [CrossRef]
117. Perreault, F.; De Faria, A.F.; Nejati, S.; Elimelech, M. Antimicrobial Properties of Graphene Oxide Nanosheets: Why Size Matters. *ACS Nano* **2015**, *9*, 7226–7236. [CrossRef] [PubMed]
118. Li, J.; Wang, G.; Zhu, H.; Zhang, M.; Zheng, X.; Di, Z.; Liu, X.; Wang, X. Antibacterial Activity of Large-Area Monolayer Graphene Film Manipulated by Charge Transfer. *Sci. Rep.* **2014**, *4*, 4359. [CrossRef]
119. Rajabi, M.; Mousa, S.A. The Role of Angiogenesis in Cancer Treatment. *Biomedicines* **2017**, *5*, 34. [CrossRef]
120. Vimalraj, S.; Pichu, S.; Pankajam, T.; Dharanibalan, K.; Djonov, V.; Chatterjee, S. Nitric Oxide Regulates Intussusceptive-like Angiogenesis in Wound Repair in Chicken Embryo and Transgenic Zebrafish Models. *Nitric Oxide* **2019**, *82*, 48–58. [CrossRef]
121. Honnegowda, T.M.; Kumar, P.; Udupa, E.G.P.; Kumar, S.; Kumar, U.; Rao, P. Role of Angiogenesis and Angiogenic Factors in Acute and Chronic Wound Healing. *Plast. Aesthetic Res.* **2015**, *2*, 243–249.
122. Dunnill, C.; Patton, T.; Brennan, J.; Barrett, J.; Dryden, M.; Cooke, J.; Leaper, D.; Georgopoulos, N.T. Reactive Oxygen Species (ROS) and Wound Healing: The Functional Role of ROS and Emerging ROS-Modulating Technologies for Augmentation of the Healing Process. *Int. Wound J.* **2017**, *14*, 89–96. [CrossRef]
123. Yong, J.M.; Fu, L.; Tang, F.; Yu, P.; Kuchel, R.P.; Whitelock, J.M.; Lord, M.S. ROS-Mediated Anti-Angiogenic Activity of Cerium Oxide Nanoparticles in Melanoma Cells. *ACS Biomater. Sci. Eng.* **2022**, *8*, 512–525. [CrossRef]
124. Galadari, S.; Rahman, A.; Pallichankandy, S.; Thayyullathil, F. Reactive Oxygen Species and Cancer Paradox: To Promote or to Suppress? *Free Radic. Biol. Med.* **2017**, *104*, 144–164. [CrossRef]
125. Breton-Romero, R.; Lamas, S. Hydrogen Peroxide Signaling in Vascular Endothelial Cells. *Redox Biol.* **2014**, *2*, 529–534. [CrossRef]
126. Yi, J.; Choe, G.; Park, J.; Lee, J.Y. Graphene Oxide-Incorporated Hydrogels for Biomedical Applications. *Polym. J.* **2020**, *52*, 823–837. [CrossRef]
127. Wei, P.; Wang, L.; Xie, F.; Cai, J. Strong and Tough Cellulose—Graphene Oxide Composite Hydrogels by Multi-Modulus Components Strategy as Photothermal Antibacterial Platform. *Chem. Eng. J.* **2022**, *431*, 133964. [CrossRef]
128. Ali, N.H.; Amin, M.C.I.M.; Ng, S.-F. Sodium Carboxymethyl Cellulose Hydrogels Containing Reduced Graphene Oxide (RGO) as a Functional Antibiofilm Wound Dressing. *J. Biomater. Sci. Polym. Ed.* **2019**, *30*, 629–645. [CrossRef]
129. Soliman, M.; Sadek, A.A.; Abdelhamid, H.N.; Hussein, K. Graphene Oxide-Cellulose Nanocomposite Accelerates Skin Wound Healing. *Res. Vet. Sci.* **2021**, *137*, 262–273. [CrossRef]

130. Wang, Y.; Shi, L.; Wu, H.; Li, Q.; Hu, W.; Zhang, Z.; Huang, L.; Zhang, J.; Chen, D.; Deng, S.; et al. Graphene Oxide—IPDI—Ag/ZnO@ Hydroxypropyl Cellulose Nanocomposite Films for Biological Wound-Dressing Applications. *ACS Omega* **2019**, *4*, 15373–15381. [CrossRef]
131. Prakash, J.; Venkataprasanna, K.S.; Bharath, G.; Banat, F.; Niranjan, R.; Venkatasubbu, G.D. In-Vitro Evaluation of Electrospun Cellulose Acetate Nanofiber Containing Graphene Oxide/TiO2/Curcumin for Wound Healing Application. *Colloids Surf. A Physicochem. Eng. Asp.* **2021**, *627*, 127166. [CrossRef]
132. Purnamasari, W.; Budiastanti, T.A.; Aminatun, A.; Rahmah, U.; Sumarsih, S.; Chang, J.-Y.; Fahmi, M.Z. Naproxen Release Behaviour from Graphene Oxide/Cellulose Acetate Composite Nanofibers. *RSC Adv.* **2022**, *12*, 8019–8029. [CrossRef]
133. Hashem, A.H.; Hasanin, M.; Kamel, S.; Dacrory, S. A New Approach for Antimicrobial and Antiviral Activities of Biocompatible Nanocomposite Based on Cellulose, Amino Acid and Graphene Oxide. *Colloids Surf. B Biointerfaces* **2022**, *209*, 112172. [CrossRef]
134. Chakraborty, S.; Ponrasu, T.; Chandel, S.; Dixit, M.; Muthuvijayan, V. Reduced Graphene Oxide-Loaded Nanocomposite Scaffolds for Enhancing Angiogenesis in Tissue Engineering Applications. *R. Soc. Open Sci.* **2018**, *5*, 172017. [CrossRef]
135. Esmaeili, E.; Eslami-Arshaghi, T.; Hosseinzadeh, S.; Elahirad, E.; Jamalpoor, Z.; Hatamie, S.; Soleimani, M. The Biomedical Potential of Cellulose Acetate/Polyurethane Nanofibrous Mats Containing Reduced Graphene Oxide/Silver Nanocomposites and Curcumin: Antimicrobial Performance and Cutaneous Wound Healing. *Int. J. Biol. Macromol.* **2020**, *152*, 418–427. [CrossRef]
136. Li, X.-X.; Dong, J.-Y.; Li, Y.-H.; Zhong, J.; Yu, H.; Yu, Q.-Q.; Lei, M. Fabrication of Ag—ZnO@ Carboxymethyl Cellulose/K-Carrageenan/Graphene Oxide/Konjac Glucomannan Hydrogel for Effective Wound Dressing in Nursing Care for Diabetic Foot Ulcers. *Appl. Nanosci.* **2020**, *10*, 729–738. [CrossRef]
137. Liu, Y.; Morishima, T.; Yatsui, T.; Kawazoe, T.; Ohtsu, M. Size Control of Sol–Gel-Synthesized ZnO Quantum Dots Using Photo-Induced Desorption. *Nanotechnology* **2011**, *22*, 215605. [CrossRef]
138. Liu, Y.; Kim, H.-I. Characterization and Antibacterial Properties of Genipin-Crosslinked Chitosan/Poly (Ethylene Glycol)/ZnO/Ag Nanocomposites. *Carbohydr. Polym.* **2012**, *89*, 111–116. [CrossRef]
139. Li, Z.; Zhang, F.; Meng, A.; Xie, C.; Xing, J. ZnO/Ag Micro/Nanospheres with Enhanced Photocatalytic and Antibacterial Properties Synthesized by a Novel Continuous Synthesis Method. *RSC Adv.* **2015**, *5*, 612–620. [CrossRef]
140. Ahmad, S.A.; Das, S.S.; Khatoon, A.; Ansari, M.T.; Afzal, M.; Hasnain, M.S.; Nayak, A.K. Bactericidal Activity of Silver Nanoparticles: A Mechanistic Review. *Mater. Sci. Energy Technol.* **2020**, *3*, 756–769. [CrossRef]
141. Matharu, R.K.; Tabish, T.A.; Trakoolwilaiwan, T.; Mansfield, J.; Moger, J.; Wu, T.; Lourenço, C.; Chen, B.; Ciric, L.; Parkin, I.P.; et al. Microstructure and Antibacterial Efficacy of Graphene Oxide Nanocomposite Fibres. *J. Colloid Interface Sci.* **2020**, *571*, 239–252. [CrossRef]
142. Shome, S.; Talukdar, A.D.; Upadhyaya, H. Antibacterial Activity of Curcumin and Its Essential Nanoformulations against Some Clinically Important Bacterial Pathogens: A Comprehensive Review. *Biotechnol. Appl. Biochem.* **2021**, *69*, 2357–2386. [CrossRef]
143. Rai, D.; Singh, J.K.; Roy, N.; Panda, D. Curcumin Inhibits FtsZ Assembly: An Attractive Mechanism for Its Antibacterial Activity. *Biochem. J.* **2008**, *410*, 147–155. [CrossRef]
144. Heil, M.; Eitenmüller, I.; Schmitz-Rixen, T.; Schaper, W. Arteriogenesis versus Angiogenesis: Similarities and Differences. *J. Cell. Mol. Med.* **2006**, *10*, 45–55. [CrossRef] [PubMed]
145. Mukherjee, S.; Sriram, P.; Barui, A.K.; Nethi, S.K.; Veeriah, V.; Chatterjee, S.; Suresh, K.I.; Patra, C.R. Graphene Oxides Show Angiogenic Properties. *Adv. Healthc. Mater.* **2015**, *4*, 1722–1732. [CrossRef] [PubMed]
146. Xie, Y.-Y.; Hu, X.-H.; Zhang, Y.-W.; Wahid, F.; Chu, L.-Q.; Jia, S.-R.; Zhong, C. Development and Antibacterial Activities of Bacterial Cellulose/Graphene Oxide-CuO Nanocomposite Films. *Carbohydr. Polym.* **2020**, *229*, 115456. [CrossRef] [PubMed]
147. Zhang, L.; Yu, Y.; Zheng, S.; Zhong, L.; Xue, J. Preparation and Properties of Conductive Bacterial Cellulose-Based Graphene Oxide-Silver Nanoparticles Antibacterial Dressing. *Carbohydr. Polym.* **2021**, *257*, 117671. [CrossRef] [PubMed]
148. Zmejkoski, D.Z.; Marković, Z.M.; Mitić, D.D.; Zdravković, N.M.; Kozyrovska, N.O.; Bugárová, N.; Todorović Marković, B.M. Antibacterial Composite Hydrogels of Graphene Quantum Dots and Bacterial Cellulose Accelerate Wound Healing. *J. Biomed. Mater. Res. Part B Appl. Biomater.* **2022**, *110*, 1796–1805. [CrossRef] [PubMed]

pharmaceutics

MDPI

Article

Investigating the Targeting Power to Brain Tissues of Intranasal Rasagiline Mesylate-Loaded Transferosomal In Situ Gel for Efficient Treatment of Parkinson's Disease

Hala N. ElShagea [1], Rana R. Makar [1], Alaa H. Salama [1,2], Nermeen A. Elkasabgy [3,*] and Emad B. Basalious [3]

1 Department of Pharmaceutics and Industrial Pharmacy, Faculty of Pharmacy, Ahram Canadian University, 6th of October City, Cairo 12451, Egypt
2 Pharmaceutical Technology Department, National Research Centre, Dokki, Cairo 12622, Egypt
3 Department of Pharmaceutics and Industrial Pharmacy, Faculty of Pharmacy, Cairo University, Kasr El-Aini Street, Cairo 11562, Egypt
* Correspondence: nermeen.ahmed.elkasabgy@pharma.cu.edu.eg

Abstract: Rasagiline mesylate (RSM) is a hydrophilic drug with poor oral bioavailability (36%) because of hepatic first-pass metabolism. The present study focuses on delivering RSM directly to the brain through its inclusion within transferosomal in situ gel administered through the intranasal (IN) route. Transferosomes were formed by the thin-film hydration method with the aid of Design-Expert® software by varying the edge activator (EA) type in the absence or presence of cholesterol. By desirability calculations, the optimum formulation was composed of phosphatidylcholine and sodium deoxycholate as an EA (5:1% *w/w*) with no cholesterol. The optimum formulation was 198.63 ± 34.98 nm in size and displayed an entrapment efficiency of 95.73 ± 0.09%. Transmission electron microscopy revealed discrete and spherical vesicles. Optimized transferosomes were further incorporated into an in situ gel composed of 0.5% pectin, 15% Pluronic® F-127, and 5% Pluronic® F-68 and tested for the in vivo performance. The systemic as well as brain kinetics were assessed in rats by comparing the IN-administered in situ gel to the IV aqueous solution. The optimum in situ gel showed safety and biocompatibility on rats' nasal mucosa with enhanced brain bioavailability (131.17%). Drug targeting efficiency and direct transport percentage indices (304.53% and 67.16%, respectively) supported successful brain targeting offering direct nose-to-brain drug delivery.

Keywords: drug delivery; nanotechnology; mucoadhesion; nose-to-brain delivery; brain kinetics

1. Introduction

Parkinson's disease is a progressive neurological disorder in which the neurons of the substantia nigra pars compacta and the nigrostriatal tract are degenerated [1]. Additionally, it is accompanied by a decrease in dopamine levels in the striatum, which causes motor dysfunction [2]. It targets about 2% of people over the age of 60 years [3]. It is thought that genetic and environmental factors play a significant role in the onset and progression of Parkinson's disease [4]. Tremors, spasms, muscle rigidity, bradykinesia, hypersensitivity, abnormal posture, and movement are among the specific motor symptoms caused by the dopaminergic neurons loss, which can affect patients' quality of life [5]. Parkinson's disease leads to a decline in life expectancy based on the severity of motor impairment. So, in order to reduce the mortality rate, several approaches are used, including effective therapy and deep brain stimulation [6].

Rasagiline mesylate (RSM) is a second-generation monoamine oxidase inhibitor [7,8]. Unlike selegiline (the first monoamine oxidase inhibitor used for Parkinson's disease treatment), RSM does not produce amphetamine-like metabolites and is not accompanied by the neurotoxic side effects caused by these metabolites [9]. However, RSM produces a neuroprotective metabolite called L-aminoindane, which in turn leads to a lower recommended therapeutic daily dose [10]. RSM was introduced into the market as oral tablets

(Azilect®) with a single daily recommended dose of 1 mg [11]. RSM possesses reduced oral bioavailability (36%) because of the extensive first-pass metabolism [12], which affects its therapeutic efficacy. Thus, altering the route of administration is one of the promising solutions to boost the drug bioavailability and efficacy.

The intranasal (IN) route of administration is considered a non-invasive path to deliver the drug directly to the central nervous system [13]. The IN route is characterized with the ease of self-administration, which in turn enhances patient compliance [14]. Additionally, it allows the direct access of the drug to the brain, bypassing the hepatic first-pass metabolism that occurs upon the conventional oral administration. Intranasally administered drugs can escape the blood–brain barrier (BBB) that limits drug transportation to the brain, leading to a significant enhancement in drug bioavailability [15–17]. Direct nose-to-brain targeting can occur through trigeminal and olfactory pathways that are found in the nasal cavity, thus reaching the brain in sufficient concentrations [18].

However, the limiting factors for IN absorption in general are the reduced capacity of the nasal cavity and rapid mucociliary clearance [19]. Hence, the use of mucoadhesive agents with or without the addition of permeation enhancers can be adopted for extending the mucociliary residence time, which in turn enhances drug absorption and bioavailability. This enhancement in drug bioavailability is mainly linked to the increased residence time in the nasal cavity [20]. In case of delivering hydrophilic drugs, another limiting factor for IN absorption is added, which is the low permeability of hydrophilic molecules [21]. This can be addressed by rendering the drug more lipophilic through the inclusion of lipophilic vesicles, which can boost the IN permeability of the hydrophilic drugs [22]. In conclusion, formulating an IN-administered formulation loaded with a hydrophilic drug with enhanced drug bioavailability is considered a challenge.

Several approaches were adopted in order to reduce the mucociliary clearance and increase the nasal residence time. Among these approaches is the preparation of in situ-forming gels [23], where the drug is administered in solution form and transforms into gel in response to some endogenous stimuli, such as the increase in temperature or pH, or the presence of ions [24,25]. Combining in situ-forming gel polymers with mucoadhesive polymers results in a greater effectiveness and higher efficiency through the prolongation of the residence time at the administration site, which in turn enhances the drug bioavailability [26–29]. An optimum concentrations selection of the used polymers is based on the sol-to-gel transition temperatures and gelation time [30]. Sherje et al. was able to formulate cyclodextrin-based in situ gel (pH-responsive) of paliperidone using different polymers, such as Carbopol 934 and hydroxypropyl methyl cellulose K4M, which were capable of transforming into gel at 34 °C after 2.1 ± 0.1 min, where the gelation time was sufficient to resist the rapid mucociliary clearance [31]. On the other hand, Liu et al. succeeded in the preparation of Pluronic-based in situ hydrogels for vaginal application of nonoxinol-9 using 18% Pluronic® F-127 and 6% Pluronic® F-68, which transformed into gel in the temperature range of 28.5–31.5 °C [32].

Nanosized drug delivery systems may also be adopted to enhance drug permeability across biological membranes due to the small particle size and large surface-area-to-mass ratio of the formed particles, which in turn improve the therapeutic efficacy [33,34]. This is in addition to their capability of carrying both hydrophilic and lipophilic drugs, making them available for various routes of administration [35]. Transferosomes are liposome-derived nanovesicles that have an ultra-flexible nature owing to the incorporation of edge activators (EA). Transferosomes have the ability to squeeze through the nasal mucosa due to their elastic nature [36]. EA are single-chain surfactants that increase the deformability of the formed vesicles through destabilization of the lipid bilayers, resulting in a higher capability to cross the biological membranes [37]. In addition to their general advantages as a nanocarrier, transferosomes are considered superior drug carriers for IN delivery as they were reported to enhance membrane permeability and decrease mucociliary clearance, as well as reduce nasal peptidase degradation, which in turn led to the enhanced drug bioavailability of IN-administered drugs [38].

The literature includes some studies addressing the direct delivery of the RSM to the brain via the IN route. One study discussed the preparation of RSM-loaded solid lipid nanoparticles by conducting a modified microemulsion method. The selected formulation possessed an entrapment efficiency value of 37.8%. The selected formulation was further incorporated into a thermosensitive mucoadhesive gel prepared using Pluronic® F-127 and hydroxypropyl methylcellulose E5. Ex vivo permeation studies showed the superiority of the solid lipid nanoparticles-loaded in situ gel over the drug suspension and free drug-loaded in situ gel. However, this study lacked the investigation of the in vivo behavior on an animal model [39]. Another study discussed the preparation of RSM-loaded deformable ethosomes. The prepared ethosomes possessed an entrapment efficiency value of 38%. The authors indicated the success of the prepared ethosomes to permeate through the nasal mucosa. Nonetheless, the study lacked the pre-clinical investigations of the proposed formulation [40]. From the previous studies, we observed that the obtained entrapment efficiency values were less than 40%, which is considered a low value and is accredited to the drug's aqueous nature [41]. On the other hand, the present study succeeded in enhancing the proportion of the entrapped drug in the prepared transferosomes to values exceeding 95%, which was considered challenging when incorporating a hydrophilic drug in lipid-based vesicles. For the authors' information, this is considered the first study discussing the loading of RSM in transferosomes intended for brain delivery through the intranasal route. Moreover, the current study avoided the use of harmful organic solvents, such as chloroform, and presented the preparation of the transferosomal formulation using ethanol. Moreover, this research is considered a comprehensive study that combines an in vitro characterization of the delivery system and in vivo investigation into an animal model (rats) to determine the efficacy of brain targeting.

This study aimed at exploring the pairing of the used lipid component (phosphatidylcholine) and EA for the formulation of RSM-loaded transferosomes. Following this, the selection of the most suitable combination of thermosensitive and mucoadhesive polymers for the preparation of an in situ gel to be later loaded with the optimum transferosomal formulation was performed. The transferosomal formulation and the loaded in situ gel are characterized for choosing the best formulation. The ability of the formed in situ gel to form gel at physiological temperature, its rheological properties, and in vitro drug release were assessed. Finally, the therapeutic efficacy of the optimum in situ gel transferosomal formulation was evaluated in vivo using Wistar Albino rats for assessing brain kinetics in addition to brain-targeting indices to ensure nose-to-brain drug targeting in sufficient concentrations.

2. Materials and Methods

2.1. Materials

Rasagiline mesylate (RSM) was kindly gifted by Marcyrl Pharmaceutical Industries (Cairo, Egypt). Phosphatidylcholine from egg yolk was obtained from Fisher Scientific (Hampton, NH, USA). Absolute ethanol, Span® 60, sodium cholate, sodium deoxycholate, Pluronics (F-68, L-31, L-35), and cholesterol were procured from Sigma-Aldrich (St. Louis, MO, USA). Potassium dihydrogen phosphate and disodium hydrogen phosphate were provided by El-Nasr Pharmaceutical Chemicals Company (Cairo, Egypt). Dialysis bag with cutoff 12–14 KDa with flat width of 25 mm was obtained from FREY scientific, Nashua, NH, USA, as well as calcium ammonium nitrate, ammonium formate, and ethyl acetate (LC-MS grade). All other chemicals were of reagent grade and used as received.

2.2. Methodology

2.2.1. Preparation of RSM-Loaded Transferosomes

RSM-loaded transferosomes were prepared by thin-film hydration technique to enhance the drug incorporation in the transferosomal vesicles [42]. In a round-bottom flask, 33.33 mg edge activator (EA), 166.66 mg phosphatidylcholine, and cholesterol, if present, were mixed and dissolved together with 10 mg RSM in 15 mL ethanol. Evaporation of the organic solvent was carried out under vacuum at 50 °C using rotary evaporator (Heidolph VV 2000, Burladingen, Germany) at rotation speed 90 rpm until a thin film was deposited on the inner wall of the round-bottom flask. The formed film was then hydrated with 10 mL phosphate-buffered saline (PBS; pH 7.4) under normal pressure and temperature 50 °C. Following, the obtained dispersions were sonicated (Elmasonic S30H, Singen, Germany) for 2 min to ensure that the formed dispersions were free from any aggregates and then stored overnight at 4 °C. Different transferosomal formulations were prepared by altering the type of EA in presence and absence of cholesterol according to a mixed factorial design ($6^1.2^1$) (Table 1). Blank transferosomes were prepared concurrently using the same weights but without the addition of drug to eliminate any interactions from the used ingredients [43].

The construction and analysis of the adopted experimental design were performed using Design-Expert® software (Stat-Ease, Inc., Minneapolis, MN, USA) so as to ascertain the impact of various variables on the characteristics of the formulated RSM-loaded transferosomes. The desirability function was used in order to determine the optimum preparation condition. The independent variables were the type of EA (sodium cholate, sodium deoxycholate, Pluronic® F-68, Pluronic® L-35, Pluronic® L-31, and Span® 60) [X1] with the presence/absence of cholesterol [X2]. On the other hand, the dependent variables were VS [Y1], ZP [Y2], and %EE [Y3]. In order to determine the optimized formulation, Y1 had to be minimized, while Y2 and Y3 had to be maximized. The formulation with the highest desirability was considered as the optimum formulation and selected for further study. The composition of the prepared transferosomal formulations is clarified in Table 2.

Table 1. Mixed factorial design for the optimization of RSM-loaded transferosomal formulations.

Independent Variables	**Levels**	
X1:Type of EA	Sodium cholate, sodium deoxycholate, Pluronic® F-68, Pluronic® L-35, Pluronic® L-31, and Span® 60	
X2:Cholesterol	Absent	Present
Dependent variables	Desirability Constraint	
Y1:VS	Minimize	
Y2:ZP	Maximize	
Y3:%EE	Maximize	

Abbreviations: EA, edge activator; VS, vesicle size; ZP, zeta potential; EE, entrapment efficiency.

Table 2. Composition and characterization of RSM-loaded transferosomal formulations.

Formulation Code	**Factor 1 X1:EA Type**	**Factor 2 X2:Cholesterol**	**Response 1 Y1:VS (nm)**	**Response 2 Y2:ZP (mV)**	**Response 3 Y3:EE%**
F1	Span® 60	Present	491.40 ± 48.79	−32.60 ± 4.94	43.25 ± 5.02
F2	Pluronic® F-68	Present	347.26 ± 56.66	−29.65 ± 0.49	52.33 ± 3.53
F3	Sodium cholate	Present	283.30 ± 8.62	−36.95 ± 1.06	54.80 ± 5.19
F4	Pluronic® L-35	Present	391.95 ± 56.17	−39.60 ± 6.36	51.73 ± 5.46
F5	Pluronic® L-31	Present	387.95 ± 52.82	−30.50 ± 1.27	48.51 ± 1.85
F6	Sodium deoxycholate	Present	248.56 ± 32.47	−35.45 ± 3.18	54.98 ± 6.52
F7	Span® 60	Absent	448.70 ± 14.84	−24.90 ± 1.13	50.68 ± 1.24
F8	Pluronic® F-68	Absent	227.51 ± 13.69	−26.25 ± 4.31	61.37 ± 0.53
F9	Sodium cholate	Absent	208.42 ± 11.95	−33.20 ± 0.28	69.40 ± 0.98
F10	Pluronic® L-35	Absent	276.00 ± 27.05	−29.20 ± 2.26	57.47 ± 2.65
F11	Pluronic® L-31	Absent	352.90 ± 15.41	−30.00 ± 0.42	55.45 ± 5.65
F12	Sodium deoxycholate	Absent	198.63 ± 34.98	−33.45 ± 4.73	95.73 ± 0.09

Abbreviations: EA, edge activator; VS, vesicle size; ZP, zeta potential; EE, entrapment efficiency. All values are represented as mean ± SD (n = 3).

2.2.2. Characterization of RSM-Loaded Transferosomes

Assessment of Vesicle Size (VS), Polydispersity Index (PDI), and Zeta Potential (ZP)

VS, PDI, and ZP are crucial parameters for the selection of the optimized transferosomal formulation, and they have an impact on the stability and quality of the formulated transferosomes. These parameters were measured using ZetaSizer Nano ZS (Malvern Instrument Ltd., Worcestershire, UK). Each of the prepared formulations was diluted with distilled water (1:10 v/v) until obtaining a faint opalescent appearance with suitable intensity for light scattering. The measurements were performed in duplicates, and the outcomes were expressed as mean ± SD.

Assessment of Entrapment Efficiency (%EE)

The incorporation of water-soluble drugs in transferosomes (lipid-rich vesicles) is one of the main challenges in the formulation of such vesicles. Assessment of %EE was carried out using the indirect method such that 1.5 mL of the prepared RSM-loaded transferosomal dispersions were ultra-centrifuged at 18,000 rpm at 4 °C for 1 h using a cooling centrifuge (Beckman, Fullerton, Canada). The supernatant was filtered through Millipore® filter (0.45 µm) and assessed spectrophotometrically at 271 nm for the determination of the amount of free RSM (unentrapped RSM) (Schimadzu spectrophotometer, model UV-1601 PC, Kyoto, Japan). The same procedures were carried out for the blank transferosomal dispersions to exclude any possible interferences [43]. The test was executed in duplicates, and the readings were stated as mean ± SD. The subsequent equation was utilized for calculating the %EE [43]:

$$\%EE = \frac{\text{Total amount of RSM} - \text{Free RSM}}{\text{Total amount of RSM}} \times 100 \quad (1)$$

2.2.3. Characterization of the Optimized Transferosomal Formulation

Fourier Transform Infrared Spectroscopy (FTIR)

FTIR spectrophotometer (IRspirit, Shimadzu, Kyoto, Japan) was used for the determination of any possible interactions between the different components of the optimized RSM-loaded transferosomal formulation. This process was carried out at ambient temperature by placing about 2–3 mg of each individual component, in addition to the freeze-dried formulation (F12), followed by scanning at the range of 4400–400 cm^{-1}. The samples were scanned with scanning number of 32 scans per sample at a resolution of 4 cm^{-1}. Freeze-drying process was carried out such that samples were placed in glass containers and frozen at −80 °C then transferred to the lyophilizer (Novalyphe-NL 500; Savant Instruments Corp, Holbrook, NY, USA). The process continued for 48 h at freezing temperature of −50 °C under vacuum pressure 0.001 mbar.

Transmission Electron Microscopy (TEM)

TEM was conducted for the detailed morphological examination of the optimized RSM-loaded transferosomal formulation by negative staining technique. One drop of the aqueous dispersion was added on carbon-coated copper grid, left to adhere for 1 min, then excess dispersion was removed with a filter paper. Following this, 1% phosphotungestic acid solution was added and left to dry with the sample at room temperature before being examined at 100 kV [44,45].

2.2.4. Preparation of RSM-Loaded Transferosomal In Situ Gels

The cold technique described by Zaki et al. [46] was followed for the preparation of in situ gel containing the optimized RSM-loaded transferosomal formulation. Different concentrations of the thermosensitive polymers, such as Pluronic® F-127 and Pluronic® F-68, in addition to the mucoadhesive pectin were used for the formulation of the in situ gel. Using a magnetic stirrer (Jenway, Staffordshire, England), 0.5% w/v of pectin was dispersed in 5 mL of the optimized transferosomal formulation, followed by the addition of a mixture of Pluronic® F-127 and Pluronic® F-68 in different concentrations with continuous stirring at 300 rpm [39]. The prepared dispersions were kept in the refrigerator overnight until clear solutions were obtained [26]. The composition of the formulated in situ gels is compiled in Table 3.

Table 3. Composition and sol-to-gel transition temperature of the formed in situ gels.

Gel Formulation Code	Composition			
	Pectin (% *w*/*v*)	Pluronic® F-127 (% *w*/*v*)	Pluronic® F-68 (% *w*/*v*)	Sol to Gel Temperature (°C)
G1	0.50	15	0	32.4 ± 0.56
G2	0.50	15	5	36.2 ± 0.28
G3	0.50	15	10	40.1 ± 1.69

2.2.5. Characterization of the Prepared RSM-Loaded Transferosomal In Situ Gels

Determination of Sol-to-Gel Transition Temperature and Gelation Time

The in situ gels were tested for their sol-to-gel transition temperature by placing 2 mL of each gel individually in a test tube, which was placed in a thermostatic water bath (oscillating thermostatically controlled shaker, GallenKamp, England), with each tube covered with Parafilm®. The temperature of the water bath was gradually raised from 25 °C to 37 °C in increments of 3 °C with a sufficient time (15 min) to equilibrate at each new temperature setting [47]. The sample gelation temperature was identified when the meniscus does not move by tilting the test tube with a 90° angle [48,49].

The sol-to-gel transition time was detected by the test tube inversion technique by transferring 1 mL of the formulated gels in a stoppered test tube and then placing the tubes in a thermostatically controlled water bath adjusted at 37 °C. The sol-to-gel transition time was estimated when the test tube was tilted every 10 s and no flow was noticed [50].

Assessment of Rheological Properties

Temperature sweep test was used for the assessment of temperature-dependent complex viscosity [51]. The rheological properties were assessed using viscoelastometer (Anton Paar, MCR301 SN80218500, Austria) with a parallel plate geometry (gap of 0.5 mm), a temperature control system (Peltier system), and Rheoplus/32 V3.40 software version (Anton Paar, Austria). This was carried out by placing the gel sample (5 mL) in a shearing jig and testing them at a frequency of 1 Hz and amplitude gamma of 1%. A gradual increase in temperature from 25 to 37 °C was made with an elevation rate of 2 °C/min [52]. Complex viscosity (*) was plotted against temperature (T) to detect the ability of the tested samples to transform into a gel at the physiological temperature, thus aiding in the choice of the optimum in situ gel formulation.

In Vitro Drug Release

Dialysis cellulose bag method was adopted for the assessment of drug release parameters. The in vitro drug release was carried out for the optimum RSM-loaded transferosomal formulation along with the formulated in situ gels loaded with the optimized transferosomal formulation. In brief, equivalent volumes of each sample (corresponding to 1 mg drug) were placed in a dialysis cellulose bag, which was pre-soaked overnight in distilled water. The packed cellulose bags were tightly secured from both ends to avoid any leakage. The secured bag was placed in a glass bottle pre-filled with 20 mL ethanolic PBS solution (10% *v*/*v*, pH 7.4) [53–55] then transferred to a thermostatically controlled shaker adjusted at 100 rpm at 37 °C ± 0.5 [56]. Aliquots (2 mL) of the release medium were withdrawn at different pre-determined time intervals (0.5, 1, 2, 3, 4, 5, 6, and 8 h) and instantly replaced by equal volume of freshly prepared release medium. The collected samples were then evaluated spectrophotometrically at λ_{max} 271 against blanks. The measured release parameters were the % drug released after 0.5 h ($Q_{0.5h}$) to assess the initial drug flush release, in addition to the % of drug released after 8 h (Q_{8h}) to ensure the sustainability of drug release upon incorporation in gel formulations. The same aforementioned procedure (without blank) was carried to assess the release of the pure drug from its dispersion for comparison purposes. The % of drug released was illustrated against time.

2.2.6. Effect of Storage

The effect of storage of the optimized RSM-loaded transferosomal formulation along with the respective optimum in situ gel containing the optimum transferosomal formulation was assessed at 4 ± 2 °C for three months [57,58]. At the end of the study period, evaluation of VS, PDI, ZP, and %EE was performed for the optimized transferosomal formulation in addition to the sol-to-gel transition temperature re-evaluation for the selected in situ gel containing the optimized RSM-loaded transferosomal formulation. In vitro drug release was performed for both the optimum transferosomal formulation as well as the optimum in situ gel formulation loaded with it. These procedures were held along with visual inspection for any physical changes, sedimentation, or aggregation [57]. The similarities between the release profiles of the freshly prepared optimum transferosomal formulation and the stored one, as well as, the optimized fresh in situ gel formulation and the stored gel, were calculated using the model-independent mathematical approach proposed by Moore and Flanner [59].

$$f_2 = 50.\log\left[\left\{1 + \left(\frac{1}{n}\right)\sum\nolimits_{t-1}^{n}(R_t - T_t)^2\right\}^{-0.5} \times 100\right] \qquad (2)$$

where n is the number of the samples withdrawn, and R and T are the percentage of RSM released from either the freshly prepared or stored formulation (F12), respectively, which is repeated for the freshly prepared and stored in situ gel formulation (G2) at time t [60,61].

2.2.7. In Vivo Studies

The in vivo animal studies were performed on male Wistar Albino rats weighing 200–250 g. Animal use was in agreement with the National Institutes of Health Guide for The Care and Use of Laboratory Animals (NIH, publication No.85–23, 1996). The study protocol was accepted by the institutional review board, Research Ethics Committee, Faculty of Pharmacy, Cairo University [PI (3043)]. The rats were housed in cages, with each containing six animals, at ambient temperature and pressure, with free entry of food and water, and a 12 h light and dark cycle.

Assessment of Formulation Biocompatibility

In order to assess the safety and the biocompatibility of the applied in situ gel formulation on the nasal epithelial cell membrane, histopathological evaluation was carried out after applying the optimum RSM-loaded transferosomal in situ gel (4 mg/kg) intranasally [62] to four male Wistar Albino rats. On the other hand, another four rats were used as control and did not receive the in situ gel. Four hours post application, the rats were mercy sacrificed, then the nasal epithelial cell membrane was dissected to be examined for any harmful effects [25,46]. Specimens were fixed in 10% neutral buffer formalin, then decalcified by 10% formic acid, trimmed, washed in water, dehydrated in ascending grade of ethyl alcohol, cleared in xylene, and lastly fixed in paraffin at 70 °C before being prepared in paraffin blocks. Thin sections (4–6 μm) were processed using microtome and stained with hematoxylin and eosin before being inspected by Olympus BX53 microscope [63].

In Vivo Pharmacokinetics

The study was performed so as to determine the pharmacokinetic parameters of the intranasally administered RSM-loaded transferosomal in situ gel (G2) compared with the intravenous (IV) RSM aqueous solution, which was administered to male Wistar Albino rats. A non-blind, one-period, randomized parallel design was applied. Sixty-six Wistar Albino rats were selected for the study. The animals were distributed over two equal groups; Group 1 received IV RSM aqueous solution and Group 2 received IN RSM-loaded transferosomal in situ gel (G2). The dose of RSM in both treatments was corresponding to 4 mg/kg drug [62]. The study was carried out over 12 h and the animals were visually examined along the study period to detect any behavioral disorder or illness. At time intervals 0 (pre-dose), 0.25, 0.5, 0.75, 1, 1.25, 1.5, 2, 4, 6, 8 and 12 h post administration of each treatment, three rats from each group were mercy sacrificed for the collection of respective plasma and brain samples. Blood samples were taken from the trunk of the sacrificed animals directly into heparinized tubes followed by centrifugation (Beckman, Fullerton, Canada) at 4000 rpm for 15 min at 25 °C to separate plasma [64], while brain tissue samples were collected by opening the sacrificed animal's skull, dissecting the brain, then removing any adhering tissues followed by homogenization with saline (three-fold its volume) using ultra Turrax homogenizer (T 25 digital ULTRA- TURRAX®, IKA, Germany) at 24,000 rpm for 1 min [65]. Both plasma and brain samples were maintained at −20 °C pending analysis.

Chromatographic Conditions

The assessment of RSM in plasma and brain tissues was carried out applying a sensitive, selective, and validated LC-MS/MS [66]. The internal standard used was clonazepam. The detector used was Triple Quarupole MS/MS (Waters Corp., Milford, MA, USA). Analyst 1.6.3 software version was utilized for data acquisition and integration. The used column was a reverse-phase column (C_{18}, 4.6 × 50 mm, 5 um, Waters Corp., Milford, MA, USA). The mobile phase was prepared by mixing calcium ammonium nitrate and 0.01 M ammonium formate in the ratio 4:1 (*v*/*v*). Isocratic chromatographic separation was carried out at 15 °C with a flow rate of 1 mL/min.

Sample Preparation

Liquid–liquid extraction was performed by adding 0.5 mL of either plasma or homogenized brain samples to 4 mL ethyl acetate and vortexing for 30 s, then centrifuging at 3000 rpm at 4 °C for 15 min. The organic layer was evaporated until dryness under a gentle nitrogen stream at 40 °C (Vacufuge 5301, Eppendorf, Hamburg, Germany), and the residue was then reconstituted with 100 µL mobile phase and vortexed for 1 min. A volume of 20 µL aliquot of the reconstituted sample was injected into the column for analysis.

Brain and Systemic Kinetic Analysis

The pharmacokinetic parameters in both plasma and brain tissue homogenates were calculated for comparative studies between IN and IV administration. For investigated plasma samples, the mean RSM plasma concentration was plotted versus time in a plasma concentration-time curve. Kinetica® software (version 5.0, 2017, Thermo Fisher Scientific, Waltham, MA, USA) was used for the calculation of peak plasma concentration (C_{max}), the time required to reach it (T_{max}) along with the area under plasma concentration-time curve over 12 h ($AUC_{0\text{-}12}$). Absolute bioavailability of RSM in plasma after IN administration was calculated relative to the IV RSM aqueous solution.

For brain samples, the mean RSM brain concentration was plotted versus time, and the pharmacokinetic parameters (C_{max}, T_{max}, and $AUC_{0\text{-}12}$) were determined following the same way previously mentioned for plasma samples. RSM bioavailability in brain tissues from IN administration was calculated relative to the IV RSM aqueous solution.

To follow RSM targeting to the brain, drug targeting efficiency (DTE) and nose-to-brain direct transport percentage (DTP) [67] were calculated as follows:

$$DTE(\%) = \left(\frac{\left(\frac{B}{P}\right)_{IN}}{\left(\frac{B}{P}\right)_{IV}} \right) \times 100 \tag{3}$$

$$DTP\ (\%) = \left(\frac{B_{IN} - B_X}{B_{IN}} \right) \times 100 \tag{4}$$

where B and P stand for $AUC_{0\text{-}12}$ in brain and plasma, correspondingly. IN and IV represent intranasal and intravenous administration, correspondingly, and B_X is the portion of the drug that reached the brain from blood–brain barrier (BBB) following IN administration. The following equation was used for the calculation of B_X [67],

$$B_X = \left(\frac{B_{IV}}{P_{IV}} \right) \times P_{IN} \tag{5}$$

Statistical Analysis

To statistically compare different formulations, either Student's *t*-test or analysis of variance (ANOVA) was conducted using Microsoft excel. Significant differences are determined when p values are < 0.05.

3. Results and Discussion

3.1. Characterization of RSM-Loaded Transferosomes

3.1.1. Assessment of Vesicle Size (VS), Polydispersity Index (PDI), and Zeta Potential (ZP)

According to Table 2, and as illustrated in Figure 1a,b, it could be demonstrated that the prepared transferosomal formulations showed VS values ranging from 198.63 ± 34.98 to 491.40 ± 48.79 nm. As illustrated in the figure, it is obvious that both the type of EA and the presence of cholesterol had a significant influence on the VS ($p < 0.0001$ and $p = 0.0001$, respectively). Regarding the type of the EA, the VS was greatly affected by either the HLB value, ionic nature, or the molecular structure of the used EA. The behavior of anionic EA was different from that of nonionic EA. Upon comparing the VS of the formulations prepared using nonionic EA, we found a significant reduction in the VS with the increase in the HLB value of the used EA. The used nonionic EA can be descendingly ordered according to their HLB values as follows: Pluronic® F-68 > Pluronic® L-35 > Pluronic® L-31 > Span® 60. The obtained VS values for the transferosomes prepared using the previously mentioned EA were 227.51 ± 13.69, 276.00 ± 27.05, 352.90 ± 15.41, and 448.70 ± 11.84 nm, respectively, in absence of cholesterol. This enhanced decrease in the obtained VS values might be attributed to the decrease in interfacial tension during vesicle formation using higher HLB values [68]. On the other hand, the obtained VS values of the formulations prepared by anionic EA (sodium cholate and sodium deoxycholate) were the smallest (208.42 ± 11.95 and 198.63 ± 34.98 nm, respectively) compared with those prepared using the nonionic EA. This enhanced decrease in the VS might be due to the steric repulsion between the charged EA molecules arranged on the surface of the vesicles causing an increase in the curvature of the vesicles membrane [69], in addition to the insignificant difference between the VS of the transferosomes prepared using sodium cholate and sodium deoxycholate owing to the nearly similar HLB values (18 and 16, correspondingly) as well as the molecular weight values (430.6 and 414.6, respectively).

Conversely, the presence of cholesterol had a significant influence on increasing the VS ($p = 0.0001$) of the formed transferosomes compared with those lacking its addition. This might be attributed to the bulky structure of cholesterol, which led to an increase in the VS of the formed vesicles [70]. The incorporation of cholesterol in the lipid bilayer might have resulted in more aqueous distribution within the vesicle due to the interference with the closed packing of the lipid bilayer [71,72]. Design expert plots representing the influence of the studied factors are demonstrated in Figure 1a,b.

PDI is an assessment of size distribution that affects the homogeneity of the tested samples. It was previously reported that PDI values < 0.7 indicate narrow vesicle size distribution [73,74]. Since PDI values ranged from 0.3 ± 0.02 to 0.68 ± 0.02, this indicated the narrow size distribution and homogenous dispersion of the formed vesicles and, hence, their better stability.

It has been reported that formulations with ZP values exceeding +30 mV or −30 mV are said to be more stable with less aggregation probability [75,76]. As demonstrated in Table 2 and Figure 1c,d, the obtained ZP values ranged from −39.60 ± 6.36 to −24.90 ± 1.13 mV.

Both the type of EA and the presence of cholesterol imparted a significant effect ($p = 0.0219$ and $p = 0.0038$) on the ZP value. Regarding the type of EA, it was previously reported that anionic EA, being negatively charged, possesses a significant effect on ZP at an EA concentration of 1 g/L [77], and since the used concentration of EA was 3.33 g/L, it obviously led to the enhancement of the negative value of ZP. On the other side, it was deduced that the presence of cholesterol increased the negative value of ZP, which might be due to the effect of cholesterol on the arrangement of EA molecules at the interface of the vesicles [78].

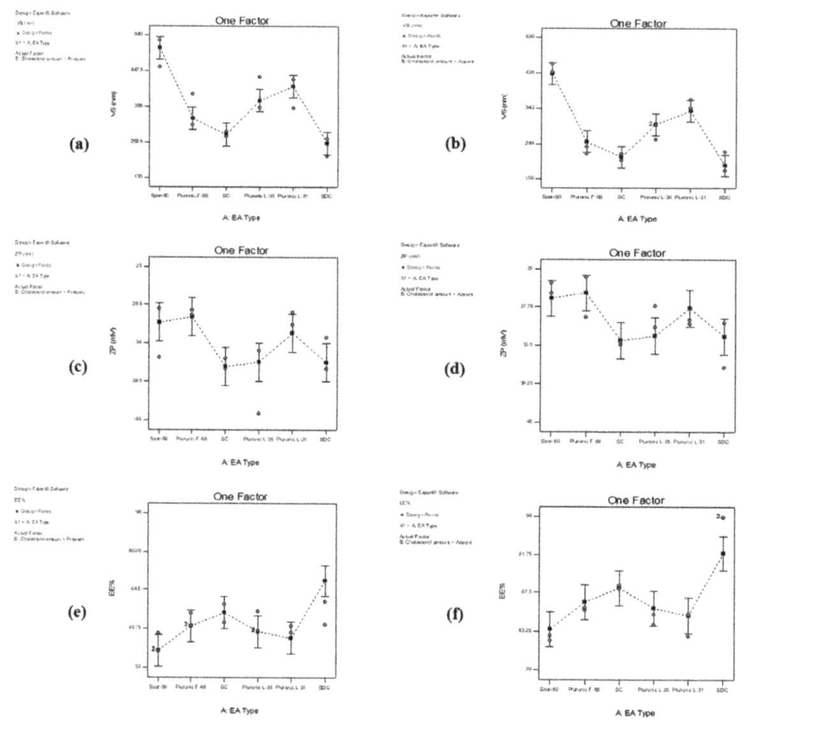

Figure 1. Line plot for the effect of EA on VS (**a**) with cholesterol, (**b**) without cholesterol; on ZP (**c**), with cholesterol, (**d**) without cholesterol; and on %EE (**e**) with cholesterol, (**f**) without cholesterol.

3.1.2. Assessment of Entrapment Efficiency (%EE)

As demonstrated in Table 2 and Figure 1e,f, the values of EE ranged from 43.25 ± 5.02 to 95.73 ± 0.09. It was shown that the type of EA affected the %EE significantly ($p = 0.002$) in the absence of cholesterol, while it imparted a non-significant difference in its presence. The ionic nature, the molecular size, and the HLB values of the used EA played a vital role in entrapping RSM effectively. Regarding the ionic nature of the used EA, it was obvious that using the anionic EA, sodium cholate, or deoxycholate showed higher EE values relative to those prepared using nonionic ones [70], which might be due to the protonation of the amino group in the propargylamine residue of the drug. This protonated amino group may have formed an electrostatic bond with the negative charge of the anionic EA [79]. Additionally, upon comparing both the anionic EAs used, it was found that the highest EE values were obtained for the vesicles formed using sodium deoxycholate. This could be attributed to the small molecular size (414.6 g/mol) of sodium deoxycholate [80,81] resulting in a less steric hindrance upon closure of the vesicles [68]. With regard to the transferosomal formulations prepared using nonionic EA, we found that the %EE increased ascendingly with the respective increase in the HLB values. The lowest and highest %EE values were noted for transferosomes formed using Span® 60 (HLB = 4.7) and Pluronic® F-68 (HLB = 29), respectively. This was in accordance to a previous study that encapsulated the hydrophilic drug N-acetyl glucosamine within niosomes. EA with higher HLB yielded vesicles with the larger aqueous spaces needed for drug entrapment within the formed lamellae and provided greater protection for drug leakage from the formed niosomes, resulting in higher encapsulation efficiency [82].

Additionally, the statistical analysis of the obtained results gave a significant effect (p = 0.0005) of the presence of cholesterol on the %EE values. It was obvious that adding cholesterol significantly decreased the %EE values for the prepared transferosomal formulations (p = 0.0005). This might be due to the steric hindrance caused by cholesterol, which limited the drug inclusion in the formed vesicles [83]. On the other hand, it is believed that the addition of cholesterol led to disruption of the linear structure of transferosomes, causing a negative impact on %EE values [70]. Furthermore, the addition of cholesterol might result in increasing the bilayer interfacial region hydrophobicity, resulting in less entrapment for the drug [84].

3.2. *Optimization of the Formulation Variables*

One formulation combining the desirable characteristics (with desirability value = 0.749) (F12, containing sodium deoxycholate as EA in the absence of cholesterol) was selected as the optimized RSM-loaded transferosomal formulation. The optimum selection of different variables was acquired by numerical optimization based on the desirability value obtained from Design-Expert® software [85]. F12 demonstrated the following values (VS: 198.635 ± 34.98 nm, PDI: 0.45 ± 0.079, ZP: −33.45 ± 4.73 mV, and %EE: 95.735 ± 0.091%). Additional characterization tests regarding its morphology and the compatibility of the drug with other used components are demonstrated below. Moreover, it was further incorporated within in situ gel formulations.

3.3. *Characterization of the Optimized Transferosomal Formulation (F12)*

3.3.1. Fourier Transform Infrared Spectroscopy (FTIR)

As shown in Figure 2a, the FTIR spectrum for pure RSM revealed characteristic sharp peaks at 3276.57 cm^{-1}, 1626.87 cm^{-1}, 1204.45 cm^{-1}, 1044.62 cm^{-1}, and 759.2 cm^{-1} owing to propargyl group ≡C–H stretching vibration, the stretching of N– H...O, symmetric and asymmetric S–O stretching, and stretching of the C–S bond, respectively.

Figure 2b shows the FTIR spectrum of phosphatidylcholine with significant peaks at 2922.65 cm^{-1} and 2837.03 cm^{-1} due to long-chain fatty acid C-H stretching [86]. Symmetric C=O stretching vibration was observed at 1729.62 cm^{-1} [87], and peaks of phosphate-groups-building phospholipid appeared at 1250.12 cm^{-1} [88].

FTIR absorption peaks for sodium deoxycholate were illustrated in Figure 2c, showing the broad band of –OH stretching vibrations that appeared at 3390.73 cm^{-1}. At 2939.78.49 and 2865.57 cm^{-1}, two bands were detected, which represented symmetric and asymmetric -CH_2 stretching vibrations, respectively. A carboxylate ester group C=O stretching vibration band was detected at 1569.78 cm^{-1} [89].

Regarding the FTIR spectra of the physical mixture (Figure 2d), the peak intensity at 3276.57 cm^{-1} significantly decreased, while the characteristic peaks of RSM were still present with the preservation of the other components peaks. On the other hand, in the optimum formulation illustrated in Figure 2e, the peak at 3276.57 cm^{-1} completely disappeared, which might be due to the inclusion of the drug inside the formed vesicles. This is in addition to the absence of the peak sharpness of the other peaks, indicating the drug incorporation in the formed transferosomes. The shifting of some peaks from 1626.87, 1044.62, and 1204.45 cm^{-1} to 1689.66, 1056.04, and 1221.58 cm^{-1} may be due to a dilution effect, which represents the achievement of drug entrapment inside the vesicles while retaining its properties [53,90]. This might indicate the absence of interaction between the components of the formulation [91].

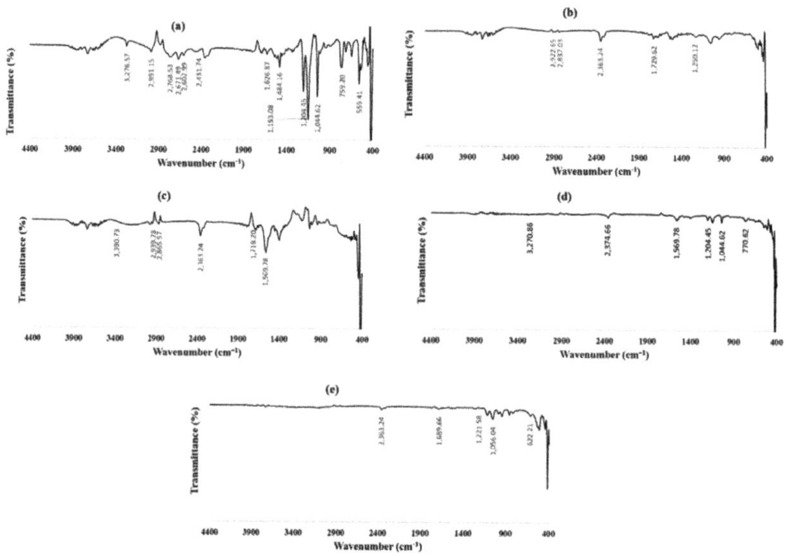

Figure 2. FTIR spectra of (**a**) RSM, (**b**) phosphatidylcholine, (**c**) sodium deoxycholate, (**d**) physical mixture of the components, and (**e**) optimized RSM-loaded transferosomes (F12).

3.3.2. Transmission Electron Microscopy (TEM)

TEM images of the optimized RSM-loaded transferosomal formulation (F12) are illustrated in Figure 3. It is obvious that the transferosomal vesicles were well-identified and spherical in shape with nearly perfect edges. The measured VS was in good correlation (~200 nm) with the results previously obtained from ZetaSizer Nano ZS.

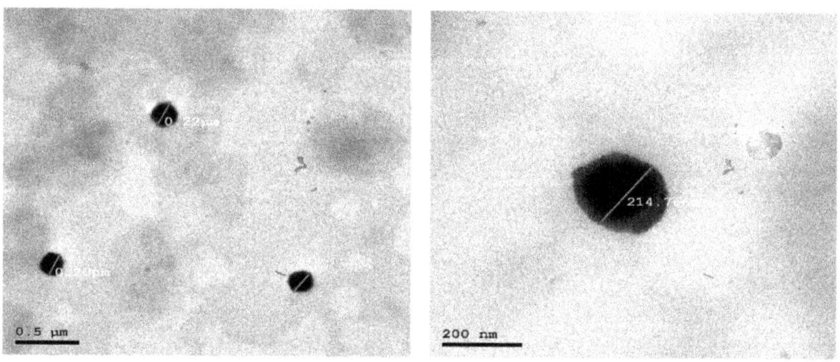

Figure 3. TEM micrographs of the optimized RSM-loaded transferosomes (F12).

3.4. Characterization of Mucoadhesive RSM-Loaded Transferosomal In Situ Gels

The in situ gel is a type of pharmaceutical formulation that is liquid (sol) outside the human body and transforms into a gel consistency inside the human body under physiological conditions [24]. The in situ gel prepared in the current study depended on the use of a mixture of thermosensitive polymers, such as Pluronic® F-127 and Pluronic® F-68, in addition to a mucoadhesive agent, such as pectin, in different concentrations.

Pectin is a natural polysaccharide capable of forming a three-dimensional network in the gel structure [92]. Optimum concentrations selection is based on the sol-to-gel transition temperatures and gelation time [30].

In this study, various concentrations of Pluronic® F-68 were added to a single concentration of both Pluronic® F-127, in addition to the mucoadhesive polymer, pectin (0.5% *w*/*v*), to prepare three in situ gels (G1, G2, and G3) containing the optimized RSM-loaded transferosomal formulation (F12) (Table 3). The cold method adopted produced homogenous yellowish dispersions that were visually inspected with no aggregates in liquid form at ambient temperature. The formulated RSM-loaded transferosomal in situ gels were assessed for their sol-to-gel transition temperature, rheological properties, and in vitro drug release for the selection of the optimum in situ gel.

3.4.1. Sol-to-Gel Transition Temperature

As shown in Table 3, it was obvious that the sol-to-gel temperature was up to 40.1 °C. By analyzing the results, it was manifested that the incorporation of Pluronic® F-68 in the composition of the in situ gel (prepared using single concentration of Pluronic® F-127; 15% *w*/*v*) significantly elevated ($p < 0.05$) the sol-to-gel transition temperature. Moreover, it was noticed that elevating the concentration of Pluronic® F-68 from 5 to 10% *w*/*v* led to a corresponding increase in the sol-to-gel transition temperature from 36.2 ± 0.282 °C to 40.1 ± 1.69 °C. This observation might be attributed to the presence of a higher PEO/PPO ratio in the structure of Pluronic® F-68 compared with Pluronic® F-127 [52]. As previously reported by Yuan et al., who explained the idea that Pluronics with high hydrophobic PPO (such as Pluronic® F-127) proportion had low sol-to-gel transition temperature, while those composed of high hydrophilic PEO (such as Pluronic® F-68) proportion demonstrated higher gelation temperatures [93]. This confirms the result that the incorporation of Pluronic® F-68 having higher PEO/PPO ratio compared with Pluronic® F-127 led to the elevation of gelation temperature [52]. By checking the results of the sol-to-gel transition time, it was obvious that the obtained values were around 15 s.

3.4.2. Rheological Study

The rheological properties assessment illustrated in Figure 4 confirmed that upon increasing the concentration of Pluronic® F-68, a relative increase in the complex viscosity occurred. The elevation of the complex viscosity was in the order that G1 (lacking Pluronic® F-68) was the first to form the gel, followed by G2 (5% *w*/*v* Pluronic® F-68) and then G3 (10% *w*/*v* Pluronic® F-68). The estimated complex viscosity values were 128.0, 99.3 and 84.2 Pa.s at 25 °C for G1, G2, and G3, while they reached 730, 1130, and 1240 Pa.s, respectively, at 37 °C. The results indicated the increased complex viscosity upon elevating the concentration of Pluronic® F-68 (G1 < G2 < G3).

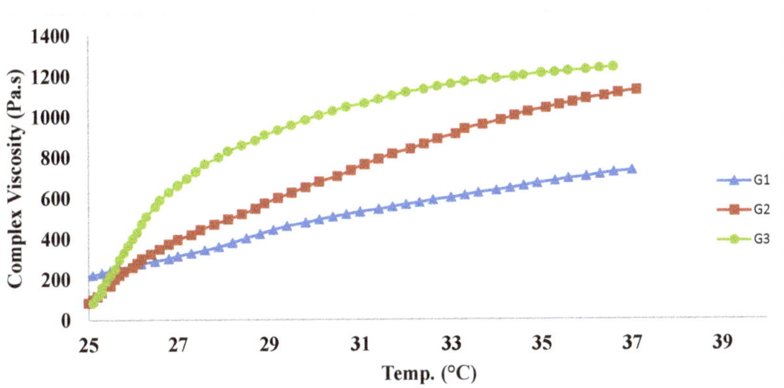

Figure 4. Relationship between temperature and complex viscosity of in situ gels: G1, G2, and G3. Composition of the in situ gels is compiled in Table 3.

3.4.3. In Vitro Drug Release

It was detected that the drug was totally released from the prepared drug dispersion in 0.5 h. Figure 5 represents the percentage of RSM released from the optimized RSM-loaded transferosomal formulation (F12) and the prepared in situ gels (G1, G2, and G3) in ethanolic PBS solution (10% v/v, pH 7.4) in addition to the drug dispersion. From the figure, it is obvious that the optimized transferosomal formulation F12 suffered from a flush release of 52.79 ± 2.1% within the first 0.5 h ($Q_{0.5\ h}$), followed by a slower release where the % of drug released after 8 h (Q_{8h}) was 100.42 ± 4.02%. This initial flush might be due to the release of the drug entrapped near the surface layers of the formed transferosomes, while the rest of the drug entrapped in the deep layers was released in a slower manner later [94]. On the other hand, the incorporation of F12 within the in situ gels controlled the initial burst release of RSM, where the $Q_{0.5h}$ values were 4.86 ± 6.87, 13.50 ± 7.64, and 22.89 ± 2.39% for G3, G2, and G1, respectively, with a significant reduction ($p < 0.05$) when compared with the free transferosomal formulation (F12). This might be due to the enhanced viscosity of the formed gels, which in turn reduced the drug release [95]. Q_{8h} values were assessed to assure the sustainability of drug release in gel formulations and evaluate the effect of Pluronic® F-68 on the gelation temperature, so by comparing the Q_{8h} values of the investigated in situ gels containing the optimized formulation, F12, it was evident that the obtained values were significantly smaller than that of the free transferosomal formulation. The obtained Q_{8h} values were 100.25 ± 0.62, 87.25 ± 4.11, and 64.42 ± 7.63% for G1, G2, and G3, respectively. Furthermore, it is obvious that the presence of Pluronic® F-68 and increasing its concentration led to a significant reduction in the % of drug released after 0.5 and 8 h. This might be due to the increased viscosity of the gel at 37 °C due to the incorporation of Pluronic® F-68, which is in accordance with Din et al. [96].

From the preceding findings, it can be deduced that the in situ gel (G2) was the best regarding its sol-to-gel transition temperature of 36.2 ± 0.282°C, as well as its controlled release behavior for RSM. The selected in situ gel formulation (G2) was investigated for further studies.

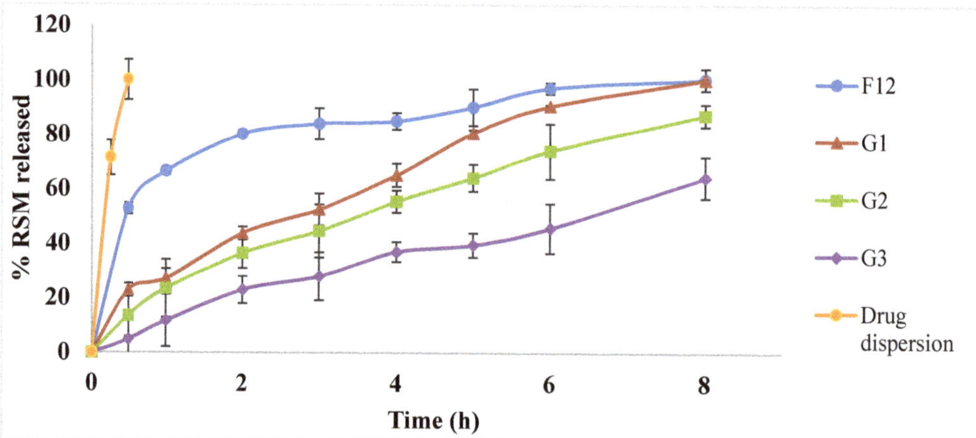

Figure 5. Release profiles of RSM from optimized RSM-loaded transferosomal formulation (F12) and prepared in situ gels (G1, G2, G3) in ethanolic phosphate-buffered saline; pH 7.4. Composition of the in situ gels is illustrated in Table 3.

3.5. *Effect of Storage*

The optimized RSM-loaded transferosomal formulation (F12) along with the respective optimum in situ gel (G2) were re-evaluated after storage for three months at 4 °C. All refrigerated gel formulations showed no sedimentation or aggregations. The stored free transferosomal formulation, F12, was re-evaluated for its VS, PDI, ZP, and %EE measurements, and the results revealed that the obtained values (294.85 ± 20.29 nm, 0.505 ± 0.021, −37.85 ± 0.77 mV, and 89.55 ± 1.62%, respectively) were insignificantly different compared with the freshly prepared formulation ($p > 0.05$). Moreover, the stored in situ gel (G2) showed an insignificant difference ($p > 0.05$) regarding the sol-to-gel transition temperature when compared with the freshly formed one, where the obtained values were 36.81 ± 0.47 versus 36.2 ± 0.282, respectively. In vitro RSM release profiles revealed an insignificant difference ($p > 0.05$) between the freshly prepared transferosomal formulation (F12) and the stored one, as well as the freshly prepared in situ gel (G2) and the stored one, as shown in Figure 6. Furthermore, to be approved by the FDA guidance for industry, the similarity factor should be above 50 in order to ensure the similarity between the dissolution profiles [59]. Since the similarity factor for the optimum formulation F12 before and after storage was 54, and that of the in situ gel formulation (G2) before and after storage was 64, the physical stability of the prepared transferosomal formulation and the corresponding in situ gel could be confirmed, with no drug leakage from the formed vesicles.

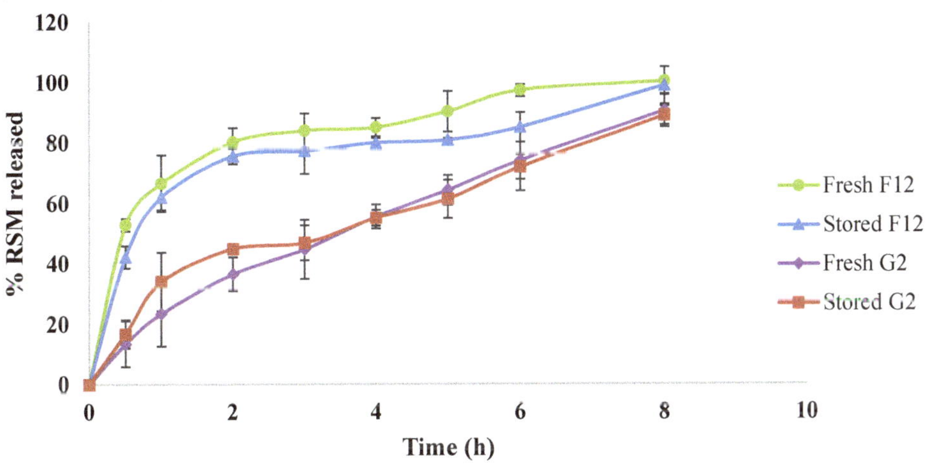

Figure 6. Release profiles of RSM from fresh optimized RSM-loaded transferosomal formulation (F12), stored (F12), fresh in situ gel (G2), stored (G2) in ethanolic phosphate-buffered saline; pH 7.4.

Composition of the in situ gels is compiled in Table 3.

3.6. In Vivo Studies

All the animals subjected to in vivo studies tolerated the drug and were alive with the same level of vitality, showing normal behavior along the whole sampling time.

3.6.1. Assessment of Formulation Biocompatibility

To detect the biocompatibility and safety of the administered IN in situ gel containing the optimum RSM-loaded transferosomal formulation (G2), a histopathological study was performed on male Wistar Albino rats. As illustrated in Figure 7, it is obvious that no significant changes could be detected in the treated group compared with the untreated control group, indicating the absence of any damaging effects on the microscopic structure of the nasal mucosa. In the treated group the nasal mucosa of the sacrificed rats remained intact with no severe signs of necrosis or hemorrhage, furthermore, the epithelial layer was intact with no change in the basal membrane and the superficial part of the submucosa. The obtained results might be attributed to the use of safe components for the formulation of the in situ gel. Several researchers studied the safety of the drug [97], as well as the used transferosomal components, such as phosphatidylcholine [36] and sodium deoxycholate [98], and the in situ-forming gel components, such as Pluronics and pectin [99,100], for IN delivery. Thus, these results indicate that RSM-loaded transferosomal in situ gel (G2) is considered as a safe and biocompatible formulation for IN administration.

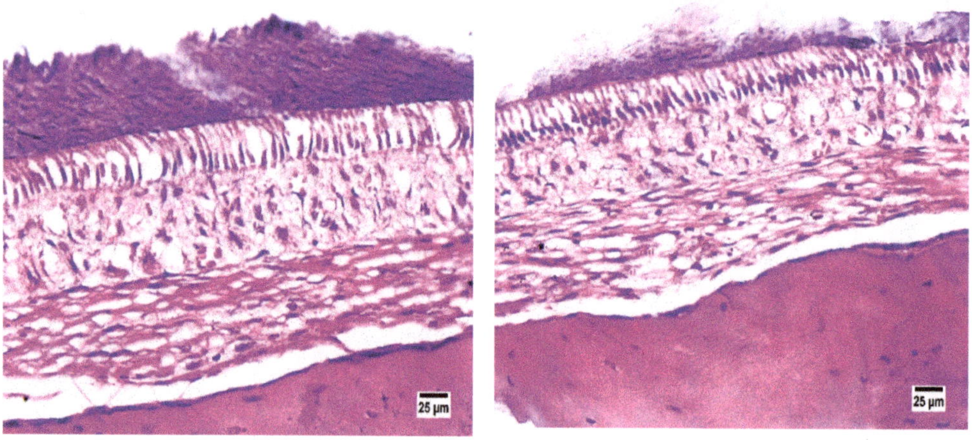

(**a**) (**b**)

Figure 7. Photomicrographs showing normal histological structure of nasal mucosa in (**a**) control group (untreated) and (**b**) intranasally administered RSM-loaded transferosomal in situ-gel-treated group (stain used is hematoxylin and eosin).

3.6.2. In Vivo Pharmacokinetics

The calibration curve of the conducted LC-MS/MS technique presented a lower limit of quantification of 0.1 ng/mL in both plasma and brain tissues, with good linearity from 0.1 to 1000 ng/mL (R^2 of the calibration curve lines were 0.9995 and 0.9993 for plasma and brain, respectively).

RSM concentrations in plasma and brain homogenates were illustrated against time, and the constructed curves were illustrated in Figure 8a,b. The calculated pharmacokinetic parameters, C_{max}, T_{max}, and $AUC_{0\text{-}12}$, are represented in Table 4.

From the RSM plasma concentration-time curve (Figure 8a), it is obvious that both the investigated samples, RSM IV aqueous solution and RSM-loaded transferosomal in situ gel (G2), possessed different shapes. It is clear that the plasma concentration-time curve of the IV sample possessed higher C_{max} than the IN-administered in situ gel formulation. Moreover, comparable T_{max} could be detected. Table 4 shows the pharmacokinetic parameters of both samples in the plasma. From the table, it is found that the obtained C_{max} values were 103.30 ± 6.95 and 14.01 ± 5.30 ng/mL after 0.25 h (T_{max}) following IV and IN administration, respectively. From the obtained values, we observed that the C_{max} value of IN-administered in situ gel (G2) was significantly lower (p = 0.0012) than that of IV aqueous solution. Alternatively, there was non-significant difference in T_{max} as C_{max} was reached after 0.25 h for both groups. Concerning the $AUC_{0\text{-}12h}$, it was clear that the calculated values for IN in situ gel (27.31 ± 5.60 ng.h/mL) was significantly less (p = 0.001) than that of IV aqueous solution (63.4 ± 3.00 ng.h/mL), which might explicate the drug availability in brain tissues rather than plasma [101]. The absolute bioavailability of the drug in plasma after IN in situ gel application was calculated to be 43.07%. This value being less than 100% might indicate the brain targeting of the drug. Further confirmations on the efficient brain targeting was indicated after the calculation of RSM concentration in the brain tissues.

By investigating the RSM concentration in the brain tissues and studying the brain concentration-time curve (Figure 8b), it is manifested that the IV aqueous solution, as well as the IN-administered in situ gel, showed differently shaped curves, where the IN-administered formulation possessed higher C_{max} and comparable T_{max} values compared with the IV aqueous solution. By comparing the calculated results of the brain kinetics parameters (Table 4), it is observed that C_{max} following IN in situ gel administration was significantly higher ($p = 0.0014$) than that following IV aqueous solution, where the obtained values were 381.58 ± 10.15 and 241.93 ± 11.41 ng/mL after 0.25 h (T_{max}) for the aforementioned treatments, respectively. From the table, the calculated $AUC_{0\text{-}12h}$ values showed significant differences ($p = 0.002$) between the IN-administered in situ gel and IV aqueous solution, where the obtained values were 586.47 ± 31.50 versus 447.08 ± 31.49 ng.h/mL for the previously mentioned treatments, respectively. The brain bioavailability of the drug from IN in situ gel was 131.17% relative to the IV aqueous solution, which could indicate that nasal application of the formulated IN in situ gel succeeded in the brain targeting of the drug.

To confirm the brain targetability of the optimized in situ gel formulation, drug targeting efficiency (DTE%) and direct transport percentage (DTP%) were used for comparing the $AUC_{0\text{-}12h}$ values obtained from the drug concentration-time curve in plasma and homogenized brain tissues. It is believed that a value of DTE% equal to 100% means that the drug concentration is in equal proportion in the brain following both IV aqueous solution and IN in situ gel administration. On the other hand, if the value of DTE% > 100%, then the drug is preferentially targeted to the brain following IN administration, and if DTE% < 100%, then the drug is preferentially targeted to the brain following IV administration [102]. Calculated DTE% was found to be 304.53%, confirming that IN administration of the in situ gel led to a better brain targeting. This might be due to the incorporation of pectin as a mucoadhesive polymer that increased the residence time in the nasal mucosa, in addition to the use of Pluronic® F-68 that might have increased the complex viscosity and gelation temperature, which was high enough to transform into gel at physiological temperature as previously mentioned, which in turn increased the $AUC_{0–12\,h}$.

The other parameter of the drug, namely DTP%, was assessed in order to determine whether the drug reached the brain through the BBB or directly from the nose-to-brain through the olfactory pathway [102]. The calculated DTP% of the tested IN in situ gel was 67.16%, suggesting the predominance of direct nose-to-brain transport following the IN in situ gel administration. The high DTE% and DTP% values confirmed the successful brain targeting of RSM.

By comparing the values of the calculated DTE% and DTP% for the developed in situ gel containing RSM-loaded transferosomes with other studies in the literature designed for the brain targeting of the drug, it is observed that the developed formulation in the current study succeeded in enhancing the brain targeting. One study tested the brain targeting of the RSM-loaded chitosan glutamate nanoparticles after intranasal administration, and the results revealed that the DTP% was calculated to be 69.27 ± 2.1% [3]. Another study addressed the preparation of RSM-loaded gellan gum transdermal patches, where the obtained DTE% and DTP% values were 193.75% and 48.15%, respectively [12].

The obtained results in the current study and the efficient brain targeting could be ascribed to the small VS of the formed transferosomes [103]. Furthermore, the Pluronic® F-127 in the formed in situ gel might have resulted in entanglement with the glycoprotein chains of the nasal mucosa, which can permit longer residence and, hence, absorption [104,105]. Finally, the presence of pectin as mucoadhesive polymer assured the reduced drug mucociliary clearance and increased the residence of the formulation onto the nasal mucosa.

Table 4. Pharmacokinetic parameters of RSM following the administration of RSM IV aqueous solution and RSM intranasal in situ gel (G2) in plasma and brain tissues.

In Plasma			
Parameter	**IV Aqueous Solution**	**IN In Situ Gel**	***p*-Value**
C_{max} (ng/mL)	103.30 ± 6.95	14.01 ± 5.30	0.0012
T_{max} (h)	0.25	0.25	-
$AUC_{0\text{-}12h}$ (ng.h/mL)	63.40 ± 3.00	27.31 ± 5.60	0.001
Absolute bioavailability (%)	–	43.07%	
In Brain			
Parameter	IV Aqueous Solution	IN In Situ Gel	*p*-Value
C_{max} (ng/mL)	241.93 ± 11.41	381.58 ± 10.15	0.0014
T_{max} (h)	0.25	0.25	-
$AUC_{0\text{-}12h}$ (ng.h/mL)	447.08 ± 31.49	586.47 ± 31.50	0.002
Brain bioavailability (%)	–	131.17%	

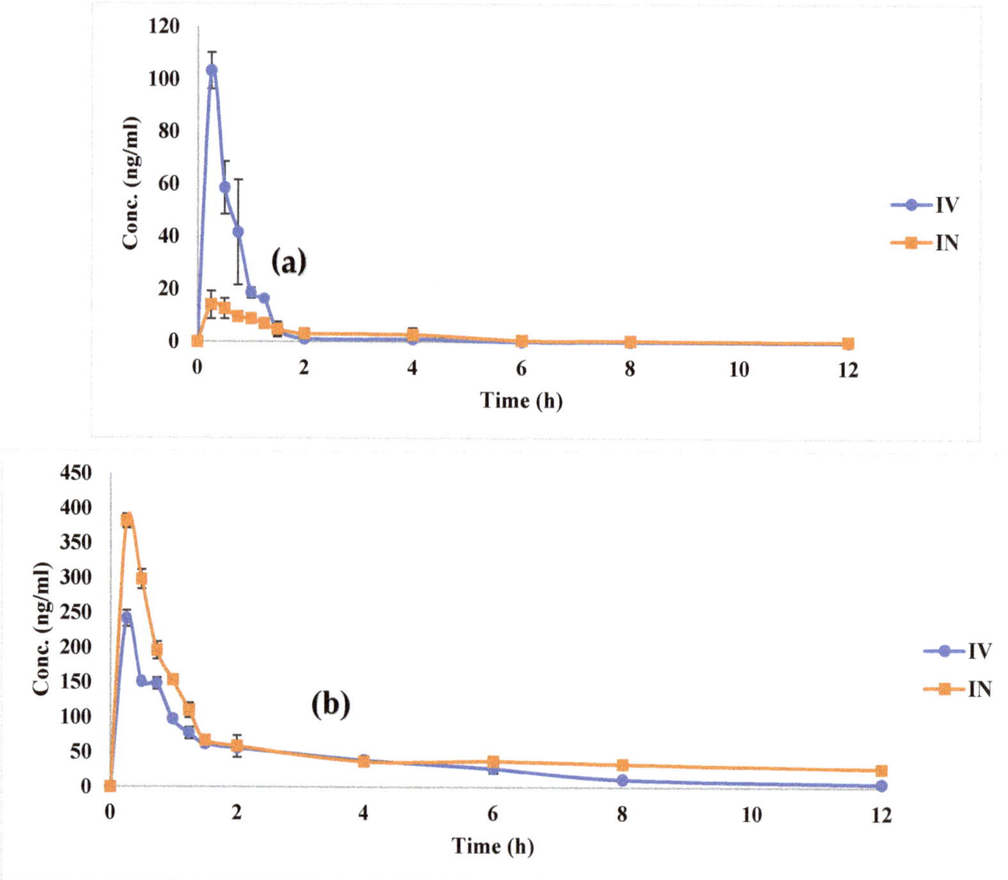

Figure 8. RSM concentration-time curve following the administration of RSM IV aqueous solution and RSM IN in situ gel (G2) in (**a**) plasma and (**b**) brain tissues.

4. Conclusions

In the present study, in situ-forming gels containing rasagiline mesylate-loaded transferosomes were successfully prepared for efficient intranasal delivery of the drug as a way to bypass the first-pass metabolism. Among the prepared transferosomal formulations and after statistical analysis of the results, it was found that the transferosomal formulation (F12) prepared using sodium deoxycholate as an EA and lacking the addition of cholesterol possessed the lowest vesicle size < 200 nm and highest entrapment efficiency value > 95%. The optimum transferosomal formulation was loaded into an in situ-forming gel prepared using a mixture of Pluronics (15% w/v Pluronic® F-127 & 5% w/v Pluronic® F-68) along with a mucoadhesive polymer—0.5% pectin. In vitro drug release studies revealed the significant effect of the prepared in situ gel on reducing the initial burst obtained from the transferosomal dispersion. The selected in situ gel possessed excellent cytocompatibility on the nasal mucosa of rats. Furthermore, a significant enhancement in the brain delivery of the drug was obtained after the intranasal delivery of the gel formulation compared with the intravenous delivery of RSM aqueous solution, where the brain bioavailability was calculated to be 131.17%. The obtained results indicated the development of a promising intranasal formulation for direct nose-to-brain drug targeting.

Author Contributions: Conceptualization, H.N.E., R.R.M., A.H.S., N.A.E. and E.B.B.; software, H.N.E., R.R.M., A.H.S., N.A.E. and E.B.B.; formal analysis H.N.E., R.R.M., A.H.S., N.A.E. and E.B.B.; investigation, H.N.E., R.R.M., A.H.S., N.A.E. and E.B.B.; resources, H.N.E., R.R.M., A.H.S., N.A.E. and E.B.B.; writing—original draft preparation, H.N.E., R.R.M., A.H.S. and N.A.E.; writing—review and editing, H.N.E., R.R.M., A.H.S., N.A.E. and E.B.B.; supervision, R.R.M., A.H.S., N.A.E. and E.B.B. All authors have read and agreed to the published version of the manuscript.

Funding: This research received no external funding.

Institutional Review Board Statement: The study protocol was approved by the institutional review board, Research Ethics Committee, Faculty of Pharmacy, Cairo University [PI (3043)].

Informed Consent Statement: Not applicable.

Data Availability Statement: The data presented in this study are available in the article.

Conflicts of Interest: The authors declare no conflict of interest.

References

1. Chougar, L.; Arsovic, E.; Gaurav, R.; Biondetti, E.; Faucher, A.; Valabrègue, R.; Pyatigorskaya, N.; Dupont, G.; Lejeune, F.X.; Cormier, F. Regional Selectivity of Neuromelanin Changes in the Substantia Nigra in Atypical Parkinsonism. *Mov. Disord.* **2022**, *37*, 1245–1255. [CrossRef] [PubMed]
2. Bartos, C.; Pallagi, E.; Szabó-Révész, P.; Ambrus, R.; Katona, G.; Kiss, T.; Rahimi, M.; Csóka, I. Formulation of levodopa containing dry powder for nasal delivery applying the quality-by-design approach. *Eur. J. Pharm. Sci.* **2018**, *123*, 475–483. [CrossRef] [PubMed]
3. Mittal, D.; Md, S.; Hasan, Q.; Fazil, M.; Ali, A.; Baboota, S.; Ali, J. Brain targeted nanoparticulate drug delivery system of rasagiline via intranasal route. *Drug Deliv.* **2016**, *23*, 130–139. [CrossRef] [PubMed]
4. Jiang, D.Q.; Wang, H.K.; Wang, Y.; Li, M.X.; Jiang, L.L.; Wang, Y. Rasagiline combined with levodopa therapy versus levodopa monotherapy for patients with Parkinson's disease: A systematic review. *Neurol. Sci.* **2020**, *41*, 101–109. [CrossRef]
5. Cereda, E.; Cilia, R.; Canesi, M.; Tesei, S.; Mariani, C.B.; Zecchinelli, A.L.; Pezzoli, G. Efficacy of rasagiline and selegiline in Parkinson's disease: A head-to-head 3-year retrospective case—Control study. *J. Neurol.* **2017**, *264*, 1254–1263. [CrossRef]
6. Müller, T. Pharmacokinetic/pharmacodynamic evaluation of rasagiline mesylate for Parkinson's disease. *Expert Opin. Drug Metab. Toxicol.* **2014**, *10*, 1423–1432. [CrossRef]
7. Chen, J.J.; Swope, D.M.; Dashtipour, K. Comprehensive review of rasagiline, a second-generation monoamine oxidase inhibitor, for the treatment of Parkinson's disease. *Clin. Ther.* **2007**, *29*, 1825–1849. [CrossRef]
8. Robakis, D.; Fahn, S. Defining the role of the monoamine oxidase-B inhibitors for Parkinson's disease. *CNS Drugs* **2015**, *29*, 433–441. [CrossRef]
9. Güneş, M.; Karavana, S.Y. Non-Oral Drug Delivery in Parkinson's Disease: Current Applications and Future. *Turk. J. Pharm. Sci.* **2022**, *19*, 343. [CrossRef]
10. Tandarić, T.; Vianello, R. Computational insight into the mechanism of the irreversible inhibition of monoamine oxidase enzymes by the antiparkinsonian propargylamine inhibitors rasagiline and selegiline. *ACS Chem. Neurosci.* **2019**, *10*, 3532–3542. [CrossRef]

11. Zubiaur, P.; Matas, M.; Martín-Vílchez, S.; Soria-Chacartegui, P.; Villapalos-García, G.; Figueiredo-Tor, L.; Calleja, S.; Navares-Gómez, M.; de Miguel, A.; Novalbos, J. Polymorphism of Drug Transporters, Rather Than Metabolizing Enzymes, Conditions the Pharmacokinetics of Rasagiline. *Pharmaceutics* **2022**, *14*, 2001. [CrossRef] [PubMed]
12. Bali, N.R.; Salve, P.S. Impact of rasagiline nanoparticles on brain targeting efficiency via gellan gum based transdermal patch: A nanotheranostic perspective for Parkinsonism. *Int. J. Biol. Macromol.* **2020**, *164*, 1006–1024. [CrossRef] [PubMed]
13. Chattopadhyay, S.; Das, S.; Sarma, K.N. Nose-to-brain drug delivery: An update to the alternative path to successful targeted antimigraine drugs. *Int. J. Appl. Pharm.* **2021**, *13*, 67–75. [CrossRef]
14. Lombardo, R.; Musumeci, T.; Carbone, C.; Pignatello, R. Nanotechnologies for intranasal drug delivery: An update of literature. *Pharm. Dev. Technol.* **2021**, *26*, 824–845. [CrossRef]
15. Dufes, C.; Olivier, J.C.; Gaillard, F.; Gaillard, A.; Couet, W.; Muller, J.M. Brain delivery of vasoactive intestinal peptide (VIP) following nasal administration to rats. *Int. J. Pharm.* **2003**, *255*, 87–97. [CrossRef]
16. Fonseca, L.C.; Lopes, J.A.; Vieira, J.; Viegas, C.; Oliveira, C.S.; Hartmann, R.P.; Fonte, P. Intranasal drug delivery for treatment of Alzheimer's disease. *Drug Deliv. Transl. Res.* **2021**, *11*, 411–425. [CrossRef]
17. Salama, A.H.; Salama, A.A.; Elhabak, M. Single step nanospray drying preparation technique of gabapentin-loaded nanoparticles-mediated brain delivery for effective treatment of PTZ-induced seizures. *Int. J. Pharm.* **2021**, *602*, 120604. [CrossRef]
18. Gartziandia, O.; Egusquiaguirre, S.P.; Bianco, J.; Pedraz, J.L.; Igartua, M.; Hernandez, R.M.; Préat, V.; Beloqui, A. Nanoparticle transport across in vitro olfactory cell monolayers. *Int. J. Pharm.* **2016**, *499*, 81–89. [CrossRef]
19. Alberto, M.; Paiva-Santos, A.C.; Veiga, F.; Pires, P.C. Lipid and Polymeric Nanoparticles: Successful Strategies for Nose-to-Brain Drug Delivery in the Treatment of Depression and Anxiety Disorders. *Pharmaceutics* **2022**, *14*, 2742. [CrossRef]
20. Erdő, F.; Bors, L.A.; Farkas, D.; Bajza, Á.; Gizurarson, S. Evaluation of intranasal delivery route of drug administration for brain targeting. *Brain Res. Bull.* **2018**, *143*, 155–170. [CrossRef]
21. Dholakia, J.; Prabhakar, B.; Shende, P. Strategies for the delivery of antidiabetic drugs via intranasal route. *Int. J. Pharm.* **2021**, *608*, 121068. [CrossRef] [PubMed]
22. Ozsoy, Y.; Gungor, S.; Cevher, E. Nasal delivery of high molecular weight drugs. *Molecules* **2009**, *14*, 3754–3779. [CrossRef] [PubMed]
23. Yurtdaş-Kırımlıoğlu, G. A promising approach to design thermosensitive in situ gel based on solid dispersions of desloratadine with Kolliphor® 188 and Pluronic® F127. *J. Therm. Anal. Calorim.* **2022**, *147*, 1307–1327. [CrossRef]
24. Vigani, B.; Rossi, S.; Sandri, G.; Bonferoni, M.C.; Caramella, C.M.; Ferrari, F. Recent advances in the development of in situ gelling drug delivery systems for non-parenteral administration routes. *Pharmaceutics* **2020**, *12*, 859. [CrossRef]
25. Tengamnuay, P.; Sahamethapat, A.; Sailasuta, A.; Mitra, A.K. Chitosans as nasal absorption enhancers of peptides: Comparison between free amine chitosans and soluble salts. *Int. J. Pharm.* **2000**, *197*, 53–67. [CrossRef]
26. Cirri, M.; Maestrelli, F.; Nerli, G.; Mennini, N.; D'Ambrosio, M.; Luceri, C.; Mura, P.A. Development of a cyclodextrin-based mucoadhesive-thermosensitive in situ gel for clonazepam intranasal delivery. *Pharmaceutics* **2021**, *13*, 969. [CrossRef]
27. Sideek, S.A.; El-Nassan, H.B.; Fares, A.R.; ElMeshad, A.N.; Elkasabgy, N.A. Different Curcumin-Loaded Delivery Systems for Wound Healing Applications: A Comprehensive Review. *Pharmaceutics* **2023**, *15*, 38. [CrossRef]
28. Salama, A.H.; AbouSamra, M.M.; Awad, G.E.A.; Mansy, S.S. Promising bioadhesive ofloxacin-loaded polymeric nanoparticles for the treatment of ocular inflammation: Formulation and in vivo evaluation. *Drug Deliv. Transl. Res.* **2021**, *11*, 1943–1957. [CrossRef]
29. AbouSamra, M.M.; Salama, A.H.; Awad, G.E.A.; Mansy, S.S. Formulation and evaluation of novel hybridized nanovesicles for enhancing buccal delivery of ciclopirox olamine. *AAPS PharmSciTech* **2020**, *21*, 283. [CrossRef]
30. Baloglu, E.; Karavana, S.Y.; Senyigit, Z.A.; Guneri, T. Rheological and mechanical properties of poloxamer mixtures as a mucoadhesive gel base. *Pharm. Dev. Technol.* **2011**, *16*, 627–636. [CrossRef]
31. Sherje, A.P.; Londhe, V. Development and evaluation of pH-responsive cyclodextrin-based in situ gel of paliperidone for intranasal delivery. *AAPS PharmSciTech* **2018**, *19*, 384–394. [CrossRef] [PubMed]
32. Liu, Y.; Yang, F.; Feng, L.; Yang, L.; Chen, L.; Wei, G.; Lu, W. In vivo retention of poloxamer-based in situ hydrogels for vaginal application in mouse and rat models. *Acta Pharm. Sin. B* **2017**, *7*, 502–509. [CrossRef] [PubMed]
33. De Jong, W.H.; Borm, P.J. Drug delivery and nanoparticles: Applications and hazards. *Int. J. Nanomed.* **2008**, *3*, 133. [CrossRef] [PubMed]
34. Kamel, R.; Afifi, S.M.; Kassem, I.A.A.; Elkasabgy, N.A.; Farag, M.A. Arabinoxylan and rhamnogalacturonan mucilage: Outgoing and potential trends of pharmaceutical, environmental, and medicinal merits. *Int. J. Biol. Macromol.* **2020**, *165*, 2550–2564. [CrossRef] [PubMed]
35. Singh, S.; Pandey, V.K.; Tewari, R.P.; Agarwal, V. Nanoparticle based drug delivery system: Advantages and applications. *Indian J. Sci. Technol.* **2011**, *4*, 177–180. [CrossRef]
36. Natsheh, H.; Touitou, E. Phospholipid vesicles for dermal/transdermal and nasal administration of active molecules: The effect of surfactants and alcohols on the fluidity of their lipid bilayers and penetration enhancement properties. *Molecules* **2020**, *25*, 2959. [CrossRef]
37. Aboud, H.M.; Ali, A.A.; El-Menshawe, S.F.; Elbary, A.A. Nanotransfersomes of carvedilol for intranasal delivery: Formulation, characterization and in vivo evaluation. *Drug Deliv.* **2016**, *23*, 2471–2481. [CrossRef]

38. Ibrahim, S.S.; Elseoud, O.G.A.; Mohamedy, M.H.; Amer, M.M.; Mohamed, Y.Y.; Elmansy, S.A.; Kadry, M.M.; Attia, A.A.; Fanous, R.A.; Kamel, M.S.; et al. Nose-to-brain delivery of chrysin transfersomal and composite vesicles in doxorubicin-induced cognitive impairment in rats: Insights on formulation, oxidative stress and TLR4/NF-kB/NLRP3 pathways. *Neuropharmacology* **2021**, *197*, 108738. [CrossRef]
39. Toksoy, M.O.; Tirnaksiz, F.F. Development of rasagiline mesylate loaded solid lipid nanoparticles in a thermosensitive mucoadhesive gel: Formulation design using DoE, in-vitro and ex-vivo characterization. *J. Res. Pharm.* **2021**, *25*, 695–707.
40. Mishra, N.; Tiwari, D.K.; Mishra, K. Development of intranasal deformable ethosomes of rasagiline mesylate for the effective management of parkinsonism. *Int. J. Pharm. Biol. Sci.* **2020**, *10*, 25–33.
41. Raj, N.D.; Rao, A.R.; Bhimanadhuni, C.N. Development of RP-HPLC method for the estimation of Rasagiline mesylate in bulk and tablet dosage forms. *Int. Curr. Pharm. J.* **2012**, *1*, 285–287. [CrossRef]
42. Yaghoobian, M.; Haeri, A.; Bolourchian, N.; Shahhosseni, S.; Dadashzadeh, S. The impact of surfactant composition and surface charge of niosomes on the oral absorption of repaglinide as a BCS II model drug. *Int. J. Nanomed.* **2020**, *15*, 8767. [CrossRef] [PubMed]
43. Balata, G.F.; Faisal, M.M.; Elghamry, H.A.; Sabry, S.A. Preparation and characterization of ivabradine HCl transfersomes for enhanced transdermal delivery. *J. Drug Deliv. Sci. Technol.* **2020**, *60*, 101921. [CrossRef]
44. Tavano, L.; Vivacqua, M.; Carito, V.; Muzzalupo, R.; Caroleo, M.C.; Nicoletta, F. Doxorubicin loaded magneto-niosomes for targeted drug delivery. *Colloids Surf. B Biointerfaces* **2013**, *102*, 803–807. [CrossRef]
45. ElKasabgy, N.A.; Elsayed, I.; Elshafeey, A.H. Design of lipotomes as a novel dual functioning nanocarrier for bioavailability enhancement of lacidipine: In-vitro and in-vivo characterization. *Int. J. Pharm.* **2014**, *472*, 369–379. [CrossRef]
46. Zaki, N.M.; Awad, G.A.; Mortada, N.D.; Abd ElHady, S.S. Enhanced bioavailability of metoclopramide HCl by intranasal administration of a mucoadhesive in situ gel with modulated rheological and mucociliary transport properties. *Eur. J. Pharm. Sci.* **2007**, *32*, 296–307. [CrossRef]
47. Jeong, B.; Choi, Y.K.; Bae, Y.H.; Zentner, G.; Kim, S.W. New biodegradable polymers for injectable drug delivery systems. *J. Control. Release* **1999**, *62*, 109–114. [CrossRef]
48. Vadnere, M.; Amidon, G.; Lindenbaum, S.; Haslam, J.L. Thermodynamic studies on the gel-sol transition of some pluronic polyols. *Int. J. Pharm.* **1984**, *22*, 207–218. [CrossRef]
49. Gilbert, J.C.; Richardson, J.L.; Davies, M.C.; Palin, K.J.; Hadgraft, J. The effect of solutes and polymers on the gelation properties of pluronic F-127 solutions for controlled drug delivery. *J. Control. Release* **1987**, *5*, 113–118. [CrossRef]
50. Liu, L.; Tang, X.; Wang, Y.; Guo, S. Smart gelation of chitosan solution in the presence of $NaHCO_3$ for injectable drug delivery system. *Int. J. Pharm.* **2011**, *414*, 6–15. [CrossRef]
51. Krtalić, I.; Radošević, S.; Hafner, A.; Grassi, M.; Nenadić, M.; Cetina-Čižmek, B.; Filipović-Grčić, J.; Pepić, I.; Lovrić, J. D-optimal design in the development of rheologically improved in situ forming ophthalmic gel. *J. Pharm. Sci.* **2018**, *107*, 1562–1571. [CrossRef]
52. Hirun, N.; Kraisit, P.; Tantishaiyakul, V. Thermosensitive Polymer Blend Composed of Poloxamer 407, Poloxamer 188 and Polycarbophil for the Use as Mucoadhesive In Situ Gel. *Polymers* **2022**, *14*, 1836. [CrossRef] [PubMed]
53. Kanwar, N.; Bhandari, R.; Kuhad, A.; Sinha, V.R. Polycaprolactone-based neurotherapeutic delivery of rasagiline targeting behavioral and biochemical deficits in Parkinson's disease. *Drug Deliv. Transl. Res.* **2019**, *9*, 891–905. [CrossRef] [PubMed]
54. Hammad, R.W.; Sanad, R.A.; Abdelmalak, N.S.; Torad, F.A.; Latif, R. New intranasal cross-linked mosapride xyloglucan pluronics micelles (MOS-XPMs) for reflux esophagitis disease: In-vitro optimization and improved therapeutic efficacy. *J. Adv. Res.* **2020**, *23*, 83–94. [CrossRef] [PubMed]
55. Hammad, R.W.; Sanad, R.A.; Abdelmalk, N.S.; Aziz, R.L.; Torad, F.A. Intranasal surface-modified mosapride citrate-loaded nanostructured lipid carriers (MOS-SMNLCs) for treatment of reflux diseases: In vitro optimization, pharmacodynamics, and pharmacokinetic studies. *AAPS PharmSciTech* **2018**, *19*, 3791–3808. [CrossRef] [PubMed]
56. Yang, Z.Z.; Zhang, Y.Q.; Wang, Z.Z.; Wu, K.; Lou, J.N.; Qi, X.R. Enhanced brain distribution and pharmacodynamics of rivastigmine by liposomes following intranasal administration. *Int. J. Pharm.* **2013**, *452*, 344–354. [CrossRef] [PubMed]
57. Albash, R.; Yousry, C.; Al-Mahallawi, A.M.; Alaa-Eldin, A.A. Utilization of PEGylated cerosomes for effective topical delivery of fenticonazole nitrate: In-vitro characterization, statistical optimization, and in-vivo assessment. *Drug Deliv.* **2021**, *28*, 1–9. [CrossRef] [PubMed]
58. Barakat, S.S.; Nasr, M.; Ahmed, R.F.; Badawy, S.S.; Mansour, S. Intranasally administered in situ gelling nanocomposite system of dimenhydrinate: Preparation, characterization and pharmacodynamic applicability in chemotherapy induced emesis model. *Sci. Rep.* **2017**, *7*, 9910. [CrossRef]
59. Moore, J.; Flanner, H. Mathematical comparison of dissolution profiles. *Pharm. Technol.* **1996**, *20*, 64–74.
60. Samaha, D.; Shehayeb, R.; Kyriacos, S. Modeling and comparison of dissolution profiles of diltiazem modified-release formulations. *Dissolution Technol.* **2009**, *16*, 41–46. [CrossRef]
61. ElShagea, H.N.; ElKasabgy, N.A.; Fahmy, R.H.; Basalious, E.B. Freeze-dried self-nanoemulsifying self-nanosuspension (snesns): A new approach for the preparation of a highly drug-loaded dosage form. *AAPS PharmSciTech* **2019**, *20*, 258. [CrossRef] [PubMed]
62. Ravi, P.R.; Aditya, N.; Patil, S.; Cherian, L. Nasal in-situ gels for delivery of rasagiline mesylate: Improvement in bioavailability and brain localization. *Drug Deliv.* **2015**, *22*, 903–910. [CrossRef] [PubMed]

63. Bancroft, J.D.; Gamble, M. *Theory and Practice of Histological Techniques*; Elsevier Health Sciences, Churchill Livingstone: London, UK, 2008.
64. El-Mahrouk, G.; Aboul-Einien, M.H.; Elkasabgy, N.A. Formulation and evaluation of meloxicam orally dispersible capsules. *Asian J. Pharm. Sci.* **2009**, *4*, 8–22.
65. Fatouh, A.M.; Elshafeey, A.H.; Abdelbary, A. Agomelatine-based in situ gels for brain targeting via the nasal route: Statistical optimization, in vitro, and in vivo evaluation. *Drug Deliv.* **2017**, *24*, 1077–1085. [CrossRef] [PubMed]
66. Ma, J.; Chen, X.; Duan, X.; Deng, P.; Wang, H.; Zhong, D. Validated LC–MS/MS method for quantitative determination of rasagiline in human plasma and its application to a pharmacokinetic study. *J. Chromatogr. B* **2008**, *873*, 203–208. [CrossRef]
67. Vyas, T.K.; Babbar, A.K.; Sharma, R.K.; Misra, A. Intranasal mucoadhesive microemulsions of zolmitriptan: Preliminary studies on brain-targeting. *J. Drug Target.* **2005**, *13*, 317–324. [CrossRef]
68. Kassem, M.A.; Aboul-Einien, M.H.; El Taweel, M.M. Dry gel containing optimized felodipine-loaded transferosomes: A promising transdermal delivery system to enhance drug bioavailability. *AAPS PharmSciTech* **2018**, *19*, 2155–2173. [CrossRef]
69. Mu, X.; Zhong, Z. Preparation and properties of poly (vinyl alcohol)-stabilized liposomes. *Int. J. Pharm.* **2006**, *318*, 55–61. [CrossRef]
70. Al-Mahallawi, A.M.; Khowessah, O.M.; Shoukri, R.A. Nano-transfersomal ciprofloxacin loaded vesicles for non-invasive trans-tympanic ototopical delivery: In-vitro optimization, ex-vivo permeation studies, and in-vivo assessment. *Int. J. Pharm.* **2014**, *472*, 304–314. [CrossRef]
71. Duangjit, S.; Pamornpathomkul, B.; Opanasopit, P.; Rojanarata, T.; Obata, Y.; Takayama, K.; Ngawhirunpat, T. Role of the charge, carbon chain length, and content of surfactant on the skin penetration of meloxicam-loaded liposomes. *Int. J. Nanomed.* **2014**, *9*, 2005. [CrossRef]
72. Adel, I.M.; ElMeligy, M.F.; Abdelrahim, M.E.; Maged, A.; Abdelkhalek, A.A.; Abdelmoteleb, A.M.; Elkasabgy, N.A. Design and characterization of spray-dried proliposomes for the pulmonary delivery of curcumin. *Int. J. Nanomed.* **2021**, *16*, 2667–2687. [CrossRef]
73. Kreuter, J. *Colloidal Drug Delivery Systems*; CRC Press: Boca Raton, FL, USA, 1994; Volume 66.
74. Salama, A.H.; Abdelkhalek, A.A.; Elkasabgy, N.A. Etoricoxib-loaded bio-adhesive hybridized polylactic acid-based nanoparticles as an intra-articular injection for the treatment of osteoarthritis. *Int. J. Pharm.* **2020**, *578*, 119081. [CrossRef]
75. Joseph, E.; Singhvi, G. Multifunctional nanocrystals for cancer therapy: A potential nanocarrier. In *Nanomaterials for Drug Delivery and Therapy*; Elsevier: Amsterdam, The Netherlands, 2019; pp. 91–116.
76. Müller, R.H.; Jacobs, C.; Kayser, O. Nanosuspensions as particulate drug formulations in therapy: Rationale for development and what we can expect for the future. *Adv. Drug Deliv. Rev.* **2001**, *47*, 3–19. [CrossRef]
77. Kosmulski, M.; Mączka, E. Zeta potential in dispersions of titania nanoparticles in moderately polar solvents stabilized with anionic surfactants. *J. Mol. Liq.* **2022**, *355*, 118972. [CrossRef]
78. Asasutjarit, R.; Lorenzen, S.I.; Sirivichayakul, S.; Ruxrungtham, K.; Ruktanonchai, U.; Ritthidej, G.C. Effect of solid lipid nanoparticles formulation compositions on their size, zeta potential and potential for in vitro pHIS-HIV-hugag transfection. *Pharm. Res.* **2007**, *24*, 1098–1107. [CrossRef]
79. Naoi, M.; Maruyama, W.; Shamoto-Nagai, M. Neuroprotective Function of Rasagiline and Selegiline, Inhibitors of Type B Monoamine Oxidase, and Role of Monoamine Oxidases in Synucleinopathies. *Int. J. Mol. Sci.* **2022**, *23*, 11059. [CrossRef]
80. Sodium Deoxycholate. Available online: https://www.sigmaaldrich.com/EG/en/search/sodium-deoxycholate?focus=products&gclid=CjwKCAiAkrWdBhBkEiwAZ9cdcMalphdZ3qU7FBfsxyfSrsQs9w2u0ToGV1kDGBhBIVXLPXcj7abd1RoCMIYQAvD_BwE&page=1&perpage=30&sort=relevance&term=sodium%20deoxycholate&type=product_name (accessed on 29 December 2022).
81. Sodium Cholate. Available online: https://www.sigmaaldrich.com/EG/en/search/sodium-cholate?focus=products&page=1&perpage=30&sort=relevance&term=sodium%20cholate&type=product_name (accessed on 29 December 2022).
82. Shatalebi, M.; Mostafavi, S.; Moghaddas, A. Niosome as a drug carrier for topical delivery of N-acetyl glucosamine. *Res. Pharm. Sci.* **2010**, *5*, 107.
83. Torres-Flores, G.; Gonzalez-Horta, A.; Vega-Cantu, Y.I.; Rodriguez, C.; Rodriguez-Garcia, A. Preparation and characterization of liposomal everolimus by thin-film hydration technique. *Adv. Polym. Technol.* **2020**, *2020*, 5462949. [CrossRef]
84. Abdelbary, G. Ocular ciprofloxacin hydrochloride mucoadhesive chitosan-coated liposomes. *Pharm. Dev. Technol.* **2011**, *16*, 44–56. [CrossRef] [PubMed]
85. Basalious, E.B.; Shawky, N.; Badr-Eldin, S.M. SNEDDS containing bioenhancers for improvement of dissolution and oral absorption of lacidipine. I: Development and optimization. *Int. J. Pharm.* **2010**, *391*, 203–211. [CrossRef] [PubMed]
86. Zhou, Y.; Dong, W.; Ye, J.; Hao, H.; Zhou, J.; Wang, R.; Liu, Y. A novel matrix dispersion based on phospholipid complex for improving oral bioavailability of baicalein: Preparation, in vitro and in vivo evaluations. *Drug Deliv.* **2017**, *24*, 720–728. [CrossRef] [PubMed]
87. Lasch, P.; Pacifico, A.; Diem, M. Spatially resolved IR microspectroscopy of single cells. *Biopolym. Orig. Res. Biomol.* **2002**, *67*, 335–338. [CrossRef] [PubMed]
88. Depciuch, J.; Sowa-Kućma, M.; Nowak, G.; Dudek, D.; Siwek, M.; Styczeń, K.; Parlińska-Wojtan, M. Phospholipid-protein balance in affective disorders: Analysis of human blood serum using Raman and FTIR spectroscopy. A pilot study. *J. Pharm. Biomed. Anal.* **2016**, *131*, 287–296. [CrossRef] [PubMed]

89. Eldeeb, A.E.; Salah, S.; Amer, M.S.; Elkasabgy, N.A. 3D nanocomposite alginate hydrogel loaded with pitavastatin nanovesicles as a functional wound dressing with controlled drug release; preparation, in-vitro and in-vivo evaluation. *J. Drug Deliv. Sci. Technol.* **2022**, *71*, 103292. [CrossRef]
90. Kaur, M.; Sharma, S.; Sinha, V. Polymer based microspheres of aceclofenac as sustained release parenterals for prolonged anti-inflammatory effect. *Mater. Sci. Eng. C* **2017**, *72*, 492–500. [CrossRef] [PubMed]
91. Adel, S.; ElKasabgy, N.A. Design of innovated lipid-based floating beads loaded with an antispasmodic drug: In-vitro and in-vivo evaluation. *J. Liposome Res.* **2014**, *24*, 136–149. [CrossRef]
92. Karavasili, C.; Fatouros, D.G. Smart materials: In situ gel-forming systems for nasal delivery. *Drug Discov. Today* **2016**, *21*, 157–166. [CrossRef]
93. Yuan, Y.; Cui, Y.; Zhang, L.; Zhu, H.P.; Guo, Y.S.; Zhong, B.; Hu, X.; Zhang, L.; Wang, X.H.; Chen, L. Thermosensitive and mucoadhesive in situ gel based on poloxamer as new carrier for rectal administration of nimesulide. *Int. J. Pharm.* **2012**, *430*, 114–119. [CrossRef]
94. Hasan, M.; Elkhoury, K.; Kahn, C.J.; Arab-Tehrany, E.; Linder, M. Preparation, characterization, and release kinetics of chitosan-coated nanoliposomes encapsulating curcumin in simulated environments. *Molecules* **2019**, *24*, 2023. [CrossRef]
95. Abo Elela, M.M.; ElKasabgy, N.A.; Basalious, E.B. Bio-shielding in situ forming gels (BSIFG) loaded with lipospheres for depot injection of quetiapine fumarate: In vitro and in vivo evaluation. *AAPS PharmSciTech* **2017**, *18*, 2999–3010. [CrossRef]
96. Din, F.U.; Mustapha, O.; Kim, D.W.; Rashid, R.; Park, J.H.; Choi, J.Y.; Ku, S.K.; Yong, C.S.; Kim, J.O.; Choi, H.G. Novel dual-reverse thermosensitive solid lipid nanoparticle-loaded hydrogel for rectal administration of flurbiprofen with improved bioavailability and reduced initial burst effect. *Eur. J. Pharm. Biopharm.* **2015**, *94*, 64–72. [CrossRef] [PubMed]
97. Hawthorne, G.H.; Bernuci, M.P.; Bortolanza, M.; Tumas, V.; Issy, A.C.; Del-Bel, E. Nanomedicine to overcome current Parkinson's treatment liabilities: A systematic review. *Neurotox. Res.* **2016**, *30*, 715–729. [CrossRef] [PubMed]
98. Salem, H.F.; Kharshoum, R.M.; Abou-Taleb, H.A.; Naguib, D.M. Nanosized transferosome-based intranasal in situ gel for brain targeting of resveratrol: Formulation, optimization, in vitro evaluation, and in vivo pharmacokinetic study. *AAPS PharmSciTech* **2019**, *20*, 181. [CrossRef] [PubMed]
99. Agrawal, M.; Saraf, S.; Saraf, S.; Dubey, S.K.; Puri, A.; Gupta, U.; Kesharwani, P.; Ravichandiran, V.; Kumar, P.; Naidu, V.G. Stimuli-responsive In situ gelling system for nose-to-brain drug delivery. *J. Control. Release* **2020**, *327*, 235–265. [CrossRef] [PubMed]
100. Bulloch, M.N.; Hutchison, A.M. Fentanyl pectin nasal spray: A novel intranasal delivery method for the treatment of breakthrough cancer pain. *Expert Rev. Clin. Pharmacol.* **2013**, *6*, 9–22. [CrossRef] [PubMed]
101. El Taweel, M.M.; Aboul-Einien, M.H.; Kassem, M.A.; Elkasabgy, N.A. Intranasal zolmitriptan-loaded bilosomes with extended nasal mucociliary transit time for direct nose to brain delivery. *Pharmaceutics* **2021**, *13*, 1828. [CrossRef] [PubMed]
102. Muntimadugu, E.; Dhommati, R.; Jain, A.; Challa, V.G.; Shaheen, M.; Khan, W. Intranasal delivery of nanoparticle encapsulated tarenflurbil: A potential brain targeting strategy for Alzheimer's disease. *Eur. J. Pharm. Sci.* **2016**, *92*, 224–234. [CrossRef]
103. Seju, U.; Kumar, A.; Sawant, K. Development and evaluation of olanzapine-loaded PLGA nanoparticles for nose-to-brain delivery: In vitro and in vivo studies. *Acta Biomater.* **2011**, *7*, 4169–4176. [CrossRef]
104. Chatterjee, B.; Amalina, N.; Sengupta, P.; Mandal, U.K. Mucoadhesive polymers and their mode of action: A recent update. *J. Appl. Pharm. Sci.* **2017**, *7*, 195–203.
105. Al Khateb, K.; Ozhmukhametova, E.K.; Mussin, M.N.; Seilkhanov, S.K.; Rakhypbekov, T.K.; Lau, W.M.; Khutoryanskiy, V.V. In situ gelling systems based on Pluronic F127/Pluronic F68 formulations for ocular drug delivery. *Int. J. Pharm.* **2016**, *502*, 70–79. [CrossRef]

pharmaceutics

MDPI

Article

Increasing Bioavailability of Trans-Ferulic Acid by Encapsulation in Functionalized Mesoporous Silica

Gabriela Petrișor [1,2,3], Ludmila Motelica [1,2,3], Denisa Ficai [2,3,4], Cornelia-Ioana Ilie [1,2,3], Roxana Doina Trușcă [1,2,3], Vasile-Adrian Surdu [1,2,3], Ovidiu-Cristian Oprea [2,3,4,5,*], Andreea-Luiza Mîrț [1,2,3,6], Gabriel Vasilievici [6], Augustin Semenescu [7], Anton Ficai [1,2,3,5] and Lia-Mara Dițu [8,9]

1 Science and Engineering of Oxide Materials and Nanomaterials, Faculty of Chemical Engineering and Biotechnologies, University POLITEHNICA of Bucharest, Gh. Polizu 1-7, 011061 Bucharest, Romania
2 National Research Center for Food Safety, University POLITEHNICA of Bucharest, Splaiul Independentei 313, 060042 Bucharest, Romania
3 National Center for Micro and Nanomaterials, University POLITEHNICA of Bucharest, Splaiul Independentei 313, 060042 Bucharest, Romania
4 Department of Inorganic Chemistry, Physical Chemistry and Electrochemistry, Faculty of Chemical Engineering and Biotechnologies, University POLITEHNICA of Bucharest, Gh. Polizu 1-7, 011061 Bucharest, Romania
5 Academy of Romanian Scientists, Ilfov Street 3, 050044 Bucharest, Romania
6 National Institute for Research & Development in Chemistry and Petrochemistry—ICECHIM, 202 Spl. Independentei, 060021 Bucharest, Romania
7 Department Engineering and Management for Transports, University POLITEHNICA of Bucharest, 060042 Bucharest, Romania
8 Department of Microbiology and Immunology, Faculty of Biology, University of Bucharest, 1-3 Aleea Portocalelor, 060101 Bucharest, Romania
9 Research Institute of the University of Bucharest, 050095 Bucharest, Romania
* Correspondence: ovidiu73@yahoo.com

Abstract: Two types of mesoporous materials, MCM-41 and MCM-48, were functionalized by the soft-template method using (3-aminopropyl)triethoxysilane (APTES) as a modifying agent. The obtained mesoporous silica materials were loaded with trans-ferulic acid (FA). In order to establish the morphology and structure of mesoporous materials, a series of specific techniques were used such as: X-ray Diffraction (XRD), Scanning Electron Microscopy (SEM), Brunauer-Emmet-Teller (BET), Fourier Transform Infrared Spectroscopy (FTIR) and thermogravimetric analysis (TGA). We monitored the in vitro release of the loaded FA at two different pH values, by using simulated gastric fluid (SGF) and simulated intestinal fluid (SIF). Additionally, *Staphylococcus aureus* ATCC 25923, *Escherichia coli* ATCC 25922, *Pseudomonas aeruginosa* ATCC 27853 and *Candida albicans* ATCC 10231 were used to evaluate the antimicrobial activity of FA loaded mesoporous silica materials. In conclusion such functionalized mesoporous materials can be employed as controlled release systems for polyphenols extracted from natural sources.

Keywords: mesoporous silica; (3-aminopropyl)triethoxysilane; trans-ferulic acid; antimicrobial activity; controlled release

1. Introduction

As many bioactive substances can often exhibit unwanted effects at high concentrations, while only scanty drug concentrations with low efficacy are arriving at target tissue, various encapsulation methods and drug carriers have been developed [1,2].

Through the morphological control and the functionalization of inorganic nanoparticles, various advances in science have been developed so that delivery systems are more efficient in the transport of different drugs [3–8]. Mesoporous silica nanoparticles (MSNs) represent a new research opportunity for the development of controlled release systems [4,9]. The improvement of the transport systems of active substances in the body led to the development of new drug delivery systems. In the development of these systems, the goal is to keep the drug dose under control, a slow release, targeted release to the area of interest [10–12]. Due to the physico-chemical properties of mesoporous silica (very high pore numbers and specific surface), it allows high loading capacity, good compatibility and easy functionalization [13].

Starting from inorganic precursors, mesoporous silica can have different structures, such as MCM (Mobile Composition of Matter), SBA (Santa Barbara Amorphous), TUD (Technische Universiteit Delft), HMS (Hollow Mesoporous Silica) or MCF (Meso Cellular Form) [14,15]. The MCM family was the first type of mesoporous material synthesized since 1992, which include among other silica types, the hexagonal mesoporous MCM-41 and the cubic mesoporous arranged MCM-48 [16]. The major difference between the two materials is related to the arrangements of the pores. If MCM-41 has the pores arranges uniaxial, the MCM-48 has the pores arranged in a three-dimensional fashion and thus, the release of the active components will be unidirectional for MCM-41 or in all directions for MCM-48 [17].

Surface functionalization of mesoporous silica is one of the methods by which the interaction between drugs and mesoporous silica is improved for better efficiency in targeted delivery [18,19]. Covalent bonding between functional groups and silica can be achieved by grafting and co-condensation, post-synthesis and direct incorporation methods [20–22]. The most common functionalization methodology of the mesoporous silica surface are made with groups such as: amine (3-aminopropyl)triethoxysilane, thiol (3-mercaptopropyl)trimethoxysilane and sulfonic acid (trimethyl[propyl]ammonium chloride) [23–26].

The structure of mesoporous silica allows it to be loaded with drugs, polyphenols or more complex natural agents such as natural extracts [27–29]. Polyphenols are given special attention due to their pharmacological properties and because they are extremely numerous found in various plants, fruits and vegetables [30–34] while their biological activity is very wide. The porous structure of the silica-based materials allows a high loading capacity with various drugs or bioactive substances (e.g., antimicrobials, polyphenols) and further facilitate the controlled release by gradual unloading into the target tissue. By achieving this slower release of the drugs from the pores of the silica particles, a steady concentration of the released substance can be maintained, ensuring a reliable biological activity for longer times [35]. Due to the proven potential of biologically active agents, such as specific polyphenols, in preventing or mitigating the onset of chronic diseases, considerable interest has been shown in the development of dietary supplements containing polyphenols and/or consumer products rich in polyphenols [36,37].

Polyphenols are extremely important components of the human diet due to their special properties such as antioxidant activity, free radical scavenging abilities and the ability to function as antibiotics (exerting anti-diarrheal, anti-ulcer, and anti-inflammatory effects) and to alleviate tissue damage induced by oxidative stress associated with chronic diseases [38–40].

Ferulic acid (FA) is part of the phenolic acid class and is a derivative of cinnamic acid frequently found in numerous plants [41,42]. One of the most important roles of FA is that it has a strong antioxidant activity, but it has multiple pharmacological activities such as antimicrobial, antibacterial, anticancer, anti-inflammatory, antidiabetic, etc. [43–48]. Ferulic acid is a powerful antioxidant ingredient found in many vegetables, fruits and grains. It absorbs UV rays and protects the skin from the harmful effects of ultraviolet radiation, especially erythema and skin irritations. If it is used together with vitamin C and vitamin E, it potentiates the antioxidant effects, the removal of their pigment spots and the stability of the cosmetic product formula.

The aim of this study was to synthesize mesoporous materials, namely MCM-41 and MCM-48, and to functionalize them by grafting with amino groups following the reaction with (3-aminopropyl)triethoxysilane (APTES). The obtained materials were loaded with trans-ferulic acid to observe the loading capacity of mesoporous silica. After obtaining all the materials, they were investigated to determine the pore volume and surface area with Brunauer-Emmet-Teller analysis and the structure of the materials with X-ray diffraction (XRD). The morphology of the synthesized, functionalized and loaded materials was analysed through Scanning Electron Microscopy (SEM), and the identification and estimation of the loading quantity with trans-ferulic acid was determined by Fourier Transform Infrared Spectroscopy (FTIR) in connection with thermogravimetric analysis (TGA). The materials loaded with trans-ferulic acid were subjected to a in vitro release study in two simulated biological fluids with different pH to observe their release profiles. The FA loaded mesoporous silica materials were tested to evaluate the antimicrobial activity on four strains *Staphylococcus aureus* ATCC 25923, *Escherichia coli* ATCC 25922, *Pseudomonas aeruginosa* ATCC 27853 and *Candida albicans* ATCC 1023. The natural agents, such as polyphenols, could be good candidates in the treatment of infections especially when the infections involve resistant bacteria and common antibiotics are not efficient. Moreover, these silica particles loaded with polyphenols have an additional advantage because the residues (faces) does not generates microbial resistance.

2. Materials and Methods

2.1. Materials

Mesoporous silica was prepared starting from tetraethyl orthosilicate (TEOS) as silica precursor, cetyltrimethylammonium bromide (CTAB) as template agent, ammonia (NH_3) and absolute ethanol, all from Merck (Darmstadt, Germany). According to the ratio between the components, two mesoporous systems (MCM41 and MCM48) were obtained as we previously presented in [35,49]. In this paper, a special attention was paid to the influence of the functionalisation and thus, both types of MCM materials were functionalized with (3-aminopropyl)triethoxysilane (APTES) purchased from Sigma Aldrich (St. Louis, MO, USA), while the loading of the mesoporous materials was done with trans-ferulic acid (FA, ≥98%) solution in acetone (both from Sigma Aldrich).

Release study was performed in simulated intestinal and gastric solutions obtained by mixing sodium chloride (NaCl) purchased from Sigma Aldrich, sodium hydroxide (NaOH, 1 N), hydrochloric acid (HCl, 2 N) purchased from S.C. Silal Trading SRL (București, Romania) and potassium dihydrogen phosphate (KH_2PO_4, ≥98%) from Carl Roth (Karlsruhe, Germany).

All the substances were used without further purification in all performed experiments together with distilled water (dw).

All strains tested in this study were obtained from the Microorganisms Collection of the Department of Microbiology, Faculty of Biology & Research Institute of the University of Bucharest.

2.2. Equipment

Mesoporous materials, of MCM-41 and MCM-48 types, and APTES functionalized mesoporous silica, as well as the trans-ferulic acid loaded mesoporous samples, were characterized by modern, usual techniques. X-ray powder diffraction (XRD) diffractograms were recorded by using $Cu_{K\alpha}$ radiation with a Panalytical X'Pert Pro MPD instrument. A Thermo IN50 MX instrument was used to record the FTIR spectra in attenuated total reflectance mode (ATR) for all the samples. The recorded spectra were used to carried out the study of the structural features of the MCM supports as well as the drug delivery systems. BET analysis (the N_2 adsorption isotherms) was performed on a NOVA 2200e Gas Sorption Analyzer (Quantachrome, Boynton Beach, FL, USA), at 77.35 K and relative pressure p/p_0 = 0.005–1.0. Before measurements, the materials were outgassed for 4 h at 110 °C under vacuum. The surface morphology of the samples was examined using a QUANTA INSPECT F electron microscope equipped with a field emission gun and an energy dispersive (EDS) detector, on samples covered with silver. Thermogravimetric analyses were recorded using a Netzsch 449C STA Jupiter instrument in the

20–900 °C temperature interval, in an open crucible, under a dynamic atmosphere of dry air (50 mL/min). A heating rate of 10 °C/min was employed.

The controlled release of trans-ferulic acid from the obtained mesoporous materials was evaluated with an Agilent 1260 Infinity High Performance Liquid Chromatograph equipped with Diode Array Detector (HPLC-DAD). Ultrapure water and acetonitrile (HPLC grade, Sigma Aldrich) were used as mobile phase and separation was performed on an Aqua C18 column (250 × 4.6 mm, 5 μm).

2.3. Preparation and Functionalization of Mesoporous Materials

Both mesoporous materials, MCM-41 and MCM-48, used as a support for functionalization and further loading, were synthesized using the soft template method starting from proper ratio of TEOS and CTAB (Figure 1). The synthesis was carried out under the same conditions, the working conditions being described in our previous work [49].

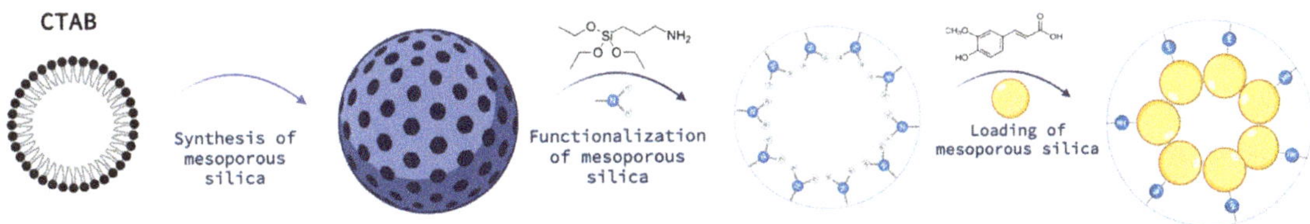

Figure 1. Synthesis of functionalized mesoporous systems loaded with ferulic acid (Created with BioRender.com).

The functionalization of mesoporous silica was done following the method [50], using (3-aminopropyl)triethoxysilane as coupling agent. One gram of each mesoporous material (MCM-41 and MCM-48), was dried in the vacuum drying oven at a temperature of 23 °C for 3 h. After drying, 100 mL ethanol was added and the suspensions were sonicated for one hour. 125 μL of APTES was added to each suspension and left to reflux for 24 h and sonicated for one hour. The obtained suspensions were filtered and left to dry.

2.4. Adsorption of Trans-Ferulic Acid

To load the obtained mesoporous materials, a saturated solution of 0.4 g of trans-ferulic acid (FA) in 4 mL of acetone was prepared. 1 g of mesoporous material was added in a glass vessel and kept under vacuum, 2 mbar, for 30 min. After this period of time, the saturated solution of trans-ferulic acid was added stepwise (in three successive steps) to enter the pores of the material. After drying at 60 °C mesoporous materials loaded trans-ferulic acid were obtained as presented in Table 1. In all cases, the FA was loaded in a 0.4:1 ratio (*w*/*w*) to the mesoporous support materials.

Table 1. Types of mesoporous material loaded with trans-ferulic acid (FA).

Sample Code	Materials Type
MCM-41	MCM-41
MCM-41_APTES	MCM-41: (3-aminopropyl)triethoxysilane
MCM-41_FA	MCM-41: trans-ferulic acid
MCM-41_APTES_FA	MCM-41: (3-aminopropyl)triethoxysilane: trans-ferulic acid
MCM-48	MCM-48
MCM-48_APTES	MCM-48: (3-aminopropyl)triethoxysilane
MCM-48_FA	MCM-48: trans-ferulic acid
MCM-48_APTES_FA	MCM-48: (3-aminopropyl)triethoxysilane: trans-ferulic acid

2.5. In Vitro Release Study

The release profiles of the materials loaded with trans-ferulic acid were evaluated in two simulated biological fluids, simulated gastric fluid (SGF, pH = 1.2) and simulated intestinal fluid (SIF, pH = 6.8) [35,51]. The release of the trans-ferulic acid from the mesoporous materials (functionalized or not with APTES) was done in SGF and SIF (140 mL) solution considering 50 mg mesoporous supports loaded with trans-ferulic acid. Throughout the study, the solutions were kept under magnetic stirring at 37 ± 2 °C. Samples were taken at predetermined time intervals and FA concentration was quantified by high performance liquid chromatography.

2.6. Antimicrobial Activity

Staphylococcus aureus ATCC 25923, *Escherichia coli* ATCC 25922, *Pseudomonas aeruginosa* ATCC 27853 and *Candida albicans* ATCC 10231 were used to evaluate the antimicrobial activity of silica mesoporous materials.

2.6.1. Quantitative Determination of Antimicrobial Activity

The minimum inhibitory concentration (MIC) evaluation was made by using the decimal microdilution method in a liquid medium: Nutrient Broth for bacterial species and Sabouraud for fungal species. In this sense, suspensions of microbial cells are made in a sterile physiological buffer (PBS) using 18–24 h cultures, reaching a standard density of 1.5×10^8 CFU/mL (colony forming units/mL) for bacterial species, respectively 3×10^8 CFU/mL for *Candida* sp. Decimal dilutions are made from each nanoparticle suspension, followed by inoculation with a standard microbial suspension (medium liquid volumetric ratio: microbial suspension = 10:1). Following the same steps, the blank/control (C) samples are performed: sterility and microbial growth. The 96-well plates are incubated at 37 °C for 24 h. The determination of MIC values was performed both by macroscopic observation and by reading at 620 nm (the suspensions are transferred to a sterile plate because the initial plate contains precipitate/NPs deposited on the bottom of the well and would interfere with the absorbance of the medium) [52–54].

2.6.2. Semi-Quantitative Evaluation of Microbial Adherence to an Inert Substratum

The evaluation of the inert substrate adhesion potential of the tested strains was carried out by the crystal violet staining method. After 24 h of incubation, 96-well plates are washed thrice with phosphate buffered saline solution and fixed with cold CH_3OH (5 min). After its removal, the dried plates are stained with 1% crystal violet solution (15 min). The excess dye is removed by washing, and in order to determine the MAIC values (minimum adhesion inhibition concentration), the dye included in the cells adhered to the walls of the well is dissolved with 33% acetic acid. Spectrophotometer readings will be performed at 490 nm with the BioTek Synergy™ HTX ELISA Multi-Mode Reader (BioTek, Winooski, VT, USA) [52–54].

3. Results and Discussions

All the materials, including pure supports as well as the loaded mesoporous materials were characterized by the appropriate physico-chemical methods.

3.1. X-ray Diffraction

All four diffraction patterns recorded at low angles on the mesoporous MCM-41 materials, Figure 2, present the typical arrangement for these materials. The strong diffraction peak from 2.43°, is attributed to the (100) crystallization plane, while the other less intense peaks correspond to the (110), (200) and (210) crystallization planes, characteristic to the hexagonal mesoporous MCM-41 structure. These peaks are consistent with literature data [55].

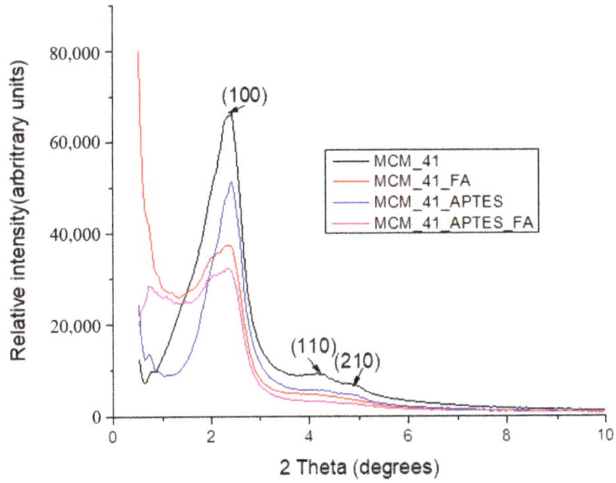

Figure 2. X-ray diffractograms for the MCM-41 based samples: MCM-41, MCM-41_FA, MCM-41_APTES and MCM-41_APTES_FA.

From the XRD data it can be seen that the functionalization of MCM-41 with APTES does not alter the ordered mesoporous structure of silica, but a slight shift and decrease in the intensity of the peak feature of the (100) crystallization plane is observed [56,57]. This is due to the formation of a silica layer bearing aminopropyl moieties on the surface and in the pores of the mesoporous material as a result of the hydrolysis and condensation reactions that take place during the functionalization reaction. At the same time, the pores of the mesoporous material decrease in size and this is also visible in XRD.

In addition, it is observed that the loading of MCM-41 and MCM-41_APTES materials with trans-ferulic acid, carried out under vacuum, does not alter the ordered mesoporous structure of the silica, but induces a considerable decrease in the intensity of the peaks and alters the shape of the peak characteristic for the (100) crystallization plane, due to the absorption of trans-ferulic acid. Due to the specific pattern of the XRD spectra it is expected that FA is mostly loaded inside the pores [35].

The X-ray diffractograms obtained for MCM-48 based materials, Figure 3, present the characteristic (211) peak at 2.52°, while the other three important peaks, (220), (420) and (332) are positioned at higher 2Θ values. This arrangement is characteristic to the cubic structure of MCM-48 [58]. The X-ray diffraction data obtained for MCM-48 materials functionalized with APTES, indicates a slight shift of the peak corresponding to the (211) crystallization plane [57,59] due to the formation of a silica layer on the surface and in the pores of the mesoporous material as a result of the reactions of hydrolysis and condensation occurring during functionalization reaction. At the same time, the pores of the mesoporous material decrease in size.

For the mesoporous materials that were loaded with ferulic acid, the XRD data indicates a considerable decrease in the intensity and the degree of crystallinity, in addition to the shift of the (220) and (211) characteristic peaks. All these information, the decrease in intensity, the crystallinity degree and the characteristic peaks shifting, may indicate the loading of polyphenols in the pores of the mesoporous material, but also a strong interaction between the two components.

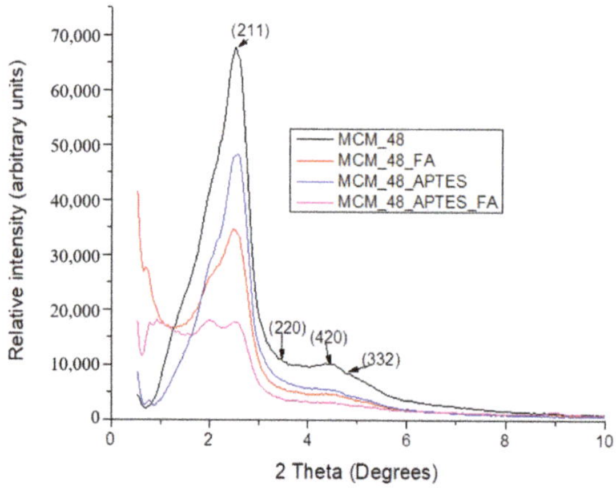

Figure 3. X-ray data for the MCM-48 based samples: MCM-48, MCM-48_FA, MCM-48_APTES and MCM-48_ APTES _FA.

3.2. Specific Surface Area—Brunauer-Emmet-Teller Adsorption Isotherms

Following the functionalization process of the mesoporous material MCM-41/48 with APTES, it can be seen from BET data (Table 2) that the specific surface area slightly decreases from 1365 m^2/g for MCM-41, to 1014 m^2/g for the material MCM-41_APTES and from 1582 m^2/g for MCM-48, to 1555 m^2/g for the material MCM-48_APTES as a result of the deposition of APTES on the surface of the mesoporous nanoparticles, which causes the material's pores to become narrower as a consequence of the functionalization. The overall surface area of these mesoporous materials has two components, the external surface area of the spherical particles, with a small contribution—less than 1 m^2/g, and the internal surface area of the cylindrical pores, which assure the very high surface area. Because during the loading process, the FA will enter inside the pores of the material, filling them, the BET determined specific surface area will drastically decrease, roughly by a factor of 3. As a consequence of the FA loading, the pore size decrease, and some of them even disappear when the loading degree is high, therefore, the overall specific surface area decreases considerable.

Table 2. BET characteristics of mesoporous materials.

Type of Material	BET Surface Area m^2/g	Langmuir Surface Area m^2/g	Volume of Pores cm^3/g
MCM-41	1365	2.294	0.783
MCM-41_APTES	1014	2.251	0.5706
MCM-41_APTES_FA	301.3	2.564	0.1931
MCM-48	1582	2.383	0.9423
MCM-48_APTES	1555	1.897	0.7371
MCM-48_APTES_FA	504.6	2.218	0.2798

In the case of MCM-41_APTES, the functionalization with APTES leads to a decrease of the determined BET surface area of 1.34 times, while after FA loading, in the case of MCM-41_APTES_FA the decrease is 3.36 times. In the case of MCM-48, a higher BET surface area is observed compared to MCM-41, but after functionalization the BET surface area for MCM-48_APTES slightly decreases (by 1.01 times). After loading with FA the BET surface area for MCM_48_APTES_FA decreases by 3.08 times.

Analysing the data from Table 2, we can conclude that the BET data are in good agreement with the XRD analysis, indicating that the FA is adsorbed inside the pores of the mesoporous materials.

3.3. Fourier Transform Infrared Spectroscopy

In order to characterize the structure, the FT-IR spectra of MCM-41, MCM-41_FA, MCM-41_APTES and MCM-41_APTES_FA (Figure 4). In the FTIR spectra of MCM-41 mesoporous materials the most important peaks of characteristic vibrations can be identified. The broad bands between ~3200–3400 cm^{-1} correspond to the associated silanol (Si-OH) surface groups and adsorbed hydrogen-bonded water molecules. The bands at 1239 cm^{-1} and 1057 cm^{-1} can be assigned to the stretching vibrations of the asymmetric Si-O-Si units, while the band from ~980 cm^{-1} is associated with silanol groups of MCM-41. The stretching vibrations of the symmetric Si-O-Si units can be identified as the band at 807 cm^{-1} and the peak from 440 cm^{-1} is generated by the Si-O-Si moiety's deformation vibrations [60,61].

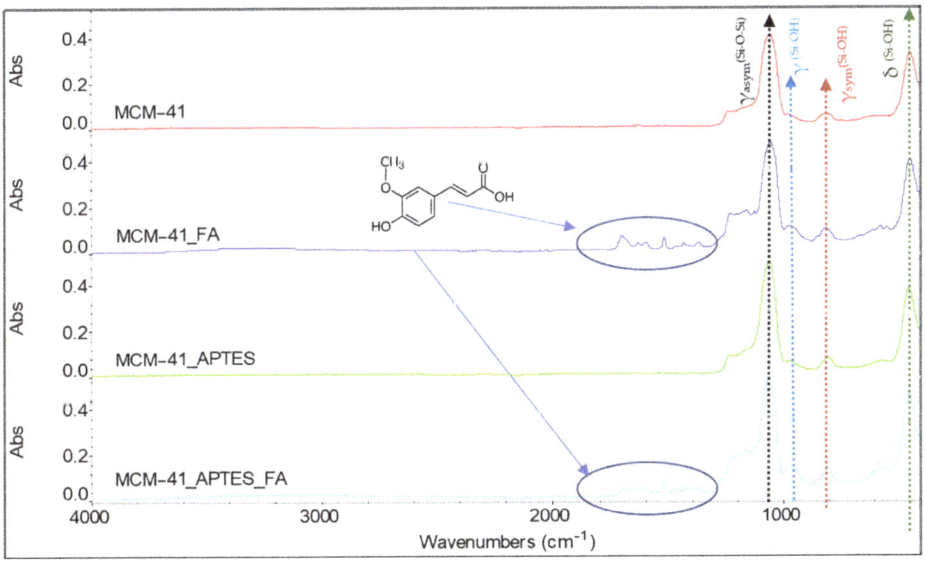

Figure 4. FTIR spectra and band assignments for the samples MCM-41, MCM-41_FA, MCM-41_APTES and MCM-41_APTES_FA.

The characteristic peaks for Si-O-Si bonds from the APTES functionalized mesoporous material, shifted to slightly higher wavelengths, can be identified in the FTIR spectrum (Figure 4). In addition, the bands characteristic of the functional groups in the APTES structure are present. The presence in the FTIR spectra of the band at 2980 cm^{-1}, characteristic of the three methylene (propyl) groups clearly proves the functionalization of MCM-41.

Unfortunately, the bands associated with NH_2 cannot be identified because of the lower molar absorptivity and lower content. Additionally, the bending vibration bands characteristic of the N–H bond normally present around 714 cm^{-1}, the symmetric bending vibration band characteristic of the $-NH_2$ group and the stretching vibration band corresponding to the C–N bond normally present around the value of 1000–1200 cm^{-1} cannot be highlighted as a result of the overlap with the vibration/stretching bands characteristic of Si–O–Si bonds in the range 1000–1130 cm^{-1} and that of $Si–CH_2$ stretching in the range of 1200–1250 cm^{-1} [58].

By loading MCM-41 and MCM-41_APTES with trans-ferulic acid, a series of new bands appear in the FTIR spectra (Figure 4), between 1300–1800 cm^{-1}, being associated with the presence of FA into the mesoporous material. The peaks from 1684 cm^{-1} and 1700 cm^{-1} are associated with the stretching vibrations of the functional groups C=O and –OH, from FA. The peaks from ~1360 cm^{-1} and 1629 cm^{-1} (for MCM-41_FA) and 1387 cm^{-1} and 1630 cm^{-1} (for MCM-41_APTES_FA) are assigned to the stretching vibration of the bond between the aromatic nucleus and the carboxyl moiety in the FA [35]. The observed shifts can be explained considering the interactions which appears between the support and trans-ferulic acid.

In the FTIR spectra recorded for the MCM-48 type mesoporous materials (Figure 5), one can also observe the most important vibration peaks, characteristic for the Si-O-Si network, at ~1239 cm^{-1}, 1054 cm^{-1}, 978 cm^{-1}, 810 cm^{-1} and 436 cm^{-1}, the other features being similar with those of MCM-41 corresponding materials.

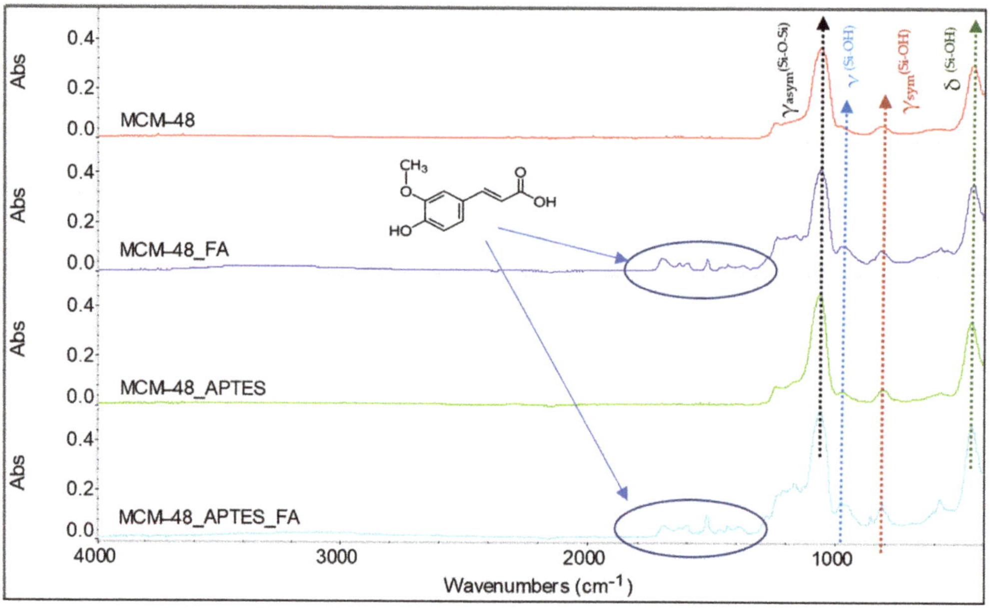

Figure 5. FTIR spectra and band assignments for the samples MCM-48, MCM-48_FA, MCM-48_APTES and MCM-48_APTES_FA.

3.4. *Scanning Electron Microscopy (SEM)*

SEM micrographs (Figure 6) recorded for the mesoporous materials based on MCM-41 indicate that particles have variable size of hundreds of nanometres and a spherical morphology. When compared to the bare MCM-41, SEM images of MCM-41_FA and MCM-41_APTES_FA show some minor heterogeneities on the external surfaces of the mesoporous silica spheres, which can be attributed to the deposition of ferulic acid. Considering their incidence, and low content, it can consider that the ferulic acid (FA) is mostly deposited into the pores of the mesoporous materials. At high magnification (100,000×), it could be clearly observed that the SEM images of the MCM-41 sample were more translucent compared to the samples modified with APTES or loaded with ferulic acid (FA). These observations are in good agreement with the XRD and FTIR data, but also with the BET analysis [35].

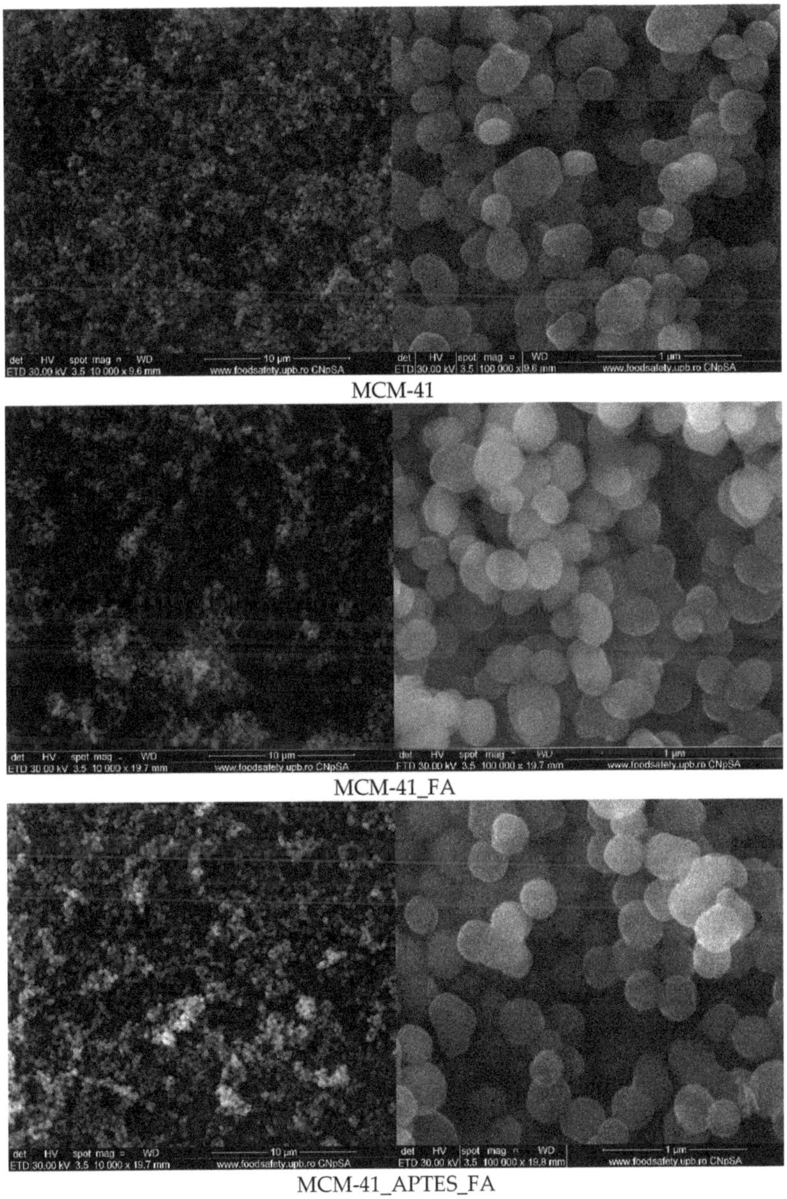

Figure 6. SEM micrographs for mesoporous materials based on MCM-41 support.

SEM micrographs (Figure 7) recorded for the mesoporous materials based on MCM-48 indicate the presence of quasi-spherical silica particles with sizes in the 150–400 nm interval. In addition, similarly to MCM-41 based samples, we can consider that FA is mainly loaded inside the pores.

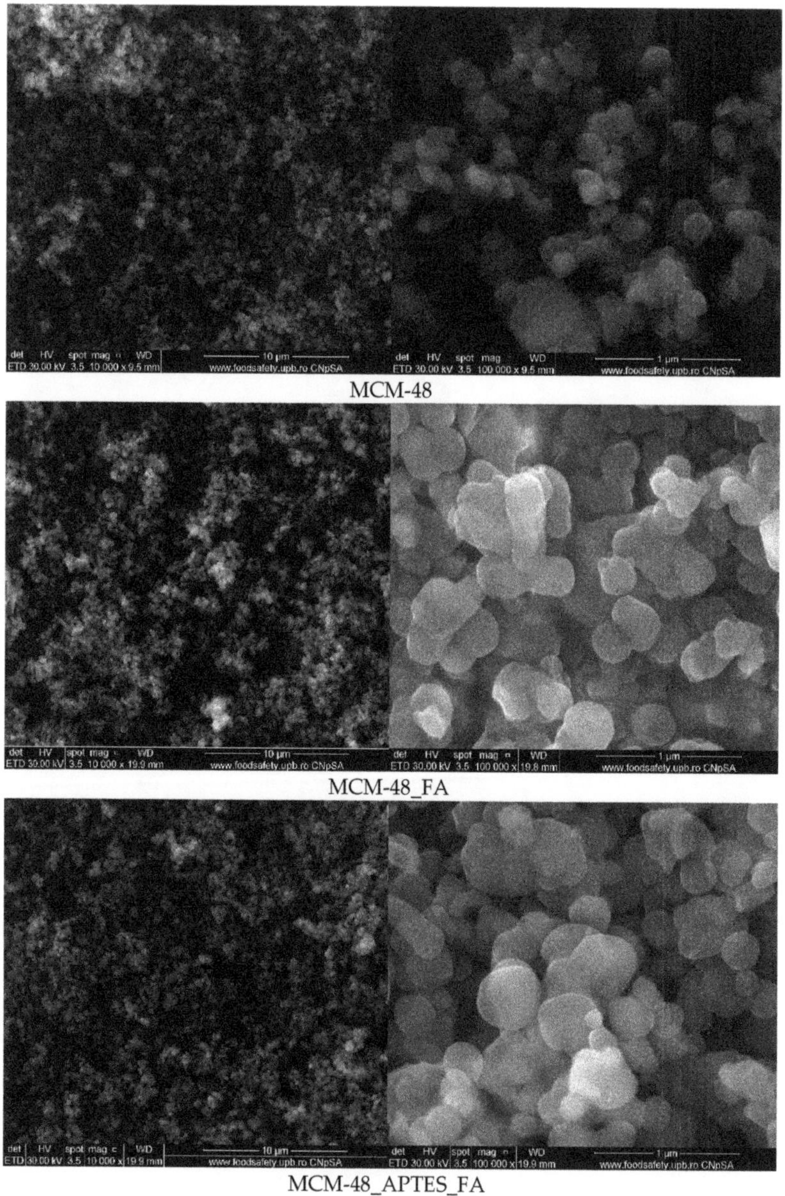

Figure 7. SEM micrographs for mesoporous materials based on MCM-48 support.

3.5. Thermogravimetric Analysis

The thermal stability of the samples, both consisting of mesoporous materials and materials loaded with polyphenols, was studied by thermogravimetric analysis. Firstly the TG curves for MCM-41 (Figure 8) and MCM-48 (Figure 9) permits the determination of some parameters like surface density of adsorbed H_2O molecules or -OH moieties, calculated as indicated in [35,49] (Table 3). The recorded mass loss up to 200 °C (1st mass loss) is generated by the elimination of physically adsorbed H_2O molecules, from particles surface or from inside the pores. The 2nd mass loss, in the interval 200–900 °C is generated by the condensation of silanol moieties (Si-OH) which leads to the silica densification.

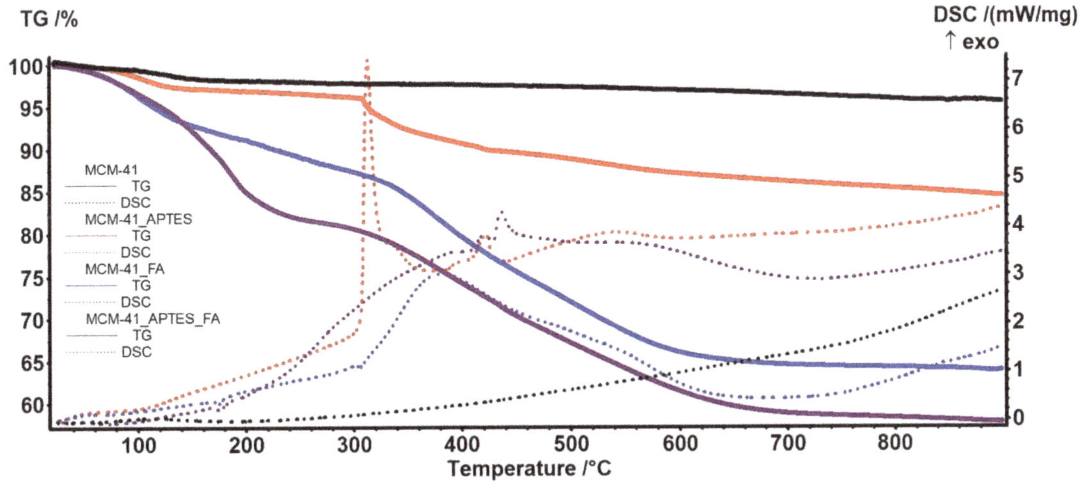

Figure 8. The TG (solid)—DSC (dotted) curves for the MCM-41 (black); MCM-41_APTES (red); MCM-41_FA (blue) and MCM-41_APTES_FA (purple).

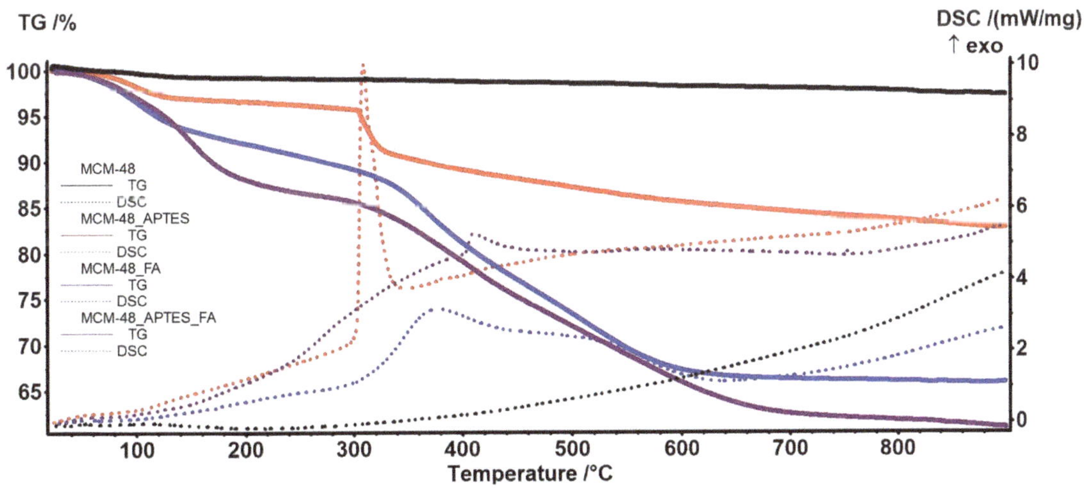

Figure 9. The TG (solid)—DSC (dotted) curves for the MCM-48 (black); MCM-48_APTES (red); MCM-48_FA (blue) and MCM-48_APTES_FA (purple).

Table 3. Surface density of adsorbed H2O molecules and -OH moieties.

Sample	1st Mass Loss (%)	2nd Mass Loss (%)	n_{H2O} (mmol/g)	n_{OH} (mmol/g)	N_{H2O} (Groups/nm^2)	N_{OH} (Groups/nm^2)
MCM-41	1.83	2.61	1.02	2.90	0.45	1.28
MCM-48	0.94	1.97	0.52	2.19	0.20	0.83

The successful functionalization of the MCM samples with APTES is indicated by the different TG/DSC curves shape for the functionalized mesoporous materials MCM-41_APTES (Figure 8) and MCM-48_APTES (Figure 9) vs. bare support. The sample are presenting a small mass loss up to 305 °C because of elimination of water molecules adsorbed on the surface of nanoparticles and condensation of –OH moieties. The process is similar with that of bare MCM-41 or MCM-48, but with higher intensity, indicating a better adsorption capacity. APTES has a boiling point of 217 °C but no thermal effect is recorded up to 300 °C, indicating the successful bonding between MCM and APTES. After 305 °C the samples are suffering a degradation process, with the main mass loss being recorded up to ~700 °C. This is an oxidation process of the organic part as indicated by the strong exothermic effects with peaks at 313 and 309 °C respectively.

The MCM-41_FA and MCM-41_APTES_FA samples present a weak endothermic peak with onset at 170.3 and 168.2 °C respectively, assigned to the melting of loaded FA. Same type of endothermic effect is present on DSC curve of MCM-48_FA sample, with onset at 170.3. For the MCM-48_APTES_FA sample the effect is not visible, only a small inflexion point at 144.8 °C being detected. The lack of a clear melting effect and the smaller temperature recorded as an inflexion on DSC curve for the MCM-48_APTES_FA sample indicates stronger interactions between FA and the mesoporous support in this case. The relevant data are presented in Table 4.

Table 4. Most important data from thermogravimetric analysis.

Sample	Mass Loss RT-305 °C (%)	Mass Loss 305–700 °C (%)	Residual Mass (%)	Estimated FA Load (%)
MCM-41_APTES	3.99	9.94	84.49	-
MCM-41_FA	12.82	22.70	63.86	33.15
MCM-41_APTES_FA	19.55	21.65	57.74	31.66
MCM-48_APTES	4.47	11.19	82.65	-
MCM-48_FA	11.08	22.77	65.81	32.26
MCM-48_APTES_FA	14.63	22.98	60.90	26.32

The results indicate that the APTES functionalization has an impact especially on estimated load on MCM-48_APTES_FA vs. MCM-48_FA, decreasing the FA loaded amount from ~32 to ~26%.

3.6. *In Vitro Release Study*

Release curves of FA from mesoporous materials and functionalized mesoporous materials are shown in Figure 10. As can be seen, all unmodified mesoporous materials loaded with FA had a fast release profile of up to 70–80% (within six hours) compared to mesoporous materials functionalized with amino groups and loaded with FA that had a slower release profile of up to 40–60% (within 24 h) [35]. From this difference between the release profiles, it can be clearly observed that the functionalization with aminopropyl groups considerably reduced the release rate of the active substance. Considering also, our previous works [35,49] it is obvious that the chemical surface modification with APTES or other silanization agents can be a good solution to induce a better tuning capacity of the release of these polyphenols for specific applications, including food supplements. As can be seen in the study, the release rate depends on the interactions of the functional group with the substance, which means that the use of different silanization agents bearing (-NH_2, -COOH, -SH) could be exploited in tuning the delivery characteristics of the trans-ferulic acid [62]. The functionalization of the mesoporous materials with aminopropyl moieties has an important impact on both the release profile and rate over the first six hours. It can see that the release is slightly increasing over this period of time and this can be, most probably explained by the development of strong hydrogen bonds between the NH_2 (amino moieties of the MCM support) and OH and COOH (of trans-ferulic acid)—also visualized in FTIR as a ~28 cm^{-1} shift of a specific band of COOH. Depending on the pH, even electrostatic interactions can appear, amino groups being susceptible to protonation, especially at pH $<$ 7.2 while carboxyl groups are susceptible to deprotonation at pH $>$ 7. As indicated by the experimental data presented in [63] the normal gastrointestinal transit time can be divided in three intervals: first 2–5 h are spent in the stomach, followed by 2–6 h of release in small intestine and 10–60 h in the large bowel. By coupling these times with the data obtained from release profiles in SGF and SIF, we can state that between 20–40% of FA will be released in the stomach (depending on actual transit time), with additional 20–40% of loaded FA being release in the small intestine. Additional FA quantities can be released in large bowel as a function of the actual transit time. In addition, after FA loading, the APTES functionalized MCM-41 or MCM-48 particles can be embedded in a mucoadhesive system [64,65], that will allow modulation of residence time and FA recovery [66]. Furthemore, by comparing with antimicrobial drugs, such as antibiotics, the negative environmental impact is low as these systems don't lead to antimicrobial resistance.

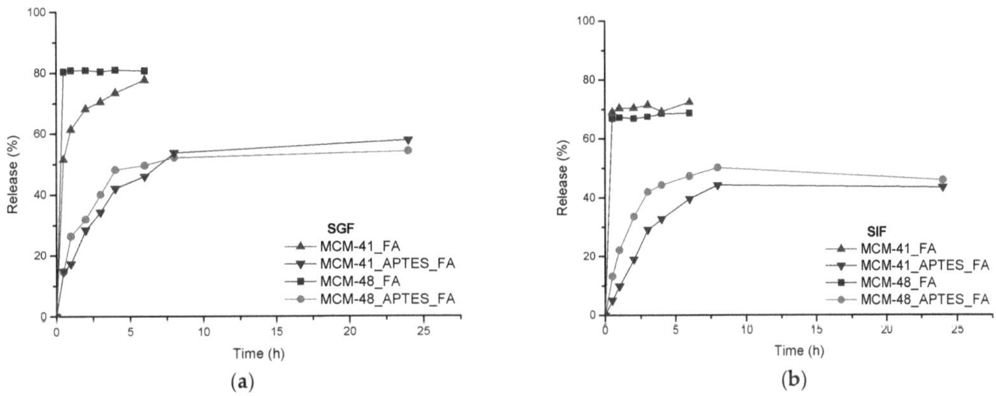

Figure 10. Release profiles for FA from the MCM-41_FA; MCM-41_APTES_FA; MCM-48_FA; MCM-48_APTES_FA samples in SGF (**a**) and SIF (**b**).

In both, SGF and SIF, even after 24 h, the cumulative release of FA from the silanized mesoporous samples remain still below that from the bare mesoporous systems at 6 h, proving that aminopropyl groups have an important impact over the release rate. In SGF, the delayed nature of the delivery of FA is also observed but the difference between the cumulative releases of FA from the silanized samples comparing with the bare mesoporous samples is lower.

By comparing the MCM-48_FA with MCM-48_APTES_FA system, the first observation is that the release curves are similar in both simulated biological fluids, SGF and SIF. Unlike the systems containing MCM-48, the systems based on MCM-41 present a different behaviour. MCM-41_FA, had a faster release profile in the simulated intestinal fluid while and MCM-41_APTES_FA had a slower release when compared to MCM-48 materials.

3.7. Antimicrobial Activity

The mesoporous silica materials were tested to evaluate the antimicrobial activity on four strains *Staphylococcus aureus* ATCC 25923, *Escherichia coli* ATCC 25922, *Pseudomonas aeruginosa* ATCC 27853 and *Candida albicans* ATCC 1023.

3.7.1. Quantitative Evaluation of Antimicrobial Activity

The lowest concentration at which the tested samples still can inhibit the microbial growth represents the minimum inhibitory concentration (MIC). The obtained values (mg/mL) are presented in Table 5.

Table 5. Determined values for minimum inhibitory concentration (MIC).

Strains	MIC (mg/mL)								
	MCM-41	MCM-41_APTES	MCM-41_FA	MCM-41_APTES_FA	MCM-48	MCM-48_APTES	MCM-48_FA	MCM-48_APTES_FA	C Ferulic Acid
S. aureus ATCC 25923	0.1	0.001	1	0.001	0.01	0.01	10	0.01	10
E. coli ATCC 25922	0.1	0.1	1	0.1	0.1	0.1	0.01	0.1	1
P. aeruginosa ATCC 27853	0.01	0.01	1	0.01	0.01	0.01	0.1	1	1
C. albicans ATCC 10231	1	0.01	1	0.001	0.01	0.1	0.1	1	100

The quantitative results for the silica-based mesoporous materials indicated the highest sensitivity against *P. aeruginosa* which is an important observation, considering that this species is frequently involved in healthcare associate infections. It can be observed that the materials loaded with ferulic acid negatively influence the growth of pathogens strains tested, compared to the controls. The MCM-41_APTES_FA and MCM-41_APTES samples determined the highest sensitivity of *S. aureus*, *P. aeruginosa* and *C. albicans*, with MIC values ranging from 0.01 and 0.001 mg/mL. The MCM-41_APTES_FA presented the best antimicrobial activity against Gram-positive and Gram-negative bacteria tested in this study. Overall, a synergic effect between mesoporous materials and ferulic acid can be observed.

A recent study [67] also observed the bacteriostatic effect of ferulic acid against Gram-positive and Gram-negative bacteria. Also, Borges et al. [45] determined the antibacterial activity of ferulic acid against *S. aureus*, *E. coli*, *P. aeruginosa* and *L. monocytes*. The MIC values are 1 mg/mL for *E. coli* and *P. aeruginosa*, and 1.25 mg/mL for *S. aureus*. Ferulic acid produced changes in membrane properties, especially hydrophobicity changes, decreasing negative charge and damage to molecular mechanisms.

3.7.2. Semi-Quantitative Assessment of Microbial Adherence to the Inert Substratum

In Table 6 are presented the minimum inhibition concentrations (mg/mL) for adherence to the inert substratum, for the silica-based mesoporous materials.

Table 6. Determination of minimum adhesion inhibition concentration (MAIC).

Strains	MAIC (mg/mL)								
	MCM-41	MCM-41_APTES	MCM-41_FA	MCM-41_APTES_FA	MCM-48	MCM-48_APTES	MCM-48_FA	MCM-48_APTES_FA	C Ferulic Acid
S. aureus ATCC 25923	0.1	0.001	0.1	0.001	0.01	0.01	1	0.01	1
E. coli ATCC 25922	0.1	0.1	1	0.1	0.1	0.1	0.01	0.1	0.1
P. aeruginosa ATCC 27853	0.01	0.01	1	0.01	0.01	0.01	0.1	1	1
C. albicans ATCC 10231	0.1	0.001	1	0.001	0.01	0.01	0.01	1	100

As indicated by the MIC and MAIC values (Tables 5 and 6), *S. aureus*, *E. coli* and *P. aeruginosa* are the most sensitive strains. The lowest values of MAIC range from 0.001 and 0.1 mg/mL in the case of silica-based mesoporous materials. Among all the studied samples, MCM-41_APTES_FA prevented the adherence of pathogen strains to the inert substratum, respectively, the development of the mature and stable biofilm, and presenting the most pronounced inhibitory effect. The samples functionalized with APTES and/or loaded with ferulic acid present a better bacteriostatic effect on the strain's growth than mesoporous silica. Accordingly, with the previous assays, it seems that ferulic acid not only determined the damage to cell growth but also MCM-41/MCM-48 functionalized with

APTES induced the hydrophobicity changes and the bacteriostatic effects. Furthermore, ferulic acid, as a dietary polyphenol, improves the modulation of gut microbiota [68,69] and the antimicrobial activity of silica-based mesoporous materials loaded with ferulic acid and, in vitro release profiles, confirms the potential for these materials as food supplements. In future, we want to continue this study with biocompatibility assay and the influence of these materials on probiotic bacteria/intestinal microbiota.

4. Conclusions

In this study, two types of functionalized mesoporous materials, MCM-41 and MCM-48, were synthesized by the soft-template method using (3-aminopropyl)triethoxysilane (APTES) as a modifying agent. The BET, TGA and XRD analyses indicate that mesoporous materials were obtained and further functionalized with APTES. The as obtained functionalized mesoporous materials were loaded with trans-ferulic acid using the vacuum assisted loading technology and found that the loading mainly occurs within the pores. The APTES functionalized mesoporous materials exhibited comparatively loading capacity when compared with the simple MCM-41, but smaller values for MCM-48. Strong interaction between the functionalized support and trans-ferulic acid are proved by a strong FTIR shift of about 28 cm^{-1} of the carboxyl group, and lower melting temperature of the loaded FA. Due to these strong interactions, the release rate of FA decreased significantly in both SIF and SGF, which can be beneficial allowing the development of sustained drug delivery systems of biological active agents, including polyphenols, for antimicrobial, antibacterial, anticancer, anti-inflammatory or antidiabetic purposes. The use of ferulic acid, instead of a specific antibiotic, has the advantage that the release into the nature of the residual polyphenol (FA not released within the gastrointestinal tract) will not have a negative environmental impact.

Author Contributions: Conceptualization, A.F. and G.P.; methodology, O.-C.O., G.P. and D.F.; validation, A.F., R.D.T. and A.S., formal analysis, V.-A.S., G.V. and C.-I.I.; investigation, L.M., D.F., C.-I.I., R.D.T., V.-A.S., A.-L.M., G.V. and L.-M.D.; writing—original draft preparation, A.F., D.F., L.M., A.-L.M. and L.-M.D.; writing—review and editing, O.-C.O., G.P., G.V. and D.F.; supervision, A.S. and A.F.; project administration, R.D.T.; funding acquisition, O.-C.O. All authors have read and agreed to the published version of the manuscript.

Funding: This work was supported by a grant of the Ministry of Research, Innovation and Digitization, CCCDI—UEFISCDI, project number PN-III-P2-2.1-PED-2021-1788, within PNCDI III; 647PED/2022 "Nutraceutice nanostructurate inovative cu bioactivități sinergice pentru protecție hepato-digestivă".

Institutional Review Board Statement: Not applicable.

Informed Consent Statement: Not applicable.

Data Availability Statement: Not applicable.

Acknowledgments: Contribution of A.-L.M. and G.V. was supported by the Ministry of Research, Innovation, and Digitization through Program 1—Development of the national research and development system, Subprogram 1.2-Institutional Performance- Projects to finance excellence in RDI, Grant no. 15PFE/2021.

Conflicts of Interest: The authors declare no conflict of interest. The funders had no role in the design of the study; in the collection, analyses, or interpretation of data; in the writing of the manuscript; or in the decision to publish the results.

References

1. Nastyshyn, S.; Stetsyshyn, Y.; Raczkowska, J.; Nastishin, Y.; Melnyk, Y.; Panchenko, Y.; Budkowski, A. Temperature-Responsive Polymer Brush Coatings for Advanced Biomedical Applications. *Polymers* **2022**, *14*, 4245. [CrossRef] [PubMed]
2. Huang, Y.Q.; Cao, L.; Parakhonskiy, B.V.; Skirtach, A.G. Hard, Soft, and Hard-and-Soft Drug Delivery Carriers Based on $CaCO_3$ and Alginate Biomaterials: Synthesis, Properties, Pharmaceutical Applications. *Pharmaceutics* **2022**, *14*, 909. [CrossRef] [PubMed]

3. Stephen, S.; Gorain, B.; Choudhury, H.; Chatterjee, B. Exploring the role of mesoporous silica nanoparticle in the development of novel drug delivery systems. *Drug Deliv. Transl. Res.* **2022**, *12*, 105–123. [CrossRef] [PubMed]
4. Porrang, S.; Davaran, S.; Rahemi, N.; Allahyari, S.; Mostafavi, E. How Advancing are Mesoporous Silica Nanoparticles? A Comprehensive Review of the Literature. *Int. J. Nanomed.* **2022**, *17*, 1803–1827. [CrossRef]
5. Motelica, L.; Ficai, D.; Oprea, O.; Ficai, A.; Trusca, R.D.; Andronescu, E.; Holban, A.M. Biodegradable Alginate Films with ZnO Nanoparticles and Citronella Essential Oil-A Novel Antimicrobial Structure. *Pharmaceutics* **2021**, *13*, 1020. [CrossRef]
6. Mihaly, M.; Comanescu, A.F.; Rogozea, E.A.; Meghea, A. Nonionic Microemulsion Extraction of Ni (II) from Wastewater. *Mol. Cryst. Liq. Cryst.* **2010**, *523*, 63–72. [CrossRef]
7. Motelica, L.; Vasile, B.S.; Ficai, A.; Surdu, A.V.; Ficai, D.; Oprea, O.C.; Andronescu, E.; Jinga, D.C.; Holban, A.M. Influence of the Alcohols on the ZnO Synthesis and Its Properties: The Photocatalytic and Antimicrobial Activities. *Pharmaceutics* **2022**, *14*, 2842. [CrossRef]
8. Ficai, D.; Ficai, A.; Vasile, B.S.; Ficai, M.; Oprea, O.; Guran, C.; Andronescu, E. Synthesis of Rod-Like Magnetite by Using Low Magnetic Field. *Dig. J. Nanomater. Bios.* **2011**, *6*, 943–951.
9. Vallet-Regi, M.; Schuth, F.; Lozano, D.; Colilla, M.; Manzano, M. Engineering mesoporous silica nanoparticles for drug delivery: Where are we after two decades? *Chem. Soc. Rev.* **2022**, *51*, 5365–5451. [CrossRef]
10. Patra, J.K.; Das, G.; Fraceto, L.F.; Campos, E.V.R.; Rodriguez-Torres, M.D.P.; Acosta-Torres, L.S.; Diaz-Torres, L.A.; Grillo, R.; Swamy, M.K.; Sharma, S.; et al. Nano based drug delivery systems: Recent developments and future prospects. *J. Nanobiotechnol.* **2018**, *16*, 71. [CrossRef]
11. Petrisor, G.; Motelica, L.; Craciun, L.N.; Oprea, O.C.; Ficai, D.; Ficai, A. Melissa officinalis: Composition, Pharmacological Effects and Derived Release Systems-A Review. *Int. J. Mol. Sci.* **2022**, *23*, 3591. [CrossRef] [PubMed]
12. Mihaly, M.; Lacatusu, I.; Meghea, A. Sulphonephtalein chromophore as molecular probe in micelle systems. *Rev. Chim.-Buchar.* **2007**, *58*, 929–932.
13. Trzeciak, K.; Chotera-Ouda, A.; Bak-Sypien, I.I.; Potrzebowski, M.J. Mesoporous Silica Particles as Drug Delivery Systems-The State of the Art in Loading Methods and the Recent Progress in Analytical Techniques for Monitoring These Processes. *Pharmaceutics* **2021**, *13*, 950. [CrossRef]
14. Kazemzadeh, P.; Sayadi, K.; Toolabi, A.; Sayadi, J.; Zeraati, M.; Chauhan, N.P.S.; Sargazi, G. Structure-Property Relationship for Different Mesoporous Silica Nanoparticles and its Drug Delivery Applications: A Review. *Front. Chem.* **2022**, *10*, 823785. [CrossRef]
15. Dolete, G.; Purcareanu, B.; Mihaiescu, D.E.; Ficai, D.; Oprea, O.C.; Birca, A.C.; Chircov, C.; Vasile, B.S.; Vasilievici, G.; Ficai, A.; et al. A Comparative Loading and Release Study of Vancomycin from a Green Mesoporous Silica. *Molecules* **2022**, *27*, 5589. [CrossRef] [PubMed]
16. Wang, Y.Z.; Sun, L.Z.; Jiang, T.Y.; Zhang, J.H.; Zhang, C.; Sun, C.S.; Deng, Y.H.; Sun, J.; Wang, S.L. The investigation of MCM-48-type and MCM-41-type mesoporous silica as oral solid dispersion carriers for water insoluble cilostazol. *Drug Dev. Ind. Pharm.* **2014**, *40*, 819–828. [CrossRef]
17. Kumar, D.; Schumacher, K.; von Hohenesche, C.D.F.; Grun, M.; Unger, K.K. MCM-41, MCM-48 and related mesoporous adsorbents: Their synthesis and characterisation. *Colloid Surf. A* **2001**, *187*, 109–116. [CrossRef]
18. Chircov, C.; Matei, M.F.; Neacsu, I.A.; Vasile, B.S.; Oprea, O.C.; Croitoru, A.M.; Trusca, R.D.; Andronescu, E.; Sorescu, I.; Barbuceanu, F. Iron Oxide-Silica Core-Shell Nanoparticles Functionalized with Essential Oils for Antimicrobial Therapies. *Antibiotics* **2021**, *10*, 1138. [CrossRef]
19. Mihaly, M.; Lacatusu, I.; Enesca, I.A.; Meghea, A. Hybride nanomaterials based on silica coated C-60 clusters obtained by microemulsion technique. *Mol. Cryst. Liq. Cryst.* **2008**, *483*, 205–215. [CrossRef]
20. Vinu, A.; Hossain, K.Z.; Ariga, K. Recent advances in functionalization of mesoporous silica. *J. Nanosci. Nanotechnol.* **2005**, *5*, 347–371. [CrossRef]
21. Narayan, R.; Gadag, S.; Garg, S.; Nayak, U.Y. Understanding the Effect of Functionalization on Loading Capacity and Release of Drug from Mesoporous Silica Nanoparticles: A Computationally Driven Study. *ACS Omega* **2022**, *7*, 8229–8245. [CrossRef] [PubMed]
22. Culita, D.C.; Simonescu, C.M.; Patescu, R.E.; Dragne, M.; Stanica, N.; Oprea, O. o-Vanillin functionalized mesoporous silica-coated magnetite nanoparticles for efficient removal of Pb(II) from water. *J. Solid State Chem.* **2016**, *238*, 311–320. [CrossRef]
23. Alswieleh, A.M. Modification of Mesoporous Silica Surface by Immobilization of Functional Groups for Controlled Drug Release. *J. Chem.* **2020**, *2020*, 9176257. [CrossRef]
24. Beagan, A.; Alotaibi, K.; Almakhlafi, M.; Algarabli, W.; Alajmi, N.; Alanazi, M.; Alwaalah, H.; Alharbi, F.; Alshammari, R.; Alswieleh, A. Amine and sulfonic acid functionalized mesoporous silica as an effective adsorbent for removal of methylene blue from contaminated water. *J. King Saud. Univ. Sci.* **2022**, *34*, 101762. [CrossRef]
25. Yang, L.M.; Wang, Y.J.; Luo, G.S.; Dai, Y.Y. Functionalization of SBA-15 mesoporous silica with thiol or sulfonic acid groups under the crystallization conditions. *Micropor. Mesopor. Mat.* **2005**, *84*, 275–282. [CrossRef]
26. Culita, D.C.; Simonescu, C.M.; Patescu, R.E.; Preda, S.; Stanica, N.; Munteanu, C.; Oprea, O. Polyamine Functionalized Magnetite Nanoparticles as Novel Adsorbents for Cu(II) Removal from Aqueous Solutions. *J. Inorg. Organomet. Polym. Mater.* **2017**, *27*, 490–502. [CrossRef]

27. Chircov, C.; Spoiala, A.; Paun, C.; Craciun, L.; Ficai, D.; Ficai, A.; Andronescu, E.; Turculet, S.C. Mesoporous Silica Platforms with Potential Applications in Release and Adsorption of Active Agents. *Molecules* **2020**, *25*, 3814. [CrossRef]
28. Florea, M.G.; Ficai, A.; Oprea, O.; Guran, C.; Ficai, D.; Pall, L.; Andronescu, E. Drug Delivery Systems Based on Silica with Prolonged Delivery of Folic Acid. *Rev. Rom. Mater.* **2012**, *42*, 313–316.
29. Szewczyk, A.; Brzezinska-Rojek, J.; Osko, J.; Majda, D.; Prokopowicz, M.; Grembecka, M. Antioxidant-Loaded Mesoporous Silica-An Evaluation of the Physicochemical Properties. *Antioxidants* **2022**, *11*, 1417. [CrossRef]
30. Abbas, M.; Saeed, F.; Anjum, F.M.; Afzaal, M.; Tufail, T.; Bashir, M.S.; Ishtiaq, A.; Hussain, S.; Suleria, H.A.R. Natural polyphenols: An overview. *Int. J. Food Prop.* **2017**, *20*, 1689–1699. [CrossRef]
31. Cutrim, C.S.; Cortez, M.A.S. A review on polyphenols: Classification, beneficial effects and their application in dairy products. *Int. J. Dairy Technol.* **2018**, *71*, 564–578. [CrossRef]
32. de Araujo, F.F.; Farias, D.D.; Neri-Numa, I.A.; Pastore, G.M. Polyphenols and their applications: An approach in food chemistry and innovation potential. *Food Chem.* **2021**, *338*, 127535. [CrossRef] [PubMed]
33. Di Lorenzo, C.; Colombo, F.; Biella, S.; Stockley, C.; Restani, P. Polyphenols and Human Health: The Role of Bioavailability. *Nutrients* **2021**, *13*, 273. [CrossRef] [PubMed]
34. Stromsnes, K.; Lagzdina, R.; Olaso-Gonzalez, G.; Gimeno-Mallench, L.; Gambini, J. Pharmacological Properties of Polyphenols: Bioavailability, Mechanisms of Action, and Biological Effects in In Vitro Studies, Animal Models, and Humans. *Biomedicines* **2021**, *9*, 1074. [CrossRef]
35. Petrisor, G.; Motelica, L.; Ficai, D.; Trusca, R.D.; Surdu, V.A.; Voicu, G.; Oprea, O.C.; Ficai, A.; Andronescu, E. New Mesoporous Silica Materials Loaded with Polyphenols: Caffeic Acid, Ferulic Acid and p-Coumaric Acid as Dietary Supplements for Oral Administration. *Materials* **2022**, *15*, 7982. [CrossRef]
36. Diaz, M.S.; Martin-Castellanos, A.; Fernandez-Elias, V.E.; Torres, O.L.; Calvo, J.L. Effects of Polyphenol Consumption on Recovery in Team Sport Athletes of Both Sexes: A Systematic Review. *Nutrients* **2022**, *14*, 4085. [CrossRef]
37. Plamada, D.; Vodnar, D.C. Polyphenols-Gut Microbiota Interrelationship: A Transition to a New Generation of Prebiotics. *Nutrients* **2022**, *14*, 137. [CrossRef]
38. Istrati, D.; Lacatusu, I.; Bordei, N.; Badea, G.; Oprea, O.; Stefan, L.M.; Stan, R.; Badea, N.; Meghea, A. Phyto-mediated nanostructured carriers based on dual vegetable actives involved in the prevention of cellular damage. *Mat. Sci. Eng. C-Mater.* **2016**, *64*, 249–259. [CrossRef]
39. Lacatusu, I.; Badea, N.; Murariu, A.; Oprea, O.; Bojin, D.; Meghea, A. Antioxidant Activity of Solid Lipid Nanoparticles Loaded with Umbelliferone. *Soft Mater.* **2013**, *11*, 75–84. [CrossRef]
40. Niculae, G.; Badea, N.; Meghea, A.; Oprea, O.; Lacatusu, I. Coencapsulation of Butyl-Methoxydibenzoylmethane and Octocrylene into Lipid Nanocarriers: UV Performance, Photostability and in vitro Release. *Photochem. Photobiol.* **2013**, *89*, 1085–1094. [CrossRef]
41. Kim, J.K.; Park, S.U. A Recent Overview on the Biological and Pharmacological Activities of Ferulic Acid. *Excli. J.* **2019**, *18*, 132–138. [CrossRef] [PubMed]
42. Marcato, D.C.; Spagnol, C.M.; Salgado, H.R.N.; Isaac, V.L.B., Correa, M.A. New and potential properties, characteristics, and analytical methods of ferulic acid: A review. *Braz. J. Pharm. Sci.* **2022**, *58*, e18747. [CrossRef]
43. Sahin, M.; Erkan, N.; Ayranci, E. Solution Behavior of p-Coumaric, Caffeic and Ferulic Acids in Methanol as Determined from Volumetric Properties: Attempts to Explore a Correlation with Antioxidant Activities. *J. Solut. Chem.* **2016**, *45*, 52–66. [CrossRef]
44. Zdunska, K.; Dana, A.; Kolodziejczak, A.; Rotsztejn, H. Antioxidant Properties of Ferulic Acid and Its Possible Application. *Skin Pharmacol. Phys.* **2018**, *31*, 332–336. [CrossRef]
45. Borges, A.; Ferreira, C.; Saavedra, M.J.; Simoes, M. Antibacterial Activity and Mode of Action of Ferulic and Gallic Acids Against Pathogenic Bacteria. *Microb. Drug Resist.* **2013**, *19*, 256–265. [CrossRef]
46. Gao, J.H.; Yu, H.; Guo, W.K.; Kong, Y.; Gu, L.N.; Li, Q.; Yang, S.S.; Zhang, Y.Y.; Wang, Y.X. The anticancer effects of ferulic acid is associated with induction of cell cycle arrest and autophagy in cervical cancer cells. *Cancer Cell Int.* **2018**, *18*, 102. [CrossRef]
47. Ohnishi, M.; Matuo, T.; Tsuno, T.; Hosoda, A.; Nomura, E.; Taniguchi, H.; Sasaki, H.; Morishita, H. Antioxidant activity and hypoglycemic effect of ferulic acid in STZ-induced diabetic mice and KK-A(y) mice. *Biofactors* **2004**, *21*, 315–319. [CrossRef]
48. Liu, Y.J.; Shi, L.; Qiu, W.H.; Shi, Y.Y. Ferulic acid exhibits anti-inflammatory effects by inducing autophagy and blocking NLRP3 inflammasome activation. *Mol. Cell. Toxicol.* **2022**, *18*, 509–519. [CrossRef]
49. Petrisor, G.; Ficai, D.; Motelica, L.; Trusca, R.D.; Birca, A.C.; Vasile, B.S.; Voicu, G.; Oprea, O.C.; Semenescu, A.; Ficai, A.; et al. Mesoporous Silica Materials Loaded with Gallic Acid with Antimicrobial Potential. *Nanomaterials* **2022**, *12*, 1648. [CrossRef]
50. Mohammadnezhad, G.; Abad, S.; Soltani, R.; Dinari, M. Study on thermal, mechanical and adsorption properties of amine-functionalized MCM-41/PMMA and MCM-41/PS nanocomposites prepared by ultrasonic irradiation. *Ultrason. Sonochem.* **2017**, *39*, 765–773. [CrossRef]
51. Pan, X.M.; Li, J.; Gan, R.; Hu, X.N. Preparation and in vitro evaluation of enteric-coated tablets of rosiglitazone sodium. *Saudi. Pharm. J.* **2015**, *23*, 581–586. [CrossRef] [PubMed]
52. Clinical and Laboratory Standards Institute. Testing. In *CLSI Supplemenent M100*; Clinical and Laboratory Standards Institute: Wayne, PA, USA, 2021.
53. Spoiala, A.; Ilie, C.I.; Trusca, R.D.; Oprea, O.C.; Surdu, V.A.; Vasile, B.S.; Ficai, A.; Ficai, D.; Andronescu, E.; Ditu, L.M. Zinc Oxide Nanoparticles for Water Purification. *Materials* **2021**, *14*, 4747. [CrossRef]

54. Ilie, C.I.; Oprea, E.; Geana, E.I.; Spoiala, A.; Buleandra, M.; Pircalabioru, G.G.; Badea, I.A.; Ficai, D.; Andronescu, E.; Ficai, A.; et al. Bee Pollen Extracts: Chemical Composition, Antioxidant Properties, and Effect on the Growth of Selected Probiotic and Pathogenic Bacteria. *Antioxidants* **2022**, *11*, 959. [CrossRef] [PubMed]
55. Brezoiu, A.M.; Prundeanu, M.; Berger, D.; Deaconu, M.; Matei, C.; Oprea, O.; Vasile, E.; Negreanu-Pirjol, T.; Muntean, D.; Danciu, C. Properties of Salvia officinalis L. and Thymus serpyllum L. Extracts Free and Embedded into Mesopores of Silica and Titania Nanomaterials. *Nanomaterials* **2020**, *10*, 820. [CrossRef] [PubMed]
56. Enache, D.F.; Vasile, E.; Simonescu, C.M.; Culita, D.; Vasile, E.; Oprea, O.; Pandele, A.M.; Razvan, A.; Dumitru, F.; Nechifor, G. Schiff base-functionalized mesoporous silicas (MCM-41, HMS) as Pb(II) adsorbents. *Rsc. Adv.* **2018**, *8*, 176–189. [CrossRef]
57. Kister, O.; Roessner, F. Synthesis and characterization of mesoporous and amorphous silica modified with silica-organo-sulfogroups. *J. Porous Mat.* **2012**, *19*, 119–131. [CrossRef]
58. Benhamou, A.; Baudu, M.; Derriche, Z.; Basly, J.P. Aqueous heavy metals removal on amine-functionalized Si-MCM-41 and Si-MCM-48. *J. Hazard. Mater.* **2009**, *171*, 1001–1008. [CrossRef]
59. Lewandowski, D.; Ruszkowski, P.; Pinska, A.; Schroeder, G.; Kurczewska, J. SBA-15 Mesoporous Silica Modified with Gallic Acid and Evaluation of Its Cytotoxic Activity. *PLoS ONE* **2015**, *10*, e0132541. [CrossRef]
60. Huang, X.Y.; Young, N.P.; Townley, H.E. Characterization and Comparison of Mesoporous Silica Particles for Optimized Drug Delivery. *Nanomater. Nanotechnol.* **2014**, *4*, 1–15. [CrossRef]
61. Enache, D.F.; Vasile, E.; Simonescu, C.M.; Razvan, A.; Nicolescu, A.; Nechifor, A.C.; Oprea, O.; Patescu, R.E.; Onose, C.; Dumitru, F. Cysteine-functionalized silica-coated magnetite nanoparticles as potential nano adsorbents. *J. Solid State Chem.* **2017**, *253*, 318–328. [CrossRef]
62. Zaharudin, N.S.; Isa, E.D.M.; Ahmad, H.; Rahman, M.B.A.; Jumbri, K. Functionalized mesoporous silica nanoparticles templated by pyridinium ionic liquid for hydrophilic and hydrophobic drug release application. *J. Saudi. Chem. Soc.* **2020**, *24*, 289–302. [CrossRef]
63. Lee, Y.Y.; Erdogan, A.; Rao, S.S.C. How to Assess Regional and Whole Gut Transit Time With Wireless Motility Capsule. *J. Neurogastroenterol.* **2014**, *20*, 265–270. [CrossRef] [PubMed]
64. Butnarasu, C.; Petrini, P.; Bracotti, F.; Visai, L.; Guagliano, G.; Pla, A.F.; Sansone, E.; Petrillo, S.; Visentin, S. Mucosomes: Intrinsically Mucoadhesive Glycosylated Mucin Nanoparticles as Multi-Drug Delivery Platform. *Adv. Healthc Mater.* **2022**, *11*, 2200340. [CrossRef] [PubMed]
65. Amin, M.K.; Boateng, J.S. Enhancing Stability and Mucoadhesive Properties of Chitosan Nanoparticles by Surface Modification with Sodium Alginate and Polyethylene Glycol for Potential Oral Mucosa Vaccine Delivery. *Mar. Drugs* **2022**, *20*, 156. [CrossRef]
66. Fan, B.; Liu, L.; Zheng, Y.; Xing, Y.; Shen, W.G.; Li, Q.; Wang, R.Y.; Liang, G.X. Novel pH-responsive and mucoadhesive chitosan-based nanoparticles for oral delivery of low molecular weight heparin with enhanced bioavailability and anticoagulant effect. *J. Drug Deliv. Sci. Tec.* **2022**, *78*, 103955. [CrossRef]
67. Ijabadeniyi, O.A.; Govender, A.; Olagunju, O.F.; Oyedeji, A.B. The antimicrobial activity of two phenolic acids against foodborne Escherichia coli and Listeria monocytogenes and their effectiveness in a meat system. *Ital. J. Food Sci.* **2021**, *33*, 39–45. [CrossRef]
68. Ozdal, T.; Sela, D.A.; Xiao, J.B.; Boyacioglu, D.; Chen, F.; Capanoglu, E. The Reciprocal Interactions between Polyphenols and Gut Microbiota and Effects on Bioaccessibility. *Nutrients* **2016**, *8*, 78. [CrossRef]
69. Liu, X.C.; Martin, D.A.; Valdez, J.C.; Sudakaran, S.; Rey, F.; Bolling, B.W. Aronia berry polyphenols have matrix-dependent effects on the gut microbiota. *Food Chem.* **2021**, *359*, 129831. [CrossRef]

pharmaceutics

Article

Green Synthesis of Highly Fluorescent Carbon Dots from Bovine Serum Albumin for Linezolid Drug Delivery as Potential Wound Healing Biomaterial: Bio-Synergistic Approach, Antibacterial Activity, and In Vitro and Ex Vivo Evaluation

Dina Saeed Ghataty [1], Reham Ibrahim Amer [2], Mai A. Amer [3], Mohamed F. Abdel Rahman [4] and Rehab Nabil Shamma [5,*]

1 Department of Pharmaceutics, Faculty of Pharmacy, October University for Modern Sciences and Arts (MSA), Giza 12451, Egypt
2 Department of Pharmaceutics and Pharmaceutical Technology, Faculty of Pharmacy, Al-Azhar University, Cairo 11754, Egypt
3 Department of Microbiology and Immunology, Faculty of Pharmacy, October University for Modern Sciences and Arts (MSA), Giza 12451, Egypt
4 Department of Biology and Biochemistry, School of Life and Medical Sciences, University of Hertfordshire Hosted by Global Academic Foundation, Cairo 4813001, Egypt
5 Department of Pharmaceutics and Industrial Pharmacy, Faculty of Pharmacy, Cairo University, Cairo 11562, Egypt
* Correspondence: rehab.shamma@pharma.cu.edu.eg; Tel.: +20-1119301245

Abstract: A simple and green approach was developed to produce novel highly fluorescent bovine serum albumin carbon dots (BCDs) via facile one-step hydrothermal treatment, using bovine serum albumin as a precursor carbon source. Inherent blue photoluminescence of the synthesized BCDs provided a maximum photostability of $90.5 \pm 1.2\%$ and was characterized via TEM, FT-IR, XPS, XRD, UV-visible, and zeta potential analyses. By virtue of their extremely small size, intrinsic optical and photoluminescence properties, superior photostability, and useful non-covalent interactions with the synthetic oxazolidinone antibiotic linezolid (LNZ), BCDs were investigated as fluorescent nano-biocarriers for LNZ drug delivery. The release profile of LNZ from the drug delivery system (LNZ–BCDs) revealed a distinct biphasic release, which is beneficial for mollifying the lethal incidents associated with wound infection. The effective wound healing performance of the developed LNZ–BCDs were evaluated through various in vitro and ex vivo assays such as MTT, ex vivo hemolysis, in vitro antibacterial activity, in vitro skin-related enzyme inhibition, and scratch wound healing assays. The examination of LNZ–BCDs as an efficient wound healing biomaterial illustrated excellent biocompatibility and low cytotoxicity against normal human skin fibroblast (HSF) cell line, indicating distinct antibacterial activity against the most common wound infectious pathogens including *Staphylococcus aureus* (ATCC® 25922) and methicillin-resistant *Staphylococcus aureus*, robust anti-elastase, anti-collagenase, and anti-tyrosinase activities, and enhanced cell proliferation and migration effect. The obtained results confirmed the feasibility of using the newly designed fluorescent LNZ–BCDs nano-bioconjugate as a unique antibacterial biomaterial for effective wound healing and tissue regeneration. Besides, the greenly synthesized BCDs could be considered as a great potential substitute for toxic nanoparticles in biomedical applications due to their biocompatibility and intense fluorescence characteristics and in pharmaceutical industries as promising drug delivery nano-biocarriers for effective wound healing applications.

Keywords: carbon dots; hydrothermal treatment; bovine serum albumin; linezolid delivery; antibacterial; wound healing

1. Introduction

The total global number of skin injury cases has substantial healthcare ramifications, as it represents almost 50% of the world's yearly expenditure in the aspect of healthcare [1].

Understandably, wound healing is well-known to be one of the most critical challenges in medical society [2]. As bacteria come in contact with the exposed skin surface area, they readily colonize in the exudative wound fluid and necrotic tissues, hence resulting in mounted inflammation and delayed wound healing [3]. The healing process of an infected wound is complicated, as the bacterial infection at the wound surface represents a major threat to public health in wound care management, which may transform normal wound healing into a chronic wound [4]. The process of healing skin wounds consists of a series of four successive phases comprising hemostasis, inflammation, cell proliferation, and tissue remodeling [2].

A wide range of advancements in biomaterials and nanomaterials-based regenerative approaches have been used to facilitate and accelerate wound healing via promoting tissue regeneration and executing an effective barrier against wound infection [2,5]. Over the last decade, carbon-based nanomaterials have been extensively used for their excellent antibacterial properties, wound healing, and sterilization applications, in addition to their great biocompatibility [5]. Among them, carbon dots (CDs), as a novel zero-dimensional (0D) nanomaterial in the carbon family, have attracted enormous interest owing to their extremely small size (<10 nm), easy surface functionalization, low toxicity, superior biocompatibility, high stability, obvious advantages in aqueous solubility, high surface area, and being eco-friendly [6,7]. Furthermore, it is extensively acknowledged that CDs exhibit unique optical, electrochemical, and fluorescent properties. As per these unique properties, CDs have displayed a promising potential use as a novel carbon nanostructure in many fields of biomedical applications for in vitro and in vivo bioimaging, wound dressing, and gene and drug delivery [5,8]. Besides, researchers reported that CDs possess intense photoluminescence following two-photon fluorescence excitation near the infrared region, hence fostering their applications in anti-stoke biosensing as well as bioimaging [8,9]. There are numerous studies as well about utilizing CDs as substrates in the structure of biosensor probes due to the CDs' high surface area, hence possibly enhancing the electrochemical signal of electrodes and presenting further active sites for aptamer immobilization [10]. In addition, CDs have displayed great capabilities to be utilized as a fluorescent imaging probe in complex biological systems. Thus their distinct optical characteristics, biocompatibility, as well as low toxicity make them a potential candidate for in vivo applications [8].

Synthetic approaches that have been developed to synthesize CDs can be divided into top-down and bottom-up techniques. The top-down technique utilizes physical and chemical approaches starting from a vast range of either natural or chemical precursors, which assemble to synthesize CDs, including pyrolysis, microwave irradiation, hydrothermal method, and ultrasonic treatment. Whereas the bottom-up technique utilizes physical approaches only to nano-fragment inorganic larger carbon precursors, including graphene, graphite, and carbon nanotubes, such as electrochemical synthesis, laser ablation, and arc discharge [11]. Among these techniques, the hydrothermal method has drawn tremendous attention as it is cost-effective, fast, facile, and a green one-step method with decreased processing severity which uses deionized (DI) water only as a solvent [12,13]. It is worth highlighting that it has been the most commonly applied method since it is convenient and efficient [14]. Notably, no surface passivation agent is required, whereas only the carbon source plays an important role in the synthesis of the CDs [13,15].

Recently tremendous attention has also been directed toward green chemistry for the development of CDs derived from crude natural materials, natural polymers, and cost-effective and biodegradable materials [11]. CDs derived from crude natural materials, including biomass waste, are green and generally better than their chemical counterparts because of the renewable recourses and lack of chemicals involved and have been synthesized via hydrothermal techniques from several precursors, including peach gum, watermelon peels, strawberries, papaya, peanut shells, spent tea, and olive pits [11,16]. Not only was biomass waste utilized to develop CDs, the use of several natural polymers, including polysaccharides and proteins to generate CDs has attracted great attention due to their inherent biocompatibility, biodegradability, and distinct physicochemical and biological properties. Natural polymer-derived CDs have been synthesized via hydrothermal techniques from many precursors, including chitosan, gelatin, lignin, xylan, and silk fibroin [16]. Among the precursors recently examined across literature, it can be inferred that proteins are potential precursors to synthesize CDs and are interesting materials due to their enhanced adsorption capacity, low toxicity, superior biodegradability, and exquisite non-immunogenicity [12,17]. The conjugation mechanism of proteins with drug molecules has shed light on various research areas and stipulated new prospects for the development of novel drugs [18]. Bovine serum albumin (BSA), a model globular protein, is a biocompatible, biodegradable, highly aqueous-soluble, inexpensive, and non-toxic carrier, which conjugates with drugs through non-covalent interactions and presents a 76% sequence homology with the three-dimensional (3D) structure of human serum albumin (HSA) [18–20]. Furthermore, BSA facilitates the drug to be delivered and transported in the body and be easily given up at the surface of the cell. The flexibility in conformation, as well as the existence of reactive groups on BSA, facilitate its attachment with other substances of different structures [20,21]. BSA nanoparticles were reported to be able to control the drug encapsulation and release as well as extend its circulation in the bloodstream [20]. Additionally, as reported earlier, BSA as a protein source is advantageous for the complex wound healing process, whilst BSA-based biomaterials have displayed remarkable cell affinity intrinsic characteristics [21].

Linezolid (LNZ) has been one of the most promising topical oxazolidinone antibiotics for treating and avoiding abundant bacterial skin infections caused by injury, abrasion, and surgery. It is a Food and Drug Administration (FDA) approved drug for treating common wound infectious bacteria such as penicillin-resistant *Streptococcus pneumonia*, methicillin-resistant *Staphylococcus aureus* (MRSA), vancomycin-resistant *Enterococci* (VRE), and glycopeptide intermediate *Staphylococcus aureus* (GISA). LNZ exerts its antibacterial activity via inhibiting the protein synthesis of bacteria through attaching to the 23S portion of the 50S ribosomal subunit, hence hindering bacterial growth. LNZ, as a topical wound healing biomaterial, treats several wounds due to burns and diabetic foot ulcers, attributed to its effectiveness [2,22].

In this study, novel highly fluorescent antibacterial bovine serum albumin CDs (BCDs) were synthesized via cost-effective and green one-step hydrothermal treatment using BSA as the precursor carbon source. The obtained BCDs were thoroughly characterized using numerous microscopic, optical, and spectroscopic techniques, including transmission electron microscopy (TEM), Fourier-transform infrared spectroscopy (FT-IR), X-ray photoelectron spectroscopy (XPS), X-ray diffraction (XRD), UV-visible, as well as photoluminescence and zeta potential measurements. Then, the BCDs were loaded with various ratios of LNZ to prepare LNZ–BCDs nano-bioconjugate complexes as efficient drug delivery nano-systems. The developed LNZ–BCDs nano-bioconjugates exhibiting promising spectroscopic, in vitro drug release and ex vivo characteristics are expected to facilitate wound healing via a bio-synergistic approach. Finally, the biocompatibility, cytotoxicity, and overall wound healing performance of the developed LNZ–BCDs nano-bioconjugate were further investigated by evaluating the survival rate, anti-elastase, anti-collagenase, and anti-tyrosinase activities, and effective wound healing properties against normal human skin fibroblast (HSF) cell line via MTT, ex vivo hemolysis, in vitro antibacterial activity by broth microdilution method, in vitro skin-related enzyme inhibition as well as scratch wound healing assays.

2. Materials

Linezolid was generously provided by Pfizer, Egypt. Bovine serum albumin (BSA), ethylenediamine tetraacetic acid (EDTA), MTT (3-(4,5-dimethylthiazol-2-yl)-2,5-diphenyltetrazolium bromide) solution, N-2-hydroxyethylpiperazine-N-2-ethane sulfonic acid (HEPES) buffer, citrate buffer, 2-furanacryloyl-l-leucylglycyl-l-prolyl-l-alanine, kojic acid, Dulbecco's modified Eagle's medium (DMEM), fetal bovine serum–Dulbecco's modified Eagle's medium (FBS-DMEM), *N*-Methoxysuccinyl-Ala-Ala-Pro-chloromethyl ketone, and *N*-Methoxysuccinyl-Ala-Ala-Pro-Val-*p*-nitroanilide were all purchased from Sigma-Aldrich Co., St. Louis, MO, USA.

Clostridium histolyticum (1 mg/mL) buffer and Dimethyl sulfoxide (DMSO) were obtained from Fisher Scientific, Loughborough, UK. Human red blood cells (HRBCs), normal human skin fibroblast (HSF) cell line, human leukocyte elastase, and mushroom tyrosinase were acquired from Nawah Scientific Inc., Cairo, Egypt. Deionized water (DI) was utilized in all the experiments. Analytical grade chemicals were used.

2.1. Methods

Synthesis of BCDs Nano-Biocarrier and LNZ–BCDs Nano-Bioconjugate

The fluorescent carbon dots (CDs) were typically synthesized via a green facile one-pot hydrothermal technique adopted by Amin et al. [23], with slight modification. Bovine serum albumin (BSA) was employed as a carbon source precursor for the development of the fluorescent bovine serum albumin carbon dots (BCDs) nano-biocarrier. Briefly, 3.6 g of BSA was dissolved in 80 mL deionized (DI) water under gentle stirring using a magnetic stirrer for 20 min until a clear solution was attained. The solution was then transferred into a 150 mL Teflon-lined hydrothermal stainless-steel autoclave reactor (OLT-150ML, OLLITAL Technology Co., Ltd., Xiamen, China) and then heated in an electrical oven at 200 °C for 6 h. After cooling down at room temperature, the resultant yellowish-brown solution was ultra-centrifuged using a 3-16KL centrifuge (Sigma, Germany) for 20 min at 15,000 rpm at 25 °C to remove large insoluble carbonaceous particles and was then filtered using a 0.22 μm membrane filter (Membrane Solutions® sterile syringe filter, Auburn, WA, USA). For further purification, the transparent filtrate was then dialyzed in the dark using a dialysis membrane (1000 Da molecular weight cut off, Frey Scientific, Nashua, NH, USA) against deionized water for 48 h, and then the final fluorescent BCDs nano-biocarrier solution was obtained and stored in a dark, cool place for further analysis.

For the conjugation of LNZ on BCDs nano-biocarrier, aqueous solutions of LNZ (0.6 mg/mL) and BCDs nano-biocarriers were mixed at different ratios (BCDs: LNZ = 4:1, 2:1, 1:1, 1:3, and 1:5) under continuous stirring using a magnetic stirrer at 25 °C for 48 h in a dark condition. Finally, the resultant LNZ–BCDs nano-bioconjugates were placed in an amber bottle and stored in a dark, cool place for further studies.

2.2. Characterization of BCDs Nano-Biocarrier and LNZ–BCDs Nano-Bioconjugate

The transmission electron microscope (TEM) image of BCDs nano-biocarrier was captured by a JEM-2100 microscope (JEOL Ltd., Japan) operating at an acceleration voltage of 200 kV. Particle size analysis was conducted by Image J software. Fourier-transform infrared (FT-IR) spectra of the LNZ molecules, BSA, as well as lyophilized samples of BCDs nano-biocarrier, and LNZ–BCDs nano-bioconjugate, were recorded on an IRAffinity-1S FT-IR spectrometer (SHIMADZU Corporation, Kyoto, Japan) to analyze the surface functional groups. X-ray photoelectron spectroscopy (XPS) was performed to investigate the elemental composition of BCDs nano-biocarrier using K-ALPHA X-ray photoelectron spectrometer (ThermoFisher Scientific, Waltham, MA, USA) with Al-K_α radiation. The crystal structure of BCDs nano-biocarrier was investigated via Bruker D8 DISCOVER X-ray diffractometer (XRD, Berlin, Germany) with Ni-filtered Cu-K_α radiation (45 kV, 40 mA, and λ = 0.15416 nm). The optical properties of LNZ, BCDs nano-biocarrier, and LNZ–BCDs nano-bioconjugate were analyzed using UV-1800 240V UV spectrophotometer (SHIMADZU Corporation, Kyoto, Japan). A Lumina LF1201005 fluorescence spectrometer (ThermoFisher Scientific, Waltham, MA, USA) was used to conduct all the fluorescence measurements of the BCDs nano-biocarrier. Excitation, as well as emission slits, were maintained at 10 nm. Finally, zeta (ζ) potential measurements were performed to determine the surface charge of LNZ, BCDs nano-biocarrier, and LNZ–BCDs nano-bioconjugate using a Nano ZS90 zeta-sizer (Malvern, Worcestershire, UK) at room temperature.

2.3. Drug Loading and Encapsulation Efficiency of LNZ–BCDs Nano-Bioconjugates

The drug loading efficiency (DLE) and drug encapsulation efficiency (DEE) of the prepared LNZ–BCDs nano-bioconjugates were estimated as per the method described by Jalali et al. [24]. Briefly, 5 mL of the LNZ–BCDs nano-bioconjugate was dialyzed in the dark against deionized water at 25 ± 0.2 °C for 48 h [25]. Afterward, the amount of free unbound LNZ drug molecules in the supernatant was quantified with UV-visible spectroscopy (SHIMADZU Corporation, Model UV-1800 240V, Japan) at 251 nm [26]. The DLE (%) and DEE (%) were estimated using the following equations:

$$DLE\ (\%) = \frac{Weight\ of\ drug\ loaded\ in\ LNZ\text{–}BCDs\ nano\text{–}bioconjugate}{Total\ weight\ of\ LNZ\text{–}BCDs\ nano\text{–}bioconjugate} \times 100 \quad (1)$$

$$DEE\ (\%) = \frac{Weight\ of\ drug\ loaded\ in\ LNZ\text{–}BCDs\ nano\text{–}bioconjugate}{Initial\ weight\ of\ drug} \times 100 \quad (2)$$

The experiment was performed in triplicate. The mean as well as standard deviation were recorded.

2.4. In Vitro Drug Release Studies of LNZ from the LNZ–BCDs Nano-Bioconjugate

The in vitro release studies of LNZ from the LNZ–BCDs nano-bioconjugate and the free LNZ drug solution were conducted using the dialysis bag diffusion method, adopted by Singh et al. [27] with slight modifications. The dissolution medium was phosphate buffer saline (PBS) (pH 7.4), which mimics physiological pH. Afterward, 3 mL of the LNZ–BCDs nano-bioconjugate and the free LNZ drug solution were placed in dialysis bags (1000 Da molecular weight cut off, Frey Scientific, Nashua, NH, USA), immersed in 80 mL PBS (pH 7.4) in separate glass vials, and placed in the Shaker Incubator apparatus (ZHICHENG ZHWY-2102C, Shanghai, China) at 100 rpm at 37 ± 0.3 °C to mimic the skin temperature. Aliquots of 3 mL were taken from the dissolution medium at predefined time points at 0.5, 1, 2, 3, 4, 5, 6, 7, 8, 10, 12, 24, 36, and finally at 48 h. The sink conditions were maintained by immediately replenishing the equivalent volume of fresh PBS (pH 7.4) after each aliquot withdrawal. The concentration of LNZ released in the aliquots withdrawn from the dissolution medium was quantified spectrophotometrically via a UV spectrophotometer (SHIMADZU Corporation, Model UV- 1800 240V, Kyoto, Japan) at 251 nm. The study was performed in triplicate and was graphically presented as the cumulative percentage of drug release versus time. Data from the in vitro drug release study was further analyzed using different kinetic models to determine the drug release pattern.

2.5. Ex Vivo Hemolysis Assay

Ex vivo hemolysis assay was conducted according to the method described by Huang et al. [28]. Freshly collected human red blood cells (HRBCs) were separated by centrifugation for 10 min at 2500 rpm and then washed three times and dispersed in 4 mL of sterile PBS (pH 7.4). Afterward, 200 µL of diluted HRBCs was added to 600 µL of sterile PBS (pH 7.4) solution with diverse concentrations (25–300 µg/mL) of the LNZ–BCDs nano-bioconjugate. Deionized water and sterile PBS (pH 7.4) were employed as positive and negative controls, respectively. All samples were then shaken and incubated at 37 °C for 2 h and then centrifuged again at 2500 rpm for 15 min. The supernatant was collected, and optical density was recorded by UV-1800 240V UV spectrophotometer (SHIMADZU Corporation, Kyoto, Japan) at 541 nm while using sterile PBS (pH 7.4) as a blank. The hemolysis percentage was estimated using the following equation:

$$Hemolysis\ percentage\ (\%) = \frac{A_s - A_n}{A_p - A_n} \times 100 \quad (3)$$

where A_s, A_n, and A_p present the absorbances of the sample, negative, and positive controls, respectively. The assay was conducted in triplicate. The mean as well as standard deviation were recorded.

2.6. Cytotoxicity Assay

The cell cytotoxicity and biocompatibility of BCDs nano-biocarrier and LNZ–BCDs nano-bioconjugate were assessed via MTT (3-(4,5-dimethylthiazol-2-yl)-2,5-diphenyltetrazolium bromide) assay against the normal human skin fibroblast (HSF) cell line, which was obtained from Nawah Scientific Inc., Egypt. Briefly, HSF cell line suspension (100 µL/well) was seeded into a 96-well plate, cultured in Dulbecco's modified Eagle's medium (DMEM) containing 100 mg/mL streptomycin, 100 units/mL penicillin, and 10% of heat-inactivated fetal bovine serum (FBS), and afterward incubated at 37 °C for 24 h under a humidified atmosphere with 5% CO_2. Afterward, the cells were treated with various concentrations of BCDs nano-biocarrier and LNZ–BCDs nano-bioconjugate (25–1000 µg/mL) and incubated for an additional 24 h. Subsequently, the culture medium was cast-off, and the cells were washed using sterile PBS (pH 7.4) three times. MTT reagent (20 µL of 5 mg/mL stock solution) was added into each well and then incubated at 37 °C for another 4 h to facilitate the formation of the violet-colored formazan. In each well, the formed crystals of formazan were thoroughly dissolved using 200 µL of dimethyl sulfoxide (DMSO). After shaking the resultant solutions for 10 min, the optical density (OD) of each solution at λ_{max} 570 nm was recorded using a multi-well FLUOstar® Omega microplate reader (BMG LABTECH, Baden-Wurttemberg, Germany). Cell viability was expressed as the percentage of survival cells using (Equation (4)) and reported as the mean values of triplicate measurements [29].

$$Cell\ viability\ (\%) = \frac{OD_t}{OD_c} \times 100 \quad (4)$$

where OD_t and OD_c represent the optical densities of the treated and control samples, respectively.

2.7. In Vitro Antibacterial Activity by Broth Microdilution Method

The minimum inhibitory concentration (MIC) of pure LNZ, BCDs, and their formulated conjugate (LNZ−BCDs) were tested against pathogens commonly causing wound infection, such as *Staphylococcus aureus* (ATCC® 25922) and methicillin-resistant *Staphylococcus aureus* (MRSA) that was previously isolated from dental clinic surface. The MIC was determined by the broth microdilution method. Stock solutions of LNZ were prepared at a concentration of 300 µg/mL and then sterilized by filtration. Stock solutions were serially diluted (2-fold) in sterile Müeller Hinton broth (MHB) with a dilution range of 0.125 to 150 µg/mL. Overnight culture turbidity was adjusted equivalent to the 0.5 McFarland standard and then diluted to give a final concentration equivalent to 10^6 CFU/mL [30]. One hundred microliters of the adjusted bacterial culture were added to an equal volume of the tested dilutions in a 96-well microtiter plate. The plates were then incubated at 37 °C for 24 h. The effect of the conjugation between LNZ and BCDs was determined by measuring the change in the MIC of the pure LNZ and unconjugated BCDs. The synergistic and antagonistic activity of this conjugation was reflected by a decrease or increase in the MIC values, respectively, compared to the unconjugated LNZ.

The MIC was recorded as the lowest concentration of an antimicrobial agent, which gave no visible growth. Isolates were classified as susceptible ($\leq$4 µg/mL), or resistant ($\geq$8 µg/mL) to LNZ according to the Clinical and Laboratory Standards Institute (CLSI) breakpoints [31]. The experiment was conducted in triplicate. The mean as well as standard deviation were recorded.

2.8. In Vitro Skin-Related Enzyme Inhibitory Assays

The anti-elastase, anti-collagenase, and anti-tyrosinase activities were assessed following the method reported by Mostafa et al. [32]. The pure LNZ, BCDs nano-biocarrier, and LNZ–BCDs nano-bioconjugate were tested for in vitro skin-related enzyme activity inhibition assays. For the anti-elastase assay, human leukocyte elastase (1 µg/mL) was incubated with N-2-hydroxyethylpiperazine-N-2-ethane sulfonic acid (HEPES) buffer (pH 7.5). Each of the tested samples or the standard inhibitor *N*-Methoxysuccinyl-Ala-Ala-Pro-chloromethyl ketone (1.4 mg/mL) was added into the 96-well plate for 20 min at 25 °C before the addition of 100 μL substrate of 1 mM *N*-Methoxysuccinyl-Ala-Ala-Pro-Val-*p*-nitroanilide. Afterward, the optical density was measured after 40 min of incubation at 405 nm against a blank well lacking the test sample/inhibitor. Various concentrations of the tested samples (25–300 μg/mL) were used.

For the anti-collagenase, collagenase type 1 from *Clostridium histolyticum* (1 mg/mL) buffer (pH 7.4) along with tested samples or standard inhibitor ethylenediamine tetraacetic acid (EDTA) (1.4 mg/mL) were incubated at 37 °C for 20 min prior to the addition of 100 μL of the substrate 2-furanacryloyl-l-leucylglycyl-l-prolyl-l-alanine (FALGPA). The mixture was then incubated at 37 °C for an additional 1 h before the addition of 200 μL of 2% ninhydrin in 200 mM citrate buffer (pH 5) and placed in a water bath for 5 min. Afterward, the solution was left to cool down completely. Afterwards 200 μL of 50% isopropanol was added, and the optical densities were analyzed at 540 nm. Various concentrations of the tested samples (25–300 μg/mL) were used.

For the anti-tyrosinase assay, mushroom tyrosinase (5600 units/mL) was incubated at 37 °C for 15 min along with tested samples or standard inhibitor kojic acid (1.4 mg/mL) before the addition of the substrate 1 mM L-DOPA. Afterward, the optical density of the formed dopachrome was analyzed at 475 nm. Various concentrations of the tested samples (75–500 μg/mL) were used. All tests were conducted in triplicate. The enzyme inhibition activity was expressed in percentage using the following equation:

$$Enzyme\ inhibition\ activity\ (\%) = \frac{Optical\ density\ of\ control - Optical\ density\ of\ sample}{Optical\ density\ of\ control} \times 100 \quad (5)$$

2.9. Scratch Wound Healing Assay

For the scratch wound healing assay, a normal human skin fibroblast (HSF) cell line, acquired from Nawah Scientific Inc. (Cairo, Egypt), was plated at a density of 2×10^5/well on a coated 12-well plate and subsequently cultured in a 5% fetal bovine serum–Dulbecco's modified Eagle's medium (FBS DMEM) at 37 °C and 5% CO_2 [33]. Afterward, the horizontal scratches were performed in the confluent monolayer, and the 12-well plate was then extensively washed using PBS (pH 7.4). The control wells were refilled with a fresh medium, whereas the test wells were treated using a fresh media of BCDs nano-biocarrier and LNZ–BCDs nano-bioconjugate for a period of 48 h. Images were taken after 0, 24, and 48 h of the incubation period via an inverted microscope (Carl Zeiss, Jena, Germany). The 12-well plate was then incubated at 37 °C and 5% CO_2 in-between time points. The obtained images were then analyzed via Mill ImageView software version 3.7. The assay was performed in triplicate. The width of the wound gap (mm) was estimated as the mean distance between the edges of performed scratches [34]. Whereas the rate of cell migration (*RM*) was estimated using the following equation:

$$RM = \frac{(W_i - W_f)}{t} \quad (6)$$

where, W_i and W_f present the mean initial and final width of the wound gap, respectively, and t presents the migration duration (h). Furthermore, the area of the wound was estimated via tracing cell-free area in the captured images via Fiji-ImageJ public domain software version 1.53 (Bethesda, MD, USA), and wound closure (%) was calculated using the following equation:

$$Wound\ closure\ (\%) = \frac{(A_{t=0} - A_{t=\Delta t})}{A_{t=0}} \times 100 \quad (7)$$

where, $A_{t=0}$ presents the mean wound area measured instantly after the scratch was performed, at time zero. $A_{t=\Delta t}$ presents the mean wound area measured some hours after the scratch was performed. Results are expressed as the mean and standard deviation of three readings.

2.10. Statistical Analysis

Statistical analysis of in vitro drug release kinetic models was carried out using one-way analysis of variance (ANOVA) followed by Tukey's Multiple Comparison post hoc test; $p \leq 0.05$. Moreover, in vitro skin-related enzyme inhibitory assays were carried out in triplicates, and results were expressed as mean ± standard deviation. A non-linear regression curve was used to calculate IC_{50}. An unpaired *t*-test was used for statistical comparison between the two groups. $p < 0.05$ is considered statistically significant. Analyses were done using GraphPad Prism 6.01 (San Diego, CA, USA).

3. Results and Discussion

3.1. Synthesis of BCDs Nano-Biocarrier and LNZ–BCDs Nano-Bioconjugate

In this study, highly fluorescent CDs derived from BSA for LNZ drug delivery were designed for effective wound healing treatment. Numerous techniques have been proposed for synthesizing CDs, among which the hydrothermal method is regarded as the best method, as it is green and offers large-scale as well as facile synthesis procedures. In this study, BCDs nano-biocarriers were synthesized via one-step hydrothermal carbonization of BSA at 200 °C, resulting in the formation of a dark yellowish-brown solution from a yellow-colored solution which provided the first sign of the successful formation of BCDs [35]. This method effectively breaks down the native three-dimensional (3D) structure of BSA and renders carboxyl and amine groups extensively exposed [17]. Purification and separation of BCDs nano-biocarriers by dialysis yielded a pale yellow-colored solution. Afterward, to investigate the potential of BCDs nano-biocarrier in the delivery of antibacterial agents for effective wound healing, LNZ was loaded onto the BCDs.

3.2. Transmission Electron Microscopy (TEM) Analysis

TEM analysis was carried out to investigate the morphology of the synthesized BCDs nano-biocarrier. The TEM image of the BCDs nano-biocarrier is shown in Figure 1a. The BCDs nano-biocarrier clearly showed monodispersed spherical-like shape with a narrow size distribution and a relatively uniform size without any apparent aggregation. The statistical particle size distribution of the BCDs nano-biocarrier ranges from $1.5 \pm 0.2 - 7.5 \pm 0.1$ nm with an average diameter of 4.5 ± 0.3 nm (Figure 1b). Selected area electron diffraction (SAED) pattern of BCDs nano-biocarrier presented diffused rings without any lattice spot or ring (Figure 1c). This corresponds to the amorphous nature of the graphitic carbon, which was further confirmed via XRD and XPS analyses [13,36]. Hence, it can be concluded that the synthesized BCDs nano-biocarrier is certainly within the quantum-sized materials [12].

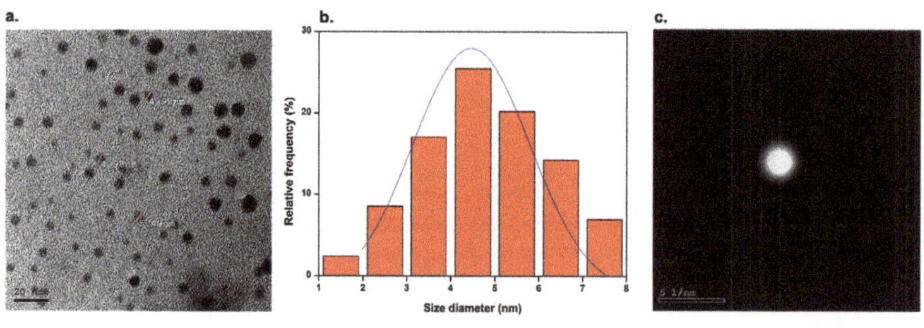

Figure 1. (**a**) Transmission electron microscope (TEM) image at the scale of 20 nm, (**b**) size distribution histogram, and (**c**) selected area electron diffraction (SAED) pattern of the BCDs nano-biocarrier.

3.3. Fourier-Transform Infrared Spectroscopy (FT-IR) Analysis

FT-IR spectroscopy was performed to characterize surface functional groups and to confirm carbonization and conjugation processes. FT-IR spectra of pure LNZ, pure

BSA, BCDs nano-biocarrier, and LNZ–BCDs nano-bioconjugate have revealed several typical characteristic bands, as presented in Figure 2 [15,17]. FT-IR spectrum of pure LNZ displayed distinctive bands at 3361 cm^{-1} for –NH group, 3057 cm^{-1} for aromatic –CH, 2978 and 2853 cm^{-1} for aliphatic –CH, and 1747 and 1675 cm^{-1} for C=O of an inner ester of five-membered ring and amide, respectively. Previous studies reported a similar FT-IR spectrum for LNZ pure drug [2,37].

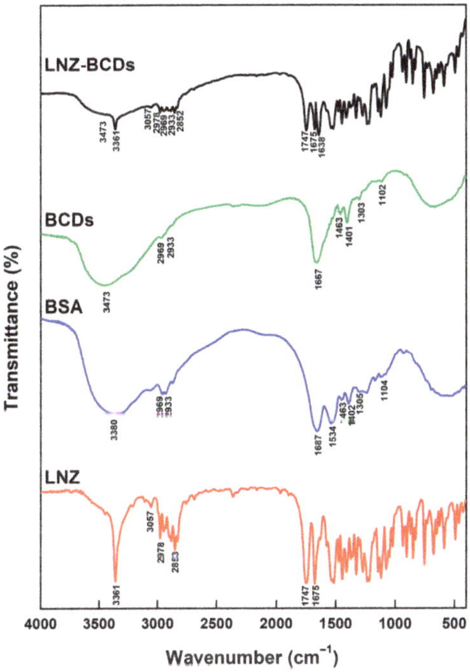

Figure 2. Fourier-transform infrared (FT-IR) spectra of the pure LNZ, pure BSA, BCDs nano-biocarrier, and LNZ–BCDs nano-bioconjugate.

At first, the FT-IR spectrum of pure BSA presented complex fingerprint bands attributed to the characteristic chemical structure of amino acids [17]. However, after the hydrothermal carbonization process, the FT-IR spectrum of BCDs nano-biocarrier became simpler and the absorption bands were slightly shifted due to the altered chemical environment (Figure 2). Many characteristic bands were still found in the FT-IR spectrum of BCDs nano-biocarrier, which correspond to –OH/–NH broadband at 3600–3299 cm^{-1}, aliphatic –CH stretching at 2969 and 2933 cm^{-1}, carbonyl (C=O) stretching at 1667 cm^{-1}, C=C stretching at 1463 cm^{-1}, C–N stretching at 1401 cm^{-1}, C–O stretching at 1303 cm^{-1}, and symmetric stretching vibration of C–O–C at 1102 cm^{-1} [38]. The absorption bands of both the carbonyl (C=O) stretching and the C–O stretching together indicate the existence of the –COO– functional group [39]. Moreover, a blue shift for the carbonyl (C=O) stretching was observed. This tendency can be attributed to the electron cloud existing between carbons; thus, oxygen atoms tend to move toward the direction of oxygen [40]. Other researchers reported similar findings for other CDs [15,39,40]. Additionally, the existence of the hydroxyl (−OH) functional group plays an important role in enhancing the antibacterial activity of BCDs nano-biocarrier, thus facilitating wound healing. Alike finding was previously reported by Pandiyan et al. [41] for CDs derived from sugarcane industrial wastes.

After capping LNZ on the surface of the BCDs nano-biocarrier, the FT-IR spectrum of LNZ–BCDs nano-bioconjugate exhibited not only the distinctive bands of BCDs nano-biocarrier, but also the distinctive bands of LNZ (Figure 2). This observation confirmed the existence of the LNZ drug molecules in the product structure. Similar findings were obtained by Arsalani et al. [42] for the polyethylene glycol passivated CDs loaded with methotrexate. Nevertheless, the carbonyl (C=O) stretching in the LNZ–BCDs nano-bioconjugate spectrum was shifted to a lower wavelength (1638 cm^{-1}). Ultimately, such reduction in the vibrational wavelength indicates the potential formation of an amide group and the successful tagging of LNZ with BCDs nano-biocarrier via non-covalent interactions [43,44]. Similar findings were previously reported by Hassan et al. [43] for ibuprofen grafted on nitrogen-doped CDs. The above-mentioned results indicate that the BCDs nano-biocarrier's surface was enriched with plentiful hydroxyl, amino, and carboxyl groups. These functional groups can potentially act as active sites for attaching extrinsic molecules through either hydrogen bonding or van der Waals interactions. Therefore, the –NH and the two C=O groups in the LNZ drug molecules tend to form hydrogen bonds with the surface functional groups of BCDs nano-biocarrier. Similar results were previously reported by Shao et al. [39] for lycorine-loaded CDs.

3.4. X-ray Photoelectron Spectroscopy (XPS)

XPS was conducted to examine the surface elemental and chemical composition, as well as the nature of bonds existing in the synthesized BCDs nano-biocarrier, as shown in Figure 3. The total XPS survey spectrum indicated the presence of three major elements of C, N, and O, with atomic percentages of 64.36, 12.76, and 22.88%, respectively [36]. The distinct binding energy peaks observed at 285.76, 400.14, and 532.03 eV correspond to C1s, N1s, and O1s, respectively (Figure 3a).

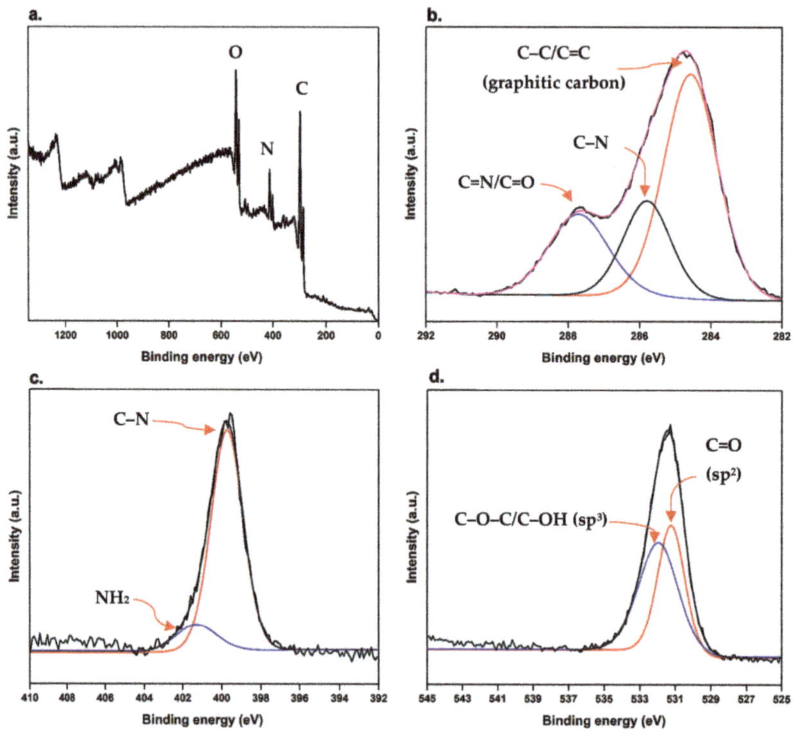

Figure 3. X-ray photoelectron (XPS) spectra of BCDs nano-biocarrier. (**a**) survey XPS spectrum and high-resolution spectra of (**b**) C1s, (**c**) N1s, and (**d**) O1s.

As demonstrated in the high-resolution XPS spectrum of C1s (Figure 3b), three main peaks were observed at 284.56, 285.79, and 287.70 eV, which correspond to C–C/C=C (for graphitic carbon), C–N, and C=N/C=O, respectively [15,36]. Similarly, the high-resolution spectrum of N1s (Figure 3c) can be deconvoluted in the presence of two characteristic peaks attributed to C–N at 399.73 eV and NH_2 at 401.30 eV [15]. High-resolution O1s spectrum (Figure 3d) revealed two distinct binding energy peaks at 531.21 and 531.93 eV ascribing to C=O (sp^2) and C–O–C/C–OH (sp^3), respectively [39]. Interestingly, the results displayed that the surface of the synthesized BCDs nano-biocarrier may be provided with hydroxyl, amide, and carbonyl functional groups. Therefore, these surface hydrophilic functional groups not only remarkably enhance the stability and solubility of BCDs nano-biocarrier in the aqueous medium but also significantly foster applications in medicine and biology [15]. These results correlate well with the results of FT-IR.

3.5. X-ray Diffraction (XRD)

The XRD was employed to investigate the crystalline nature of BCDs nano-biocarrier. As shown in Figure 4, the XRD pattern reveals a distinct broad diffraction peak located at $2\theta = 24.01°$, corresponding to interlayer spacing in graphite (0.34 nm) [15]. This finding indicates the amorphous carbon phase of BCDs nano-biocarrier without any crystalline phases and could attribute to the introduction of more oxygen-containing groups [1,45]. Furthermore, the results confirm that the BCDs nano-biocarrier exhibit graphitic nature with highly disordered carbon atoms, hence containing graphite-like structures [14,46]. These results are in good agreement with the data of XPS. Similar findings were reported by Rahmani et al. [47] and Hu et al. [15] for nitrogen doped CDs and albumin CDs, respectively

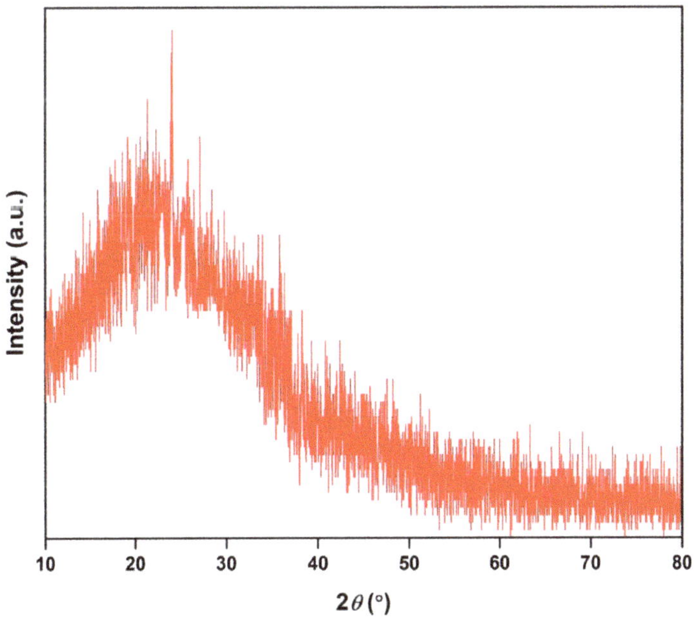

Figure 4. X-ray diffraction (XRD) pattern of BCDs nano-biocarrier.

3.6. UV-Visible Spectroscopy

The optical properties of the pure LNZ, BCDs nano-biocarrier, and LNZ–BCDs nano-bioconjugate were characterized via analyzing their UV–visible absorption spectra. As shown in Figure 5a, the UV–visible absorption spectrum of pure LNZ exhibits a strong absorbance peak located at 251 nm, indicating the λ_{max} of the pure drug molecules [2]. It can be obviously seen that the UV-visible absorption spectrum of BCDs nano-biocarrier displays a distinct absorbance peak centered at about 280 nm (Figure 5a). This absorbance peak typically corresponds to π–π* electronic transition of C=C bonds, hence indicating the existence of aromatic π orbitals in the BCDs nano-biocarrier and corresponding to the characteristic feature of the protein α-helical structure [20,48]. A similar finding was reported by Amin et al. [23] for nitrogen-doped CDs using date kernel. Visually, it can be easily seen that the aqueous solution of BCDs nano-biocarrier shows a transparent, uniform, and pale-yellow colored solution in daylight and emits an obvious intense bright blue fluorescence under the UV light excitation at 365 nm (Figure 5b). This indicates the formation of BCDs nano-biocarrier exhibiting a relatively high quantum yield, similar to previously reported studies [12,46]. On the other hand, LNZ–BCDs nano-bioconjugate's UV–visible absorption spectrum revealed that the absorbance peaks of both LNZ and BCDs nano-biocarrier were retained at 251 nm and 280 nm, respectively, thus confirming successful conjugation and attachment of LNZ drug molecules on the surface of BCDs nano-biocarrier. A similar finding was reported by Sun et al. [7] for the doxorubicin entrapped CDs.

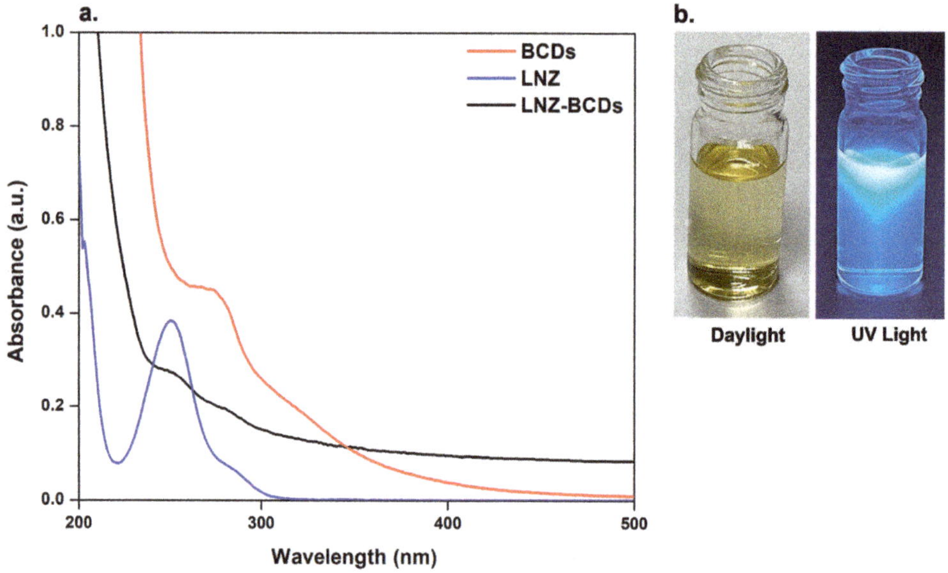

Figure 5. (**a**) UV-visible absorption spectra of pure LNZ, BCDs nano-biocarrier, and LNZ–BCDs nano-bioconjugate, and (**b**) photographic images of BCDs nano-biocarrier in daylight and under UV light excitation at 365 nm.

3.7. Fluorescence Spectroscopy

The fluorescence properties of the BCDs nano-biocarrier were investigated using fluorescence spectroscopy. It is worth noting that the BSA chain by itself is regarded as a fluorescent molecule, owing to the presence of two different types of tryptophan (Trp–134 and Trp–213) residues localized on the surface of the protein in domain I and in the hydrophobic cavity of domain II, respectively, which can interact or attach to other molecules [49].

As shown in Figure 6a, the fluorescence excitation and emission spectra of the BCDs nano-biocarrier present a distinct maximum emission peak centered at about 425 ± 1.2 nm when excited at an optimal wavelength of around 320 ± 1 nm. This can be ascribed to the amino acid residues present in the BCDs nano-biocarrier, including tryptophan (Trp), tyrosine (Tyr), and phenylalanine (Phe) [50]. The mechanism of the fluorescence emission for BCDs nano-biocarrier is due to band gap-transition. This is reasonably attributed to the fact that the maximum excitation peak centered at 320 nm (Figure 6a) is so near to the absorbance peak of the BCDs nano-biocarrier at a wavelength around 280 nm (Figure 5a), as previously reported [49]. Interestingly, the functional groups (–COOH, –OH, and –NH_2) present on the BCDs nano-biocarrier surface, which were previously confirmed via FT-IR analysis, can result in a series of emissive traps that is of pronounced importance for the strong fluorescent properties displayed by the BCDs nano-biocarrier [46]. Furthermore, the fluorescence emission spectrum of the BCDs nano-biocarrier exhibits an obvious good symmetry with a narrow full width at half maximum (FWHM) of 89 nm. This indicates a narrow size distribution and monodispersed BCDs nano-biocarrier [25,51]. Notably, these results correlate well with results obtained from the TEM analysis. Similar findings were reported by other researchers [15,52].

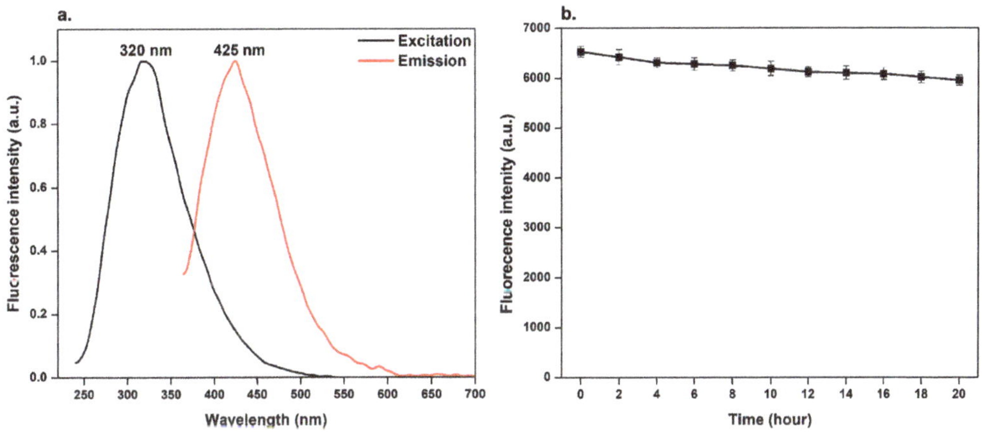

Figure 6. Fluorescence measurements for BCDs nano-biocarrier. (**a**) Fluorescence maximum excitation ($\lambda_{excitation}$ = 380 nm) and emission ($\lambda_{emission}$ = 480 nm) spectra, and (**b**) fluorescence intensity upon continuous excitation with UV-lamp at wavelength 365 nm.

3.8. Photostability

The photostability of BCDs nano-biocarrier was investigated upon continuous exposure to UV light irradiation for 20 h using Vilber VL-6 LC UV-lamp (France) at wavelength 365 nm [15,28]. It was observed that the fluorescence intensity of the BCDs nano-biocarrier displays no significant change in the intensity and still preserves around 90.5 $\pm$ 1.2% after 20 h, as presented in Figure 6b. This tendency confirms that the BCDs nano-biocarrier exhibit high photostability and great resistance to photobleaching, as well as providing a potential alternative chemical for bioimaging applications [28]. Similar findings were reported by other researchers [15,28].

3.9. Zeta Potential

The zeta (ζ) potential measurements were carried out to investigate the surface charge and assess the stability of the florescent BCDs nano-biocarrier against aggregation, as well as to confirm the conjugation of the BCDs nano-biocarrier with the synthetic antibiotic, LNZ [23]. The ζ-potential value of the BCDs nano-biocarrier was found to be -25.0 ± 0.7 mV (Figure 7), hence indicating good electrostatic stabilization ascribed by the high negative charge, which prevents agglomeration via strong inter-particulate electrostatic repulsion forces [20,40]. The high negatively charged surface of the BCDs nano-biocarrier can be attributed to the abundance of hydroxyl, carboxyl, and amino characteristic functional groups anchoring on the surface of BCDs nano-biocarrier, in consistency with the FT-IR and XPS data [13,42]. The remarkable electrostatic stability of BCDs nano-biocarrier confirms their convenience for several applications [53].

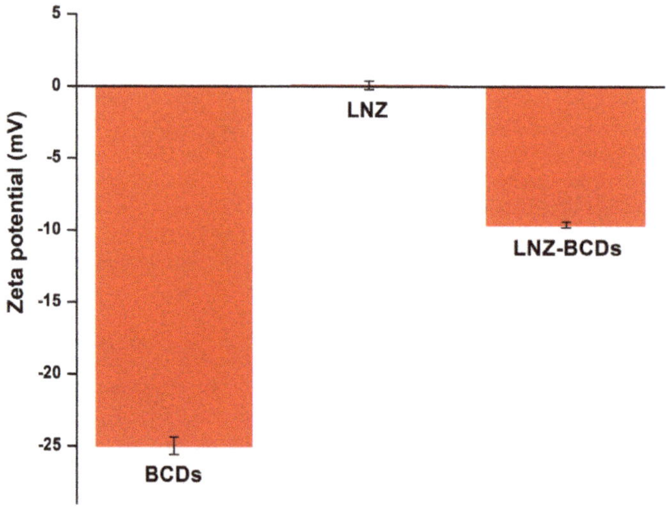

Figure 7. The ζ-potential measurements for BCDs nano-biocarrier, LNZ drug molecules, and LNZ–BCDs nano-bioconjugate.

Interestingly, the physical conjugation of the electrically neutral LNZ on the surface of the negatively charged BCDs nano-biocarrier was demonstrated through a shift in ζ-potential value from -25.0 ± 0.7 mV to -9.6 ± 0.2 mV (Figure 7). This decrease in the surface charge confirmed the formation of LNZ–BCDs nano-bioconjugate complexes with a ζ-potential value of -9.6 ± 0.2 mV. This can be ascribed to the physical interactions between LNZ and BCDs nano-biocarrier via strong π–π interactions among the benzene structures, where the BCDs exhibit sp^2-carbon network that can load the aromatic structure of LNZ [54]. Thus, LNZ presents a high affinity for the negatively charged BCDs nano-biocarrier. Similar findings were previously reported in the literature for other CDs [7,54].

3.10. Drug Loading and Encapsulation Efficiency of LNZ–BCDs Nano-Bioconjugates

The developed LNZ–BCDs nano-bioconjugates were designed to facilitate wound healing and promote tissue regeneration. LNZ, as a model synthetic oxazolidinone antibiotic with low aqueous solubility, was selected to study the drug loading efficiency (DLE) and drug encapsulation efficiency (DEE) of the BCDs nano-biocarrier [2]. As presented in Table 1, the DEE and DLE efficiency substantially increased as the ratio of BCDs:LNZ increased up to 1:1. DEE/DLE were $91.8 \pm 1.3/20.7 \pm 0.69$, $92.5 \pm 1.4/21.1 \pm 0.19$, and $97.2 \pm 1.0/22.5 \pm 0.23\%$ when the ratio of BCDs:LNZ was 4:1, 2:1, and 1:1, respectively (Table 1). A similar result was reported for piperine-loaded BSA/oxidized gum Arabic nanocomposites in which DEE and DLE increased upon increasing the concentration of piperine [24]. Moreover, Rahmani et al. [47] prepared pH-responsive doxorubicin-loaded chitosan-montmorillonite-nitrogen-doped CDs for targeted treatment of cancer cells with high entrapment and loading efficiency of 91 and 49%, respectively. Higher ratios of BCDs:LNZ (1:3 and 1:5) were counterproductive, whereas the DEE/DLE declined to $88.1 \pm 1.9/19.8 \pm 0.36$ and $85.3 \pm 1.1/18.6 \pm 0.47\%$, respectively. This was probably attributed to the drug precipitation [55]. Overall, the maximum DEE/DLE that could be obtained was $97.2 \pm 1.0/22.5 \pm 0.23\%$ when the ratio of BCDs to LNZ was 1:1. Hence, this might be ascribed to the possible hydrogen bonding and π-π stacking interactions [20,45].

Table 1. Data of drug loading and encapsulation efficiency of LNZ–BCDs nano-bioconjugates.

BCDs:LNZ	DEE (%)	DLE (%)
4:1	91.8 ± 1.3	20.7 ± 0.69
2:1	92.5 ± 1.4	21.1 ± 0.19
1:1	97.2 ± 1.0	22.5 ± 0.23
1:3	88.1 ± 1.9	19.8 ± 0.36
1:5	85.3 ± 1.1	18.6 ± 0.47

Results are expressed as mean ± SD.

3.11. In Vitro Drug Release Studies of LNZ from the LNZ–BCDs Nano-Bioconjugate

An ideal wound healing biomaterial must postulate complete drug release over a long period of up to 24 to 48 h [2]. The cumulative release profile of the LNZ–BCDs nano-bioconjugate in comparison to the free LNZ drug solution was studied for 48 h, as shown in Figure 8. It was observed that the percentage LNZ released from the free drug solution was almost 98 ± 0.5% after 6 h. This resembles a fast and uncontrolled release manner. Nevertheless, the release of LNZ from the LNZ–BCDs nano-bioconjugate displayed a controlled release manner since the percentage of LNZ released after 6 h did not exceed 52 ± 1.3% [56]. The LNZ–BCDs nano-bioconjugate achieved almost complete drug release within 48 h in comparison to that of free LNZ drug solution within 6 h only (Figure 8). These findings indicate that LNZ–BCDs nano-bioconjugate significantly controlled LNZ release from the synthesized LNZ–BCDs nano-bioconjugate.

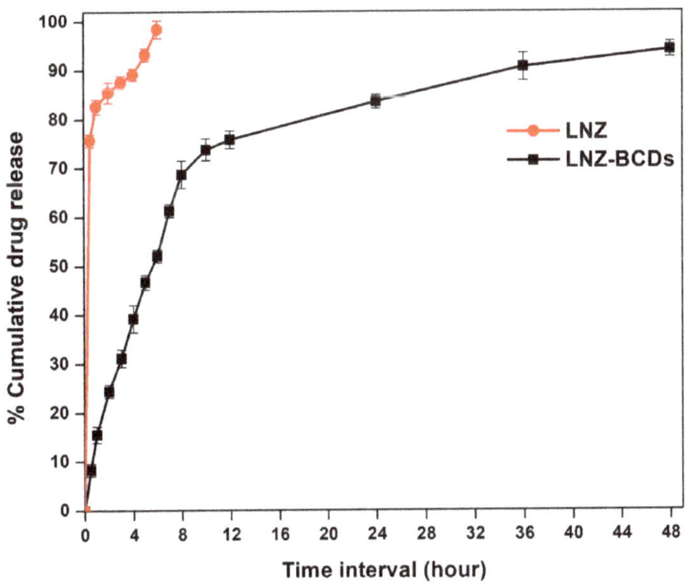

Figure 8. In vitro release profile of the LNZ–BCDs nano-bioconjugate in comparison to the LNZ drug solution in PBS (pH 7.4) at 37 ± 0.2 °C for up to 48 h.

The release profile of LNZ from the LNZ–BCDs nano-bioconjugate during the experiment displayed a biphasic release pattern, including a relatively fast-release property in the first 12 h, subsequently followed by a sustained release for a prolonged time for 48 h of the experimental period. A similar finding was reported by Karami et al. for isophethalaldoxime palladacycle complex-loaded BSA nanoparticles with a cumulative release profile over a period of 45 h in PBS pH 7.4 at 37 °C [20]. In the initial fast-release phase, almost 75 ± 1.8% of the drug was released from the LNZ–BCDs nano-bioconjugate within 12 h. This is due to the constant release rate of LNZ in the dissolution medium attributed to the weakly stacked drug molecules on the superficial zones of the graphene-like structures of the BCDs nano-biocarrier, which were controlled by a diffusion process due to the π–π interactions [20,54]. This behavior is first and foremost advantageous to exert the antibacterial action in the wound bed throughout the first few hours via drawing mesenchymal cells [2]. Subsequently, in the sustained LNZ release phase, the rate of LNZ release from the LNZ–BCDs nano-bioconjugate was gradual and much slower. This can be ascribed to the increasing diffusion pathways' distances and to the remaining LNZ drug fraction entrapped in the inner core of the LNZ–BCDs nano-bioconjugate, which consistently diffused slowly from the matrix to the dissolution medium [20,25]. This tendency prevents recolonization and stimulates tissue renovation in the subsequent phases of the wound healing mechanism. Hence, this postulates a potentially mesmerizing opportunity for the synthesized LNZ–BCDs nano-bioconjugate for regenerative medicine. A similar finding was reported by Mehta et al. for lisinopril-loaded CDs derived from pasteurized milk with a cumulative release profile over 48 h in PBS pH 5.2, 6.2, and 7.4 at 37 °C [25].

An interesting point that is noteworthy to highlight is the influence of the negative ζ-potential value of the LNZ–BCDs nano-bioconjugate (−9.6 ± 0.2 mV) on the drug release profile. It was found that negative ζ-potential facilitates the drug delivery process and aids in wound healing via allowing the LNZ–BCDs nano-bioconjugate to easily penetrate through the cellular membrane and progressively increase the percentage LNZ released to accumulate in the cytoplasm and exert its therapeutic effect [53]. Of interest, the total percentage LNZ released from the LNZ–BCDs nano-bioconjugate by the end of the 48 h was approximately 95 ± 1.6%. This confirmed the proper loading efficiency of the LNZ drug molecules within the LNZ–BCDs nano-bioconjugate. This finding is in good correlation with previously reported studies [20,43].

Kinetic profile analysis for the LNZ–BCDs nano-bioconjugate release data was carried out according to zero order, first order, second order, Higuchi diffusion, Hixon-Crowel, and Baker-Lonsdal mathematical functions. To determine the drug release kinetics, cumulative release data of LNZ from LNZ–BCDs nano-bioconjugate were fitted in various models (Figure S1 and Table 2). According to the correlation coefficient (R^2) value attained for each of the above-mentioned kinetic models, it was observed that the release of LNZ from the drug delivery system (LNZ–BCDs) seemed to be best fitting to the Second order model order kinetics as the plots revealed the prime linearity (R^2 value = 0.985).

Table 2. Parameters and R^2 values of each kinetic model for estimating the release of LNZ from (1:1) LNZ–BCDs nano-bioconjugate.

	Kinetic Model					
	Zero Order	**First Order**	**Second Order**	**Higuchi Diffusion**	**Hixon-Crowel**	**Baker-Lonsdal**
R^2	0.804 $K_0 = 0.02714$	0.956 $K_1 = 0.00094$	0.985 $K_2 = 0.00005$	0.915 $K_P = 1.872038$	0.912 $K_\beta = 0.000917$	0.957 $K_C = 0.00012$

3.12. Ex Vivo Hemolysis Assay

The hemolysis assay was performed to further investigate ex vivo blood biocompatibility. It is one of the most important properties that should be evaluated for any biomaterial intended to be in contact with blood elements to prevent serious adverse effects for in vivo drug-delivery applications [57,58]. In the current study, the potential hemolytic activity induced by the synthesized LNZ–BCDs nano-bioconjugate wound healing biomaterial was investigated as the indication of ex vivo blood biocompatibility [58]. As shown in Figure 9a, the solution in deionized water was used as a positive control and turned red color due to hemolysis resulting in the release of hemoglobin (Hb) from the red blood cells (RBCs), whereas the negative control (PBS solutions) did not show any hemolysis [59]. The hemolytic images presented in Figure 9a show no obvious hemolysis in the PBS solutions with different LNZ–BCDs nano-bioconjugate concentrations (25–300 μg/mL). Although the hemolytic activity slightly increased at higher LNZ–BCDs nano-bioconjugate concentration, the hemolysis percentage was retained less than 5% even at concentrations up to 300 μg/mL (Figure 9b). It is worth highlighting that the LNZ–BCDs biomaterial is regarded as a non-toxic, non-hemolytic, and feasible blood-contacting material with favorable biocompatibility with RBCs, hence intended for secure in vivo drug-delivery applications, as the ISO 10993-4 precisely outlines safe biomaterials as having a hemolysis percentage ≤5% [57,60]. Of interest, it was previously reported that the hemolysis percentage of plain LNZ drug molecules was found to be 14% [59]. Hence, the less hemolysis of the LNZ–BCDs nano-bioconjugate overcame the high hemolysis percentage associated with plain LNZ drug molecules, which portrays their potential for drug delivery. Therefore, the results of the ex vivo hemolysis assay suggest that the LNZ–BCDs biomaterial is proper for medical application and potentially feasible for facilitating wound healing through blood circulation, similar to previously reported studies [58,61].

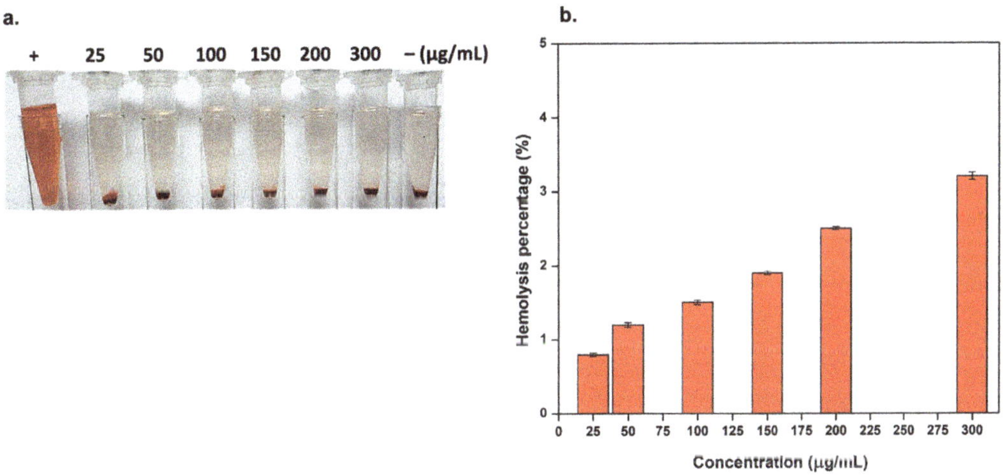

Figure 9. Hemolytic activity of LNZ–BCDs nano-bioconjugate. (**a**) Hemolytic images after treatment with LNZ–BCDs nano-bioconjugate of different concentrations (25–300 μg/mL). Particularly, (–) and (+) signs correspond to the negative and positive controls, respectively, and (**b**) hemolysis percentage induced by the LNZ–BCDs nano-bioconjugate.

3.13. Cytotoxicity Assay

MTT assay was carried out against the HSF cell line to evaluate the biocompatibility and cytotoxicity of the synthesized BCDs and LNZ–BCDs nano-biomaterials. As shown in Figure 10, the cell viability of both BCDs and LNZ–BCDs nano-biomaterials displayed no noticeable toxicity to the HSF cell line after incubation for 24 h, confirming that these nano-biomaterials exhibit excellent biocompatibility. By comparing the cytotoxicity results of the BCDs nano-biocarrier with that of LNZ–BCDs nano-bioconjugate, the LNZ-loaded BCDs presented slightly higher cell cytotoxicity than the plain BCDs nano-biocarrier. However, the LNZ–BCDs nano-bioconjugate still maintained high cell viability above 91% even at a high concentration of 1000 μg/mL. This indicates that LNZ–BCDs nano-bioconjugate presented excellent biocompatibility and extremely low cytotoxicity and provides further proof as a promising potent drug delivery nano-system [7,42]. These findings postulate that LNZ–BCDs nano-bioconjugate could be an ideal candidate for escaping the dose-dependent side effects of the free LNZ, including gastrointestinal disorders, skin rashes, and allergic reactions, due to their relatively small mean particle size and shielding effects, and confirm the potential secure biomedical applications [40,42]. Similar studies [55,62] revealed that

LNZ-loaded nano-systems exhibit higher antibacterial activity and lower cytotoxicity as compared with the conventional free LNZ, indicating their potential therapeutic effects.

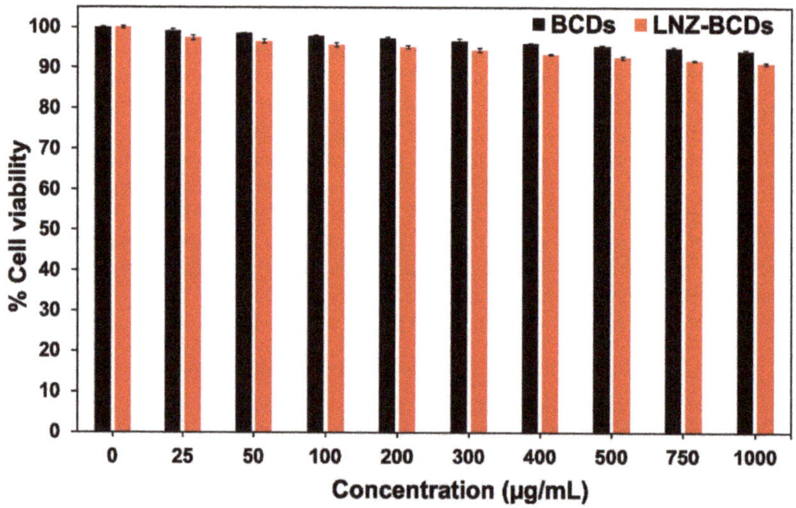

Figure 10. Cell viability percentage of HSF cell line against BCDs nano-biocarrier and LNZ−BCDs nano-bioconjugate at various concentrations for 24 h.

3.14. *In Vitro Antibacterial Activity by Broth Microdilution Method*

The MIC of pure LNZ, BCDs nano-biocarrier, and their formulated nano-bioconjugate LNZ−BCDs was detected against MRSA and *Staphylococcus aureus* (ATCC® 25922). Both isolates were sensitive to pure LNZ and their MIC was 4 µg/mL, as shown in Table 3. The BCDs nano-biocarrier showed a slight antibacterial activity against both MRSA and *Staphylococcus aureus* (ATCC® 25922) (Table 3). This finding correlates well with the data mentioned in the FT-IR analysis, indicating that the existence of a hydroxyl (−OH) functional group in the structure of BCDs nano-biocarrier plays an important role in enhancing its antibacterial activity. Previous studies [63,64] have also shown that CDs exhibit antibacterial activity.

Table 3. Results of MIC of LNZ, BCDs nano-biocarrier, and LNZ−BCDs nano-bioconjugate against different bacterial strains.

Bacterial Strain	Minimum Inhibitory Concentration (MIC)		
	LNZ (µg/mL)	BCDs (mg/mL)	LNZ−BCDs (µg/mL)
Staphylococcus aureus (ATCC® 25922)	4 ± 0.00 (S) *	11.25 ± 0.43	2 ± 0.00 (S)
Methicillin-resistant *Staphylococcus aureus* (MRSA)	4 ± 0.00 (S)	11.25 ± 0.43	0.25 ± 0.09 (S)

* S: sensitive.

Interestingly, the conjugation between LNZ drug molecules and BCDs nano-biocarrier in the formulated nano-bioconjugate LNZ−BCDs significantly reduced the MIC of LNZ and increased the bacterial sensitivity. The conjugation showed synergistic antibacterial activity subscribed to both LNZ and BCDs bio-nanocarrier together in the LNZ–BCDs nano-bioconjugate in comparison with their singular use, where the MIC of LNZ was distinctively reduced against *Staphylococcus aureus* (ATCC® 25922) by 2-fold and against MRSA by 16-fold (Table 3). Therefore, it is worth highlighting that the nano-bioconjugated formula of both LNZ and BCDs nano-biocarrier possessed synergistic antibacterial activity and declined the growth of both MRSA and *Staphylococcus aureus* (ATCC® 25922), which are major causes for wound infections. Furthermore, the formulated nano-bioconjugate LNZ−BCDs displayed even better antibacterial activity as the amino functional groups on the surface, positive surface charge, as well as small particle size facilitated the quick binding to the bacteria (negative charge on the surface), thus destroying the surface charge and eventually entering the bacteria [61]. Accordingly, the nano-bioconjugate LNZ−BCDs has the potential for use as a wound healing biomaterial to diminish bacterial load and avoid colonization at the wound bed, and hence facilitate the wound healing process.

3.15. *In Vitro Skin-Related Enzyme Inhibitory Assays*

The present study performed a screening of pure LNZ, BCDs nano-biocarrier, and LNZ–BCDs nano-bioconjugate regarding their in vitro inhibition of different skin-related enzymes, namely tyrosinase, collagenase, and elastase. The effect of pure LNZ, BCDs nano-biocarrier, and LNZ–BCDs nano-biomaterials on the percentage enzyme inhibition activity along with the IC_{50} (μg/mL) of various skin-related enzymes in comparison to their corresponding positive controls is presented in Table 4.

Table 4. Effect of LNZ, BCDs nano-biocarrier, and LNZ–BCDs nano-bioconjugate on the percentage enzyme inhibition activity along with the IC_{50} (μg/mL) of various skin-related enzymes in comparison to their corresponding positive controls.

Test Sample	Anti-Elastase		Anti-Collagenase		Anti-Tyrosinase	
	% Inhibition	**IC_{50} (μg/mL)**	**% Inhibition**	**IC_{50} (μg/mL)**	**% Inhibition**	**IC_{50} (μg/mL)**
LNZ–BCDs	$95.92 \pm 2.21^{a,b}$	$30.01 \pm 1.13^{a,b,c}$	$93.23 \pm 1.65^{a,c}$	$208.31 \pm 3.08^{a,b,c}$	$85.12 \pm 1.50^{a,b,c}$	$180.01 \pm 2.12^{a,c}$
LNZ	88.00 ± 1.35	57.20 ± 2.88	65.05 ± 1.48	335.34 ± 2.09	65.00 ± 1.63	363.50 ± 2.08
BCDs	91.34 ± 1.47	45.50 ± 2.17	92.02 ± 1.25	253.66 ± 2.51	80.23 ± 1.41	180.40 ± 5.09
+ve control	92.52 ± 4.63	44.92 ± 1.71	79.82 ± 2.63	315.12 ± 2.21	76.52 ± 0.83	321.65 ± 3.41

Results are presented as mean ± standard deviation. [a], [b], and [c] represent significant difference from LNZ, BCDs nano-biocarrier, and +ve control, respectively.

Results revealed that LNZ–BCDs nano-bioconjugate had a significantly higher anti-elastase activity compared to each of LNZ (p = 0.006) and BCDs nano-biocarrier (p = 0.04) and a significantly higher anti-collagenase activity compared to LNZ ($p < 0.0001$) and positive control (p = 0.0017) (Table 4). Furthermore, LNZ–BCDs nano-bioconjugate illustrated a significantly higher anti-tyrosinase activity than LNZ, BCDs nano-biocarrier, and positive control ($p < 0.0001$, p = 0.0147, and p = 0.001, respectively). It is worth highlighting that the LNZ–BCDs nano-bioconjugate showed a significantly lower IC_{50} for the different skin-related enzymes than all other samples (all $p < 0.01$). The only exception was the anti-tyrosinase IC_{50} of BCDs nano-biocarrier, which was equal to the LNZ–BCDs nano-bioconjugate IC_{50} (p = 0.908) (Table 4). Therefore, the LNZ–BCDs nano-bioconjugate exhibited the highest and most robust anti-elastase, anti-collagenase, and anti-tyrosinase activities compared with pure LNZ and BCDs nano-biocarrier. These results indicate the synergistic effect subscribed to both LNZ and BCDs nano-biocarrier together in the LNZ–BCDs nano-bioconjugate in comparison with their singular use.

The strong anti-elastase and anti-collagenase activities of LNZ–BCDs nano-bioconjugate potentially plays a vital role in re-epithelialization and shortening the duration of the wound healing process. Previous researchers [65] reported in the literature that elastase and collagenase may potentiate deprivation of the extracellular matrix and growth factors that prolong the inflammatory phase, thus delaying the wound healing process. Hence, preventing unnecessary elastase and collagenase at the wound site is relatively important. Moreover, the great anti-tyrosinase activity presented by LNZ–BCDs nano-bioconjugate would be beneficial in the treatment of hyperpigmentation observed during and after the wound healing process [66]. Hence, the LNZ–BCDs nano-bioconjugate showed a promising wound healing potential and a melanogenesis-inhibiting activity.

3.16. Scratch Wound Healing Assay

The evaluation of the effectiveness of BCDs and LNZ–BCDs nano-biomaterials in the wound healing process was determined in vitro using normal human skin fibroblast (HSF) cell line. In the current study, the scratch wound healing assay was selected as it is considered to mimic an incision wound in vitro [19]. The prime advantage of this assay is its relative feasibility and simplicity. The classic scratch wound primarily heals via the proliferation and migration of cells along with contraction and closure of the wound gap; thus, it is necessary to closely monitor the wound healing rate by imaging to confirm the complete wound healing process and tissue regeneration [34]. Changes in the width of wounds for treated and untreated HSF cell lines were assessed at 24 h and 48 h, and images are presented in Figure 11a,b. The wound closure percentages for treated and untreated HSF cell lines are graphically represented in Figure 11c.

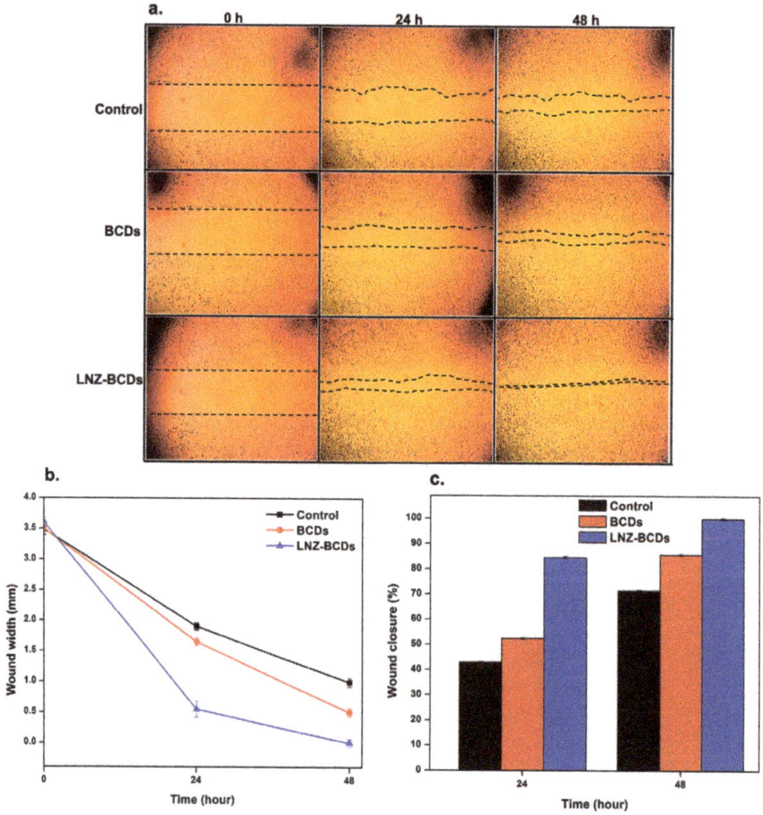

Figure 11. (**a**) Images at 1 mm scale bar, (**b**) profile of changes in the width of wounds with time, and (**c**) wound closure percentages of untreated control and treated normal human skin fibroblast (HSF) cell line with BCDs nano-biocarrier and LNZ–BCDs nano-bioconjugate at 24 and 48 h.

During the assay, significant differences in the improvement of the wound status for the treated cells with BCDs and LNZ–BCDs nano-biomaterials from the untreated control cells were witnessed. Cells treated with BCDs nano-biocarrier illustrated considerably higher contraction and closure of the wound gap compared to untreated control cells throughout the assay. After 48 h, BCDs nano-biocarrier allowed faster wound closure than untreated control cells with approximately 85.75 ± 0.03% wound closure, while the wound width was reduced to 0.5 ± 0.04 mm of the initial wound width (3.50 ± 0.08 mm). On the other hand, cells treated with LNZ–BCDs nano-bioconjugate illustrated a significantly higher contraction and closure of the wound gap with approximately 84.53 ± 0.13% wound closure compared with both the untreated control and BCDs nano-biocarrier treated cells after 24 h. Wound closure analysis revealed complete closure of the scratch wound gap for the LNZ–BCDs nano-bioconjugate treated cells (99.97 ± 0.02%) compared with both untreated control (71.43 ± 0.02%) and BCDs nano-biocarrier treated (85.75 ± 0.03%) cells, which failed to heal completely after 48 h. These differences confirm the synergistic effect and excellent healing efficiency subscribed to both LNZ and BCDs nano-biocarrier together in the LNZ–BCDs nano-bioconjugate in comparison with the singular use of BCDs nano-biocarrier. Similar to the skin-related enzyme inhibition results, the LNZ–BCDs nano-bioconjugate combining both LNZ and BCDs nano-biocarrier exhibited robust anti-elastase, anti-collagenase, and anti-tyrosinase activities, thus accelerating wound healing and tissue regeneration processes.

It is interesting to shed light on the rate of cell migration analysis, which illustrated that LNZ–BCDs nano-bioconjugate enabled a higher rate of cell migration of 75.21 ± 0.02 μm than other BCDs nano-biocarrier treated and untreated control cells of 62.50 ± 0.02 and 52.08 ± 0.03 μm, respectively, by 48 h. This indicates that the developed LNZ–BCDs nano-bioconjugate was capable of remarkably enhancing and promoting the fibroblasts proliferation and migration favoring the wound healing mechanism due to the presence of both LNZ and BCDs nano-biocarrier together as compared to BCDs nano-biocarrier treated and untreated control cells, which presents promising wound healing properties. These findings are consistent with the results of Rohiwal et al. [34] for bovine serum albumin (BSA)-dextran bio-nanoconjugate.

4. Conclusions

A highly fluorescent BCDs nano-biocarrier was successfully synthesized via green, facile, and one-step hydrothermal treatment without any further chemical modification. The developed BCDs nano-biocarrier, emitting bright blue fluorescence, illustrated extremely small size (1.5 ± 0.2–7.5 ± 0.1 nm), easy surface functionalization, intrinsic optical and fluorescence properties, high water solubility, superior photostability, and distinctive antibacterial activity. An innovative biphasic release BCDs of LNZ, which retains the intrinsic characteristics that meet the desirable properties of an ideal wound healing biomaterial, was successfully developed at an optimum ratio of 1:1, which showed a high drug encapsulation and loading efficiency of 97.2 ± 1.0% and 22.5 ± 0.23%, respectively. The developed LNZ–BCDs drug delivery nano-system did not impose any significant cytotoxicity with HSF cells and maintained high cell viability >91%, thus might be utilized as a potential candidate in many fields of biomedical applications. The in vitro and ex vivo results confirmed that the LNZ–BCDs nano-bioconjugate possessed excellent biocompatibility with HRBCs with hemolysis percentage <5%, distinct antibacterial activity against the most common wound infectious pathogens, including *Staphylococcus aureus* (ATCC® 25922) and methicillin-resistant *Staphylococcus aureus*, robust anti-elastase, anti-collagenase, and anti-tyrosinase activities, and an overall promising wound healing performance with accelerated wound closure and improved tissue regeneration. To our knowledge, this is the first reported study to synthesize highly fluorescent CDs derived from BSA for LNZ drug delivery, which displays great potential for future in vivo and clinical applications. Given the results of this study, it can be speculated that the synthesized novel LNZ–BCDs drug delivery nano-system could bring a paradigm shift in the use of biomaterials for biomedical applications such as biosensing, bioimaging, photocatalysis, and for potential theranostic applications as a promising agent that synchronously recognizes, delivers therapeutic cargo, and assesses the response to treatment. Uniformity and size control of CDs are critical steps and remain a challenge to attain stable properties and better performance for specific applications. However, several investigations have been done until now to achieve uniform and homogeneous CDs via either synthesis or post-treatment.

Supplementary Materials: The following supporting information can be downloaded at: https://www.mdpi.com/article/10.3390/pharmaceutics15010234/s1, Figure S1: Drug release kinetics of (a) Zero order, (b) First order, (c) Second order, (d) Higuchi diffusion, (e) Hixon-Crowel, and (f) Baker-Lonsdal kinetic models for the release of LNZ from (1:1) LNZ–BCDs nano-bioconjugate.

Author Contributions: Conceptualization, R.I.A.; Methodology, D.S.G., M.A.A. and M.F.A.R.; Validation, R.I.A.; Formal analysis, D.S.G.; Investigation, D.S.G., M.A.A., M.F.A.R. and R.N.S.; Resources, R.I.A.; Data curation, M.A.A.; Writing—original draft, D.S.G.; Writing—review & editing, R.I.A. and R.N.S.; Visualization, R.N.S.; Supervision, R.I.A. and R.N.S. All authors have read and agreed to the published version of the manuscript.

Funding: This research received no external funding.

Institutional Review Board Statement: No animals were involved in this study.

Informed Consent Statement: No human subjects were involved in this study.

Data Availability Statement: Data are available upon request.

Conflicts of Interest: The authors declare no conflict of interest.

References

1. Fadilah, N.I.M.; Maarof, M.; Motta, A.; Tabata, Y.; Fauzi, M.B. The Discovery and Development of Natural-Based Biomaterials with Demonstrated Wound Healing Properties: A Reliable Approach in Clinical Trials. *Biomedicines* **2022**, *10*, 2226. [CrossRef]
2. Ghataty, D.S.; Amer, R.I.; Wasfi, R.; Shamma, R.N. Novel Linezolid Loaded Bio-Composite Films as Dressings for Effective Wound Healing: Experimental Design, Development, Optimization, and Antimicrobial Activity. *Drug Deliv.* **2022**, *29*, 3168–3185. [CrossRef] [PubMed]
3. Wei, S.-C.; Nain, A.; Lin, Y.-F.; Wu, R.-S.; Srivastava, P.; Chang, L.; Huang, Y.-F.; Chang, H.-T.; Chuang, K.-T.; Huang, C.-C. Light Triggered Programmable States of Carbon Dot Liposomes Accelerate Chronic Wound Healing via Photocatalytic Cascade Reaction. *Carbon* **2023**, *201*, 952–961. [CrossRef]
4. Shanmugapriya, K.; Kang, H.W. Engineering Pharmaceutical Nanocarriers for Photodynamic Therapy on Wound Healing: Review. *Mater. Sci. Eng. C* **2019**, *105*, 110110. [CrossRef]
5. Omidi, M.; Yadegari, A.; Tayebi, L. Wound Dressing Application of PH-Sensitive Carbon Dots/Chitosan Hydrogel. *RSC Adv.* **2017**, *7*, 10638–10649. [CrossRef]
6. Mou, C.; Wang, X.; Liu, Y.; Xie, Z.; Zheng, M. Positively Charged BODIPY@carbon Dot Nanocomposites for Enhanced Photomicrobicidal Efficacy and Wound Healing. *J. Mater. Chem. B* **2022**, *10*, 8094–8099. [CrossRef] [PubMed]
7. Sun, Y.; Zheng, S.; Liu, L.; Kong, Y.; Zhang, A.; Xu, K.; Han, C. The Cost-Effective Preparation of Green Fluorescent Carbon Dots for Bioimaging and Enhanced Intracellular Drug Delivery. *Nanoscale Res. Lett.* **2020**, *15*, 55. [CrossRef] [PubMed]
8. Behboudi, H.; Mehdipour, G.; Safari, N.; Pourmadadi, M.; Saei, A.; Omidi, M.; Tayebi, L.; Rahmandoust, M. Carbon Quantum Dots in Nanobiotechnology. In *Nanomaterials for Advanced Biological Applications*; Rahmandoust, M., Ayatollahi, M.R., Eds.; Advanced Structured Materials; Springer International Publishing: Cham, Switzerland, 2019; pp. 145–179. [CrossRef]
9. Aayanifard, Z.; Alebrahim, T.; Pourmadadi, M.; Yazdian, F.; Dinani, H.S.; Rashedi, H.; Omidi, M. Ultra PH-Sensitive Detection of Total and Free Prostate-Specific Antigen Using Electrochemical Aptasensor Based on Reduced Graphene Oxide/Gold Nanoparticles Emphasis on TiO2/Carbon Quantum Dots as a Redox Probe. *Eng. Life Sci.* **2021**, *21*, 739–752. [CrossRef]
10. Dadkhah, S.; Mehdinia, A.; Jabbari, A.; Manbohi, A. Rapid and Sensitive Fluorescence and Smartphone Dual-Mode Detection of Dopamine Based on Nitrogen-Boron Co-Doped Carbon Quantum Dots. *Microchim. Acta* **2020**, *187*, 569. [CrossRef]
11. Nocito, G.; Sciuto, E.L.; Franco, D.; Nastasi, F.; Pulvirenti, L.; Petralia, S.; Spinella, C.; Calabrese, G.; Guglielmino, S.; Conoci, S. Physicochemical Characterization and Antibacterial Properties of Carbon Dots from Two Mediterranean Olive Solid Waste Cultivars. *Nanomaterials* **2022**, *12*, 885. [CrossRef]
12. Huang, C.; Dong, H.; Su, Y.; Wu, Y.; Narron, R.; Yong, Q. Synthesis of Carbon Quantum Dot Nanoparticles Derived from Byproducts in Bio-Refinery Process for Cell Imaging and In Vivo Bioimaging. *Nanomaterials* **2019**, *9*, 387. [CrossRef] [PubMed]
13. Sachdev, A.; Gopinath, P. Green Synthesis of Multifunctional Carbon Dots from Coriander Leaves and Their Potential Application as Antioxidants, Sensors and Bioimaging Agents. *Analyst* **2015**, *140*, 4260–4269. [CrossRef] [PubMed]
14. Wang, M.; Wan, Y.; Zhang, K.; Fu, Q.; Wang, L.; Zeng, J.; Xia, Z.; Gao, D. Green Synthesis of Carbon Dots Using the Flowers of *Osmanthus fragrans* (Thunb.) Lour. as Precursors: Application in Fe^{3+} and Ascorbic Acid Determination and Cell Imaging. *Anal. Bioanal. Chem.* **2019**, *411*, 2715–2727. [CrossRef] [PubMed]
15. Hu, X.; An, X.; Li, L. Easy Synthesis of Highly Fluorescent Carbon Dots from Albumin and Their Photoluminescent Mechanism and Biological Imaging Applications. *Mater. Sci. Eng. C* **2016**, *58*, 730–736. [CrossRef]
16. Chu, K.-W.; Lee, S.L.; Chang, C.-J.; Liu, L. Recent Progress of Carbon Dot Precursors and Photocatalysis Applications. *Polymers* **2019**, *11*, 689. [CrossRef]

17. Yang, Q.; Wei, L.; Zheng, X.; Xiao, L. Single Particle Dynamic Imaging and Fe3+ Sensing with Bright Carbon Dots Derived from Bovine Serum Albumin Proteins. *Sci. Rep.* **2015**, *5*, 17727. [CrossRef]
18. Reshma; Vaishanav, S.K.; Yadav, T.; Sinha, S.; Tiwari, S.; Satnami, M.L.; Ghosh, K.K. Antidepressant Drug-Protein Interactions Studied by Spectroscopic Methods Based on Fluorescent Carbon Quantum Dots. *Heliyon* **2019**, *5*, e01631. [CrossRef]
19. Zhang, F.; Yang, H.; Yang, Y.; Wang, H.; Li, X.; Wu, X. Stretchable and Biocompatible Bovine Serum Albumin Fibrous Films Supported Silver for Accelerated Bacteria-Infected Wound Healing. *Chem. Eng. J.* **2021**, *417*, 129145. [CrossRef]
20. Karami, K.; Jamshidian, N.; Hajiaghasi, A.; Amirghofran, Z. BSA Nanoparticles as Controlled Release Carriers for Isophethalaldoxime Palladacycle Complex; Synthesis, Characterization, in Vitro Evaluation, Cytotoxicity and Release Kinetics Analysis. *New J. Chem.* **2020**, *44*, 4394–4405. [CrossRef]
21. Phan, V.H.G.; Le, T.M.D.; Janarthanan, G.; Ngo, P.-K.T.; Lee, D.S.; Thambi, T. Development of Bioresorbable Smart Injectable Hydrogels Based on Thermo-Responsive Copolymer Integrated Bovine Serum Albumin Bioconjugates for Accelerated Healing of Excisional Wounds. *J. Ind. Eng. Chem.* **2021**, *96*, 345–355. [CrossRef]
22. Patil, K.D.; Bagade, S.B.; Bonde, S.C. Biodistribution, Pharmacokinetics and Toxicity Evaluation of Mannosylated Gelatin Nanoparticles of Linezolid for Anti-Tubercular Therapy. *Mater. Technol.* **2022**, *37*, 95–103. [CrossRef]
23. Amin, N.; Afkhami, A.; Hosseinzadeh, L.; Madrakian, T. Green and Cost-Effective Synthesis of Carbon Dots from Date Kernel and Their Application as a Novel Switchable Fluorescence Probe for Sensitive Assay of Zoledronic Acid Drug in Human Serum and Cellular Imaging. *Anal. Chim. Acta* **2018**, *1030*, 183–193. [CrossRef] [PubMed]
24. Jalali, E.S.; Shojaosadati, S.A.; Hamedi, S. Green Synthesis of Bovine Serum Albumin/Oxidized Gum Arabic Nanocomposite as PH-Responsive Carrier for Controlled Release of Piperine and the Molecular Docking Study. *Int. J. Biol. Macromol.* **2023**, *225*, 51–62. [CrossRef] [PubMed]
25. Mehta, V.N.; Chettiar, S.S.; Bhamore, J.R.; Kailasa, S.K.; Patel, R.M. Green Synthetic Approach for Synthesis of Fluorescent Carbon Dots for Lisinopril Drug Delivery System and Their Confirmations in the Cells. *J. Fluoresc.* **2017**, *27*, 111–124. [CrossRef]
26. Ri, A.; Ge, Y.; Ra, M.; Am, F. Pharmaceutical and Pharmacological Evaluation of the Effect of Nano-Formulated Spironolactone and Progesterone on Inflammation and Hormonal Levels for Managing Hirsutism Experimentally Induced in Rats. *AAPS PharmSciTech* **2021**, *22*, 204. [CrossRef]
27. Singh, I.; Swami, R.; Pooja, D.; Jeengar, M.K.; Khan, W.; Sistla, R. Lactoferrin Bioconjugated Solid Lipid Nanoparticles: A New Drug Delivery System for Potential Brain Targeting. *J. Drug Target.* **2016**, *24*, 212–223. [CrossRef]
28. Huang, G.; Chen, X.; Wang, C.; Zheng, H.; Huang, Z.; Chen, D.; Xie, H. Photoluminescent Carbon Dots Derived from Sugarcane Molasses: Synthesis, Properties, and Applications. *RSC Adv.* **2017**, *7*, 47840–47847. [CrossRef]
29. Jiang, X.; Shi, Y.; Liu, X.; Wang, M.; Song, P.; Xu, F.; Zhang, X. Synthesis of Nitrogen-Doped Lignin/DES Carbon Quantum Dots as a Fluorescent Probe for the Detection of Fe3+ Ions. *Polymers* **2018**, *10*, 1282. [CrossRef]
30. Andrews, J.M.; Wise, R. In Vitro Susceptibility Testing of BMS-284756 by the BSAC Standardized Disc Testing Method. *J. Antimicrob. Chemother.* **2001**, *48*, 322–324. [CrossRef]
31. *CLSI Document M100-S21*; Performance Standards for Antimicrobial Susceptibility Testing. Twenty-First Informational Supplement; CLSI. Clinical and Laboratory Standards Institute: Wayne, PA, USA, 2020.
32. Mostafa, E.S.; Maher, A.; Mostafa, D.A.; Gad, S.S.; Nawwar, M.A.M.; Swilam, N. A Unique Acylated Flavonol Glycoside from *Prunus persica* (L.) Var. Florida Prince: A New Solid Lipid Nanoparticle Cosmeceutical Formulation for Skincare. *Antioxidants* **2021**, *10*, 436. [CrossRef]
33. Zmejkoski, D.Z.; Marković, Z.M.; Budimir, M.D.; Zdravković, N.M.; Trišić, D.D.; Bugárová, N.; Danko, M.; Kozyrovska, N.O.; Špitalský, Z.; Kleinová, A.; et al. Photoactive and Antioxidant Nanochitosan Dots/Biocellulose Hydrogels for Wound Healing Treatment. *Mater. Sci. Eng. C* **2021**, *122*, 111925. [CrossRef] [PubMed]
34. Rohiwal, S.S.; Ellederova, Z.; Tiwari, A.P.; Alqarni, M.; Elazab, S.T.; Batiha, G.E.-S.; Pawar, S.H.; Thorat, N.D. Self-Assembly of Bovine Serum Albumin (BSA)–Dextran Bio-Nanoconjugate: Structural, Antioxidant and in Vitro Wound Healing Studies. *RSC Adv.* **2021**, *11*, 4308–4317. [CrossRef] [PubMed]
35. Tungare, K.; Bhori, M.; Racherla, K.S.; Sawant, S. Synthesis, Characterization and Biocompatibility Studies of Carbon Quantum Dots from Phoenix Dactylifera. *3 Biotech* **2020**, *10*, 540. [CrossRef] [PubMed]
36. Ankireddy, S.R.; Vo, V.G.; An, S.S.A.; Kim, J. Solvent-Free Synthesis of Fluorescent Carbon Dots: An Ecofriendly Approach for the Bioimaging and Screening of Anticancer Activity via Caspase-Induced Apoptosis. *ACS Appl. Bio Mater.* **2020**, *3*, 4873–4882. [CrossRef] [PubMed]
37. Shah, S.; Maheshwari, H.; Soniwala, M.; Chavda, J. Pulmonary Delivery of Linezolid Nanoparticles for Treatment of Tuberculosis: Design, Development, and Optimization. *J. Pharm. Innov.* **2022**, *17*, 46–59. [CrossRef]
38. Sahu, V.; Khan, F. Synthesis of Bovine Serum Albumin Capped Boron-Doped Carbon Dots for Sensitive and Selective Detection of Pb(II) Ion. *Heliyon* **2020**, *6*, e03957. [CrossRef]
39. Shao, Y.; Zhu, C.; Fu, Z.; Lin, K.; Wang, Y.; Chang, Y.; Han, L.; Yu, H.; Tian, F. Green Synthesis of Multifunctional Fluorescent Carbon Dots from Mulberry Leaves (*Morus Alba* L.) Residues for Simultaneous Intracellular Imaging and Drug Delivery. *J. Nanoparticle Res.* **2020**, *22*, 229. [CrossRef]
40. Nezhad-Mokhtari, P.; Arsalani, N.; Ghorbani, M.; Hamishehkar, H. Development of Biocompatible Fluorescent Gelatin Nanocarriers for Cell Imaging and Anticancer Drug Targeting. *J. Mater. Sci.* **2018**, *53*, 10679–10691. [CrossRef]

41. Pandiyan, S.; Arumugam, L.; Srirengan, S.P.; Pitchan, R.; Sevugan, P.; Kannan, K.; Pitchan, G.; Hegde, T.A.; Gandhirajan, V. Biocompatible Carbon Quantum Dots Derived from Sugarcane Industrial Wastes for Effective Nonlinear Optical Behavior and Antimicrobial Activity Applications. *ACS Omega* **2020**, *5*, 30363–30372. [CrossRef]
42. Arsalani, N.; Nezhad-Mokhtari, P.; Jabbari, E. Microwave-Assisted and One-Step Synthesis of PEG Passivated Fluorescent Carbon Dots from Gelatin as an Efficient Nanocarrier for Methotrexate Delivery. *Artif. Cells Nanomed. Biotechnol.* **2019**, *47*, 540–547. [CrossRef]
43. Hassan, H.; Almarjeh, R.A.B.; Atassi, Y. In-Vitro Ibuprofen Release Monitoring Using Carbon Quantum Dots. *J. Fluoresc.* **2021**, *31*, 289–303. [CrossRef] [PubMed]
44. D'souza, S.L.; Chettiar, S.S.; Koduru, J.R.; Kailasa, S.K. Synthesis of Fluorescent Carbon Dots Using Daucus Carota Subsp. Sativus Roots for Mitomycin Drug Delivery. *Optik* **2018**, *158*, 893–900. [CrossRef]
45. Zhang, Z.; Lei, Y.; Yang, X.; Shi, N.; Geng, L.; Wang, S.; Zhang, J.; Shi, S. High Drug-Loading System of Hollow Carbon Dots–Doxorubicin: Preparation, in Vitro Release and PH-Targeted Research. *J. Mater. Chem. B* **2019**, *7*, 2130–2137. [CrossRef] [PubMed]
46. Zou, W.-S.; Kong, W.-L.; Zhao, Q.-C.; Zhang, J.; Zhao, X.; Zhao, D.; Wang, Y.-Q. A Composite Consisting of Bromine-Doped Carbon Dots and Ferric Ions as a Fluorescent Probe for Determination and Intracellular Imaging of Phosphate. *Microchim. Acta* **2019**, *186*, 576. [CrossRef] [PubMed]
47. Rahmani, E.; Pourmadadi, M.; Ghorbanian, S.A.; Yazdian, F.; Rashedi, H.; Navaee, M. Preparation of a PH-Responsive Chitosan-Montmorillonite-Nitrogen-Doped Carbon Quantum Dots Nanocarrier for Attenuating Doxorubicin Limitations in Cancer Therapy. *Eng. Life Sci.* **2022**, *22*, 634–649. [CrossRef] [PubMed]
48. Athinarayanan, J.; Periasamy, V.S.; Alshatwi, A.A. Phoenix Dactylifera Lignocellulosic Biomass as Precursor for Nanostructure Fabrication Using Integrated Process. *Int. J. Biol. Macromol.* **2019**, *134*, 1179–1186. [CrossRef]
49. Wee, S.S.; Ng, Y.H.; Ng, S.M. Synthesis of Fluorescent Carbon Dots via Simple Acid Hydrolysis of Bovine Serum Albumin and Its Potential as Sensitive Sensing Probe for Lead (II) Ions. *Talanta* **2013**, *116*, 71–76. [CrossRef]
50. Bronze-Uhle, E.S.; Costa, B.C.; Ximenes, V.F.; Lisboa-Filho, P.N. Synthetic Nanoparticles of Bovine Serum Albumin with Entrapped Salicylic Acid. *Nanotechnol. Sci. Appl.* **2016**, *10*, 11–21. [CrossRef]
51. Xie, Y.; Filchakova, O.; Yang, Q.; Yesbolatov, Y.; Tursynkhan, D.; Kassymbek, A.; Bouhrara, M.; Wang, K.; Balanay, M.; Fan, H. Inhibition of Cancer Cell Proliferation by Carbon Dots Derived from Date Pits at Low-Dose. *ChemistrySelect* **2017**, *2*, 4079–4083. [CrossRef]
52. Luo, J.; Kong, H.; Zhang, M.; Cheng, J.; Sun, Z.; Xiong, W.; Zhu, Y.; Zhao, Y.; Qu, H. Novel Carbon Dots-Derived from Radix Puerariae Carbonisata Significantly Improve the Solubility and Bioavailability of Baicalin. *J. Biomed. Nanotechnol.* **2019**, *15*, 151–161. [CrossRef]
53. Athinarayanan, J.; Periasamy, V.S.; Alshatwi, A.A. Unveiling the Biocompatible Properties of Date Palm Tree (*Phoenix Dactylifera* L.) Biomass-Derived Lignin Nanoparticles. *ACS Omega* **2022**, *7*, 19270–19279. [CrossRef]
54. Fahmi, M.Z.; Haris, A.; Permana, A.J.; Wibowo, D.L.N.; Purwanto, B.; Nikmah, Y.L.; Idris, A. Bamboo Leaf-Based Carbon Dots for Efficient Tumor Imaging and Therapy. *RSC Adv.* **2018**, *8*, 38376–38383. [CrossRef]
55. Guo, P.; Buttaro, B.A.; Xue, H.Y.; Tran, N.T.; Wong, H.L. Lipid-Polymer Hybrid Nanoparticles Carrying Linezolid Improve Treatment of Methicillin-Resistant Staphylococcus Aureus (MRSA) Harbored inside Bone Cells and Biofilms. *Eur. J. Pharm. Biopharm.* **2020**, *151*, 189–198. [CrossRef] [PubMed]
56. Nemr, A.A.; El-Mahrouk, G.M.; Badie, H.A. Hyaluronic Acid-Enriched Bilosomes: An Approach to Enhance Ocular Delivery of Agomelatine via D-Optimal Design: Formulation, in Vitro Characterization, and in Vivo Pharmacodynamic Evaluation in Rabbits. *Drug Deliv.* **2022**, *29*, 2343–2356. [CrossRef] [PubMed]
57. Chen, J.; Wu, Q.; Luo, L.; Wang, Y.; Zhong, Y.; Dai, H.-B.; Sun, D.; Luo, M.-L.; Wu, W.; Wang, G.-X. Dual Tumor-Targeted Poly(Lactic-Co-Glycolic Acid)–Polyethylene Glycol–Folic Acid Nanoparticles: A Novel Biodegradable Nanocarrier for Secure and Efficient Antitumor Drug Delivery. *Int. J. Nanomed.* **2017**, *12*, 5745–5760. [CrossRef] [PubMed]
58. Salami, M.S.; Bahrami, G.; Arkan, E.; Izadi, Z.; Miraghaee, S.; Samadian, H. Co-Electrospun Nanofibrous Mats Loaded with Bitter Gourd (Momordica Charantia) Extract as the Wound Dressing Materials: In Vitro and in Vivo Study. *BMC Complement. Med. Ther.* **2021**, *21*, 111. [CrossRef] [PubMed]
59. Patil, K.D.; Bagade, S.B.; Bonde, S.C. In-Vitro and Ex-Vivo Characterization of Novel Mannosylated Gelatin Nanoparticles of Linezolid by Quality-by-Design Approach. *J. Drug Deliv. Sci. Technol.* **2020**, *60*, 101976. [CrossRef]
60. Xie, X.; Hou, Z.; Duan, G.; Zhang, S.; Zhou, H.; Yang, Z.; Zhou, R. Boron Nitride Nanosheets Elicit Significant Hemolytic Activity via Destruction of Red Blood Cell Membranes. *Colloids Surf. B Biointerfaces* **2021**, *203*, 111765. [CrossRef]
61. Cui, F.; Sun, J.; Ji, J.; Yang, X.; Wei, K.; Xu, H.; Gu, Q.; Zhang, Y.; Sun, X. Carbon Dots-Releasing Hydrogels with Antibacterial Activity, High Biocompatibility, and Fluorescence Performance as Candidate Materials for Wound Healing. *J. Hazard. Mater.* **2021**, *406*, 124330. [CrossRef] [PubMed]
62. Carreño, G.; Marican, A.; Vijayakumar, S.; Valdés, O.; Cabrera-Barjas, G.; Castaño, J.; Durán-Lara, E.F. Sustained Release of Linezolid from Prepared Hydrogels with Polyvinyl Alcohol and Aliphatic Dicarboxylic Acids of Variable Chain Lengths. *Pharmaceutics* **2020**, *12*, 982. [CrossRef]

63. Mandal, S.; Prasad, S.R.; Mandal, D.; Das, P. Bovine Serum Albumin Amplified Reactive Oxygen Species Generation from Anthrarufin-Derived Carbon Dot and Concomitant Nanoassembly for Combination Antibiotic–Photodynamic Therapy Application. *ACS Appl. Mater. Interfaces* **2019**, *11*, 33273–33284. [CrossRef] [PubMed]
64. Chatzimitakos, T.; Stalikas, C. Chapter 14-Antimicrobial Properties of Carbon Quantum Dots. In *Nanotoxicity*; Rajendran, S., Mukherjee, A., Nguyen, T.A., Godugu, C., Shukla, R.K., Eds.; Micro and Nano Technologies; Elsevier: Amsterdam, The Netherlands, 2020; pp. 301–315. [CrossRef]
65. Yadav, E.; Singh, D.; Yadav, P.; Verma, A. Antioxidant and Anti-Inflammatory Properties of Prosopis Cineraria Based Phenolic Rich Ointment in Wound Healing. *Biomed. Pharmacother.* **2018**, *108*, 1572–1583. [CrossRef] [PubMed]
66. Lee, S.-Y.; Won, K.-J.; Kim, D.-Y.; Kim, M.-J.; Won, Y.-R.; Kim, N.-Y.; Lee, H.-M. Wound Healing-Promoting and Melanogenesis-Inhibiting Activities of Angelica Polymorpha Maxim. Flower Absolute In Vitro and Its Chemical Composition. *Molecules* **2021**, *26*, 6172. [CrossRef] [PubMed]

pharmaceutics

MDPI

Review

Electrospinning Nanofibers as a Dressing to Treat Diabetic Wounds

Eun Jo Jang [1,†], Rajkumar Patel [2,†] and Madhumita Patel [3,*]

1 Nano Science and Engineering, Integrated Science and Engineering Division (ISED), Underwood International College, Yonsei University, Songdogwahak-ro, Yeonsu-gu, Incheon 21983, Republic of Korea
2 Energy & Environmental Science and Engineering (EESE), Integrated Science and Engineering Division (ISED), Underwood International College, Yonsei University, 85 Songdogwahak-ro, Yeonsu-gu, Incheon 21938, Republic of Korea
3 Department of Chemistry and Nanoscience, Ewha Womans University, 52 Ewhayeodae-gil, Seodaemun-gu, Seoul 03760, Republic of Korea
* Correspondence: madhurk29@gmail.com or madhurk30@ewha.ac.kr
† These authors contributed equally to this work.

Abstract: Globally, diabetic mellitus (DM) is a common metabolic disease that effectively inhibits insulin production, destroys pancreatic β cells, and consequently, promotes hyperglycemia. This disease causes complications, including slowed wound healing, risk of infection in wound areas, and development of chronic wounds all of which are significant sources of mortality. With an increasing number of people diagnosed with DM, the current method of wound healing does not meet the needs of patients with diabetes. The lack of antibacterial ability and the inability to sustainably deliver necessary factors to wound areas limit its use. To overcome this, a new method of creating wound dressings for diabetic patients was developed using an electrospinning methodology. The nanofiber membrane mimics the extracellular matrix with its unique structure and functionality, owing to which it can store and deliver active substances that greatly aid in diabetic wound healing. In this review, we discuss several polymers used to create nanofiber membranes and their effectiveness in the treatment of diabetic wounds.

Keywords: electrospun nanofiber; diabetic mellitus; wound healing; wound dressing; polymers

1. Introduction

Diabetes mellitus (DM) is one of the most diagnosed metabolic diseases that predominately causes hyperglycemia [1,2]. Without proper treatment, diabetes causes many complications, such as slowed wound healing and the development of ulcers, resulting in increased morbidity and mortality. Wound sites create a breeding ground for various bacteria, due to their high levels of glucose, and exhibit decreased neovascularization and consequently, impaired wound healing [3].

Wound dressings are crucial for the healing of diabetic wounds. Various dressings can protect the wound area from external risk factors and provide a suitable environment for accelerated wound healing [4]. To provide the wound area with the most benefits, an ideal wound dressing should have the ability to absorb exudate, protect the wound from infection, maintain the moisture level, facilitate gas exchange, remain biocompatible and degradable, promote tissue regeneration, and be easy to remove from the wound [5,6]. Currently, many modern wound dressings are available in the market; however, they all have their own limitations. Wound dressings, such as gauze, are inexpensive but can damage the wound site upon removal [7]. Semi-permeable films permit gas exchange, although they have a low absorption capacity [8]. In contrast, foam dressings possess a larger absorption capacity; however, their long residence time leads to dryness of the wound area [9]. Furthermore, although hydrogel dressings are capable of maintaining a moist microenvironment surrounding the wound, they can increase the risk of bacterial infection [9,10]. As a result, it is imperative to develop effective dressings capable of sustainable medication release for improving diabetic wound care. Recently, many efforts have been made to create better dressings, including the addition of nanofiber membranes [11–14]. These wound dressings have shown efficacy in treating diabetic wounds, promoting tissue and vascular regeneration, and accelerating wound closure [15,16].

1.1. Nanofiber Dressing

Wound dressings made of nanofibers have been developed predominantly through electrospinning [17], blow spinning [18], microfluidic spinning [19], and centrifugal spinning techniques [20]. Of these techniques, electrostatic spinning is the most widely used because of its ability to create diameter ranges of the order of microns or nanometers, which have noticeable benefits [21]. Nanofiber wound dressings prepared via electrospinning have several advantages. First, the developed structure and function is similar to the innate extracellular matrix (ECM), which creates the ideal environment for adhesion, proliferation, migration, and differentiation of cells [22,23]. Second, the created matrix can incorporate the biocompatibility of natural polymers along with the enhanced mechanical properties that synthetic polymers provide [24]. Furthermore, its large surface area and porous structure facilitate loading of various bioactive molecules, which can be sustainably released into the wound area. The rate at which molecules are released from dressings can be controlled by modifying the structure and size of the pores, thereby accelerating wound healing [25]. Hence, electrospun nanofibers are a great alternative to the current methods of diabetic wound treatment, owing to their various benefits (Figure 1). To better understand the current state of research on the use of electrospun nanofiber membranes for diabetic wound healing, we searched Scopus for "electrospinning nanofiber for diabetic wound healing". The search results are shown in Figure 2. The number of articles published on this topic has increased, indicating that wound healing in diabetes has attracted widespread attention. In the last few years, several reviews have been published on this topic [26–28]. Liu et al. and Yan et al. reviewed the development of electrospinning technology, and Gao et al. summarized bioactive compound loaded nanofibers for diabetic wound healing. In this review, we discussed the common polymers used to fabricate electrospun nanofibers, particularly for diabetic wound healing. We summarized the latest developments in diabetic wound healing, which can offer new ideas and insights into the improved treatment of diabetic wounds.

1.2. Diabetic Wounds

Diabetic wounds are severe injuries which are common in patients with diabetes. These wounds are chronic, susceptible to infection, and require extended repair time. The healing process is delayed by various internal factors such as microvascular dysfunction, peripheral neuropathy, and hypoxia, which disrupt the normal healing phases of hemostasis, inflammation, proliferation, and remodeling [29,30]. Peripheral neuropathy, the most common type of diabetic neuropathy, often damages nerve tissue. As a result of diabetic peripheral neuropathy, wound healing is delayed due to sensory, motor, and autonomic dysfunction. Sensory neuropathy leads to a loss or absence of pain sensation, while autonomic neuropathy affects skin temperature, sweat production, and blood flow in the foot [30,31].

Additionally, diabetic wounds have increased levels of reactive oxygen species (ROS), matrix metalloproteinases (MMPs), and pro-inflammatory cytokines [including tumor necrosis factor-α (TNF-α) and Interleukin-6 (IL-6)], in comparison with nondiabetic wounds [32,33]. As a result of excess inflammatory factors and active substances such as cytokines, growth factors, and antibiotics, the ECM deteriorates rapidly, delaying stages such as re-epithelialization and disrupting diabetic wound healing. Diabetic wound healing times may also be prolonged because pro-inflammatory macrophage "M1" cannot be converted to the healing-promoting macrophage "M2", which reduces the expression of anti-inflammatory cytokines (IL-10) [34].

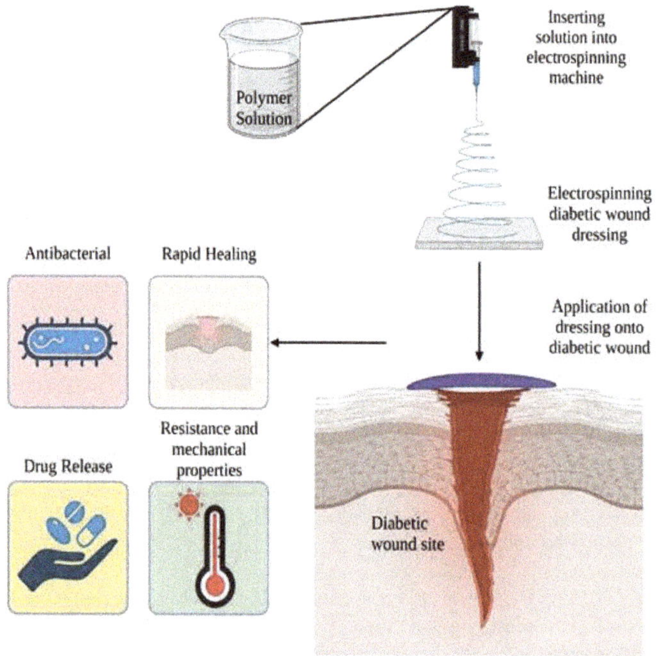

Figure 1. Schematic diagram showing electrospun nanofibers for diabetic wound healing. Created with BioRender.com.

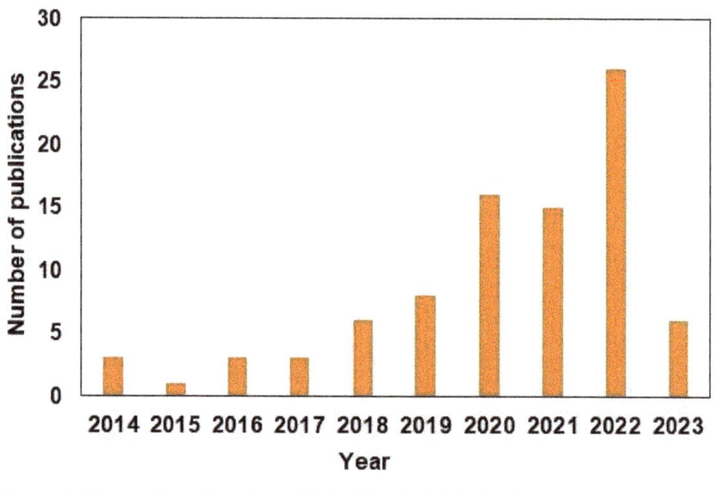

Figure 2. The number of articles published in the field of "Electrospinning nanofiber for diabetic wound healing" (source Scopus).

2. Polymeric Nanofibers for Wound Dressing

Wound dressings are essential for achieving better and faster wound closures [35]. Electrospinning is predominantly used in the development of dressing materials because of its simplicity and flexibility in creating polymers from different materials. Polymers are broadly divided into two categories: synthetic and natural. Natural polymers exhibit better biocompatibility, degradation, and lower immune responses, whereas synthetic polymers exhibit excellent mechanical strength, stiffness, and flexibility. Blending these polymers is advisable to obtain maximum benefits.

2.1. Synthetic Polymers

Synthetic polymers are artificially synthesized and customized to obtain essential properties. Their electrospun fibers are mechanically strong and stable, and they can be directly applied for diabetic wound treatment. Table 1 lists the synthetic polymers commonly used for electrospun fibers to improve diabetic wound healing.

Table 1. Synthetic polymers used for electrospun nanofibers to promote diabetic wound healing.

Polymer Used for Electrospun Fiber	Active Ingredient	Highlights	References
PCL/F-127		Modifiable size and depth enhanced angiogenesis and collagen deposition	[36]
PCL/Col	Bioactive glass nanoparticles	Improved cell attachment, proliferation and upregulated angiogenesis	[37]
PCL/Col1	Dimethyloxalylglycine	Regulation in release of DMOG and ability to stabilize HIF-1α levels and increase angiogenesis and re-epithelialization	[38]
PCL	Dimethyloxalylglycine	Increased wound closure rate, re-epithelization, and angiogenesis	[39]
Steviol glycosides polyurethane/PCL	-	Commendable mechanical characteristics, and high biocompatibility	[40]
PCL/Gum tragacanth	Curcumin	Improved antibacterial properties against *Staphylococcus aureus*, extended spectrum β lactamase, increased angiogenesis and wound closure	[41]
PCL/Col1	Calreticulin	Stimulated fibroblasts proliferation and allowed for keratinocyte migration	[42]
PCL/Col1	Melilotus officinalis extract	Improved re-epithelization and wound closure	[43]
PCL/Gelatin	Pioglitazone	Enhanced mechanical properties, cell proliferation, angiogenesis, and wound closure	[44]
Collagen/PLGA	Glucophage	Promoted wound healing rate, collagen levels, and downregulation of metalloproteinase 9	[45]
PLGA	Platelet-derived growth factor/Vancomycin or Gentamicin	Accelerated healing process, reduced phosphatase, and tensin content,	[46]
HA/PLGA	Epigallocatechin-3-O-gallate	Rapid decrease in wound area, improved re-epithelization and vasculiarzation	[47]
PLGA/Gelatin PDO/Gelatin	LL-37-mimic peptide W379	Accelerated wound healing, increased cell infiltration, vascularization, and re-epithelization	[48]
PLLA	Dimethyloxalylglycine	Improved vascularization, collagen deposition and re-epithelization Rapid stimulation of angiogenesis	[49]
Methacrylated gelatin/PLLA	*Salvia miltiorrhiza Bunge-Radix Puerariae*	Increased antibacterial properties against *S. aureus* and *E. coli*, Enhanced healing rate of the wound area	[50]
PLA/HA	Valsartan, ascorbic acid	Accelerated wound healing and re-epithelization	[51]
PLA/PVA	Cerium oxide nanoparticles	Improved in mechanical strength and biocompatibility. Enhanced wound healing rate through growth, adhesion and proliferation rate of fibroblasts	[52]

Table 1. *Cont.*

Polymer Used for Electrospun Fiber	Active Ingredient	Highlights	References
PLA/Gelatin	Epidermal growth factor	Antibacterial properties against *E. coli* and *S. aureus*, improved curative activities	[53]
PVA/chitosan	Desferrioxamine	Sustained release of desferrioxamine improved upregulation of Hif-1α and vascular growth factor. Increased cell proliferation and vessel formation	[54]
PLA/PVA	Gum tragacanth	Exhibited tissue repair and regeneration as well as collagen formation. Enhanced mechanical properties and young modulus.	[55]
PVA/Chitosan	-	Decreased in epidermal gap and rapid wound healing process	[56]
PVA/Chitosan	Zinc oxide	Enhanced antibacterial properties against *E. coli*, *P. aeruginosa*, *B. subtilis*, and *S. aureus* and increased rate of healing.	[57]
Pyrrolidine/m-PEG	Gentiopicroside, thymoquinone	Enhanced antibacterial effects against *P. aeruginosa*. Rapid wound closure rate through stimulation of cell growth, proliferation and inhibit inflammatory reaction	[58]
Polyvinylpyrrolidone	Pioglitazone	Inhibition of inflammation, management of skin condition through sustained release of pioglitazone	[59]

2.1.1. Poly (ε-caprolactone) (PCL)

PCL is a widely used biocompatible and degradable polymer that minimizes environmental impact upon degradation. PCL is an FDA approved material that is applied in wound dressings due to its outstanding spinnability and mechanical strength. Chen et.al. fabricated PCL electrospun nanofiber scaffolds with custom 3D shapes, and either radial or vertical organizations. Bone marrow-derived mesenchymal stem cells (BMSCs) laden on the nanofibers facilitate tissue development, angiogenesis, and enhanced collagen (Col1) deposition. It can also switch immune responses to help generate tissue by inhibiting the formation of M1 macrophages and pro-inflammatory cytokines while activating M2 macrophages, leading to anti-inflammatory cytokine production. This membrane promotes the immune system and facilitates wound healing [36]. The use of ECM biomimetic structures has been of constant interest for diabetic wound healing. Using ECM components Col, PCL, and bioactive glass nanoparticles, Gao et al. developed a scaffold (CPB) that could aid in endothelial cell proliferation and angiogenesis in vivo. The scaffold showed notable improvements in the expression of angiogenic factors (VEGF, Hif-1α, Col I, and α-SMA) and Col deposition compared with control group. Additionally, the scaffold improved the differentiation process and accelerated wound healing [37]. Ways to inhibit the effects of hypoxia-inducible factor 1 α (HIF-1α) are being investigated to promote diabetic wound healing. Releasing dimethyloxalylglycine (DMOG), a competitive inhibitor of prolyl hydroxylases (PHDs), near the wound area can readily stabilize HIF-1α and accelerate wound healing. The sustained release of DMOG from PCL/type I collagen (Col I) electrospun core-sheath fibers enhanced the migration and expression of wound healing genes in vitro. Furthermore, DMOG stabilizes HIF-1α levels and improves the healing process in vivo [38]. The PCL mesh with DMOG additionally enhanced the expression of growth factors (e.g., IGF-1, HB-EGF, and NGF) and anti-inflammatory factors (e.g., transforming growth factor (TGF)-β1 and IL-4) while decreasing expression levels of pro-inflammatory factors (e.g., IL-1β and IL-6) in vitro. The mesh increased the wound closure rate, re-epithelialization, maturation, and deposition of Col in vivo, two weeks after implantation [39].

A hybrid scaffold of polyurethane (PU) and PCL (PU/PCL) showed potential as a wound dressing material for diabetic wound areas. The dressing showed great permeability to oxygen and had a good degree of swelling and water content; its biocompatibility towards L-929 cells was assessed to be 86.9% when applied. Combined with its low cost, the PU/PCL dressing is an alternative to existing dressing materials for diabetic wound healing [40]. Loading curcumin (Cur) into the matrix of PCL/gum tragacanth (GT) (PCL/GT/Cur) nanofibers has been shown to accelerate the healing process of diabetic wounds, in addition to having the ability to remain resistant against *Staphylococcus aureus* and spectrum of β –lactamase. In vivo application of PCL/GT/Cur to diabetic wounds resulted in excellent granulation and cellular proliferation, Col deposition, and re-epithelization of the tissue compared with the control wounds. The developed scaffold showed an increase in angiogenesis, granulation of the tissue area, a number of fibroblasts, and a decreased epithelial gap [41]. Similarly, loading bixin with PCL nanofibers showed an improvement over innate PCL nanofiber dressings. In vitro assessment of the nanofibers showed that bixin could be released from the matrix over a two-week period, showing its sustained drug release ability. An in vivo study in diabetic mice showed that bixin plays a successful role in accelerating the wound-healing process and reducing scar tissue [60]. Calreticulin (CRT), an endoplasmic reticulum chaperone protein, enhances wound healing. In a study by Stack et al., CRT incorporated within the PCL/Col 1 nanofibers achieved a sustained release, which stimulated faster keratinocyte migration and cell polarization in vitro. In addition, the scaffold upregulated TGF-β1 protein and resulted in remarkable mechanical properties and integrity, with protection against degradation exhibiting therapeutic potential against diabetic foot ulcers [42]. In another study, glutathione, a biomolecule immobilized on PCL meshes, reduced wound-healing times in diabetic rats. Sustained release of glutathione from the mesh for up to 20 days exhibited antibacterial activity and showed its potential to be used as a wound healing material for diabetic patients [61]. A three-layered scaffold built with PCL, PCL/Col, and Col nanofibers could hold the *Melilotus officinalis* extract within its matrix. The inner Col layer was able to absorb wound exudates and promote angiogenesis, the PCL-Col middle layer improved the mechanical strength, and the outer layer protected the wound from contamination. The extract-loaded dressings exhibited proper re-epithelialization of diabetic wounds and Col production and deposition in the newly formed skin [43]. Metformin hydrochloride (MH) loaded within hyaluronic acid (HA)-keratin-polyethylene oxide and PCL nanofiber can be used to treat diabetic wounds. The sustained release of MH for over 20 days prolonged its bioactivity near diabetic wounds. The nanofibers showed excellent biocompatibility and notable mechanical and chemical properties that assisted in diabetic wound healing [62].

The organization of fibers or scaffolds remains an area of research, as their orientation has been shown to play a role in the effectiveness of diabetic wound treatments. In a study by Sun et al., nanofibrous scaffolds of PCL/Col1 with basketweave-like patterns mimicked the natural Col arrangement. Compared with aligned or randomly oriented nanofibrous scaffolds, the basketweave patterns showed the greatest improvements and enhancements in their ability to heal wounds in diabetic rats. The patterns also accelerated fibroblast migration and promoted angiogenesis, and the inflammation levels noticeably decreased [63]. The use of asymmetric wettable dressings to treat diabetic wounds is another promising approach. An asymmetric wettable dressing developed by Yu et al. using PCL by electrospinning pioglitazone-incorporated gelatin (Gel-pio) to form a hydrophobic outer layer while creating a hydrophilic layer on the inside. The outer layer acted as a water barrier for the wound area to remain dehydrated, whereas the inner layer protected against bacterial growth or infection. The in vitro results showed that gelatin (GEL) nanofibers incorporated with a pioglitazone accelerated cell proliferation and migration. In vivo, the composite dressings enhanced diabetic wound healing by enhancing cell proliferation and angiogenesis, while modulating the expression of VEGF, MIP-2, IL-1β, IL-6, TNF-α, MMP-9, and TGF-β (Figure 3) [44].

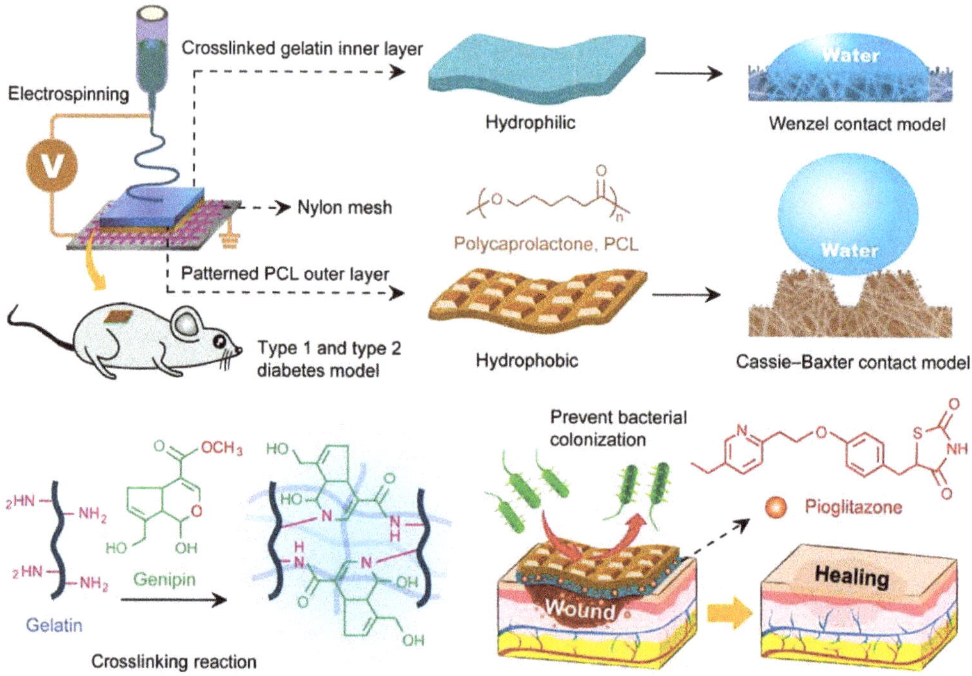

Figure 3. Graphical representation of the asymmetric wettable preparation for wound dressings. Reproduced with permission from Ref. [44]. Copyright 2020, American Chemical Society.

2.1.2. Poly(lactic-co-glycolic acid) (PLGA)

PLGA, a copolymer of poly (L-lactic acid (PLA) and polyglycolic acid (PGA), has a low toxicity toward humans. PLGA is another attractive biocompatible polymer because it is FDA approved and is used in the development of nanofiber matrices. [64]. PLGA has been used in various hybrid scaffolds for diabetic wound treatments [65].

Utilization of Col/poly-D-L-lactide-glycolide (PLGA) nanofibers to release of glucophages is a potential diabetic wound treatment approach. The PLGA/Col membrane released glucophages into the wound area over a three-week period. In addition to its sustainable drug release ability, increasing the amount of retained water promoted effective healing of diabetic wounds, enhanced Col content, and induced faster wound healing [45]. Furthermore, PLGA-Col nanofibrous scaffolds could hold and sustainably release recombinant human platelet-derived growth factor (rhPDGF) to promote diabetic wound healing. The scaffold exhibited a remarkable water retaining capacity while allowing more Col to form near the damaged area. In addition, the scaffold promoted re-epithelialization of the wound, which allowed the wound to heal at a faster rate and decreased the healing period [65]. New methods of aiding wound healing in patients with diabetes are continuously being developed. Nanofibrous PLGA scaffolds incorporating antibiotics such as vancomycin and gentamicin, and platelet-derived growth factor (PDGF) accelerated wound healing. The release of PDGF and antibiotics allowed the wound area to clear any infections and accelerated the healing process. The membrane induced higher expression of the angiogenesis marker CD31, indicating that the film could accelerate the growth of new tissue around the area [46]. Similarly, Lee et al. developed a method to deliver metformin (Met) by incorporating it into the wound dressing of PLGA nanofibers. The nanofiber scaffold that contained Met within its matrix could be released over a three-week period and had greater hydrophilicity, while also having better water retaining abilities than regular PLGA fibers. In combination with the drug release system, an in vivo application of PLGA with Met resulted in an enhancement in diabetic wound healing and helped re-epithelialize the wound area (Figure 4) [66]. In another study, the impregnation of epigallocatechin-3-O-gallate (EGCG) into an HA-PLGA scaffold released EGCG over four weeks, demonstrating its ability to treat wounds in the long term. The HA/PLGA/EGCG membrane showed an increased number of fibroblasts that were able to attach to the matrices compared to the HA/PLGA membrane. Moreover, the scaffold showed greater Col deposition, re-epithelialization, and neovascularization than the control and HA/PLGA membranes [47]. In a study by John et al., a PLGA/GEL fiber aerogel containing the LL-37-mimic peptide W379 enhanced proliferation and migration of keratinocytes and fibroblasts, while the introduction of macrochannels within the aerogel improved cell penetration. Moreover, the patterned macrochannels together with the incorporation of W379 greatly increased the healing time of diabetic wounds through re-epithelization by upregulating p38 mitogen-activated protein kinase expression [48]. Membranes from living cells have attracted attention as a new way of improving the bioactivity of living materials. A PLGA scaffold along with lipopolysaccharide/interferon-γ, an activated macrophage cell membrane, enhanced proliferation and migration of keratinocytes while speeding up wound closure, re-epithelialization, and angiogenesis when loaded with BMMSCs (RCM-fiber-BMMSCs). In addition, the scaffolds upregulated the expression of 449 genes related to wound healing compared to the nanofibers without cell membranes [67].

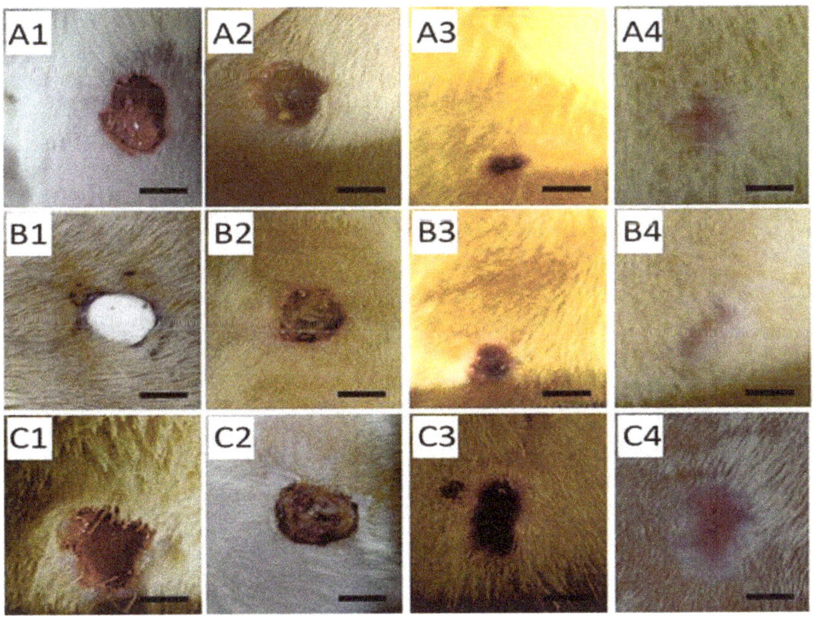

Figure 4. Wound healing on day 0 (1), 3 (2), 7 (3), and 14 (4) post treatment: (**A**) the PLGA with metformin group; (**B**) virgin PLGA; (**C**) the conventional gauze sponge group. Scale bar = 5 mm. Reproduced with permission from Ref. [66]. Copyright 2014, American Chemical Society.

2.1.3. Poly (L-lactic acid) (PLA)

PLA has excellent mechanical properties, biocompatibility, and degradability [68]. PLA has shown potential for use in biomedical applications such as wound healing, drug delivery, and tissue engineering, and it has been approved by the FDA [69]. Recently, it was shown that electrospun PLA scaffolds could be used as alternatives to promote cell migration and proliferation, and Col formation [70]. Alignment of porous poly-L-lactide (PLLA) membranes with DMOG loaded mesoporous silica nanoparticles (DS) enhanced angiogenesis in diabetic wounds. The fibers were oriented toward a single direction and contained nano-pores that could contain DMOG and Si ions. These porous characteristics allow for the controlled release of the drug contained within the fibrous matrix. The DS-PL membrane enhanced proliferation, migration, and angiogenesis in diabetic wounds, while also improving vascularization and epithelialization of the wounds. The fibers were able to control inflammation levels, which could further improve wound healing (Figure 5) [49].

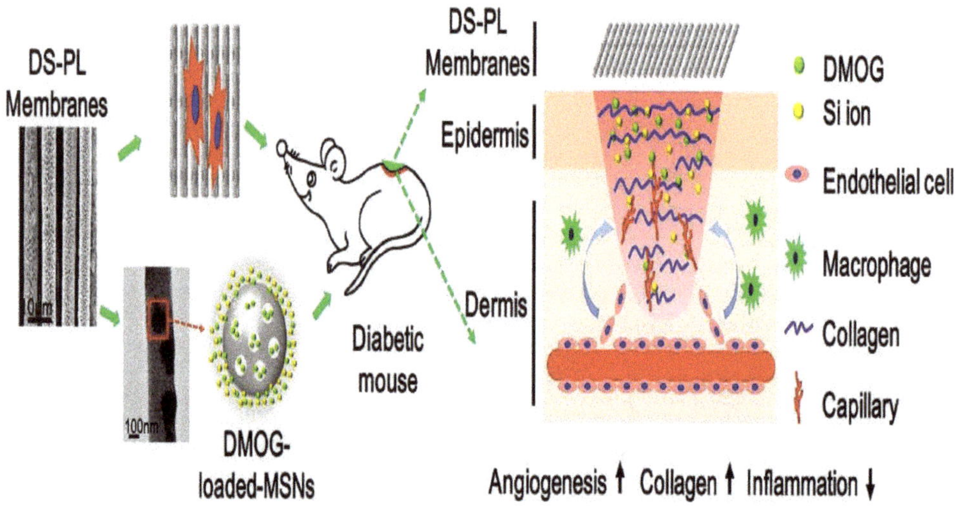

Figure 5. Graphical representation of electrospun membranes containing DMOG-loaded mesoporous silica nanoparticles (DS) for diabetic wound healing. Reproduced with permission from Ref. [49]. Copyright 2014, Elsevier.

The orientation of the electrospun nanofibers significantly affected their mechanical properties. Wu et al. designed electrospun methacrylated gelatine (MeGel)/PLLA radially oriented nanofiber mats (RNMs) as dressing patches. Dressing patches, in combination with *Salvia miltiorrhiza Bunge-Radix puerariae* (SRHC), a herbal compound, showed improvements in the closure and healing of diabetic wounds, as they promoted the proliferation and migration of human dermal fibroblasts (HDFs) compared to simple medical gauzes. When loaded with SRHC, the dressings exhibited excellent hemostatic performance, and they presented antibacterial properties against *Escherichia.coli* and *S. aureus*. Furthermore, the 10% SRHC-loaded dressing reduced inflammation and promoted vascularization and regeneration of hair follicles (Figure 6) [50].

The utilization of NIR-assisted oxygen delivery along with black phosphorus (BP) nanosheets, hemoglobin (Hb), and PLLA has been discussed as a new way of dealing with harsh hypoxic microenvironments (HMEs) in diabetic wounds. When BP is exposed to NIR radiation, it can generate heat, allowing Hb to release oxygen into the wound site. This offers antibacterial activity along with accelerated wound healing phases in both angiogenesis and cell migration. The wound area exhibited antibacterial activity against methilicillin-resistant *S. aureus and* E. coli, while exhibiting great mechanical strength to support its use in diabetic wound healing [71]. Furthermore, PLLA nanofibers promoted skin immunity, neutrophil migration, and fibroblast regulation by releasing GM18. The dressing was able to release GM18 over seven days, enabling controlled and sustained release of GM18. The released GM18 targeted the integrin $\alpha4\beta1$, which inhibited EDA-fibronectin- $\alpha4\beta1$ binding and promoted signaling of the ERK1/2 pathways, leading to improvement of the healing process. The controlled release of such substances can achieve dressing longevity and accelerate the wound healing process [72].

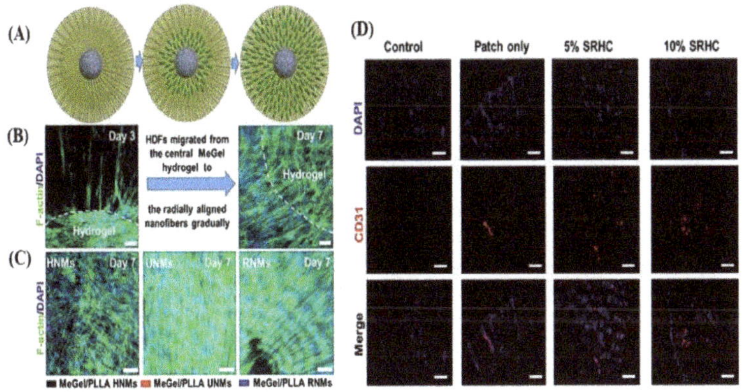

Figure 6. (**A**) Graphical representation of the cell migration process of HDFs on the MeGel/PLLA RNMs. (**B**) Fluorescent images of HDFs on the MeGel/PLLA radially oriented nanofiber mats (RNMs) at day 3 and 7. (**C**) Fluorescent images of HDFs on MeGel/PLLA uniaxially oriented nanofiber mats (UNM), haphazardly oriented nanofiber mats (HNM), and RNMs on day 7. Scale bars = 100 μm. (**D**) Fluorescent images of the regenerated skin tissue stained with CD31 (red) and DAPI (blue) 18 days post-surgery. Scale bars = 50 μm. Reproduced with permission from Ref. [50]. Copyright 2022, Elsevier.

To aid tissue formation in patients with diabetes, the combination of connective tissue growth factor (CTGF) in porous shell fibers (PLA-PVA) achieved better wound healing. These scaffolds facilitated rapid cell proliferation, migration, and angiogenesis. The release of CTGF from the porous shell fibers allowed cells in the wound area to receive CTGF over a long period [73]. In another study, PLA electrospun with HA, valsartan, and ascorbic acid was found to be an effective scaffold for diabetic wounds. The mechanical properties of the nanofibers closely matched those of the human skin. Moreover, the porous scaffold exhibited high drug solubility, oxygen permeability, and fluid uptake, and sustainably released valsartan from matrix. Compared with the traditional and existing methods of treating diabetic wounds, the release of valsartan from its nanofiber scaffold showed a much greater re-epithelization rate of up to 85.5%. Overall, the incorporation of valsartan allowed for much faster healing of the wound area, whereas the PLA/HA nanofibrous scaffolding provided a release mechanism and protection from the outside [51]. Cerium oxide nanoparticles ($nCeO_2$), which are ROS scavengers within a trilayer membrane of PLA/PVA/PLA, mimic the nature of ECM. The controlled release of $nCeO_2$ enhances diabetic wound healing by increasing cell adhesion, growth, and proliferation. In addition, the mechanical, thermal, and morphological properties were enhanced by the introduction of $nCeO_2$ [52]. Wound dressings, along with their antibacterial properties, improved diabetic wound healing, which was achieved through the incorporation of selenium (Se), graphene oxide (GO), and clarithromycin in PLA nanofibers. The mesh enhanced the healing capabilities by promoting cell adhesion and migration while being mechanically and chemically stable. Furthermore, their antibacterial properties are beneficial for the potential use of dressings [74]. Similarly, PLA/GEL nanofiber scaffolds showed antibacterial properties when combined with epidermal growth factor (EGF). The scaffold was effective in combating *E. Coli* and *S. aureus* infections. In addition, the dressings exhibited excellent mechanical properties, including maximum elongation, tensile strength, and tensile modulus. Furthermore, their ability to promote the proliferation of L929 fibroblasts cells assisted in diabetic wound healing and re-epithelization [53].

2.1.4. Polyvinyl Alcohol (PVA)

PVA is soluble in water, easy to manufacture, biocompatible, and degradable, and has excellent mechanical and chemical properties [75]. Its solubility in water provides an easy way to process and cross-link polymers; it is being investigated as an alternative for creating diabetic wound dressings.

To further enhance the properties of PVA and increase its efficiency in diabetic wound treatment, it would be beneficial to incorporate it into various other natural polymers. For example, mats made of PVA, in addition to non-mulberry SF (NMSF), growth factors, and LL-37 antimicrobial peptides, showed greater healing properties than mulberry SF-based dressings. NMSF-based dressings exhibited faster tissue development, enhanced angiogenesis, re-epithelization, and Col deposition in the wound area. The results suggested the potential for application of NMSF-based dressings in diabetic wounds [76]. A new way of putting deferrioxamine (DFO) into the PVA matrix of hydrogel nanofibrous scaffolds is to further improve the angiogenesis of wound areas in diabetic patients. The hydrogel scaffold held and sustainably released DFO for up to 72 h, thereby accelerating the initial healing process. These scaffolds increased neovascularization and promoted cell proliferation and vessel formation. In addition, the scaffolds upregulated Hif-1α and vascular endothelial growth factor expression to enhance wound healing. Usage of DFO with hydrogel nanofibrous scaffolds show its ability to inhibit prolyl-hydroxylase cofactors while upregulating the expression of Hif1-α, significantly helping the wound healing process (Figure 7) [54]. Similarly, scaffolds with GT, PCL, and PVA have the potential to be used as dressing materials for diabetic wounds. PCL/GT/PVA showed acceptable tensile strength and Young's modulus of 2.7 and 5.6 MPa, respectively, and exhibited the ability to attach to cell tissues. This allows for successful and fast proliferation of cells, and experiments on diabetic rats have shown increased epithelization and wound repair [55].

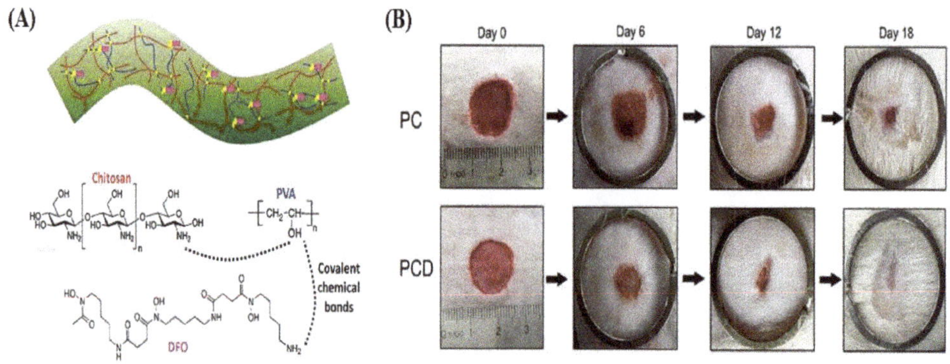

Figure 7. Hydrogel electrospun fibers' structure and the covalent chemical bonds among CS, PVA, and DFO drug (**A**), photographs of the wound healing at days 0, 6, 12, and 18 post-treatment (**B**). Reproduced with permission from Ref. [54]. Copyright 2016, Wiley.

Another nanofiber mat made of PLA along with PVA, MH, and fish sarcoplasmic protein (FSP) exhibited decreased crystallinity. The ability of nanofibers to sustainably release drugs enhanced diabetic wound healing. The nanofibers exhibited properties suitable for the adhesion and proliferation of HaCaT cells in vitro [77]. Propolis is commonly used for treating inflammatory dermal diseases. Alberti et al. incorporated propolis into a PVA scaffold that showed excellent wound treatment capabilities and no cytotoxicity in fibroblasts. Comparing untreated and treated wounds, PVA and propolis showed the highest wound closure rate at 68% after seven days. Its ability to continuously release propolis into the wound area allowed for faster treatment and healing of the wound area [78].

Due to its biodegradability, biocompatibility, antimicrobial properties, cellular binding ability, and wound healing effects, Chitosan (CS), a polysaccharide, is often blended with PVA [79]. Majd et al. designed a wound dressing made of PVA and CS, which allowed for a high moisture transmission rate and antimicrobial activity that stimulated the wound healing process. In addition, the dressing exhibited an excellent odor inhibition capacity and no noticeable cytotoxicity. In an in vivo study on diabetic rats, the dressings showed accelerated wound healing capabilities [56]. Furthermore, a wound dressing with a combination of ursolic acid (UA) and CS/PVA exhibited excellent hydrophilicity and wettability, and reduced inflammation around the wound area. The systematic release of UA helps with wound treatment, decreasing the release levels of TNF-α and IL-6 inflammatory factors. It improves the wound closure rate, promotes revascularization and re-epithelialization, and helps to regenerate hair follicles [80]. Similarly, the incorporation of zinc oxide (ZnO) within the matrix of PVA and CS allowed for the development of effective diabetic wound dressings. The sustained release of ZnO into the wound area resulted in antibacterial properties against *E. coli*, *P. aeruginosa*, *Bacillus subtilis*, and *S. aureus*, which was an improvement over the innate CS/PVA nanofiber membrane. Furthermore, the higher antioxidant properties of mats increased the performance of wound contraction within a time interval of 12 days [57]. A PVA nanofiber wound dressing combined with CS and anemoside B4 (ANE) also promoted rapid closure of the diabetic wound, accelerating re-epithelization and deposition of the Col matrix. The nanofiber matrix incorporating ANE was able to inhibit inflammatory responses and facilitated reduction of ROS generation and cytokine release (TNF-α and IL-6) both in vitro and in vivo. Additionally, the nanofiber matrix showed better water absorption, mechanical properties, and hemostatic properties [81]. Enteromorpha polysaccharide (EPP), which has antibacterial and antioxidant activities when blended with PVA, improves the repair process of skin wounds in diabetic mice. The dressing inhibits the inflammatory response while accelerating the healing process. While remaining biocompatible, the dressing achieved a high water absorption capacity, demonstrating its potential for use as a diabetic wound dressing [82].

Natural products play important roles in wound healing. The antibacterial properties of Cur derivatives (CD) in PVA nanofibers were effective against *S. aureus*, thereby preventing potential infections around the diabetic wound area. CD enhanced wound healing by activating glycogen synthase kinase-3 beta and TGF-β1 kinase domain signaling pathways [83]. PVA nanofibers containing neomycin sulfate (NS) and *Malva sylvestris* extract (MS) exhibited excellent water uptake and tensile strength, while releasing NS for 60 h and MS for 84 h. The sustained release of MS exerted antibacterial activity against *S. aureus* and *E. coli*, leading to a diabetic wound healing rate of 96.08% by day 14 in vivo [84]. Astragalus polysaccharide (APS) and astragaloside IV (AS) with polyvinyl alcohol (PVA) dressings have been developed to treat diabetic foot ulcers. The matrix facilitates sustained release of molecules and the subsequent inhibition of wound inflammation. Moreover, the dressing helped create an environment for faster deposition of Col fibers and re-epithelialization in diabetic rat wounds [85].

2.1.5. Polyvinylpyrrolidone (PVP)

PVP is a water-soluble and biocompatible polymer with good solubility in various organic solvents, making it suitable for developing nanofibers through electrospinning. The addition of gentiopicroside (GPS), thymoquinone (TQ), and methyl ether polyethylene glycol (m-PEG) to the PVP nanofiber matrix accelerated diabetic wound healing. The nanofiber mats exhibited antibacterial properties against P. aeruginosa, which is a problematic bacterium for wound treatment, while also exhibiting anti-inflammatory properties [58]. Similarly, the sustained release of pioglitazone (PGZ), an antidiabetic drug, from PVP fibers accelerated diabetic wound healing and showed anti-inflammatory properties. The released PGZ also showed a high retention rate on the skin, minimizing contact with the blood circulation [59]. Similarly, pioglitazone hydrochloride (PHR)-loaded PVP/PCL fibers increased fibroblast proliferation and epidermal regeneration while reducing oedema, neutrophil infiltration, and inflammation. The fibrous mat successfully accelerated diabetic wound healing both in vitro and in vivo [86]. To overcome the limited water absorption of conventional dressings, a combination of gelation fabrics were used as a hydrophilic layer, and polyvinyl butyral (PVB) along with PVP were used as a hydrophobic layer to create a double-layered dressing that pumps the exudate from the wound area. This leads to a low inflammatory response and moisturization of the wound area, improving the wound healing quality and accelerating the healing process [87].

2.2. Natural Polymers

Natural polymers have excellent biocompatibility and low immune responses. However, these materials exhibit poor mechanical properties. To overcome this disadvantage, natural polymers can be blended with synthetic polymers to greatly expand their applications. Table 2 lists the natural polymers that are widely used to create electrospun fibers that improve diabetic wound healing.

Table 2. Natural polymer used to create electrospun nanofibers to promote diabetic wound healing.

Polymer Used for Electrospun Fiber	Active Ingredient	Highlights	References
Gelatin/Arabinoxylan ferulate	Silver sulfadiazine	Enhanced mechanical properties and delivery of silver sulfadiazine over time enhanced antibacterial properties against *S. aureus, E. faecalis, P. aeruginosa.*	[88]
Gelatin/Bacterial cellulose	Metformin, glybenclamide	Sustained release of metformin or glybenclamide improved healing rate.	[89]
Gelatin/Poly-3-hydroxybutyrate	-	Improved fibroblasts cells adhesion and increased hair follicles and sweat glands	[90]
Silk fibroin/ Poly-(L-lactide-co-caprolactone)	Huangbai Liniment	Improved antibacterial properties, mechanical properties, and wound closure rate. Downregulate the inflammatory factors	[91]
Corn zein	Sodium citrate	Sustained release of sodium citrate enhanced the healing rate, increased thermal and mechanical properties, and exhibited higher biocompatibility	[92]
Cellulose acetate/Zein	Sesamol	Inhibited chronic inflammation and promoted fibroblast proliferation	[93]

2.3. Gelatin(GEL)

GEL shows great potential as a diabetic wound dressing, owing to its various properties. It exhibits excellent mechanical and biological properties, allows structural modification, and is biocompatible and degradable [94]. Furthermore, GEL from Col has ECM-like properties and is known to enhance epithelialization and tissue formation, thereby being beneficial for diabetic wound treatment [95]. Despite these properties, GEL alone is not sufficient as a dressing material, owing to its poor compatibility with electrospinning processes that creates poor-quality nanofibers [96]. Arabinoxylan ferulate (AXF) and GEL at different ratios were impregnated with silver to demonstrate sustained drug release and antibacterial properties. Overall, the 4:1 ratio of GEL to AXF showed the best mechanical properties, and its porosity was the highest at 95.6%, showing successful release of silver over a period. To evaluate the antibacterial properties of silver, the membrane was tested against bacteria such as *P. aeruginosa, S. aureus,* and *Enterococus faecalis* to demonstrate its antibacterial activity against both gram-negative and gram-positive bacteria. Despite its mechanical and antibacterial properties, researchers have noted that this form of treatment should only serve as a secondary wound matrix rather than a primary treatment. The GEL-AXF mats degraded in aqueous media because of the instability of GEL/AXF in aqueous environments, which limited their long-term usage as a primary wound dressing [88]. Developing protein-based dressings is important for the treatment of diabetic wounds, as they are unlikely to cause an immunologic response and are relatively biocompatible. Cam et al. developed a dressing composed of a combination of GEL and bacterial cellulose (BC) to create a natural polymer scaffold. The combined GEL/BC polymers were further electrospun with Met or glybenclamide (Gb) to evaluate their ability to increase cell proliferation. When compared side-to-side, the GEL-BC-Gb system showed a greater healing effect on the wound than the GEL-BC-Met system. Successful re-epithelization and granulation of the tissue were observed in wounds treated with the GEL-BC-Gb compared to those treated with the Gel-BC-Met system. Overall, the sustained release of Gb and Met from wound dressings showed their ability to accelerate the healing process of diabetic wounds, whereas the GEL-BC polymer exhibited its ability to release drugs and remain biocompatible with minimal side effects [89].

A scaffold developed with poly-3-hydroxybutyrate (PHB) microfibers and GEL nanofibers showed excellent characteristics in wound healing, promoting fibroblast assessment and tissue creation. The membrane also disallowed skin contraction and increased the healing rate while aiding hypodermis formation. The PHB-microfibers helped in linking the GEL nanofibers with each other, while GEL nanofibers worked as a reinforcing material to stop the membrane from shrinking. These synergistic effects of both fibers allowed GEL-PHB fibers to be successful in healing diabetic wounds (Figure 8). Mice treated with these fibers had a higher number of hair follicles and sweat glands while having a lower content of fibroblasts [90]. The development of two nanofiber series from polyurethane (PU) with cinnamon essential oil (CEO) and polyvinyl alcohol-gelatin (PVA/GEL) with nanoceria ($nCeO_2$) resulted in improved mechanical and thermal properties. The nanofibers increased the cell population when used on a diabetic wound while inhibiting the growth of *S. aureus* and *E. coil* [97].

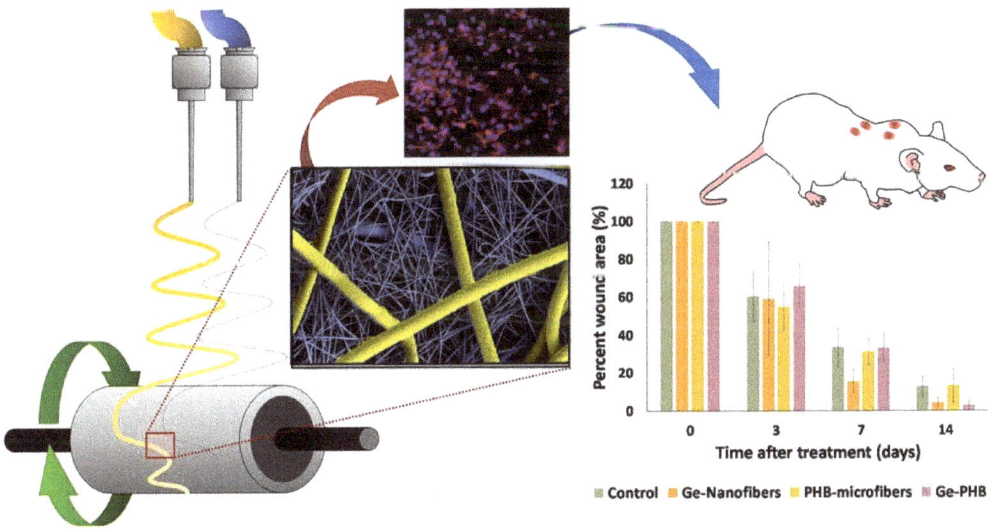

Figure 8. Graphical representation of PHB and Ge nanofibers as wound dressings. Reproduced with permission from Ref. [90]. Copyright 2021, Elsevier.

3. Silk

Silk fibroin is a natural polymer obtained from silkworm cocoons (*Bombyx mori*). It has been used in various areas of tissue regeneration, drug delivery and biomedical applications due to its excellent mechanical properties, biocompatibility, degradability, and nontoxicity.

The incorporation Cur into the matrix of electrospun SF, PCL, and PVA nanofibers shows its potential for use as a diabetic wound dressing. The scaffold could sustainably release Cur into the wound area over several hours, and its excellent mechanical properties, such as tensile strength, made it an acceptable material for use as a wound dressing. Cur acted as both an antioxidant and anti-inflammatory substance in the wound area and accelerated the healing process. Furthermore, experiments on diabetic mice showed its rapid wound healing properties compared to traditional and existing healing methods [98]. The utilization of bioactive molecules in the dressings of diabetic wounds has been extensively investigated. To effectively control potential infection in the area, the use of vitamin K3 carnosine peptide (VKC) with a laden silk fibroin scaffold (SF-VKC) showed excellent cell viability and biocompatibility while exhibiting antibacterial properties against *S.aureus, E.coli,* and *P. aeruginosa*, showing that it is effective against both gram-positive and gram-negative bacteria. Furthermore, these dressings exhibited significant mechanical properties, including drug release, water uptake, and adhesiveness, while being relatively inexpensive to produce. The overall characteristics of the scaffolding helped increase the speed of cell migration and repair of diabetic wounds, showing its great potential as a wound-treating dressing material (Figure 9) [99].

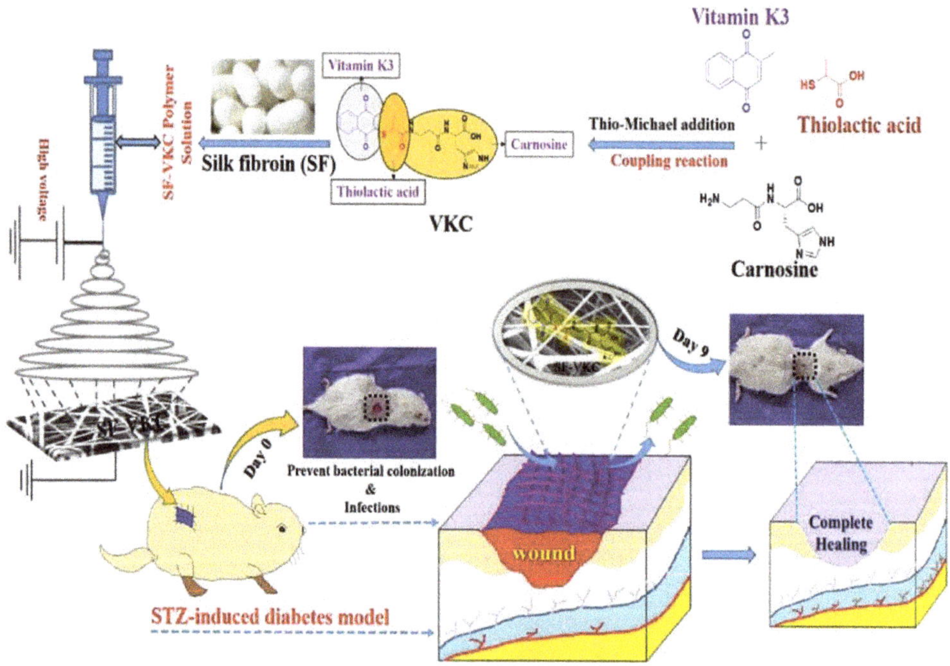

Figure 9. Schematic representation of the SF and VKC antibacterial agents used in electrospun fiber fabrication for STZ-induced diabetic wound healing applications. Reproduced with permission from Ref. [99]. Copyright 2021, American Chemical Society.

A combination of Huangbai Liniment (Compound Phellodendron Liquid, CPL) with SF and poly-(L-lactide-co-caprolactone) (PLCL) was observed to aid in diabetic wound healing. With the sustained release of the drug over a long period, the bandages were able to achieve antimicrobial activity against *S. aureus* and *E. coli.* In addition, cell proliferation improved and expression levels of TGF-β signaling pathway components and Col increased. Through animal experimentation, these bandages ensured that the membrane worked as intended and inhibited inflammatory factors [91]. SF nanofibers, menstrual blood-derived mesenchymal stem cells (MenSCs), and human amniotic membrane (AM) used as bilayer scaffolding (bSC) showed potential for use as a diabetic wound dressings. The dressings exhibited the highest epidermal and dermal regeneration rates when bSC was combined with MenSCs. Furthermore, they facilitated the upregulation of expression of genes that are critically associated with wound healing compared to the expression of genes associated with the innate AM and bSC scaffolds [100]. Similarly, an SF nanofiber matrix containing hydroxyapatite (HAp) and Cur was effective in treating diabetic wounds. The SF/HAp-Cur nanofibers exhibited much better mechanical and water uptake properties than the innate SF/HAp nanofibers. Moreover, the sustained release of Cur into the wound area exerted its antibacterial properties against *S. aureus* and *E. coli* in addition to its healing action. The dressing achieved a wound closure rate of 99.6% on day 21, whereas the innate SF/HAp nanofiber achieved a wound closure rate of 67.7%. The addition of Cur helped achieve antibacterial, antioxidant, and mechanical properties while retaining biocompatibility with the tissue [101].

4. Zein

Zein is a naturally occurring protein polymer readily found in corn. Owing to its biocompatibility, degradability, flexibility, antibacterial, and oxidative properties, it has been widely used in biomedical applications such as tissue regeneration, drug delivery processes, and wound treatment [102,103].

To sustainably release sodium citrate or other drugs into the wound area, it is necessary to secure and protect the wound area and release the drugs. To achieve such functionality with added economic benefits, a method for developing nanofibrous dressings from corn zein was developed. Air jet spinning of the nanofibers enabled synthesis via a sustainable and economically beneficial drug release system that could be used to assist wound healing in patients with diabetes. Owing to significant experimentation performed to ensure that biocompatibility is not an issue, corn zein nanofibers have the potential to become reliable and sustainable drug release systems [92].

The use of cellulose acetate (CA) with zein and sesamol produced CA/zein nanofiber membranes that acted as a delivery system for the controlled release of sesamol. To create the most effective membrane for delivery, it was determined that the ratio of CA to zein should be 12:8 to create the best membrane with a small diameter and uniform distribution. The created membrane exhibited an enhanced healing speed, as the membrane with sesamol promoted the creation of fibroblasts and inhibited chronic inflammation in the wounds (Figure 10) [93].

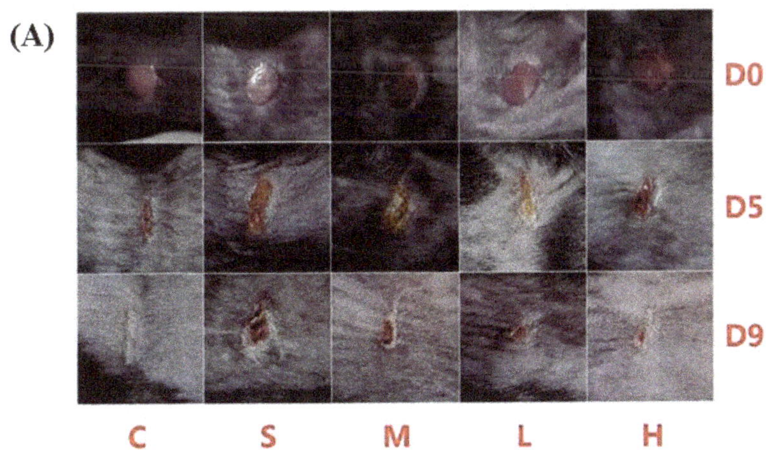

Figure 10. *Cont.*

(B)

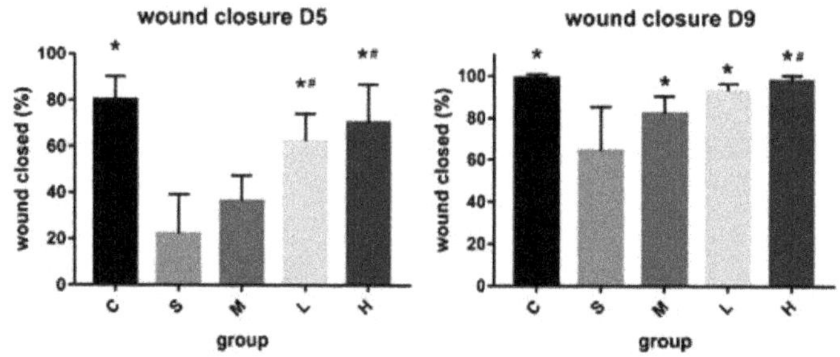

Figure 10. (**A**) Wound images at 0, 5, and 9 days (D0, D5, and D9). **H** Diabetic, 5% sesamol-CA/Zein composite nanofiber membrane; **S** Diabetic, no intervention; **M** Diabetic, CA/Zein blended nanofiber membrane; **L** Diabetic, 2% sesamol-CA/Zein composite nanofiber membrane; and **C** Normal. (**B**) Quantitative analysis of wound closure in diabetic mice at day 5 (D5) and day 9 (D9). * Statistically significant, $p < 0.05$ vs. group C, # Statistically significant, $p < 0.05$ vs. group S. Reproduced with permission from Ref. [93]. Copyright 2020, Elsevier.

5. Conclusions and Future Perspectives

Diabetic wounds are complications in patients with diabetes that take a long time to resolve. These wounds produce high levels of inflammatory cytokines and ROS, which further damage normal cells and tissues. Furthermore, diabetic wounds exhibit repeated bacterial infections, owing to their hyperglycemic environments, which cause great suffering to patients and lead to a significant burden on health care systems. The development of wound dressings is necessary to protect and accelerate wound closure. Electrospun nanofibers are a better choice for diabetic wound closure because of their structural similarity to the ECM, which induces cell adhesion, proliferation, and migration, and subsequently, new tissue formation. Compared to conventional wound dressing materials, electrospun nanofiber dressing patches have high porosity and high moisture permeability, and they provide an effective barrier against external pathogen invasion [104,105]. They exhibit a remarkable potential for encapsulating and delivering active substances that promote wound healing. In a recent study, herbal compound (SRHC)-loaded electrospun MeGEL/PLLA dressing patches accelerated the wound healing rate compared to medical gauze in vivo [50]. Similarly, bioflavonoid (quercetin)-loaded zein-based nanofibers enhanced functional recovery in diabetic neuropathy [106].

Loading small molecules, drugs, and cells can accelerate the recovery process, but single drug loading may not achieve the desired outcome. Dual loading of bioactive agents, such as zinc nanoparticles and oregano essential oil, exhibits synergistic action in diabetic wound healing [106]. Combining multiple drugs or inorganic particles may provide a potential strategy for achieving the desired treatment. Recently, wound bandages with nanomaterials have shown great potential in improving diabetic wound healing. nCeO2-loaded poly(3-hydroxybutyrate-co-3-hydroxyvalerate) (PHBV) electrospun membranes enhance vascularization and cell proliferation in vivo [107]. Wound dressing containing silver nanoparticles (Acticoat®) are the first commercial product that may pave the way for novel approaches in diabetic wound healing [108]. Multilayer electrospun scaffolds may offer another method for improving diabetic wound healing [50]. Hydrogel fiber wound dressings, which have the advantage of good air permeability and liquid absorption, may provide an opportunity for the treatment of diabetic wounds.

Despite all the efforts taken to manage diabetic wounds, the intended therapeutic outcomes have not been achieved yet. Notably, diabetic wound healing studies rely heavily on in vivo animal experiments, and the healing effect is mostly determined by the healing time, whereas analyses of the diabetic wound healing process and tissue sections are limited. Furthermore, the lack of research on the biocompatibility and degradability of electrospun fibers makes safety evaluations difficult.

Funding: This research received no external funding.

Conflicts of Interest: The authors declare no conflict of interest.

References

1. Hussain, Z.; Thu, H.E.; Shuid, A.N.; Katas, H.; Hussain, F. Recent Advances in Polymer-based Wound Dressings for the Treatment of Diabetic Foot Ulcer: An Overview of State-of-the-art. *Curr. Drug Targets* **2018**, *19*, 527–550. [CrossRef]
2. Liu, Y.; Zeng, S.; Ji, W.; Yao, H.; Lin, L.; Cui, H.; Santos, H.A.; Pan, G. Emerging Theranostic Nanomaterials in Diabetes and Its Complications. *Adv. Sci.* **2022**, *9*, 2102466. [CrossRef]
3. Pawar, K.B.; Desai, S.; Bhonde, R.R.; Bhole, R.P.; Deshmukh, A.A. Wound with Diabetes: Present Scenario and Future. *Curr. Diabetes Rev.* **2021**, *17*, 136–142. [CrossRef] [PubMed]
4. Shi, C.; Wang, C.; Liu, H.; Li, Q.; Li, R.; Zhang, Y.; Liu, Y.; Shao, Y.; Wang, J. Selection of Appropriate Wound Dressing for Various Wounds. *Front. Bioeng. Biotechnol.* **2020**, *8*, 182. [CrossRef]
5. Fahimirad, S.; Ajalloueian, F. Naturally-derived electrospun wound dressings for target delivery of bio-active agents. *Int. J. Pharm.* **2019**, *566*, 307–328. [CrossRef] [PubMed]
6. Liu, X.; Xu, H.; Zhang, M.; Yu, D.G. Electrospun Medicated Nanofibers for Wound Healing: Review. *Membranes* **2021**, *11*, 770. [CrossRef]
7. Sood, A.; Granick, M.S.; Tomaselli, N.L. Wound Dressings and Comparative Effectiveness Data. *Adv. Wound Care* **2014**, *3*, 511–529. [CrossRef]
8. Wei, S.; You, Y.; Ma, Y.; Huang, W.; Liang, X.; Zhang, A.; Lin, Y. Bi-layer supramolecular polydimethylsiloxane elastomer film: Synthesis, characterization, and application in wound dressing on normal and diabetic rat. *React. Funct. Polym.* **2019**, *141*, 21–32. [CrossRef]
9. Laurano, R.; Boffito, M.; Ciardelli, G.; Chiono, V. Wound dressing products: A translational investigation from the bench to the market. *Eng. Regen.* **2022**, *3*, 182–200. [CrossRef]
10. Darkovich, S.L.; Brown-Etris, M.; Spencer, M. Biofilm hydrogel dressing: A clinical evaluation in the treatment of pressure sores. *Ostomy/Wound Manag.* **1990**, *29*, 47–60.
11. Samadian, H.; Zamiri, S.; Ehterami, A.; Farzamfar, S.; Vaez, A.; Khastar, H.; Alam, M.; Ai, A.; Derakhshankhah, H.; Allahyari, Z.; et al. Electrospun cellulose acetate/gelatin nanofibrous wound dressing containing berberine for diabetic foot ulcer healing: In vitro and in vivo studies. *Sci. Rep.* **2020**, *10*, 8312. [CrossRef]
12. Suliman Maashi, M.; Felemban, S.G.; Almasmoum, H.A.; Jarahian, M. Nicaraven-loaded electrospun wound dressings promote diabetic wound healing via proangiogenic and immunomodulatory functions: A preclinical investigation. *Drug Deliv. Transl. Res.* **2023**, *13*, 222–236. [CrossRef]
13. Chen, L.; Zhang, L.; Zhang, H.; Sun, X.; Liu, D.; Zhang, J.; Zhang, Y.; Cheng, L.; Santos, H.A.; Cui, W. Programmable immune activating electrospun fibers for skin regeneration. *Bioact. Mater.* **2021**, *6*, 3218–3230. [CrossRef] [PubMed]
14. Shahriar, S.M.S.; Mondal, J.; Hasan, M.N.; Revuri, V.; Lee, D.Y.; Lee, Y. K. Electrospinning Nanofibers for Therapeutics Delivery. *Nanomaterials* **2019**, *9*, 532. [CrossRef]
15. Xie, Z.; Paras, C.B.; Weng, H.; Punnakitikashem, P.; Su, L.C.; Vu, K.; Tang, L.; Yang, J.; Nguyen, K.T. Dual growth factor releasing multi-functional nanofibers for wound healing. *Acta Biomater.* **2013**, *9*, 9351–9359. [CrossRef] [PubMed]
16. Sheng, Z.; Xu, Y.; Tong, Z.; Mao, Z.; Zheng, Y. Dual functional electrospun nanofiber membrane with ROS scavenging and revascularization ability for diabetic wound healing. *Colloids Interface Sci. Commun.* **2022**, *48*, 100620. [CrossRef]
17. Ramakrishna, S.; Fujihara, K.; Teo, W.-E.; Yong, T.; Ma, Z.; Ramaseshan, R. Electrospun nanofibers: Solving global issues. *Mater. Today* **2006**, *9*, 40–50. [CrossRef]
18. Monsores, K.G.d.C.; Oliveira da Silva, A.; Oliveira, S.d.S.A.; Weber, R.P.; Dias, M.L. Production of nanofibers from solution blow spinning (SBS). *J. Mater. Res. Technol.* **2022**, *16*, 1824–1831. [CrossRef]
19. Zhang, M.; Peng, X.; Fan, P.; Zhou, Y.; Xiao, P. Recent Progress in Preparation and Application of Fibers Using Microfluidic Spinning Technology. *Macromol. Chem. Phys.* **2022**, *223*, 2100451. [CrossRef]
20. Weitz, R.T.; Harnau, L.; Rauschenbach, S.; Burghard, M.; Kern, K. Polymer Nanofibers via Nozzle-Free Centrifugal Spinning. *Nano Lett.* **2008**, *8*, 1187–1191. [CrossRef]
21. Xue, J.; Wu, T.; Dai, Y.; Xia, Y. Electrospinning and Electrospun Nanofibers: Methods, Materials, and Applications. *Chem. Rev.* **2019**, *119*, 5298–5415. [CrossRef] [PubMed]
22. Lan, X.; Liu, Y.; Wang, Y.; Tian, F.; Miao, X.; Wang, H.; Tang, Y. Coaxial electrospun PVA/PCL nanofibers with dual release of tea polyphenols and ε-poly (L-lysine) as antioxidant and antibacterial wound dressing materials. *Int. J. Pharm.* **2021**, *601*, 120525. [CrossRef] [PubMed]
23. Bonferoni, M.C.; Rossi, S.; Sandri, G.; Caramella, C.; Del Fante, C.; Perotti, C.; Miele, D.; Vigani, B.; Ferrari, F. Bioactive Medications for the Delivery of Platelet Derivatives to Skin Wounds. *Curr. Drug Deliv.* **2019**, *16*, 472–483. [CrossRef] [PubMed]
24. Keshvardoostchokami, M.; Majidi, S.S.; Huo, P.; Ramachandran, R.; Chen, M.; Liu, B. Electrospun Nanofibers of Natural and Synthetic Polymers as Artificial Extracellular Matrix for Tissue Engineering. *Nanomaterials* **2021**, *11*, 21. [CrossRef]
25. Augustine, R.; Rehman, S.R.U.; Ahmed, R.; Zahid, A.A.; Sharifi, M.; Falahati, M.; Hasan, A. Electrospun chitosan membranes containing bioactive and therapeutic agents for enhanced wound healing. *Int. J. Biol. Macromol.* **2020**, *156*, 153–170. [CrossRef]

26. Liu, Y.; Li, C.; Feng, Z.; Han, B.; Yu, D.-G.; Wang, K. Advances in the Preparation of Nanofiber Dressings by Electrospinning for Promoting Diabetic Wound Healing. *Biomolecules* **2022**, *12*, 1727. [CrossRef] [PubMed]
27. Liu, Y.; Zhou, S.; Gao, Y.; Zhai, Y. Electrospun nanofibers as a wound dressing for treating diabetic foot ulcer. *Asian J. Pharm. Sci.* **2019**, *14*, 130–143. [CrossRef]
28. Gao, Z.; Wang, Q.; Yao, Q.; Zhang, P. Application of Electrospun Nanofiber Membrane in the Treatment of Diabetic Wounds. *Pharmaceutics* **2021**, *14*, 6. [CrossRef]
29. Iacob, A.-T.; Drăgan, M.; Ionescu, O.-M.; Profire, L.; Ficai, A.; Andronescu, E.; Confederat, L.G.; Lupașcu, D. An Overview of Biopolymeric Electrospun Nanofibers Based on Polysaccharides for Wound Healing Management. *Pharmaceutics* **2020**, *12*, 983. [CrossRef]
30. Patel, S.; Srivastava, S.; Singh, M.R.; Singh, D. Mechanistic insight into diabetic wounds: Pathogenesis, molecular targets and treatment strategies to pace wound healing. *Biomed. Pharmacother.* **2019**, *112*, 108615. [CrossRef]
31. Chakraborty, R.; Borah, P.; Dutta, P.P.; Sen, S. Evolving spectrum of diabetic wound: Mechanistic insights and therapeutic targets. *World J. Diabetes* **2022**, *13*, 696–716. [CrossRef] [PubMed]
32. Khanna, S.; Biswas, S.; Shang, Y.; Collard, E.; Azad, A.; Kauh, C.; Bhasker, V.; Gordillo, G.M.; Sen, C.K.; Roy, S. Macrophage dysfunction impairs resolution of inflammation in the wounds of diabetic mice. *PLoS ONE* **2010**, *5*, e9539. [CrossRef] [PubMed]
33. Nwomeh, B.C.; Yager, D.R.; Cohen, I.K. Physiology of the chronic wound. *Clin. Plast. Surg.* **1998**, *25*, 341–356. [CrossRef] [PubMed]
34. Louiselle, A.E.; Niemiec, S.M.; Zgheib, C.; Liechty, K.W. Macrophage polarization and diabetic wound healing. *Transl. Res. J. Lab. Clin. Med.* **2021**, *236*, 109–116. [CrossRef] [PubMed]
35. Khan, A.U.R.; Huang, K.; Khalaji, M.S.; Yu, F.; Xie, X.; Zhu, T.; Morsi, Y.; Jinzhong, Z.; Mo, X. Multifunctional bioactive core-shell electrospun membrane capable to terminate inflammatory cycle and promote angiogenesis in diabetic wound. *Bioact. Mater.* **2021**, *6*, 2783–2800. [CrossRef]
36. Chen, S.; Wang, H.; Su, Y.; John, J.V.; McCarthy, A.; Wong, S.L.; Xie, J. Mesenchymal stem cell-laden, personalized 3D scaffolds with controlled structure and fiber alignment promote diabetic wound healing. *Acta Biomater.* **2020**, *108*, 153–167. [CrossRef]
37. Gao, W.; Jin, W.; Li, Y.; Wan, L.; Wang, C.; Lin, C.; Chen, X.; Lei, B.; Mao, C. A highly bioactive bone extracellular matrix-biomimetic nanofibrous system with rapid angiogenesis promotes diabetic wound healing. *J. Mater. Chem. B* **2017**, *5*, 7285–7296. [CrossRef]
38. Gao, W.; Sun, L.; Fu, X.; Lin, Z.; Xie, W.; Zhang, W.; Zhao, F.; Chen, X. Enhanced diabetic wound healing by electrospun core–sheath fibers loaded with dimethyloxalylglycine. *J. Mater. Chem. B* **2018**, *6*, 277–288. [CrossRef]
39. Zhang, Q.; Oh, J.-H.; Park, C.H.; Baek, J.-H.; Ryoo, H.-M.; Woo, K.M. Effects of Dimethyloxalylglycine-Embedded Poly(ε-caprolactone) Fiber Meshes on Wound Healing in Diabetic Rats. *ACS Appl. Mater. Interfaces* **2017**, *9*, 7950–7963. [CrossRef]
40. Mehteroğlu, E.; Çakmen, A.B.; Aksoy, B.; Balcıoğlu, S.; Köytepe, S.; Ateş, B.; Yılmaz, İ. Preparation of hybrid PU/PCL fibers from steviol glycosides via electrospinning as a potential wound dressing materials. *J. Appl. Polym. Sci.* **2020**, *137*, 49217. [CrossRef]
41. Ranjbar-Mohammadi, M.; Rabbani, S.; Bahrami, S.H.; Joghataei, M.T.; Moayer, F. Antibacterial performance and in vivo diabetic wound healing of curcumin loaded gum tragacanth/poly(ε-caprolactone) electrospun nanofibers. *Mater. Sci. Eng. C* **2016**, *69*, 1183–1191. [CrossRef] [PubMed]
42. Stack, M.E.; Mishra, S.; Parimala Chelvi Ratnamani, M.; Wang, H.; Gold, L.I.; Wang, H. Biomimetic Extracellular Matrix Nanofibers Electrospun with Calreticulin Promote Synergistic Activity for Tissue Regeneration. *ACS Appl. Mater. Interfaces* **2022**, *14*, 51683–51696. [CrossRef] [PubMed]
43. Derakhshan, M.A.; Nazeri, N.; Khoshnevisan, K.; Heshmat, R.; Omidfar, K. Three-layered PCL-collagen nanofibers containing melilotus officinalis extract for diabetic ulcer healing in a rat model. *J. Diabetes Metab. Disord.* **2022**, *21*, 313–321. [CrossRef]
44. Yu, B.; He, C.; Wang, W.; Ren, Y.; Yang, J.; Guo, S.; Zheng, Y.; Shi, X. Asymmetric Wettable Composite Wound Dressing Prepared by Electrospinning with Bioinspired Micropatterning Enhances Diabetic Wound Healing. *ACS Appl. Bio Mater.* **2020**, *3*, 5383–5394. [CrossRef] [PubMed]
45. Lee, C.H.; Chang, S.H.; Chen, W.J.; Hung, K.C.; Lin, Y.H.; Liu, S.J.; Hsieh, M.J.; Pang, J.H.; Juang, J.H. Augmentation of diabetic wound healing and enhancement of collagen content using nanofibrous glucophage-loaded collagen/PLGA scaffold membranes. *J. Colloid Interface Sci.* **2015**, *439*, 88–97. [CrossRef] [PubMed]
46. Lee, C.-H.; Liu, K.-S.; Cheng, C.-W.; Chan, E.-C.; Hung, K.-C.; Hsieh, M.-J.; Chang, S.-H.; Fu, X.; Juang, J.-H.; Hsieh, I.C.; et al. Codelivery of Sustainable Antimicrobial Agents and Platelet-Derived Growth Factor via Biodegradable Nanofibers for Repair of Diabetic Infectious Wounds. *ACS Infect. Dis.* **2020**, *6*, 2688–2697. [CrossRef]
47. Shin, Y.C.; Shin, D.M.; Lee, E.J.; Lee, J.H.; Kim, J.E.; Song, S.H.; Hwang, D.Y.; Lee, J.J.; Kim, B.; Lim, D.; et al. Hyaluronic Acid/PLGA Core/Shell Fiber Matrices Loaded with EGCG Beneficial to Diabetic Wound Healing. *Adv. Healthc. Mater.* **2016**, *5*, 3035–3045. [CrossRef]
48. John, J.V.; Sharma, N.S.; Tang, G.; Luo, Z.; Su, Y.; Weihs, S.; Shahriar, S.M.S.; Wang, G.; McCarthy, A.; Dyke, J.; et al. Nanofiber Aerogels with Precision Macrochannels and LL-37-Mimic Peptides Synergistically Promote Diabetic Wound Healing. *Adv. Funct. Mater.* **2022**, *33*, 2206936. [CrossRef]
49. Ren, X.; Han, Y.; Wang, J.; Jiang, Y.; Yi, Z.; Xu, H.; Ke, Q. An aligned porous electrospun fibrous membrane with controlled drug delivery—An efficient strategy to accelerate diabetic wound healing with improved angiogenesis. *Acta Biomater.* **2018**, *70*, 140–153. [CrossRef]

50. Wu, S.; Zhao, W.; Sun, M.; He, P.; Lv, H.; Wang, Q.; Zhang, S.; Wu, Q.; Ling, P.; Chen, S.; et al. Novel bi-layered dressing patches constructed with radially-oriented nanofibrous pattern and herbal compound-loaded hydrogel for accelerated diabetic wound healing. *Appl. Mater. Today* **2022**, *28*, 101542. [CrossRef]
51. Ilomuanya, M.O.; Okafor, P.S.; Amajuoyi, J.N.; Onyejekwe, J.C.; Okubanjo, O.O.; Adeosun, S.O.; Silva, B.O. Polylactic acid-based electrospun fiber and hyaluronic acid-valsartan hydrogel scaffold for chronic wound healing. *Beni-Suef Univ. J. Basic Appl. Sci.* **2020**, *9*, 31. [CrossRef]
52. Hussein, M.A.M.; Su, S.; Ulag, S.; Woźniak, A.; Grinholc, M.; Erdemir, G.; Erdem Kuruca, S.; Gunduz, O.; Muhammed, M.; El-Sherbiny, I.M.; et al. Development and In Vitro Evaluation of Biocompatible PLA-Based Trilayer Nanofibrous Membranes for the Delivery of Nanoceria: A Novel Approach for Diabetic Wound Healing. *Polymers* **2021**, *13*, 3630. [CrossRef]
53. Xu, F.; Wang, H.; Zhang, J.; Jiang, L.; Zhang, W.; Hu, Y. A facile design of EGF conjugated PLA/gelatin electrospun nanofibers for nursing care of in vivo wound healing applications. *J. Ind. Text.* **2022**, *51*, 420S–440S. [CrossRef]
54. Chen, H.; Jia, P.; Kang, H.; Zhang, H.; Liu, Y.; Yang, P.; Yan, Y.; Zuo, G.; Guo, L.; Jiang, M.; et al. Upregulating Hif-1α by Hydrogel Nanofibrous Scaffolds for Rapidly Recruiting Angiogenesis Relative Cells in Diabetic Wound. *Adv. Healthc. Mater.* **2016**, *5*, 907–918. [CrossRef] [PubMed]
55. Ranjbar Mohammadi, M.; Kargozar, S.; Bahrami, S.H.; Rabbani, S. An excellent nanofibrous matrix based on gum tragacanth-poly (Ɛ-caprolactone)-poly (vinyl alcohol) for application in diabetic wound healing. *Polym. Degrad. Stab.* **2020**, *174*, 109105. [CrossRef]
56. Ahmadi Majd, S.; Rabbani Khorasgani, M.; Moshtaghian, S.J.; Talebi, A.; Khezri, M. Application of Chitosan/PVA Nano fiber as a potential wound dressing for streptozotocin-induced diabetic rats. *Int. J. Biol. Macromol.* **2016**, *92*, 1162–1168. [CrossRef] [PubMed]
57. Ahmed, R.; Tariq, M.; Ali, I.; Asghar, R.; Noorunnisa Khanam, P.; Augustine, R.; Hasan, A. Novel electrospun chitosan/polyvinyl alcohol/zinc oxide nanofibrous mats with antibacterial and antioxidant properties for diabetic wound healing. *Int. J. Biol. Macromol.* **2018**, *120*, 385–393. [CrossRef]
58. Almukainzi, M.; El-Masry, T.A.; Negm, W.A.; Elekhnawy, E.; Saleh, A.; Sayed, A.E.; Ahmed, H.M.; Abdelkader, D.H. Co-delivery of gentiopicroside and thymoquinone using electrospun m-PEG/PVP nanofibers: In-vitro and In vivo studies for antibacterial wound dressing in diabetic rats. *Int. J. Pharm.* **2022**, *625*, 122106. [CrossRef]
59. Obaidat, R.; Shameh, A.A.; Aljarrah, M.; Hamed, R. Preparation and Evaluation of Polyvinylpyrrolidone Electrospun Nanofiber Patches of Pioglitazone for the Treatment of Atopic Dermatitis. *AAPS PharmSciTech* **2022**, *23*, 51. [CrossRef]
60. Pinzón-García, A.D.; Cassini-Vieira, P.; Ribeiro, C.C.; de Matos Jensen, C.E.; Barcelos, L.S.; Cortes, M.E.; Sinisterra, R.D. Efficient cutaneous wound healing using bixin-loaded PCL nanofibers in diabetic mice. *J. Biomed. Mater. Res. Part B Appl. Biomater.* **2017**, *105*, 1938–1949. [CrossRef]
61. Khandaker, M.; Alkadhem, N.; Progri, H.; Nikfarjam, S.; Jeon, J.; Kotturi, H.; Vaughan, M.B. Glutathione Immobilized Polycaprolactone Nanofiber Mesh as a Dermal Drug Delivery Mechanism for Wound Healing in a Diabetic Patient. *Process* **2022**, *10*, 512. [CrossRef]
62. Tao, W.; Wang, G.; Pei, X.; Sun, W.; Wang, M. Chitosan Oligosaccharide Attenuates Lipopolysaccharide-Induced Intestinal Barrier Dysfunction through Suppressing the Inflammatory Response and Oxidative Stress in Mice. *Antioxidants* **2022**, *11*, 1384. [CrossRef] [PubMed]
63. Sun, L.; Gao, W.; Fu, X.; Shi, M.; Xie, W.; Zhang, W.; Zhao, F.; Chen, X. Enhanced wound healing in diabetic rats by nanofibrous scaffolds mimicking the basketweave pattern of collagen fibrils in native skin. *Biomater. Sci.* **2018**, *6*, 340–349. [CrossRef] [PubMed]
64. Foraida, Z.I.; Kamaldinov, T.; Nelson, D.A.; Larsen, M.; Castracane, J. Elastin-PLGA hybrid electrospun nanofiber scaffolds for salivary epithelial cell self-organization and polarization. *Acta Biomater.* **2017**, *62*, 116–127. [CrossRef]
65. Lee, C.-H.; Chao, Y.-K.; Chang, S.-H.; Chen, W.-J.; Hung, K.-C.; Liu, S.-J.; Juang, J.-H.; Chen, Y.-T.; Wang, F.-S. Nanofibrous rhPDGF-eluting PLGA–collagen hybrid scaffolds enhance healing of diabetic wounds. *RSC Adv.* **2016**, *6*, 6276–6284. [CrossRef]
66. Lee, C.H.; Hsieh, M.J.; Chang, S.H.; Lin, Y.H.; Liu, S.J.; Lin, T.Y.; Hung, K.C.; Pang, J.H.; Juang, J.H. Enhancement of diabetic wound repair using biodegradable nanofibrous metformin-eluting membranes: In vitro and in vivo. *ACS Appl. Mater. Interfaces* **2014**, *6*, 3979–3986. [CrossRef]
67. Gao, S.; Chen, T.; Wang, Z.; Ji, P.; Xu, L.; Cui, W.; Wang, Y. Immuno-activated mesenchymal stem cell living electrospun nanofibers for promoting diabetic wound repair. *J. Nanobiotechnol.* **2022**, *20*, 294. [CrossRef]
68. Drumright, R.E.; Gruber, P.R.; Henton, D.E. Polylactic Acid Technology. *Adv. Mater.* **2000**, *12*, 1841–1846. [CrossRef]
69. Elsayed, R.E.; Madkour, T.M.; Azzam, R.A. Tailored-design of electrospun nanofiber cellulose acetate/poly(lactic acid) dressing mats loaded with a newly synthesized sulfonamide analog exhibiting superior wound healing. *Int. J. Biol. Macromol.* **2020**, *164*, 1984–1999. [CrossRef]
70. Sharma, K.; Bullock, A.; Ralston, D.; MacNeil, S. Development of a one-step approach for the reconstruction of full thickness skin defects using minced split thickness skin grafts and biodegradable synthetic scaffolds as a dermal substitute. *Burn. J. Int. Soc. Burn Inj.* **2014**, *40*, 957–965. [CrossRef]
71. Zhao, Y.; Tian, C.; Liu, Y.; Liu, Z.; Li, J.; Wang, Z.; Han, X. All-in-one bioactive properties of photothermal nanofibers for accelerating diabetic wound healing. *Biomaterials* **2023**, *295*, 122029. [CrossRef] [PubMed]
72. Baldassarro, V.A.; Giraldi, V.; Giuliani, A.; Moretti, M.; Pagnotta, G.; Flagelli, A.; Clavenzani, P.; Lorenzini, L.; Giardino, L.; Focarete, M.L.; et al. Poly(l-lactic acid) Scaffold Releasing an α4β1 Integrin Agonist Promotes Nonfibrotic Skin Wound Healing in Diabetic Mice. *ACS Appl. Bio Mater.* **2023**, *6*, 296–308. [CrossRef]

73. Augustine, R.; Zahid, A.A.; Hasan, A.; Wang, M.; Webster, T.J. CTGF Loaded Electrospun Dual Porous Core-Shell Membrane For Diabetic Wound Healing. *Int. J. Nanomed.* **2019**, *14*, 8573–8588. [CrossRef] [PubMed]
74. Ciftci, F.; Ayan, S.; Duygulu, N.; Yilmazer, Y.; Karavelioglu, Z.; Vehapi, M.; Cakır Koc, R.; Sengor, M.; Yılmazer, H.; Ozcimen, D.; et al. Selenium and clarithromycin loaded PLA-GO composite wound dressings by electrospinning method. *Int. J. Polym. Mater. Polym. Biomater.* **2022**, *71*, 898–909. [CrossRef]
75. Peresin, M.S.; Habibi, Y.; Vesterinen, A.-H.; Rojas, O.J.; Pawlak, J.J.; Seppälä, J.V. Effect of Moisture on Electrospun Nanofiber Composites of Poly(vinyl alcohol) and Cellulose Nanocrystals. *Biomacromolecules* **2010**, *11*, 2471–2477. [CrossRef] [PubMed]
76. Chouhan, D.; Janani, G.; Chakraborty, B.; Nandi, S.K.; Mandal, B.B. Functionalized PVA-silk blended nanofibrous mats promote diabetic wound healing via regulation of extracellular matrix and tissue remodelling. *J. Tissue Eng. Regen. Med.* **2018**, *12*, e1559–e1570. [CrossRef]
77. Sena, S.; Sumeyra, K.N.; Ulkugul, G.; Sema, A.; Betul, K.; Muge, S.B.; Sayip, E.M.; Muhammet, U.; Cevriye, K.; Mahir, M.; et al. Controlled Release of Metformin Hydrochloride from Core-Shell Nanofibers with Fish Sarcoplasmic Protein. *Medicina* **2019**, *55*, 682. [CrossRef] [PubMed]
78. Alberti, T.B.; Coelho, D.S.; de Prá, M.; Maraschin, M.; Veleirinho, B. Electrospun PVA nanoscaffolds associated with propolis nanoparticles with wound healing activity. *J. Mater. Sci.* **2020**, *55*, 9712–9727. [CrossRef]
79. Jayakumar, R.; Prabaharan, M.; Kumar, P.S.; Nair, S.; Tamura, H.J.B.A. Biomaterials based on chitin and chitosan in wound dressing applications. *Biotechnol. Adv.* **2011**, *29*, 322–337. [CrossRef]
80. Lv, H.; Zhao, M.; Li, Y.; Li, K.; Chen, S.; Zhao, W.; Wu, S.; Han, Y. Electrospun Chitosan–Polyvinyl Alcohol Nanofiber Dressings Loaded with Bioactive Ursolic Acid Promoting Diabetic Wound Healing. *Nanomaterials* **2022**, *12*, 2933. [CrossRef]
81. Zhang, H.; Zhang, M.; Wang, X.; Zhang, M.; Wang, X.; Li, Y.; Cui, Z.; Chen, X.; Han, Y.; Zhao, W. Electrospun multifunctional nanofibrous mats loaded with bioactive anemoside B4 for accelerated wound healing in diabetic mice. *Drug Deliv.* **2022**, *29*, 174–185. [CrossRef]
82. Guo, L.; Guan, N.; Miao, W.; Zhao, W.; Li, Q. An Electrospun Scaffold Loaded with an Enteromorpha Polysaccharide for Accelerated Wound Healing in Diabetic Mice. *Mar. Drugs* **2022**, *20*, 95. [CrossRef] [PubMed]
83. Alabdali, A.Y.M.; Khalid, R.; Kzar, M.; Ezzat, M.O.; Huei, G.M.; Hsia, T.W.; Mogana, R.; Rahman, H.; Razik, B.M.A.; Issac, P.K.; et al. Design, synthesis, in silico and antibacterial evaluation of curcumin derivatives loaded nanofiber as potential wound healing agents. *J. King Saud Univ. Sci.* **2022**, *34*, 102205. [CrossRef]
84. Monirul Islam, M.; Hemmanahalli Ramesh, V.; Durga Bhavani, P.; Goudanavar, P.S.; Naveen, N.R.; Ramesh, B.; Fattepur, S.; Narayanappa Shiroorkar, P.; Habeebuddin, M.; Meravanige, G.; et al. Optimization of process parameters for fabrication of electrospun nanofibers containing neomycin sulfate and Malva sylvestris extract for a better diabetic wound healing. *Drug Deliv.* **2022**, *29*, 3370–3383. [CrossRef]
85. Yue, Y.; Liu, X.; Pang, L.; Liu, Y.; Lin, Y.; Xiang, T.; Li, J.; Liao, S.; Jiang, Y. Astragalus Polysaccharides/PVA Nanofiber Membranes Containing Astragaloside IV-Loaded Liposomes and Their Potential Use for Wound Healing. *Evid.-Based Complement. Altern. Med.* **2022**, *2022*, 9716271. [CrossRef]
86. Cam, M.E.; Yildiz, S.; Alenezi, H.; Cesur, S.; Ozcan, G.S.; Erdemir, G.; Edirisinghe, U.; Akakin, D.; Kuruca, D.S.; Kabasakal, L.; et al. Evaluation of burst release and sustained release of pioglitazone-loaded fibrous mats on diabetic wound healing: An in vitro and in vivo comparison study. *J. R. Soc. Interface* **2020**, *17*, 20190712. [CrossRef] [PubMed]
87. Zhou, L.; Xu, P.; Dong, P.; Ou, X.; Du, X.; Chen, Y.; Zhang, X.; Guo, W.; Gao, G. A self-pumping dressing with in situ modification of non-woven fabric for promoting diabetic wound healing. *Chem. Eng. J.* **2023**, *457*, 141108. [CrossRef]
88. Aduba, D.C.; An, S.-S.; Selders, G.S.; Yeudall, W.A.; Bowlin, G.L.; Kitten, T.; Yang, H. Electrospun gelatin–arabinoxylan ferulate composite fibers for diabetic chronic wound dressing application. *Int. J. Polym. Mater. Polym. Biomater.* **2019**, *68*, 660–668. [CrossRef]
89. Cam, M.E.; Crabbe-Mann, M.; Alenezi, H.; Hazar-Yavuz, A.N.; Ertas, B.; Ekentok, C.; Ozcan, G.S.; Topal, F.; Guler, E.; Yazir, Y.; et al. The comparision of glybenclamide and metformin-loaded bacterial cellulose/gelatin nanofibres produced by a portable electrohydrodynamic gun for diabetic wound healing. *Eur. Polym. J.* **2020**, *134*, 109844. [CrossRef]
90. Sanhueza, C.; Hermosilla, J.; Bugallo-Casal, A.; Da Silva-Candal, A.; Taboada, C.; Millán, R.; Concheiro, A.; Alvarez-Lorenzo, C.; Acevedo, F. One-step electrospun scaffold of dual-sized gelatin/poly-3-hydroxybutyrate nano/microfibers for skin regeneration in diabetic wound. *Mater. Sci. Eng. C* **2021**, *119*, 111602. [CrossRef]
91. Xu, X.; Wang, X.; Qin, C.; Khan, A.U.R.; Zhang, W.; Mo, X. Silk fibroin/poly-(L-lactide-co-caprolactone) nanofiber scaffolds loaded with Huangbai Liniment to accelerate diabetic wound healing. *Colloids Surf. B Biointerfaces* **2021**, *199*, 111557. [CrossRef]
92. Gough, C.R.; Bessette, K.; Xue, Y.; Mou, X.; Hu, X. Air-Jet Spun Corn Zein Nanofibers and Thin Films with Topical Drug for Medical Applications. *Int. J. Mol. Sci.* **2020**, *21*, 5780. [CrossRef] [PubMed]
93. Liu, F.; Li, X.; Wang, L.; Yan, X.; Ma, D.; Liu, Z.; Liu, X. Sesamol incorporated cellulose acetate-zein composite nanofiber membrane: An efficient strategy to accelerate diabetic wound healing. *Int. J. Biol. Macromol.* **2020**, *149*, 627–638. [CrossRef] [PubMed]
94. Gaspar-Pintiliescu, A.; Stanciuc, A.M.; Craciunescu, O. Natural composite dressings based on collagen, gelatin and plant bioactive compounds for wound healing: A review. *Int. J. Biol. Macromol.* **2019**, *138*, 854–865. [CrossRef] [PubMed]
95. Yang, X.; Chen, M.; Li, P.; Ji, Z.; Wang, M.; Feng, Y.; Shi, C. Fabricating poly(vinyl alcohol)/gelatin composite sponges with high absorbency and water-triggered expansion for noncompressible hemorrhage and wound healing. *J. Mater. Chem. B* **2021**, *9*, 1568–1582. [CrossRef]

96. Duconseille, A.; Astruc, T.; Quintana, N.; Meersman, F.; Sante-Lhoutellier, V. Gelatin structure and composition linked to hard capsule dissolution: A review. *Food Hydrocoll.* **2015**, *43*, 360–376. [CrossRef]
97. Mohamady Hussein, M.A.; Gunduz, O.; Sahin, A.; Grinholc, M.; El-Sherbiny, I.M.; Megahed, M. Dual Spinneret Electrospun Polyurethane/PVA-Gelatin Nanofibrous Scaffolds Containing Cinnamon Essential Oil and Nanoceria for Chronic Diabetic Wound Healing: Preparation, Physicochemical Characterization and In-Vitro Evaluation. *Molecules* **2022**, *27*, 2146. [CrossRef]
98. Agarwal, Y.; Rajinikanth, P.S.; Ranjan, S.; Tiwari, U.; Balasubramnaiam, J.; Pandey, P.; Arya, D.K.; Anand, S.; Deepak, P. Curcumin loaded polycaprolactone-/polyvinyl alcohol-silk fibroin based electrospun nanofibrous mat for rapid healing of diabetic wound: An in-vitro and in-vivo studies. *Int. J. Biol. Macromol.* **2021**, *176*, 376–386. [CrossRef]
99. Kandhasamy, S.; Liang, B.; Yang, D.P.; Zeng, Y. Antibacterial Vitamin K3 Carnosine Peptide-Laden Silk Fibroin Electrospun Fibers for Improvement of Skin Wound Healing in Diabetic Rats. *ACS Appl. Bio Mater.* **2021**, *4*, 4769–4788. [CrossRef]
100. Mirzadegan, E.; Golshahi, H.; Saffarian, Z.; Darzi, M.; Khorasani, S.; Edalatkhah, H.; Saliminejad, K.; Kazemnejad, S. The remarkable effect of menstrual blood stem cells seeded on bilayer scaffold composed of amniotic membrane and silk fibroin aiming to promote wound healing in diabetic mice. *Int. Immunopharmacol.* **2022**, *102*, 108404. [CrossRef]
101. Yang, M.; Yu, S.; Zhao, P.; Xie, L.; Lyu, G.; Yu, J. Fabrication of homogeneously-aligned nano-fillers encapsulated silk fibroin electrospun nanofibers for improved fibroblast attachment, epithelialization, and collagen depositions: In vitro and in vivo wound healing evaluation. *J. Biomater. Sci. Polym. Ed.* **2022**, *33*, 878–899. [CrossRef] [PubMed]
102. Pedram Rad, Z.; Mokhtari, J.; Abbasi, M. Calendula officinalis extract/PCL/Zein/Gum arabic nanofibrous bio-composite scaffolds via suspension, two-nozzle and multilayer electrospinning for skin tissue engineering. *Int. J. Biol. Macromol.* **2019**, *135*, 530–543. [CrossRef] [PubMed]
103. Pedram Rad, Z.; Mokhtari, J.; Abbasi, M. Fabrication and characterization of PCL/zein/gum arabic electrospun nanocomposite scaffold for skin tissue engineering. *Mater. Sci. Eng. C Mater. Biol. Appl.* **2018**, *93*, 356–366. [CrossRef] [PubMed]
104. Qi, Y.; Zhai, H.; Sun, Y.; Xu, H.; Wu, S.; Chen, S. Electrospun hybrid nanofibrous meshes with adjustable performance for potential use in soft tissue engineering. *Text. Res. J.* **2021**, *92*, 1537–1549. [CrossRef]
105. Gao, C.; Zhang, L.; Wang, J.; Jin, M.; Tang, Q.; Chen, Z.; Cheng, Y.; Yang, R.; Zhao, G. Electrospun nanofibers promote wound healing: Theories, techniques, and perspectives. *J. Mater. Chem. B* **2021**, *9*, 3106–3130. [CrossRef]
106. Thipkaew, C.; Wattanathorn, J.; Muchimapura, S. Electrospun Nanofibers Loaded with Quercetin Promote the Recovery of Focal Entrapment Neuropathy in a Rat Model of Streptozotocin-Induced Diabetes. *BioMed Res. Int.* **2017**, *2017*, 2017493. [CrossRef]
107. Augustine, R.; Hasan, A.; Patan, N.K.; Dalvi, Y.B.; Varghese, R.; Antony, A.; Unni, R.N.; Sandhyarani, N.; Moustafa, A.-E.A. Cerium Oxide Nanoparticle Incorporated Electrospun Poly(3-hydroxybutyrate-co-3-hydroxyvalerate) Membranes for Diabetic Wound Healing Applications. *ACS Biomater. Sci. Eng.* **2020**, *6*, 58–70. [CrossRef]
108. Neema, S.; Chatterjee, M. Nano-silver dressing in toxic epidermal necrolysis. *Indian J. Dermatol. Venereol. Leprol.* **2017**, *83*, 121–124. [CrossRef]

pharmaceutics

MDPI

Article

Casein-Based Nanoparticles: A Potential Tool for the Delivery of Daunorubicin in Acute Lymphocytic Leukemia

Nikolay Zahariev [1,2], Milena Draganova [2,3], Plamen Zagorchev [2,4] and Bissera Pilicheva [1,2,*]

1 Department of Pharmaceutical Sciences, Faculty of Pharmacy, Medical University of Plovdiv, 15A Vassil Aprilov Blvd, 4002 Plovdiv, Bulgaria
2 Research Institute, Medical University of Plovdiv, 15A Vassil Aprilov Blvd, 4002 Plovdiv, Bulgaria
3 Department of Medical Biology, Medical Faculty, Medical University of Plovdiv, 15A Vassil Aprilov Blvd, 4002 Plovdiv, Bulgaria
4 Department of Medical Physics and Biophysics, Faculty of Pharmacy, Medical University of Plovdiv, 15A Vassil Aprilov Blvd, 4002 Plovdiv, Bulgaria
* Correspondence: bisera.pilicheva@mu-plovdiv.bg

Abstract: The aim of this study was to develop casein-based nanoscale carriers as a potential delivery system for daunorubicin, as a pH-responsive targeting tool for acute lymphocytic leukemia. A coacervation technique followed by nano spray-drying was used for the preparation of drug-loaded casein nanoparticles. Four batches of drug-loaded formulations were developed at varied drug–polymer ratios using a simple coacervation technique followed by spray-drying. They were further characterized using scanning electron microscopy, dynamic light scattering, FTIR spectroscopy, XRD diffractometry, and differential scanning calorimetry. Drug release was investigated in different media (pH 5 and 7.4). The cytotoxicity of the daunorubicin-loaded nanoparticles was compared to that of the pure drug. The influence of the polymer-to-drug ratio on the nanoparticles' properties such as their particle size, surface morphology, production yield, drug loading, entrapment efficiency, and drug release behavior was studied. Furthermore, the cytotoxicity of the drug-loaded nanoparticles was investigated confirming their potential as carriers for daunorubicin delivery.

Keywords: casein; nanoparticles; daunorubicin; acute lymphocytic leukemia; targeted drug delivery; nano spray-drying; Reh cell line; cytotoxicity

1. Introduction

One of the leading causes of death worldwide is cancer and its related complications. By the end of the 20th century, the most common therapeutic approach to cancer treatment was surgery [1]. Nowadays, along with surgery, chemotherapy is considered the basis for the treatment of the most common cancers (breast, lung, liver, prostate, stomach, cervical, and thyroid cancers), including hematological malignancies [2]. Despite their high therapeutic efficacy, conventional chemotherapeutics are characterized by a lack of selectivity for accumulation in the tumor cells and by a number of serious side effects observed during treatment. These side effects are related to inadequate biodistribution of the chemotherapeutics, which leads to accumulation in healthy tissues. Therefore, one of the main challenges facing chemotherapy is the development of drug delivery systems that are effective and provide high selectivity, minimizing side effects and achieving maximum antitumor effect [1]. In recent decades, the advancement in the field of nanotechnology and oncology has led to the development of innovative chemotherapeutic drug delivery systems for targeted therapy. Such systems can specifically target tumor cells without affecting healthy tissues [3]. However, to be used as targeting drug carriers, these systems must meet certain criteria regarding their structure, particle size, biocompatibility, toxicity, and immunogenicity. Effective chemotherapeutic delivery requires the carrier to remain stable in the circulation, then pass across specific biological membranes and reach the target site. Moreover, it should be able to avoid clearance by the reticuloendothelial system and achieve a high degree of drug accumulation in the tumor tissue or specific binding to target cells, which can be accomplished either by active or passive targeting [4].

Advances in nanotechnology have led to the possibility of developing drug delivery systems based on polymer nanoparticles, which have the property to target specific tissues and therefore reduce dose-dependent side effects. Over the last decades, biopolymers have been the subject of serious scientific interest due to their specific characteristics and numerous advantages over synthetic polymers such as low immunogenicity, high biocompatibility, biodegradability, and low toxicity [5]. Biopolymers such as peptides and polysaccharides have been widely used to formulate nanoparticulate drug delivery systems that can provide controlled and targeted release, improving the biodistribution of the encapsulated drug and minimizing its side effects [6]. Compared to polysaccharides, proteins are preferred as structure-forming biopolymers for targeted delivery because of their ability to produce small-sized particulate systems with enhanced cell penetration [5,7]. Proteins can bind to different active molecules, protect them and control their release at the desired site within the body. There are numerous reports for the use of proteins such as gelatin, collagen, whey proteins, and casein for the preparation of microparticles, nanoparticles, or hydrogel delivery systems for drugs, nutrients, bioactive peptides, and probiotic organisms. Due to their nutritional and functional properties, milk proteins are widely used in the food and pharmaceutical industry [8,9].

Among the proteins used for the formulation of nanoparticulate carriers, casein has been found to have optimal structural and physicochemical properties for the development of targeted drug delivery systems with pH-dependent behavior. Casein, one of the major milk proteins, is biodegradable, non-toxic, highly stable, and inexpensive. Surfactant and stabilizing properties, the ability to bind ions and small molecules, as well as emulsification, self-assembly, and pH-responsive gelation properties make casein a suitable biopolymer for the development of targeted drug delivery systems [8]. Casein from bovine milk consists of four amphiphilic peptides—αs1, αs2, β, and k, which have a molecular weight between 19 and 25 kDa and an isoelectric point (pI) between 4,6 and 4,8 [10]. Due to their amphiphilic properties, the tendency to bind calcium phosphate and the formation of electrostatic, hydrogen, and hydrophobic interactions, caseins can self-assemble and form casein micelles with an average diameter of 50 to 500 nm [11]. Micelles exhibit pH-dependent behavior because their structure tightens with the decreasing negative surface charge of casein molecules and expands with increasing surface charge, leading to electrostatic repulsion between molecules [12–14].

Given the high degree of biocompatibility and biodegradability, the low extent of immunogenicity and toxicity of casein, as well as its pH-dependent behavior and amphiphilic properties, it is obvious why this natural polymer is preferred for the preparation of chemotherapeutic nanoparticulate drug delivery systems.

Various methods have been reported for the preparation of chemotherapeutic-loaded casein nanoparticles, including the self-assembled micellization/lyophilization technique [15], emulsification–ionic gelation [16,17], emulsion-precipitation [18], self-assembled micellization/dialysis [19–21], self-micellization/spray-drying [16,22,23], polyelectrolyte complexation [24], non-covalent polymerization [25], and Maillard conjugation [26].

A commonly used method for the preparation of protein nanoparticles for drug delivery is spray-drying. However, the separation and collection of such particles is known to be extremely challenging due to the low collection efficiency for fine particles smaller than 2 μm. To improve the effectiveness of the spray-drying process and to generate mainly nanosized particles, Swiss Büchi Labortechnik AG developed a revolutionary spray-dryer (Nano Spray-dryer B-90) [27]. Thanks to the innovative piezoelectric vibrating spray mesh head, which allows for the formation of fine droplets, and the novel electrostatic particle collector, it is possible to generate particles in the size range from 300 nm to 5 μm. Spray-drying of protein nanoparticles has been reported in numerous scientific papers [28–31], but no data were found in the literature on the nano spray-drying of casein nanoparticles loaded with chemotherapeutic agents. In this study, the encapsulation of the chemotherapeutic agent daunorubicin hydrochloride (DRB) in casein nanoparticles was demonstrated using a nanospray-drying technique.

Anthracycline antibiotics are among the most effective chemotherapeutic agents and are still considered major components of first-line chemotherapy in the treatment of solid and hematological malignancies [32]. Daunorubicin, an anthracycline antibiotic that possesses antineoplastic activity, is commonly used to treat acute myeloid leukemia (AML) and acute lymphocytic leukemia (ALL) [33]. Its antimitotic and cytotoxic effects result from the generation of free radicals and the inhibition of cell reproduction by the formation of complexes with DNA. The interaction between the base pairs inhibits the activity of topoisomerase II by stabilizing the DNA topoisomerase II complex, preventing the ligation–religation reaction that topoisomerase II catalyzes [34]. Despite its high activity, clinical use of DRB is limited due to multiple drug resistance (MDR) and its serious side effects, including cardiotoxicity, myelosuppression, and the occurrence of oral ulcers [33]. MDR results from the overexpression of P-glycoprotein efflux pumps on the surface of cancer cell membranes. This protein makes cells resistant to drug therapy by reducing the amount of drug entering cancer cells. Technological strategies for tumor-targeted delivery and thus reduced side effects can be accomplished in two ways: by the development of nanosized carriers that improve biodistribution within tumor tissues or by conjugation of anthracyclines to a carrier that specifically binds to ligands overexpressed on the cell membrane of the tumor cells [32].

The aim of this study was to develop nanosized casein-based carriers of daunorubicin, as a potential delivery tool for acute lymphocytic leukemia.

2. Materials and Methods

Daunorubicin hydrochloride (Mw 563.98 g/mol), sodium caseinate (from bovine milk), $CaCl_2{\cdot}2H_2O$ (Mw 147.01 g/mol), phosphoric acid 85%, sodium dodecyl sulfate, penicillin, streptomycin, fetal bovine serum (FBS), MTT (3-(4,5-dimethylthiazol-2-yl)-2,5-diphenyltetrazolium bromide), poly-D-lysine, and dimethyl sulfoxide (DMSO) were purchased from Sigma-Aldrich (St. Louis, MO, USA). The acetonitrile (HPLC grade) was supplied from Fisher Chemical, Lough-borough, UK. The Reh cell line (ATCC CRL-8286) was kindly provided by Dr. Tino Schenk (University of Jena). The RPMI-1640 culture medium was purchased from PAN Biotech, Aidenbach, Germany. Seahorse XFp Base medium (pH 7.4) was supplied by Agilent (Santa Clara, CA, USA). All other reagents were of analytical grade.

2.1. Preparation of DRB-Loaded Casein Nanoparticles

The coacervation technique followed by spray-drying using a Büchi B-90 nano spray-dryer (Büchi Labortechnik AG, Flawil, Switzerland) was employed for the preparation of drug-loaded casein nanoparticles. Casein solutions were prepared at varied concentrations by dissolving sodium caseinate in deionized water (pH 5.8). After the complete dissolution of sodium caseinate, 5 mg daunorubicin hydrochloride was added. The mixture was stirred on a magnetic stirrer for 60 min in order to achieve maximum incorporation of the drug. Then, the crosslinking agent calcium chloride dihydrate (2 μL/mL) was added dropwise under high-speed homogenization at 25,000 rpm (Miccra MiniBatch D-9, MICCRA GmbH, Heitersheim, Germany) for 15 min, which resulted in the formation of casein micelles. Finally, the obtained nanosuspension of casein micelles was spray dried using a Büchi B-90 nano spray-dryer under the following conditions: a mesh size of 4.0 μm, an inlet temperature of 40 °C, a solution feed rate of 60%, a spray intensity of 60%, a drying gas speed of 120 L/min, and a pressure of 30 nbar. Four batches of drug-loaded formulations were developed at varied drug–polymer ratios. The composition of the batches is presented in Table 1.

Table 1. Composition of DRB-loaded casein nanoparticles of different batches.

Sample Code	Sodium Caseinate (%)	Daunorubicin HCL (mg)	Polymer:Drug Ratio
Cas4-DRB-5	2.0	5.0	100:1
Cas3-DRB-5	1.5	5.0	75:1
Cas2-DRB-5	1.0	5.0	50:1
Cas1-DRB-5	0.5	5.0	25:1

2.2. Characterization of the Obtained DRB-Loaded Nanoparticles

2.2.1. Production Yields, Drug Loading, and Entrapment Efficiency

The production yields of the obtained nanoparticles from different batches were calculated according to Equation (1):

$$\text{Production yield (\%)} = \frac{\text{Spray dried nanoparticles (mg)}}{\text{Drug (mg)} + \text{Polymer (mg)}} \times 100 \quad (1)$$

Drug loading (DL) and entrapment efficiency (EE) were determined by HPLC analysis. Ten milligrams of each batch of nanoparticles were dissolved in 5 mL mobile phase and sonicated for 5 min into an ultrasonic bath (Sonorex Bandelin electronic, Berlin, Germany) until dissolution of the particles and extraction of DRB was achieved. The blend was then centrifuged at 5000 rpm for 15 min and filtered (0.22 µm, Chromafil®, Macherey-Nagel, Düren, Germany). The supernatant was recovered and the concentration of DRB was determined via HPLC (UltiMate 3000, Thermo Scientific, Waltham, MA, USA) under the following conditions: a 254 nm wavelength; a 5 µL injection volume; an Inertsil® ODS-3 HPLC column of 5 µm, 150 × 4.6 mm (GL Sciences, Tokyo, Japan); a 1 mL/min flow rate; a 25 °C oven temperature; a 20 °C sampler temperature; and mobile phase: 0.29% sodium dodecyl sulfate in 0.2% aqueous solution of phosphoric acid:acetonitril (1:1). The drug loading and entrapment efficiency were calculated using Equations (2) and (3), respectively.

$$\text{DL (\%)} = \frac{\text{Drug amount in the formulation}}{\text{Amount of nanoparticles}} \times 100 \quad (2)$$

$$\text{EE (\%)} = \frac{\text{Actual drug content}}{\text{Theoretical drug content}} \times 100 \quad (3)$$

2.2.2. Particle Size Analysis, Size Distribution, and Zeta Potential

The particle size of the DRB-loaded casein nanoparticles was analyzed by dynamic light scattering (Microtrac, York, PA, USA). The system measures the particle size in the range of 0.8 nm to 6.5 µm with non-invasive backscattering technology using a 3 mW helium/neon laser at a 780 nm wavelength. The system allows measurements of ζ-potential in the range from −200 mV to +200 mV. All analyses were performed in triplicates at 25 °C.

2.2.3. Scanning Electron Microscopy

Visualization of the obtained particles was performed using scanning electron microscopy (Prisma E SEM, Thermo Scientific, Waltham, MA, USA). The samples were loaded on a copper sample holder and sputter coated with carbon followed by gold using a vacuum evaporator (BH30). The images were recorded at 15 kV acceleration voltage at various magnifications using an ETD (Everhart–Thornley) detector.

2.2.4. Thermogravimetry Differential Thermal Analysis (TG/DTA)

For the thermal analysis, 3–6 mg samples were placed in Al_2O_3 crucibles and heated from 20 to 250 °C, in a static air atmosphere, with a heating rate of 10 °C min^{-1} using a SetSYS-2400 calorimeter system (Setaram Instrumentation, Caluire-et-Cuire, France).

2.2.5. X-ray Diffraction (XRD)

The degree of crystallinity of the synthesized nanoparticles was studied by X-ray powder diffractometry. The diffraction patterns of blank and DRB-loaded casein nanoparticles were recorded at a 2θ range from 5° to 90° using an Empyrean X-ray powder diffractometer (Malvern Panalytical, Malvern, UK), equipped with a TTK 600 low-temperature chamber (Anton Paar, Graz, Austria). All the measurements were performed at a voltage of 40 kV and 30 mA.

2.2.6. Fourier Transform Infrared Spectroscopy (FTIR)

FTIR spectroscopy was used to investigate possible drug/polymer interactions. The spectra were collected in the range from 600 cm^{-1} to 4000 cm^{-1} with a resolution 4 nm and 16 scans, using a Nicolet iS 10 FTIR spectrometer (Thermo Fisher Scientific, Pittsburg, PA, USA). The instrument is equipped with a diamond attenuated total reflection (ATR) accessory and the spectra were analyzed with the OMNIC® software package (Version 7.3, Thermo Electron Corporation, Madison, WI, USA).

2.3. In Vitro Drug Release

In vitro release of DRB from the casein nanoparticles was performed using the dialysis bag method. A dialysis membrane (Sigma, MWCO 12 kDa) was hydrated in distilled water for 24 h. An accurately weighed amount of nanoparticles (equivalent to 1.5 mg DRB) was dispersed in 5 mL from dissolution media and then transferred to the dialysis bag, which was closed using a plastic clamp. Each bag was placed into a beaker containing 20 mL of each fresh dissolution medium and kept under constant mild agitation on an electromagnetic stirrer at (37.0 ± 0.5) °C. Aliquots (2 mL) were taken and subsequently replaced at predetermined time intervals with fresh medium. Each sample was filtered through a 0.45 µm membrane filter (Chromafil®, Macherey-Nagel, Düren, Germany) and the pH was adjusted to pH 2 using phosphoric acid. The analysis for drug content was performed by HPLC as described in Section 2.2.1. The drug release study was performed in two different dissolution media (PBS pH 5 and PBS pH 7.4) for 30 h. The mean results of triplicate measurements and standard deviations were reported.

2.4. In Vitro Cytotoxicity

2.4.1. Cell Culture

Lymphoblastic cell line Reh (CRL-8286™, ATCC, Manassas, VA, USA), isolated from a patient with acute lymphocytic leukemia, was cultivated in RPMI-1640 media containing 10% FBS, 1% penicillin/streptomycin in cell culture incubator at (37.0 ± 0.5) °C, 5% CO_2, and high humidity. The plates were pre-coated with poly-D-lysine to ensure cell adhesion. The cells were seeded at a density of 2×10^5 cells per well into 96-well plates and in Seahorse XF plates depending on the required analysis. The cells were then treated with DRB-free and DRB-loaded casein nanoparticles and incubated for 3, 24, or 72 h, after which the assays were performed. Prior to the analyses, the cells were observed under an inverted microscope to ensure that a monolayer was formed.

2.4.2. MTT Assay

After different incubation periods, an MTT cytotoxicity test was performed. The MTT dye (3-(4,5-dimethyl-2-thiazolyl)-2,5-diphenyl-2H-tetrazolium bromide) was dissolved in PBS and added to each of the 96 wells to obtain a final concentration of 500 µg/mL After a 2 h incubation process at (37.0 ± 0.5) °C, 100 µL of the extracting agent DMSO was added. The results were measured spectrophotometrically at a 620 nm wavelength on an ELISA reader and presented as a percentage (%) of the vitality of treated cells compared to control cells. Each experiment was triplicated, and the results were calculated as mean values.

2.4.3. Analysis of Mitochondrial Function

To assess mitochondrial function, a Mito stress test on a Seahorse XFp analyzer (Agilent, Santa Clara, CA, USA) was performed. The entire culture media was replaced with Seahorse XFp Base medium (pH 7.4). Following the manufacturer's protocol, the mitochondrial inhibitors oligomycin, FCCP (trifluoromethoxy carbonyl cyanide phenylhydrazone), and rotenone/antimycin A were consecutively injected into the ports of the cartridge. Injection of the first chemical, known as an ATP synthase inhibitor, determines the production of ATP. FCCP makes the inner mitochondrial membrane permeable to protons and allows maximum electron flux through the electron transport chain (ETC). Thus, collapse of the inner membrane gradient is induced, driving mitochondria to respire at the maximum rate. The latter of the chemicals directly inhibits Complex I of the ETC and shuts mitochondrial respiration down (Figure 1). Such a combination of inhibitors allows for the assessment of several parameters: basal and maximal respiration, ATP levels, and spare respiratory capacity, as well as other mitochondrial characteristics such as proton leak, and non-mitochondrial respiration (Figure 2). For each experiment, the oxygen consumption rate (OCR) was measured, and the data were analyzed using Seahorse Wave Desktop Software v2.6.0 (Agilent, Santa Clara, CA, USA).

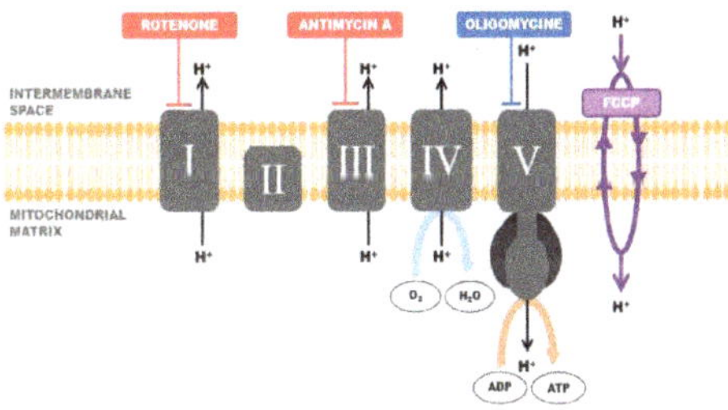

Figure 1. The effect of inhibitors on the mitochondrial respiratory chain in the Mito stress test. Created with Adobe Illustrator.

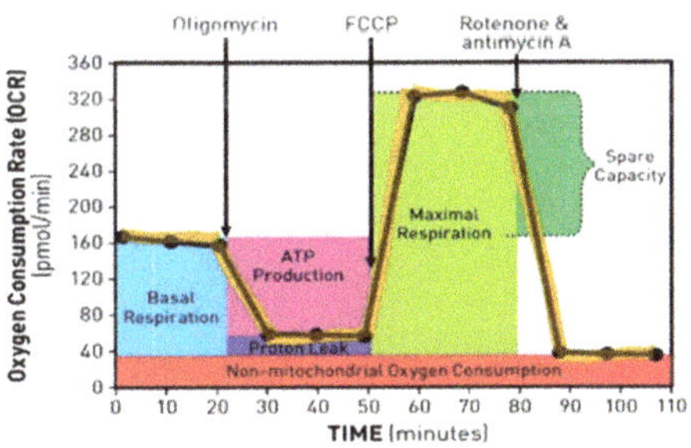

Figure 2. The main parameters of mitochondrial function are presented on the Mito stress test profile [35].

2.5. In Vitro Fluorescence Microscopy

To investigate the cellular penetration and intracellular distribution of DRB, fluorescence imaging was performed with a fluorescence microscope Axio Scope A1 (Carl Zeiss Microscopy GmbH, Jena, Germany). Prior to microscopic analysis, the cells were fixed as follows: after treatment for 3 h and 24 h, the Reh cells were washed twice with PBS, centrifuged, and the cell pellet was treated with 4% paraformaldehyde. After an additional centrifugation step, it was redispersed in PBS and the cells were placed on microscopic slides, covered with coverslips, and excited at 545 nm using a 50 W Hg lamp. The samples were observed at ×400 magnification using a filter of 570 nm.

2.6. Statistical Analysis

Pre-processing of raw OCR and ECAR data was carried out using Seahorse XF Mito Stress report generators [36]. GraphPad Prism v.6 (GraphPad Software, San Diego, CA, USA) was used for figure preparation and statistical analysis for Seahorse and MTT data. One-way ANOVA followed by a Bonferroni post-hoc test and a two-tailed t-test for multiple group comparisons were used. Probability levels of 0.05 were considered as statistically significant ($p < 0.05$). The statistical analysis represents the data as a mean value ± SEM (SEM—standard error of the mean).

3. Results and Discussion

3.1. Synthesis and Characterisation of DRB-Loaded Casein Nanoparticles

Casein nanoparticles loaded with DRB were synthesized using a simple coacervation technique followed by spray-drying. The influence of the polymer-to-drug ratio on the nanoparticles' properties such as their particle size, surface morphology, production yield, drug loading, entrapment efficiency, and drug release behavior was studied. For this purpose, four batches of drug-loaded nanoparticles were prepared and further characterized. The results are presented in Table 2. The nanoparticle production yields ranged widely from 37.67% for batch Cas4-DRB-5 to 81.12% in batch Cas1-DRB-5, steadily increasing when lower casein concentrations were used. Probably, it was the larger amount of polymer in Cas4-DRB-5 that led to increased viscosity of the feeding suspension, hindering free passage through the spray mesh of the spray-dryer. Another plausible explanation for this phenomenon could be the disruption of micellar integrity due to the displacement of calcium phosphate and the formation of precipitate prior to spray-drying [37].

Table 2. Characteristics of DRB-loaded casein nanoparticles (PDI = polydispersity index, ζ = zeta potential, DL = drug loading, and EE = entrapment efficiency); n = 3.

Sample Code	Particle Size ± SD (nm)	PDI ± SD	ζ ± SD (mV)	DL ± SD (%)	EE ± SD (%)	Yield ± SD (%)
Cas4-DRB-5	167 ± 38	29.10 ± 3.88	−33.21 ± 3.98	2.14 ± 0.07	42.80 ± 0.32	37.67 ± 1.32
Cas3-DRB-5	162 ± 37	25.06 ± 4.02	−25.53 ± 5.64	2.38 ± 0.06	47.60 ± 0.09	46.91 ± 1.27
Cas2-DRB-5	142 ± 13	27.4 ± 3.43	−21.52 ± 3.41	2.97 ± 0.07	59.04 ± 0.22	79.63 ± 1.45
Cas1-DRB-5	127 ± 42	7.65 ± 2.02	−18.63 ± 3.37	3.09 ± 0.11	61.80 ± 0.16	81.12 ± 1.58

The drug entrapment efficiency ranged from 42.80% to 61.80% and the drug loading was in the range from 2.14% to 3.09%. Considering the polymer-to-drug ratios during formulation, such low values for drug loading were not unexpected. The lowest values for drug loading and entrapment efficiency were established in batch Cas4-DRB-5, which was prepared at a 100:1 ratio. It could be assumed that due to the high concentration of casein (2%), the concentration of calcium chloride as a crosslinker was not sufficient for effective crosslinking, leading to the formation of unstable structures. Morphological analysis performed by scanning electron microscopy confirmed this hypothesis (Figure 3). No clearly defined structures were observed in the scanning electron micrographs. On the contrary, numerous agglomerates with irregular structures were found. A similar phenomenon was reported by Sinaga and co-workers and was thoroughly described [38]. Decreasing the polymer-to-drug ratio from 100:1 to 25:1 resulted in an almost two-fold increase in DL and EE (Table 2). Reduction of the casein concentration from 2% to 0.5% at a constant calcium chloride concentration allowed more efficient polymer crosslinking, leading to the formation of well-defined stable structures with DL of 3.09% and EE of 61.80% (batch Cas1-DRB-5; 25:1 ratio). The latter suggests that not only the polymer concentration and the polymer-to-drug ratio but also the polymer/crosslinker ratio determine the main characteristics of the formulated nanoparticles.

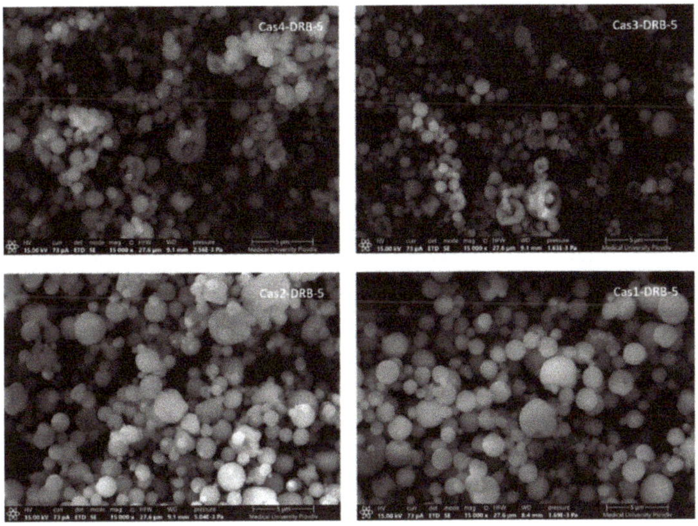

Figure 3. SEM micrographs of DRB-loaded casein nanoparticles of various batches at ×15,000 magnification.

The median size of the obtained particles ranged from 127 nm to 167 nm (Table 2) indicating a clear tendency for size reduction with the decrease in polymer concentration. The histogram of batch Cas4-DRB-5 (Figure 4) displays a bimodal particle size distribution suggesting the presence of aggregates, as hypothesized from DL and EE determination. The zeta potential of the four batches ranged from −18.63 mV to −33.21 mV, indicating the formation of a stable colloid suspension (Table 2). The negative charges on the surface of the particles resulted from the net electrostatic charge at pH values above the isoelectric point (4.6), where the casein carboxylic groups become negatively charged [39].

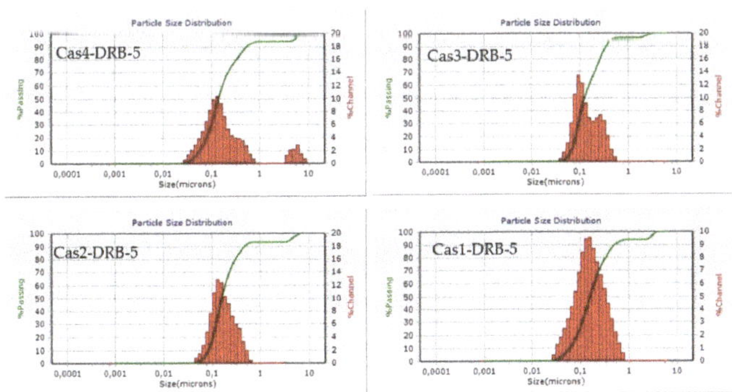

Figure 4. Dynamic light scattering histograms of DRB-loaded casein nanoparticles of different batches.

The surface morphology of the obtained particles was studied using scanning electron microscopy (Figure 3). Two types of morphologies were observed, namely solid dense and toroidal (doughnut-shaped) particles. Solid dense particles were formed at higher concentrations of the polymer—2% and 1.5% (batches Cas4-DRB-5 and Cas3-DRB-5, respectively). Generally, higher concentrations of polymer solution lead to the formation of denser droplets, due to the increased surface energy inside the droplets, which in turn results in the formation of more stable particles [36]. The results were supported by the DLS analysis where these two batches demonstrated zeta potential values −33.21 mV and −25.53 mV, respectively. In batches Cas2-DRB-5 and Cas1-DRB-5, probably due to the formation of smaller droplets, the airflow rate led to destabilization of the droplet shape and the formation of toroidal particles upon solvent evaporation. This type of morphology may also be attributed to the larger amount of water that must be evaporated in the spray-drying process. Evaporation of water from the surface of the generated droplets into the gas stream can cause thermophoretic displacement of the particles inside the droplet, leading to stronger deformation of the droplet and the formation of toroid-shaped particles [40].

The physical state of the drug before and after incorporation in the casein nanoparticles was investigated using TG/DTA. Casein thermogram displayed a broad endothermic peak at around 85 °C due to the evaporation of water from the sample (Figure 5). Daunorubicin, on the other hand, being crystalline in nature, is characterized by its melting point at around 180 °C. The DRB-free casein nanoparticles exhibited a sharp endothermic peak at 178.79 °C. After incorporation of the drug into the nanoparticles, the sharp peak corresponding to the melting point of DRB disappeared and the thermograms resembled those of the blank casein nanoparticles, which implies molecular dispersing of the drug into the protein matrix. Similar results were reported by Elzoghby et al. [16] and Puthli et al. [41].

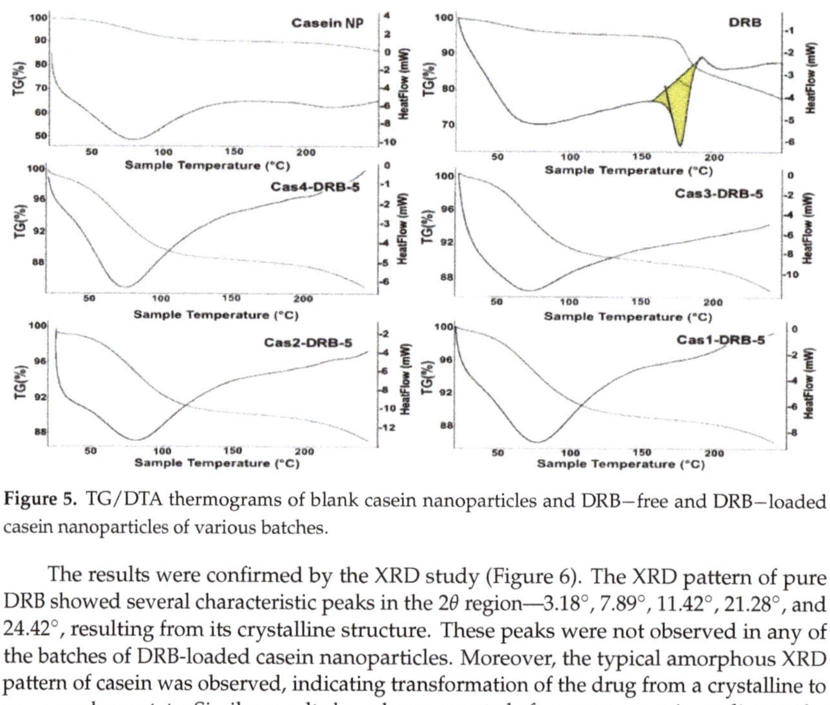

Figure 5. TG/DTA thermograms of blank casein nanoparticles and DRB−free and DRB−loaded casein nanoparticles of various batches.

The results were confirmed by the XRD study (Figure 6). The XRD pattern of pure DRB showed several characteristic peaks in the 2θ region—3.18°, 7.89°, 11.42°, 21.28°, and 24.42°, resulting from its crystalline structure. These peaks were not observed in any of the batches of DRB-loaded casein nanoparticles. Moreover, the typical amorphous XRD pattern of casein was observed, indicating transformation of the drug from a crystalline to an amorphous state. Similar results have been reported after spectroscopic studies on the interaction of the γ-cyclodextrin–daunorubicin inclusion complex [42].

In the FTIR spectra of blank casein nanoparticles (Figure 7), two distinct peaks were found at 1646 cm^{-1} in the amide I region and 1530 cm^{-1} in the amide II region, corresponding to the stretching of the carbonyl group (C=O) and to the symmetric stretching of N-C=O bonds, respectively. The peak at 1077 cm^{-1} could be due to interactions of monocationic phosphates with Na^+ while the band at 977 cm^{-1} corresponds to bionic phosphate, confirming interactions with Ca^{2+}. Two characteristic peaks of DRB were observed in the spectrum of drug-loaded casein nanoparticles. The first peak is shown at 1616.48 cm^{-1} due to C=O stretching of hydrogen-bonded quinone carbonyl groups, and the second peak is at 1581.44 cm^{-1} and attributed to C=C stretching [43], indicating successful drug incorporation into the polymer matrix. In all of the batches of drug-loaded nanoparticles, no shifts in the characteristic peaks of DRB and casein were observed, indicating the absence of interactions between the molecules.

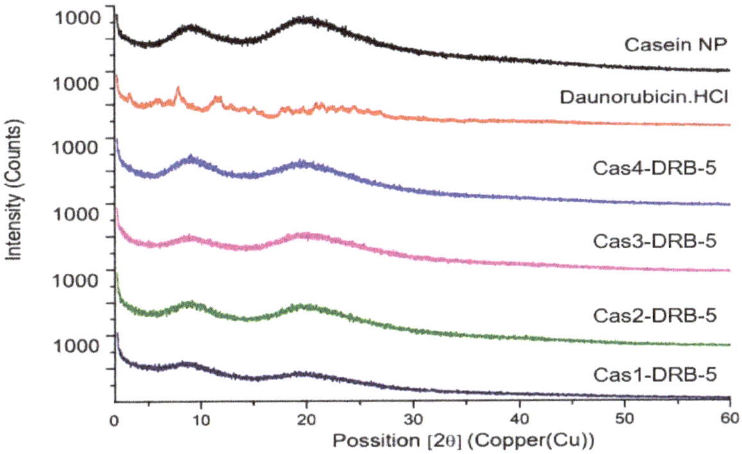

Figure 6. X-ray diffraction patterns of blank casein nanoparticles and DRB-free and DRB-loaded casein nanoparticles of different batches.

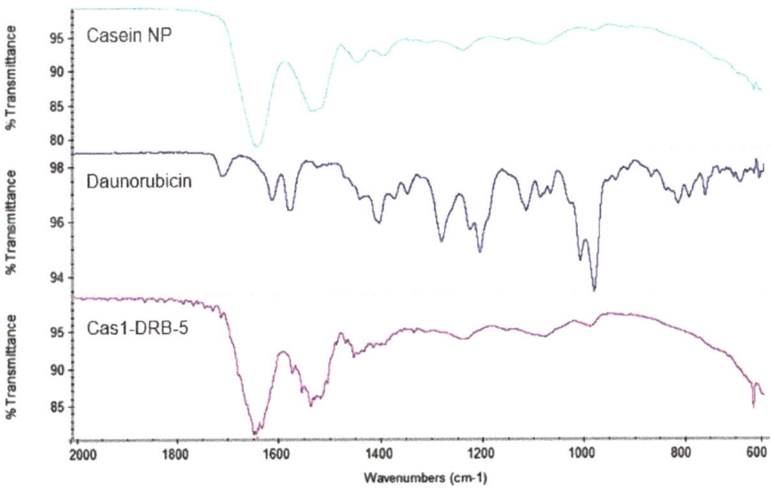

Figure 7. ATR-FTIR spectra of blank casein nanoparticles and DRB-free and DRB-loaded casein nanoparticles of batch Cas1-DRB-5.

3.2. In Vitro Drug Release

To simulate the physiological conditions, the drug release study was carried out in a neutral medium (PBS, pH 7.4). Additionally, the test was performed in a slightly acidic medium (PBS, pH 5) to mimic the environment of tumor cells and to investigate how pH might affect the release rate of DRB from the nanoparticles.

All four batches showed prolonged release profiles in both PBS buffers (Figure 8). At pH 7.4, incomplete drug release (43.73% ± 4.72%) was observed during the first 6 h from the batch Cas4-DRB-5, which was probably due to the higher polymer content and hindered drug diffusion. A similar release pattern was found for batch Cas3-DRB-5 (38.57% ± 7.45%). In batch Cas2-DRB-5, the trend was maintained (26.53% ± 3.19% within 6 h), but additional amounts of DRB were released between hours 9 and 24, which was not observed in the previous batches. The batch Cas1-DRB-5 showed higher release after 6 h (44.02% ± 3.05%) compared to the other three batches, which may be related to higher drug loading and the accumulation of DRB in the periphery of the nanoparticles in the process of spray-drying. Furthermore, DRB release was biphasic with a clearly distinguished burst release phase (20.17% ± 3.80% within the first hour) followed by sustained release of more than 70% after 24 h of testing (71.10% ± 2.22%). A statistically significant difference ($p < 0.01$) was observed in the released drug between 6h and 24 h for batches Cas2-DRB-5 and Cas1-DRB-5, whereas for the batches Cas3-DRB-5 and Cas4-DRB-5, the difference was insignificant, suggesting that the polymer-to-drug ratio played a key role in drug incorporation mode. Probably, at high casein-DRB ratios (100:1 and 75:1), the drug was incorporated deep into the core of the nanoparticles unable to undergo diffusion through the polymer and ensure complete drug release. On the other hand, when larger amounts of DRB were used (50:1 and 25:1), the drug molecules were probably distributed evenly in the internal core and the periphery of the nanoparticles allowing a more complete dissolution for the same test period. Moreover, the results could be associated with the smaller size of these particles and the shorter path for drug diffusion within the casein matrix. Cumulative drug release at pH 7.4 was analyzed for statistically significant differences between the four batches. No statistically significant difference was observed in the released DRB between the samples at either hour 1 or hour 3. A slight decrease was demonstrated for batch Cas2-DRB-5 at hour 6 (26.53% ± 3.19%) compared to the other three batches which released about 40% on average. The trend persisted at hour 9, after which drug release from batches Cas3-DRB-5 and Cas4-DRB-5 stopped, the cumulative DRB was about 55% on average, and Cas1-DRB-5 was the only sample that continued to release the drug and showed a statistically significant difference in DRB release at 24 h. Based on these results, batch Cas1-DRB-5 was considered optimal in terms of in vitro biopharmaceutical performance, whereas Cas2-DRB-5 did not meet the desired release pattern.

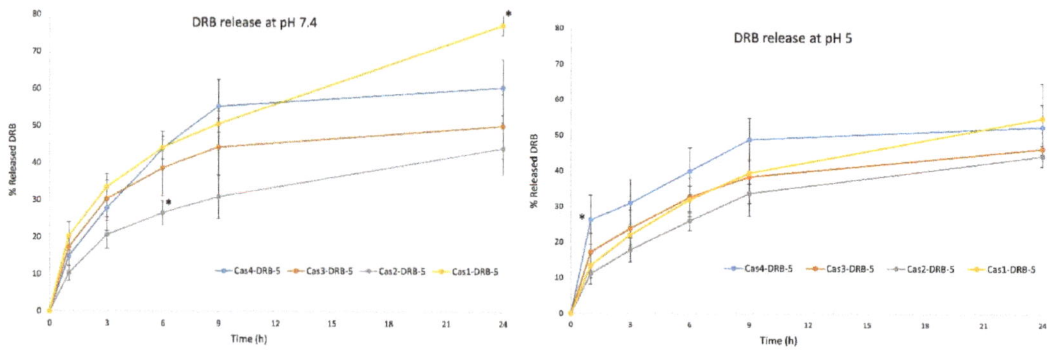

Figure 8. DRB release profiles from batches Cas4-DRB-5, Cas3-DRB-5, Cas2-DRB-5, and Cas1-DRB-5 at pH 7.4 and pH 5 (n = 6, *—statistically significant difference between models at the same time points, $p < 0.01$).

At pH 5, similar drug release patterns were obtained. DRB release was incomplete and delayed by about 3 h compared to DRB release at pH 7.4. For example, batch Cas4-DRB-5 released 43.73% ± 4.72% after 6 h at pH 7.4 whereas a similar amount (48.86% ± 6.00%) was released from the same batch at pH 5 after 9 h. The same trend was observed with batch Cas3-DRB-5 (38.57% ± 7.45% at pH 7.4/6 h vs. 38.45% ± 4.84% at pH 5/9 h). Batch Cas2-DRB-5 followed similar release patterns with only 33.79% ± 2.70% DRB released after 9 h of study. All three samples showed no significant change in DRB release after 9 h. The only model that continued to release DRB in the 9–24 h interval was Cas1-DRB-5. Moreover, the release profile was smooth and lacked an initial burst release. DRB release was incomplete, reaching 39.50% ± 12.10% after 9 h, but it was the only sample that demonstrated statistically significant drug release in the 9–24 h interval, with it reaching

54.90% ± 9.95% DRB release. Comparison of the cumulative drug release at pH 5 between the four batches at the same time points revealed a statistically significant difference only for sample Cas4-DRB-5. This batch demonstrated the highest drug release rate (almost 30% DRB was released within 1 h and the trend was maintained until the end of the study).

Statistical analysis of drug release patterns obtained at different pH values (7.4 and 5) showed no significant difference in the DRB release behavior for batches Cas4-DRB-5, Cas3-DRB-5, and Cas2-DRB-5 regardless of the sampling time for both of the dissolution media tested (7.4 or 5). The only standout batch was Cas1-DRB-5, which demonstrated differences in drug release behavior immediately after the first hour of the study. This result confirmed the potential of this batch for further research and application for drug delivery.

It can be assumed that the difference in the release profiles at the pH values studied is due to alterations in the structure and size of the particles. It is well known that casein particles have a pH-dependent swelling behavior [44,45]. At a pH close to the isoelectric point of casein (4.6), hydrophobic interactions lead to a reduction in repulsion between casein molecules, causing the formation of more compact structures with reduced size, leading to more controlled release of DRB [46,47]. Increasing the pH to 5 does not result in a swelling effect [48], but further alkalization leads to a gradual change in particle size due to loss of structural integrity. This effect was most evident for small particles (batch Cas1-DRB-5), suggesting a relationship between particle size and the swelling behavior of casein nanoparticles.

3.3. *In Vitro Cytotoxiciny*

3.3.1. MTT Test for Cell Viability

The results of the MTT test were used to assess cell viability and determine the half-maximal inhibitory concentration (IC50) value (Figure 9A). On the 3rd hour after treatment, all of the cells maintained their viability close to the control cells ($p < 0.05$). After 24 h, the cell viability decreased and allowed for the determination of IC50—5 μg/mL daunorubicin. At 72 h, the results of the MTT test demonstrated a dramatic decrease of cell viability to 25%.

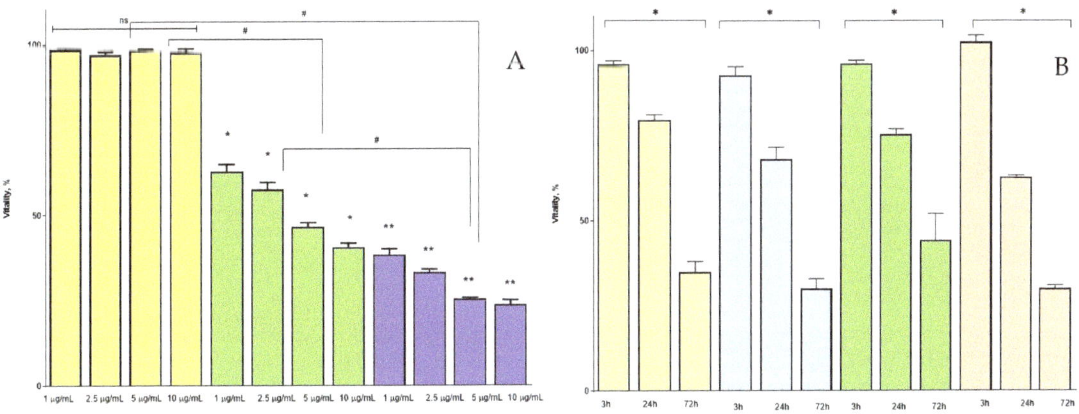

Figure 9. Cytotoxicity assay based on the viability of Reh cells treated with: (**A**)—increasing concentrations of DRB after 3 h (yellow bars), 24 h (green bars), and 72 h (blue bars) (n = 12, ns—no significant difference, $p > 0.05$; #—statistically significant difference between the groups, $p < 0.05$; *—statistically significant difference within the group treated for 24 h, $p < 0.05$); **—statistically significant difference within the group treated for 72 h, $p < 0.05$); (**B**)—casein nanoparticles of models Cas4-DRthe B-5 (yellow bars), Cas3-DRB-5 (blue bars), Cas2-DRB-5 (green bars), and Cas1-DRB-5 (orange bars) containing DRB equivalent of IC50 (5 μg/mL) 3 h, 24 h, and 72 h after treatment (n = 12, *—statistically significant difference within groups, $p < 0.05$).

To determine the effect of casein-based nanoparticles on the Reh cell line, DRB-loaded nanoparticles from batches Cas4-DRB-5, Cas3-DRB-5, Cas2-DRB-5, and Cas1-DRB-5 were used at concentrations corresponding to IC50 (Figure 9B). At 3 h, the viability was close to that of the control cells, but at 24 and 72 h it decreased to 30%. Blank casein nanoparticles that were used as a negative control had no statistically significant effect on cell viability. Since casein is known to have a cytoprotective effect [49], this may explain the higher viability of cells treated with casein nanoparticles compared to the DRB-free casein nanoparticles. According to the results obtained, the batch that had the most significant effect on cell vitality was Cas1-DRB-5.

3.3.2. Seahorse Assay

The mitochondrial metabolism of the Reh cell line was analyzed with a Seahorse XFp instrument (Agilent Technologies, Santa Clara, CA, USA) and the oxygen consumption rate (OCR) was measured. To investigate the potential mechanism of effect of the casein nanoparticles on mitochondrial activity, a Mito stress test was performed according to the manufacturer's protocol. The panel shows that the Reh cells exposed to nanoparticles of batch Cas1-DRB-5 demonstrated reduced levels of oxygen consumption, indicative of mitochondrial dysfunction. A decrease in maximal respiration, ATP production, and spare respiratory capacity was found. Statistical comparisons were performed based on control cells and a p-value < 0.05 was considered a statistically significant difference. Casein-treated cells were used as a control. The Reh cells were found to have a typical OCR mitochondrial profile, but it was reduced after nanoparticle treatment compared to the control cells as early as the 3rd hour. After one day, the results were dramatically lower (Figure 10A).

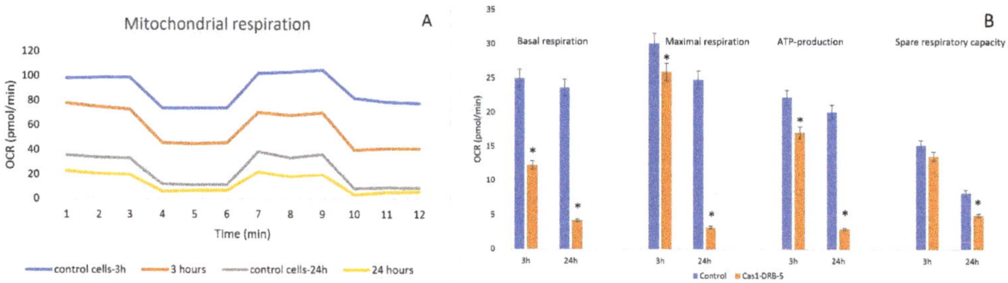

Figure 10. Effect of daunorubicin-loaded casein nanoparticles on cellular energetics, determined by Seahorse assay: (**A**)—representative diagram of the mitochondrial profile of the controls and the Cas1-DRB-5-treated Reh cells on the 3rd and on the 24th hour; (**B**)—bioenergetic parameters extracted from the OCR plot. Statistical analysis of the data represents the data as a mean value ± SEM; n = 3, *—$p \leq 0.05$.

Treatment with batch Cas1-DRB-5 resulted in a statistically significant decrease in basal respiration (from 25 to 12.3 pmol/min on the 3rd and from 23.6 to 4.2 pmol/min on the 24th hour), maximal respiration (from 30.1 to 25.9 pmol/min on the 3rd and from 24.8 to 3.2 pmol/min on the 24th hour), and ATP production (from 22.2 pmol/min to 17.1 pmol/min on the 3rd and from 20.1 to 3.2 pmol/min after 24 h). The decrease in spare respiratory capacity from 15.2 to 13.6 pmol/min was not significant after 3 h of treatment but after 24 h, decreased levels from 8.2 pmol/min to 5 pmol/min were found (Figure 10B).

In the Reh cells, DRB-loaded casein nanoparticles were found to alter the parameters of mitochondrial respiration and ATP production; furthermore, all of the observed effects were significantly pronounced. Daunorubicin is one of the most effective anticancer drugs that induces cytotoxicity by activating various mechanisms, including inhibition of DNA/RNA synthesis, heterochromatinization, oxidative stress, etc. [50]. Topoisomerase II, an enzyme that is present in both the nucleus and mitochondria of human cells, could also be inhibited. It can be assumed that the formulated casein-based nanoparticles induce an effect at the mitochondrial level. Casein, on the other hand, as a natural drug carrier, shows high efficiency for drug delivery because of its lack of toxicity and ability to improve drug bioavailability and efficacy [51]. Due to their energy-independent penetration through the plasma membrane, casein-based nanoparticles possess the ability to easily cross membranes and enhance permeability in ex vivo experiments [52]. Combining the cytotoxic potential of DRB with the advantages of casein as a carrier in the formulated DRB-loaded casein-based nanoparticles not only provides prolonged drug release but also increases permeability across the cell membranes and induces mitochondrial dysfunction, leading to a cytotoxic effect on the Reh cell line. Our results can be explained by the activation of different cytotoxic mechanisms such as increasing the generation of reactive oxygen species (ROS) and/or disrupting the integrity of the mitochondrial membrane. This leads to disruption of mitochondrial potential, inhibition of cell viability and proliferation, and ultimately cell death.

3.3.3. In Vitro Fluorescence Microscopy

In vitro fluorescence microscopy of Reh cells treated with daunorubicin-free and daunorubicin-loaded casein nanoparticles demonstrated different patterns of drug-associated fluorescence (Figure 11). During the first 3 h, strong fluorescence was observed throughout the cytoplasm and in the nucleus. Localized areas of more intense fluorescence in the cytoplasm were likely due to drug accumulation in cell organelles such as endosomes or mitochondria. The Reh cells treated with DRB-loaded casein nanoparticles demonstrated punctate, less intense fluorescence within the cytoplasm and the nucleus compared to the drug-free casein nanoparticles which correlates to the results obtained in the in vitro drug release study.

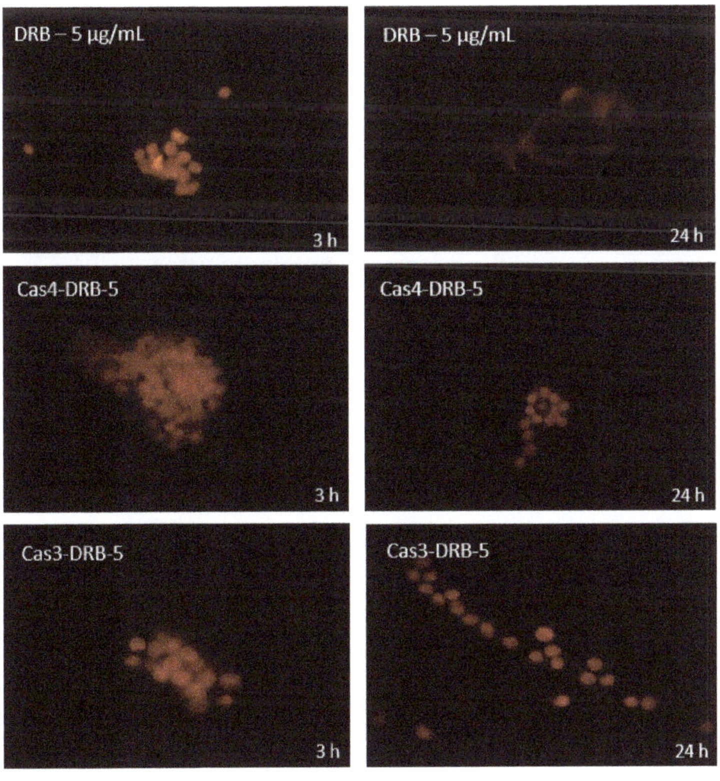

Figure 11. *Cont.*

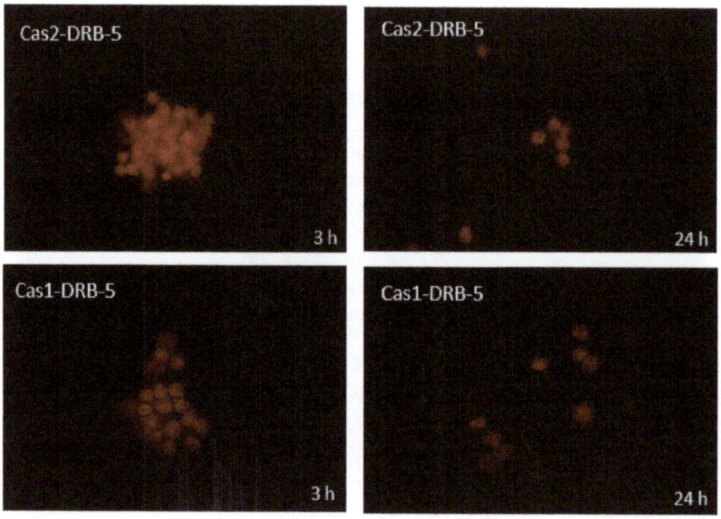

Figure 11. Fluorescence microscopy of Reh cells treated in vitro for 3 h and 24 h with daunorubicin-free (5 μg/mL) and daunorubicin-loaded casein nanoparticles of batches Cas4-DRB-5, Cas3-DRB-5, Cas2-DRB-5, and Cas1-DRB-5 (400× magnification).

Between the 3rd and 24th hour of treatment, increased fluorescence was observed and loss of the punctate appearance in the cytoplasm and the nucleus. The nucleus seemed to be more fluorescent than the cytoplasm, and the distribution of fluorescence throughout each cell resembled that of the DRB-free casein nanoparticles. Compared to the drug-free casein nanoparticles, the DRB-loaded nanoparticles demonstrated increased fluorescence in tumor cells after 24 h of treatment. Similar results were reported by Forssen et al. [53].

4. Conclusions

Within the goal of this study, daunorubicin-loaded casein nanoparticles were developed using the coacervation method followed by nano spray-drying. The particle sizes varied between 127 and 167 nm. The entrapment efficiency was highly dependent on the polymer-to-drug ratios and increased with decreasing casein concentration. The drug release was pH dependent, which confirmed our hypothesis that casein particles are suitable to be used as carriers for prolonged DRB delivery. The nanoparticles were found to alter the parameters of mitochondrial respiration and ATP production, and pronounced cytotoxicity was observed in the Reh lymphoblastic cell line.

Author Contributions: Conceptualization, B.P. and N.Z.; methodology, N.Z., M.D. and P.Z.; investigation, N.Z., M.D. and P.Z.; data curation, B.P. and P.Z.; writing—original draft preparation, N.Z. and M.D.; writing—review and editing, B.P.; visualization, N.Z., M.D. and P.Z.; supervision, B.P.; project administration, B.P.; funding acquisition, B.P. All authors have read and agreed to the published version of the manuscript.

Funding: The authors appreciate the financial support of the Medical University of Plovdiv via Project HO-15/2020 for providing the chemicals and consumables.

Institutional Review Board Statement: Not applicable.

Informed Consent Statement: Not applicable.

Data Availability Statement: The data presented in this study are available on request from the corresponding author.

Acknowledgments: The authors acknowledge Project BG05M2OP001-1.002-0005-C01 Centre of competence for Personalized Innovative Medicine PERIMED for providing access to the scientific infrastructure and sophisticated equipment for this work.

Conflicts of Interest: The authors declare no conflict of interest.

References

1. Elbialy, N.S.; Fathy, M.M.; Khalil, W.M. Doxorubicin loaded magnetic gold nanoparticles for in vivo targeted drug delivery. *Int. J. Pharm.* **2015**, *490*, 190–199. [CrossRef]
2. Caley, A.; Jones, R. Principles of cancer treatment by chemotherapy. *Surgery* **2012**, *30*, 186–190. [CrossRef]
3. Tewabe, A.; Abate, A.; Tamrie, M.; Seyfu, A.; Abdela Siraj, E. Targeted Drug Delivery—From Magic Bullet to Nano-medicine: Principles, Challenges, and Future Perspectives. *J. Multidiscip. Healthc.* **2021**, *14*, 1711–1724. [CrossRef] [PubMed]
4. Attia, M.F.; Anton, N.; Wallyn, J.; Omran, Z.; Vandamme, T.F. An overview of active and passive targeting strategies to improve the nanocarriers efficiency to tumour sites. *J. Pharm. Pharmacol.* **2019**, *71*, 1185–1198. [CrossRef]
5. Sundar, S.; Kundu, J.; Kundu, S.C. Biopolymeric nanoparticles. *STAM* **2010**, *11*, 13. [CrossRef] [PubMed]
6. Couvreur, P.; Gref, R.; Andrieux, K.; Malvy, C. Nanotechnology for drug delivery: Application to cancer and autoimmune diseases. *Prog. Solid State Chem.* **2016**, *34*, 231–235. [CrossRef]
7. Jacob, J.; Haponiuk, J.; Thomas, S.; Gopi, S. Biopolymer based nanomaterials in drug delivery systems: A review. *Mater. Today Chem.* **2018**, *9*, 43–55. [CrossRef]
8. Hong, S.; Choi, D.W.; Kim, H.N.; Park, C.G.; Lee, W.; Park, H.H. Protein-Based Nanoparticles as Drug Delivery Systems. *Pharmaceutics* **2020**, *12*, 604. [CrossRef]
9. Liu, Q.; Sun, Y.; Cheng, J.; Guo, M. Development of whey protein nanoparticles as carriers to deliver soy isoflavones. *Lebensm. Wiss. Technol.* **2022**, *155*, 112953. [CrossRef]
10. Elzoghby, A.O.; Elgohary, M.M.; Kamel, N.M. Implications of protein- and Peptide-based nanoparticles as potential vehicles for anticancer drugs. *Adv. Protein. Chem. Struct. Biol.* **2015**, *98*, 169–221.
11. Elzoghby, A.O.; El-Fotoh, W.S.; Elgindy, N.A. Casein-based formulations as promising controlled release drug delivery systems. *J. Control. Release* **2011**, *153*, 206–216. [CrossRef] [PubMed]
12. Liu, Y.; Guo, R. pH-dependent structures and properties of casein micelles. *Biophys. Chem.* **2008**, *136*, 67–73. [CrossRef] [PubMed]
13. Liu, Z.; Juliano, P.; Williams, R.P.; Niere, J.; Augustin, M.A. Ultrasound effects on the assembly of casein micelles in reconstituted-skim milk. *J. Dairy Res.* **2014**, *81*, 146–155. [CrossRef]
14. Liu, C.; Yao, W.; Zhang, L.; Qian, H.; Wu, W.; Jiang, X. Cell-penetrating hollow spheres based on milk protein. *Chem. Commun.* **2010**, *46*, 7566–7568. [CrossRef] [PubMed]
15. Bachar, M.; Mandelbaum, A.; Portnaya, I.; Perlstein, H.; Even-Chen, S.; Barenholz, Y.; Danino, D. Development and characterization of a novel drug nanocarrier for oral delivery, based on self-assembled β-casein micelles. *J. Control. Release* **2012**, *160*, 164–171. [CrossRef]
16. Elzoghby, A.O.; Helmy, M.W.; Samy, W.M.; Elgindy, N.A. Novel ionically crosslinked casein nanoparticles for flutamide delivery: Formulation, characterization, and in vivo pharmacokinetics. *Int. J. Nanomed.* **2013**, *8*, 1721–1732. [CrossRef]
17. Elzoghby, A.O.; Saad, N.I.; Helmy, M.W.; Samy, W.M.; Elgindy, N.A. Ionically-crosslinked milk protein nanoparticles as flutamide carriers for effective anticancer activity in prostate cancer-bearing rats. *Eur. J. Pharm. Biopharm.* **2013**, *85 Pt A*, 444–451. [CrossRef]
18. Narayanan, S.; Pavithran, M.; Viswanath, A.; Narayanan, D.; Mohan, C.C.; Manzoor, K.; Menon, D. Sequentially releasing dual-drug-loaded PLGA-casein core/shell nanomedicine: Design, synthesis, biocompatibility and pharmacokinetics. *Acta Biomater.* **2014**, *10*, 2112–2124. [CrossRef]
19. Shapira, A.; Assaraf, Y.G.; Epstein, D.; Livney, Y.D. Beta-casein nanoparticles as an oral delivery system for chemotherapeutic drugs: Impact of drug structure and properties on co-assembly. *Pharm. Res.* **2010**, *27*, 2175–2186. [CrossRef]
20. Shapira, A.; Davidson, I.; Avni, N.; Assaraf, Y.; Livney, Y.D. β-Casein nanoparticle-based oral drug delivery system for potential treatment of gastric carcinoma: Stability, target-activated release and cytotoxicity. *Eur. J. Pharm. Biopharm.* **2012**, *80*, 298–305. [CrossRef]
21. Shapira, A.; Markman, G.; Assaraf, Y.G.; Livney, Y.D. β-casein–based nanovehicles for oral delivery of chemotherapeutic drugs: Drug-protein interactions and mitoxantrone loading capacity. *Nanomed. NBM* **2010**, *6*, 547–555. [CrossRef] [PubMed]
22. Elzoghby, A.; Helmy, M.; Samy, W.; Elgindy, N. Spray-dried casein-based micelles as a vehicle for solubilization and controlled delivery of flutamide: Formulation, characterization, and in vivo pharmacokinetics. *Eur. J. Pharm. Biopharm.* **2013**, *84*, 487–496. [CrossRef] [PubMed]
23. Pan, K.; Zhong, Q.; Baek, S.J. Enhanced dispersibility and bioactivity of curcumin by encapsulation in casein nanocapsules. *J. Agric. Food Chem.* **2013**, *61*, 6036–6043. [CrossRef]
24. Razmi, M.; Divsalar, A.; Saboury, A.A.; Izadi, Z.; Haertlé, T.; Mansuri-Torshizi, H. Beta-casein and its complexes with chitosan as nanovehicles for delivery of a platinum anticancer drug. *Colloids Surf. B* **2013**, *112*, 362–367. [CrossRef]
25. Zhen, X.; Wang, X.; Xie, C.; Wu, W.; Jiang, X. Cellular uptake, antitumor response and tumor penetration of cisplatin-loaded milk protein nanoparticles. *Biomaterials* **2013**, *34*, 1372–1382. [CrossRef] [PubMed]
26. Xue, J.; Tan, C.; Zhang, X.; Feng, B.; Xia, S. Fabrication of epigallocatechin-3-gallate nanocarrier based on glycosylated casein: Stability and interaction mechanism. *J. Agric. Food Chem.* **2014**, *62*, 4677–4684. [CrossRef]
27. Available online: www.buchi.com/en/products/instruments/nano-spray-dryer-b-90-hp (accessed on 29 July 2022).

28. Marante, T.; Viegas, C.; Duarte, I.; Macedo, A.S.; Fonte, P. An overview on spray-drying of protein-loaded polymeric nanoparticles for dry powder inhalation. *Pharmaceutics* **2020**, *12*, 1032. [CrossRef]
29. Moslehi, M.; Mortazavi, S.; Azadi, A.; Fateh, S.; Hamidi, M.; Foroutan, S.M. Preparation, optimization and characterization of chitosan-coated liposomes for solubility enhancement of furosemide: A model BCS IV Drug. *IJPR* **2020**, *19*, 366–382.
30. Gu, B.; Linehan, B.; Tseng, Y.C. Optimization of the Büchi B-90 spray drying process using central composite design for preparation of solid dispersions. *Int. J. Pharm.* **2015**, *491*, 208–217. [CrossRef]
31. Bürki, K.; Jeon, I.; Arpagaus, C.; Betz, G. New insights into respirable protein powder preparation using a nano spray dryer. *Int. J. Pharm.* **2011**, *408*, 248–256. [CrossRef]
32. Simeonova, M.; Ivanova, G.; Enchev, V.; Markova, N.; Kamburov, M.; Petkov, C.; Devery, A.; O'Connor, R.; Brougham, D. Physicochemical characterization and in vitro behavior of daunorubicin-loaded poly(butylcyanoacrylate) nanoparticles. *Acta Biomater.* **2009**, *5*, 2109–2121. [CrossRef]
33. Wang, J.; Chen, B.; Chen, J.; Cai, X.; Xia, G.; Liu, R.; Chen, P.; Zhang, Y.; Wang, X. Synthesis and antitumor efficacy of daunorubicin-loaded magnetic nanoparticles. *Int. J. Nanomed.* **2011**, *6*, 203–211.
34. Lotfi, K.; Zackrisson, A.L.; Peterson, C. Comparison of idarubicin and daunorubicin regarding intracellular uptake, induction of apoptosis, and resistance. *Cancer Lett.* **2002**, *178*, 141–149. [CrossRef]
35. Available online: www.agilent.com/cs/library/usermanuals/public/XFp_Cell_Mito_Stress_Test_Kit_User_Guide.pdf (accessed on 1 July 2022).
36. Available online: www.agilent.com/en/product/cell-analysis/real-time-cell-metabolic-analysis/xf-software/seahorse-xf-cell-mito-stress-test-report-generators-740899?fbclid=IwAR2K0AdgiaVBUtrcWsfD0MagKj4KGCIzKUG-Nr9VgEKOedjB8TZyZWVdX6g (accessed on 1 September 2022).
37. Rose, D.; Tessier, H. Effect of Various Salts on the Coagulation of Casein. *J. Dairy Sci.* **1959**, *42*, 989–997. [CrossRef]
38. Sinaga, H.; Bansal, N.; Bhandari, B. Effects of milk pH alteration on casein micelle size and gelation properties of milk. *Int. J. Food Prop.* **2017**, *20*, 179–197. [CrossRef]
39. Madan, J.R.; Ansari, I.N.; Dua, K.; Awasthi, R. Formulation and *In Vitro* Evaluation of Casein Nanoparticles as Carrier for Celecoxib. *Adv. Pharm. Bull.* **2020**, *10*, 408–417. [CrossRef] [PubMed]
40. Iskandar, F.; Gradon, L.; Okuyama, K. Control of the morphology of nanostructured particles prepared by the spray drying of a nanoparticle sol. *J. Colloid Interface Sci.* **2003**, *265*, 296–303. [CrossRef] [PubMed]
41. Puthli, S.; Vavia, P. Gamma irradiated micro system for long-term parenteral contraception: Alternative to synthetic polymers. *Eur. J. Pharm. Sci.* **2008**, *35*, 307–317. [CrossRef]
42. Xu, D.; Wang, X.; Ding, L. Spectroscopic studies on the interaction of γ-cyclodextrin–daunorubicin inclusion complex with herring sperm DNA. *Carbohydr. Polym.* **2011**, *83*, 1257–1262. [CrossRef]
43. Bloom, H.; Briggs, L.H.; Cleverley, B. Physical properties of anthraquinone and its derivatives. Part 1. Infrared spectra. *J. Chem. Soc.* **1959**, 178–185. [CrossRef]
44. Rehan, F.; Ahemad, N.; Islam, R.A.; Gupta, M.; Gan, S.H.; Chowdhury, E.H. Optimization and formulation of nanostructured and self-assembled caseinate micelles for enhanced cytotoxic effects of paclitaxel on breast cancer cells. *Pharmaceutics* **2020**, *12*, 984. [CrossRef]
45. Coskun, A.E.I.; Sağlam, D.; Venema, P.; van der Linden, E.; Scholten, E. Preparation, structure and stability of sodium caseinate and gelatin micro-particles. *Food Hydrocoll.* **2015**, *45*, 291–300. [CrossRef]
46. Ghorbani Gorji, S.; Ghorbani Gorji, E.; Mohammadifar, M.A. Effect of pH on turbidity, size, viscosity and the shape of sodium caseinate aggregates with light scattering and rheometry. *J. Food Sci. Technol.* **2015**, *52*, 1820–1824. [CrossRef] [PubMed]
47. Schulte, J.; Stöckermann, M.; Gebhardt, R. Influence of pH on the stability and structure of single casein microparticles. *Food Hydrocoll.* **2020**, *105*, 105741. [CrossRef]
48. Gu, T.; Yao, C.; Zhang, K.; Li, C.; Ding, L.; Huang, Y.; Wu, M.; Wang, Y. Toxic effects of zinc oxide nanoparticles combined with vitamin C and casein phosphopeptides on gastric epithelium cells and the intestinal absorption of mice. *RSC Adv.* **2018**, *8*, 26078–26088. [CrossRef] [PubMed]
49. Gandhi, S.; Roy, I. Doxorubicin-loaded casein nanoparticles for drug delivery: Preparation, characterization and in vitro evaluation. *Int. J. Biol. Macromol.* **2019**, *121*, 6–12. [CrossRef] [PubMed]
50. Firouzi Niaki, E.; Van Acker, T.; Imre, L.; Nánási, P., Jr.; Tarapcsák, S.; Bacsó, Z.; Vanhaecke, F.; Szabó, G. Interactions of Cisplatin and Daunorubicin at the Chromatin Level. *Sci. Rep.* **2020**, *10*, 1107. [CrossRef]
51. Semwal, R.; Joshi, S.K.; Semwal, R.B.; Semwal, D.K. Recent Developments and Potential for Clinical Use of Casein as a Drug Carrier. *Curr. Drug Deliv.* **2023**, *20*, 250–260. [CrossRef] [PubMed]
52. Głąb, T.K.; Boratyński, J. Potential of Casein as a Carrier for Biologically Active Agents. *Top. Curr. Chem.* **2017**, *375*, 71. [CrossRef]
53. Forssen, E.A.; Malé-Brune, R.; Adler-Moore, J.P.; Lee, M.J.; Schmidt, P.G.; Krasieva, T.B.; Shimizu, S.; Tromberg, B.J. Fluorescence imaging studies for the disposition of daunorubicin liposomes (DaunoXome) within tumor tissue. *Cancer Res.* **1996**, *56*, 2066–2075.

pharmaceutics

MDPI

Article

A Nanocomposite with Extracellular Vesicles from *Lactobacillus paracasei* as a Bioinspired Nanoantibiotic Targeting *Staphylococcus aureus*

Atanu Naskar †, Hyejin Cho † and Kwang-sun Kim *

Department of Chemistry and Chemistry Institute for Functional Materials, Pusan National University, Busan 46241, Korea
* Correspondence: kwangsun.kim@pusan.ac.kr; Tel.: +82-51-510-2241
† These authors contributed equally to this work.

Abstract: The utilization of biomimetic materials that merge functional nanoparticles (NPs) with a cell-derived nanosized membrane is a state-of-the-art approach to harnessing cellular properties for biomedical applications. However, the development of biocompatible and species-selective biomimetic agents against hazardous pathogens threatening human health is still in its early stages. Herein, we report the synthesis and functional analysis of a novel nanoplatform in which a PEGylated MoS_2-ZnO (MZ) nanocomposite was cloaked with a generally regarded as safe (GRAS)-grade *Lactobacillus paracasei*-derived extracellular vesicle (LPEV) for MZ-LPEV nanocomposite and evaluated its activity against *Staphylococcus aureus*. The MZ nanocomposite was characterized via X-ray diffraction, transmission electron microscopy, and X-ray photoelectron spectroscopy. The coating of MZ with LPEV was confirmed through nanoparticle tracking analysis and zeta potential measurements. MZ-LPEV exhibited 5- to 20-fold higher antibacterial activity than that of ZO NPs and MZ nanocomposite against *S. aureus*. Reactive oxygen species (ROS) production and bacterial membrane disruption were confirmed as antibacterial mechanisms of MZ-LPEV. Finally, MZ-LPEV exhibited enhanced biocompatibility and selectivity for *S. aureus*. All our results showed that LPEV could be utilized for developing synergistic nanoantibiotics against *S. aureus*.

Keywords: extracellular vesicles; *Staphylococcus aureus*; nanocomposite; nanoantibiotic; biocompatibility; biomimetic material; *Lactobacillus paracasei*

1. Introduction

Staphylococcus is a large genus of Gram-positive bacteria that can colonize human tissue asymptomatically but may also cause simple skin infections or even lead to life-threatening illnesses [1]. Within this genus, *Staphylococcus aureus* is the leading life-threatening environmental infection owing to its ability to both effective colonization on environmental surfaces, air, skin, and mucous membranes and rapid transmission ability to the community [2–5]. The longitudinal association between persistent methicillin-resistant *S. aureus* (MRSA) colonization, environmental contamination, and recurrent human infections result in epidemics within various hospital settings and the rapid development of antibiotic resistance [6]. The currently available therapeutics or remediations for fighting *S. aureus* infections are limited [7]. Therefore, novel environmental remediation strategies are urgently needed.

Nanomaterials have attracted considerable interest due to their potential application in various domains, including healthcare. Since they act via a distinct mechanism of action from that of currently used antibiotics [8], nanomaterials have been regarded as alternatives to antibiotics that do not give rise to resistant strains [9]. However, certain nanomaterials tend to exhibit toxicity, with prolonged exposure to nanomaterials potentially having an adverse effect on human health [10]. Therefore, further research on the development of nanomaterial-based antibiotics should be conducted to overcome the above-described limitations and avoid the production of detrimental environmental contaminants. For this purpose, researchers have extensively developed novel biomimetic nanoparticles (NPs) coated with various cell-derived membranes for non-hazardous and environmentally friendly applications within the biomedical, environmental, and food industries [11]. In this regard, NPs enveloped with cell membranes not only retain the adjustable physicochemical features of synthetic NPs, but also the bio-interfacial properties and beneficial activities of biological membranes. NP-coated membranes from red blood cells [12], leukocytes [13], platelet [14], cancer cells [15], and bacteria [11] have been investigated for the aforementioned applications.

Among the cellular membranes utilized for cloaking NP-associated platforms, bacteria-derived extracellular vesicles (EVs), including outer membrane vesicles (OMVs) from Gram-negative bacteria or nanovesicles (NVs) from Gram-positive bacteria, are comparatively novel options. OMVs were previously considered to be derived from Gram-negative bacteria only due to their outer membrane layer [16]. However, NVs from Gram-positive bacteria cells, including *S. aureus* [17], *Streptomyces lividans* [18], *Listeria monocytogenes* [19], *Bacillus subtilis* [20], *Lactobacillus plantarum* [21], *L. reuteri* DSM 17938 [22], *L. paracasei* [23], and other species, have also been isolated.

The importance of bacterial membrane-cloaked nanoplatforms has been highlighted in vaccine development as these membranes are enriched in bioactive proteins, toxins, virulence factors, and immunogenic materials, which can stimulate bacteria-host interactions [11]. In addition, EVs with identical membrane structures to that of parental bacteria are non-replicative [24]. Furthermore, the poor cell-penetrating ability of nanomaterials can be readily enhanced by OMVs, since bacterial cells recognize OMVs as their own constituents [11]. In principle, while EV-coated NPs harbor the great potential for the targeted killing of bacterial cells, only a few pathogen-derived EV-coated NPs have been reported to show desired properties for antibacterial agents, which include specificity, low toxicity, and stimuli responsiveness [25,26].

Even though pathogen-derived EVs are regarded as safe following detoxification, their potential effects on human health remain unclear [27,28]. EVs sourced from generally regarded as safe (GRAS)-grade bacteria may overcome these limitations. *Lactobacillus* species are one of the most widely used non-pathogenic GRAS-grade probiotic species [29]. For instance, these bacteria have been used for fermentation in the food production industry for decades due to their ability to grow aerobically and anaerobically, in addition to their lactic acid-fermenting metabolism. The beneficial effects of *Lactobacillus* have fostered their use in various applications, including environmental issues [30,31]. It should be noted that *Lactobacillus* species and their EVs harbor innate antibacterial activity against *S. aureus* [21,32,33]. Therefore, *Lactobacillus*-derived EVs coated with functionalized antibacterial NPs can be a promising platform for developing agents against *S. aureus*.

The potential use of metals (e.g., Ag and Au) and metal oxides (e.g., ZnO and CuO) for antibacterial applications has been extensively reported [34]. In particular, ZnO (ZO) NPs have been utilized for antibacterial activity due to their ability to generate reactive oxygen species (ROS) and disrupt the bacterial cell membrane [35]. However, their toxic nature within nano-range concentrations hinders clinical application in the absence of modifications [36]. In recent years, two-dimensional (2D) layered materials such as graphene [37,38] and black phosphorus [35,39] have emerged as promising antibacterial platforms owing to their distinctive physiochemical properties. Molybdenum disulfide (MoS_2), another 2D nanomaterial, has exhibited considerable antibacterial activity mediated via physical damage to cells [40]. In addition, coating the surface of NPs with polyethylene glycol (PEG) (PEGylation) and MoS_2 could improve antibacterial activity and biocompatibility [41]. However, only a few studies have investigated the antibacterial activity of functionally modified MoS_2 nanosheets to date [40,41].

Inspired by the above-described advantageous characteristics of EVs from *Lactobacillus*, as well as the antibacterial properties of ZnO and functionally modified MoS_2 nanosheets, we sought to fabricate a PEGylated MoS_2 nanosheet-ZO NP (MZ) nanocomposite cloaked with *Lactobacillus*-derived EVs and employ it for the selective eradication of *S. aureus* pathogens that threaten human and ecosystem. The MZ nanocomposite was synthesized and fully characterized through X-ray diffraction (XRD), transmission electron microscopy (TEM), and X-ray photoelectron spectroscopy (XPS) analysis. Further, MZ coated with *Lactobacillus*-derived EVs was synthesized, and its antibacterial activity was determined via the 96-well-based microbroth dilution method. Among *Lactobacillus*-derived EVs, only *L. paracasei*-derived EVs coated onto the MZ nanocomposite (MZ-LPEV) stimulated the activity and selectivity of MZ against *S. aureus*, with enhanced ROS generation and membrane disruption when compared to those achieved with other parental NPs and nanocomposites. Furthermore, the MZ-LPEV nanocomposite exhibited greater biocompatibility when compared to that of the ZO NPs and MZ nanocomposites. Taken together, our newly developed MZ-LPEV is the first example that LPEV could be utilized for the preparation of a biocompatible and synergistic nanoantibiotic in killing *S. aureus*.

2. Materials and Methods

2.1. Synthesis of ZO NPs

ZO NP synthesis was performed as described in a previous report [42] with a low-temperature precipitation process. Initially, an approximate amount of sodium hydroxide (NaOH, 95%, Junsei, Tokyo, Japan) was added dropwise onto the aqueous solution of $Zn(NO_3)_2{\cdot}6H_2O$, (98%, Sigma-Aldrich, St. Louis, MO, USA) with continuous stirring. Then, the solution mixture was stirred for 6 h at 80 °C until transferred to an ice bath to stop the reaction. Finally, after washing with DW and ethanol, the precipitate was centrifuged and dried overnight in an air oven at 60 °C.

2.2. Synthesis of MZ Nanocomposite

The synthesis of MZ nanocomposite was accomplished through 3 steps: (1) preparation of MoS_2 nanosheets via aqueous exfoliation of MoS_2 powder, (2) PEGylation of MoS_2 nanosheets, and (3) loading of ZO NPs onto the PEG-modified MoS_2 nanosheets to obtain the functionalized MZ nanocomposite.

1st step: A previously developed method was utilized to prepare the MoS_2 nanosheets via the ultrasonication-assisted aqueous exfoliation of MoS_2 powder (<2 mm, 99%; Sigma Aldrich) [43]. Initially, ~100 mg of MoS_2 was added to 20 mL of 1-methyl-2-pyrrolidinone (NMP, 99%; Sigma-Aldrich, Saint Louis, MO, USA) solvent. Next, ultrasonication (~6 h) was employed to achieve direct exfoliation of MoS_2 in an ice bath ultrasonicator (60 Hz; UltraSonic Cleaner 100H, Shinhan-Sonic, Incheon, Korea) to prevent overheating. Subsequently, centrifugation (2000 rpm for 10 min, 4 °C) was utilized to remove the unexfoliated MoS_2, and the supernatant was centrifuged again at 10,000 rpm for 10 min at 4 °C. Finally, the directly exfoliated MoS_2 nanosheets (3.5 $mg{\cdot}mL^{-1}$) were stored in DW for further use after discarding the sediment.

2nd step: To prepare PEGylated MoS_2 nanosheets, 2 mL of MoS_2 nanosheets (3.5 $mg{\cdot}mL^{-1}$) was mixed with 100 mg of PEG 8000 (Sigma-Aldrich, Saint Louis, MO, USA) in 30 mL DW under continuous stirring for ~4 h at 25 °C. Thereafter, the PEG-modified MoS_2 nanosheets were collected via centrifugation and directly used in the next step.

3rd step: The collected PEGylated MoS_2 nanosheets were redispersed in 30 mL DW. Then, 100 mg of synthesized ZO NPs was also dispersed in the same reaction mixture and continuously stirred overnight. Finally, the MZ nanocomposite was collected via centrifugation and dried inside a vacuum air oven at 60 °C for 4 h.

2.3. Material Properties

XRD was employed to assess the diffraction patterns of ZO NPs and the MZ nanocomposite. An X-ray diffractometer (D8 Advance with DAVINCI design X-ray diffraction unit, Bruker, Berlin, Germany) with a nickel-filtered Cu Kα radiation source (λ = 1.5406 Å) in the 2θ range of 5–80° was utilized for the same. In addition, microstructural analysis of the representative sample MZ was performed via TEM (Bruker Nano GmbH, Berlin, Germany) using carbon-coated 300-mesh Cu grids. The AXIS Supra XPS microprobe surface analysis system was utilized to assess the MZ nanocomposite. The binding energy range of 200–1200 eV was used for the scanning to determine the chemical state of elements. The C 1s peak position at 284.5 eV was used as the binding energy reference.

2.4. Bacterial Strains

Acinetobacter baumannii (ATCC 19606), *Escherichia coli* (ATCC 25922), *L. paracasei* subsp. *tolerans* (ATCC 25599), *Pseudomonas aeruginosa* (ATCC 27853), *S. aureus* (ATCC 25923), *S. epidermidis* (ATCC 12228), and *S. saprophyticus* (ATCC 15305) were purchased from American Type Culture Collection (ATCC, Manassas, VA, USA; www.atcc.org, accessed on 23 October 2022). *L. acidophilus* (KCTC 3164), *L. fructosus* (KCTC 3544), and *L. plantarum* (KCTC 3107) were purchased from Korean Collection for Type Cultures (KCTC, Jeong-eup, Korea; https://kctc.kribb.re.kr, accessed on 23 October 2022).

2.5. Preparation of Bacteria-Derived EVs

L. acidophilus (KCTC 3164), *L. fructosus* (KCTC 3544), *L. plantarum* (KCTC 3107), and *L. paracasei* subsp. *tolerans* (ATCC 25599) cells were cultured in BD Difco^{TM} *Lactobacilli* MRS broth (Thermo Fisher Scientific, Waltham, MA, USA) at 37 °C with shaking at 230 rpm to an optical density at 600 nm (OD_{600}) of 1.5. The bacterial cultures were pelleted at 4000× *g* for 30 min at 4 °C. The cell-free supernatants were collected and filtered using a 0.22 μm Syringe Filter (Biofact, Daejeon, Korea). EVs from the supernatants were isolated using the ExoBacteria^{TM} OMV Isolation Kit (System Biosciences, Palo Alto, CA, USA) according to the manufacturer's instructions, and the final product was resuspended in PBS buffer. EVs were stored at 4 °C until use.

2.6. Evaluation of Antibacterial Activity

The minimum inhibitory concentration (MIC) of samples was determined *in vitro* using a 96-well plate format microbroth dilution method as previously described [35,44]. Bacterial cells of various concentrations were grown in Mueller–Hinton Broth (MHB) at 37 °C for 16 h with shaking for each MIC measurement. To evaluate the antibacterial activity of GRAS-grade bacteria-derived EVs against *S. aureus*, a standard zone of inhibition (ZOI) assay was performed as described in a previous report [45]. Here, 20 μL (10 mg·mL^{-1}) EVs and Mueller–Hinton Broth (MHB) agar plates inoculated with bacterial cell suspensions (0.5 McFarland turbidity) were used. The bactericidal activity of materials was characterized by spotting aliquots of sample-treated bacterial cultures on Luria Bertani (LB)-agar plates [39]. Checkerboard assays were employed to verify the synergistic action of materials by determining the fractional inhibitory concentration index/indices (FICI) [35,44]. A representative from triplicate experiments is shown.

2.7. Preparation of MZ-Lactobacillus-Derived EVs

The same volumes (100 μL) of MZ nanocomposite and EVs at a concentration of 2 mg·mL^{-1} were mixed in a microcentrifuge tube to adjust the MZ nanocomposite concentration at 1 mg·mL^{-1}. In order to obtain MZ-*Lactobacillus*-derived EVs, the dispersion was sonicated in a water-bath ultrasonicator for 3 min before further use for evaluating antibacterial activity. Coating was performed as described in previous work [25]. MZ-*Lactobacillus*-derived EVs were named MZ-LPEV: *L. paracasei*-derived extracellular vesicle-cloaked MZ; MZ-LMEV: *L. plantarum*-derived extracellular vesicle-cloaked MZ; MZ-LFEV: *L. fructosus*-derived extracellular vesicle-cloaked MZ; MZ-LAEV: *L. acidophilus*-derived extracellular vesicle-cloaked MZ.

2.8. Characterization of LPEV and MZ-LPEV

The size (diameter) of MZ, LPEV, and MZ-LPEV was determined via nanoparticle tracking analysis (NTA) using NanoSight NS300 (Malvern Panalytical, Malvern, UK) with a 532 nm light source according to manufacturer's instructions [46]. The physical properties of samples as zeta potential (millivolts, mV) were analyzed using a Nanopartica SZ-100 (Horiba Ltd., Kyoto, Japan) according to the manufacturer's instructions. The electrophoretic mobility μ at 25 °C in 1 mM NaCl was determined using Smoluchowski's equation $\zeta = \mu\eta/\varepsilon$, where η is the medium viscosity and ε the medium dielectric constant. Zeta potential values shown for individual samples are the means of at least three measurements with standard deviation ($p < 0.05$).

2.9. Morphological Characterization of Bacteria

The morphological changes of *S. aureus* bacterial cells [35] were examined after treatment with MZ, LPEV, and MZ-LPEV samples. For this purpose, all nanomaterials at a fixed concentration (sublethal MIC) were added to the bacterial cell suspensions, as described in Section 2.6. Thereafter, the bacterial cells were incubated at 37 °C for 16 h. The resulting cultures were collected via centrifugation at 12,000 rpm for 1 min, followed by resuspension in 500 µL of phosphate-buffered saline (PBS), pH 7, containing 2% formaldehyde and 1% glutaraldehyde. Cell morphology was fixed by incubating samples for 5 min at room temperature. The cell pellets were obtained via centrifugation, washed twice with DW, and resuspended in 1 mL of DW. A 5 µL aliquot was collected from the suspension, deposited on a silicon wafer (5 × 5 mm, Namkang Hi-Tech Co., Ltd., Seongnam, Korea), and allowed to dry at room temperature. VEGA3, a versatile tungsten thermionic emission scanning electron microscopy (SEM) system (TESCAN, Fuveau, France), was used to analyze the dried wafer according to the manufacturer's protocol.

2.10. Measurement of ROS Production

ROS production capacity of the MZ-LPEV nanocomposite against *S. aureus* was evaluated based on the previous report [39]. Initially, bacterial cells of 0.5 McFarland turbidity in PBS were treated with MZ, LPEV, and MZ-LPEV samples at 2.5 $\mu g \cdot mL^{-1}$ in the presence of 2′,7′-dichlorodihydrofluorescin diacetate (DCFH-DA) (Sigma-Aldrich, Burlington, MA, USA) at a final concentration of 30 µM in PBS. Next, the 96 well plate containing bacterial cell cultures was incubated at 37 °C for 2 h with vigorous shaking (500 rpm). The amount of ROS was determined based on fluorescence intensity with excitation and emission wavelengths of 485 and 520 nm, respectively, using FLUOstar Omega (BMG Labtech, Ortenberg, Germany). A bacterial cell suspension in PBS without treatment was used as a control. MARS Data Analysis software (ver. 3.02 R2, BMG Labtech, Ortenberg, Germany) was used to further analyze the samples. The measurements were taken in triplicate, and the relative ROS production of treated samples was compared to the control; the averaged values with standard deviation ($p < 0.05$) are shown.

2.11. In Vitro Cytotoxicity Assay

The cytotoxicity of ZO NP, MZ, and MZ-LPEV was evaluated via the colorimetric WST-1 Cell Proliferation assay using a WST assay kit (Ez-Cytox; Dogenbio, Seoul, Korea), according to the vendor's protocol [35]. Human embryonic kidney (HEK 293) cells were used, purchased from the ATCC (Manassas, VA, USA; www.atcc.org, accessed on 23 October 2022) and maintained in RPMI1640 medium (Thermo Fisher Scientific, Waltham, MA, USA) with 10% of fetal bovine serum (Thermo Fisher Scientific, Waltham, MA, USA) at 37 °C and 5% CO_2. Cells were seeded into 96-well plates at a density of 5000 cells per well and incubated for 24 h at 37 °C. Thereafter, cells were further incubated for 48 h in the presence of MZ and MZ-LPEV samples at the concentration of 10 and 25 $\mu g \cdot mL^{-1}$ (4–10 times MIC of MZ-LPEV) in 0.1% dimethyl sulfoxide. Subsequently, the cells were incubated with WST-1 reagent (one-tenth of the medium volume). A spectrophotometric microplate reader (BMG LABTECH GmbH, Ortenber, Germany) was then used to determine the amount of formazan dye formed by measuring the absorbance at 450 nm. The mean values of triplicate measurements with standard deviation ($p < 0.05$) are shown.

3. Results and Discussion

3.1. Material Properties

3.1.1. Phase Structure

Figure 1 shows the crystalline structure of synthesized ZnO (ZO) nanoparticles (NPs) and functionalized MZ nanocomposites, as determined via XRD characterization. The XRD pattern of the ZO sample shows diffraction peaks, which correspond well with hexagonal ZnO [JCPDS 36-1451] [38]. The ZO NPs maintained fine crystalline structures in the MZ nanocomposite. Moreover, some additional diffraction peaks were also visible in the MZ sample, corresponding to the (002), (100), (103), (006), (105), (110), (008) crystal planes of few-layer MoS_2 nanosheets (ICDD card No.37-1492) [47] and marked with '#' marker to distinguish itself from the peaks of ZO NPs. Taken together, the successful formation of the MZ nanocomposite was confirmed based on XRD characterization results.

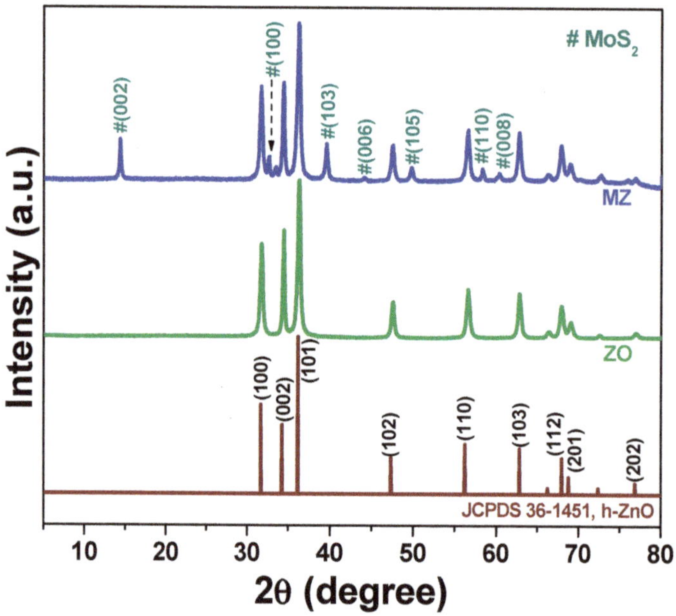

Figure 1. X-ray diffraction (XRD) patterns of ZO and MZ samples.

3.1.2. Morphology and Microstructure

The morphology of the synthesized MZ nanocomposite was characterized via TEM and is illustrated in Figure 2. Figure 2a–c depicts TEM images of the MZ nanocomposite, where the ZO NPs are clearly distributed on the MoS_2 nanosheets. The existence of distinct lattice fringes with an interplanar distance of 0.28 nm in the high-resolution TEM (HRTEM; Figure 2d) image of the representative MZ nanocomposite can correspond to the (100) plane of ZnO [42], confirming the presence of ZO NPs in the nanocomposite. Elemental mapping images of the MZ nanocomposite are also depicted in the figure and showed a good distribution of Zn (Figure 2e), O (Figure 2f), Mo (Figure 2g), and S (Figure 2h). Hence, the successful formation of the MZ nanocomposite was confirmed based on TEM and HRTEM results, which corroborated those obtained via XRD.

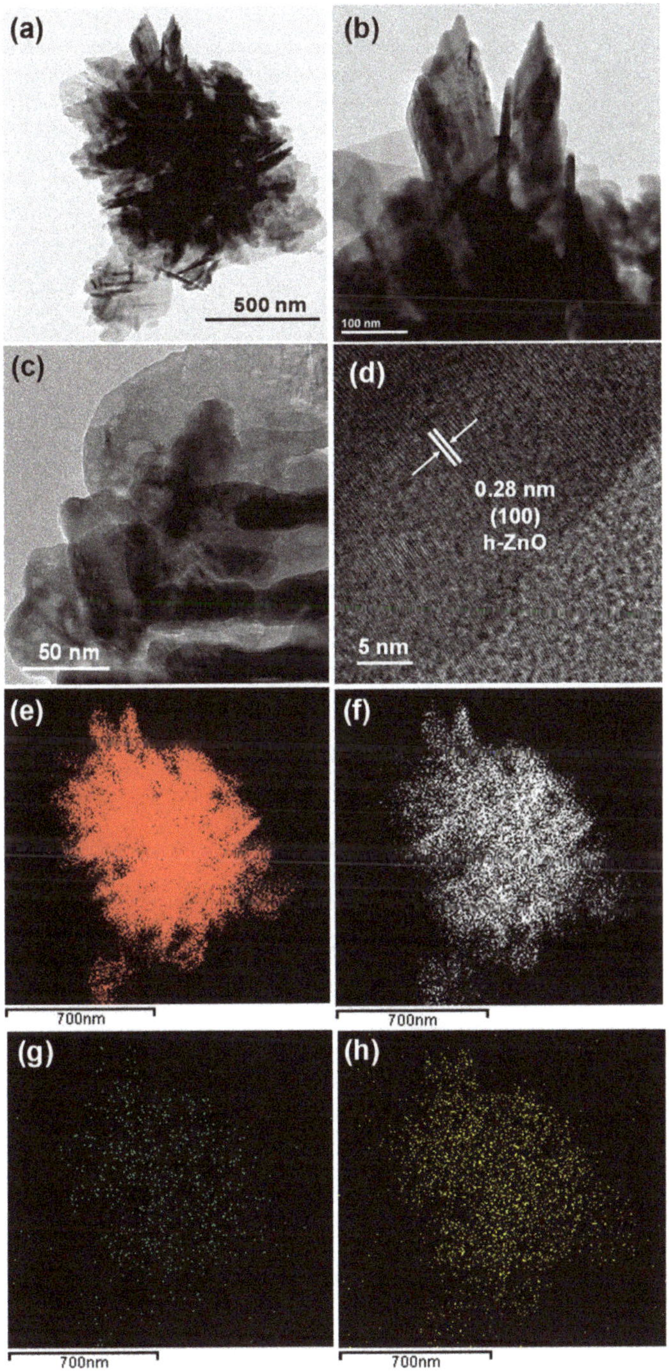

Figure 2. Transmission electron microscopy (TEM) images (**a–c**), (**d**) corresponding high-resolution TEM image, and elemental mapping of (**e**) Zn, (**f**) O, (**g**) Mo, and (**h**) S for the MZ nanocomposite.

3.1.3. XPS Results

XPS was employed to confirm the chemical composition of the MZ nanocomposite as well as the valence states of elements present in the sample; results are shown in Figure 3. Figure 3a depicts the Zn 2p spectrum, where two strong peaks at binding energies of 1021.7 and 1044.8 eV are visible and can be assigned to Zn $2p_{3/2}$ and Zn $2p_{1/2}$, respectively [37]. In addition, the energy difference between the Zn $2p_{3/2}$ and Zn $2p_{1/2}$ binding energies is ~23.1 eV, proving the presence of a Zn^{2+} valence state [37] in the MZ nanocomposite. Results presented in Figure 3b, which shows the Gaussian fitting of the Mo 3d spectrum, reveal two characteristic peaks at 229.0 and 232.1 eV. These can be assigned to Mo $3d_{5/2}$ and Mo $3d_{3/2}$, respectively [48]. Besides, an additional peak at 226.5 eV was also observed, which corresponds to the S 2s. Likewise, two peaks at 161.8 and 162.9 eV in the S 2p spectrum can also be seen and assigned to S $2p_{3/2}$ and S $2p_{1/2}$, respectively [48]. Therefore, the XPS result confirmed the successful formation of the MZ nanocomposite and was in agreement with the XRD result (Figure 1) and TEM (Figure 2) data.

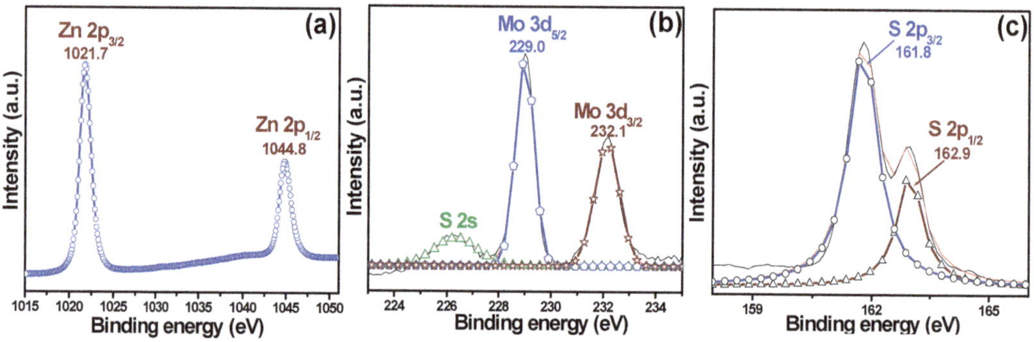

Figure 3. X-ray photoelectron spectroscopy (XPS) results for the MZ nanocomposite: (**a**) Zn 2p spectrum and Gaussian-fitted (**b**) Mo 3d and (**c**) S 2p spectra.

3.2. Characterization of MZ-LPEV

To characterize the particle size change of the MZ-LPEV sample after coating, we employed NTA, a method for visualizing and analyzing particles in liquids that relates the rate of Brownian motion to particle size using a microscope camera [46]. We subjected LPEV and MZ-LPEV to NTA while comparing them with each other. The mean values obtained by comparing sizes from D90 samples (90% of the total volume of material in the sample is contained) [46,49] of triplicate capturing were 160.4 and 465.2 nm for LPEV, and MZ-LPEV, respectively (Table 1). This indicated that the size of MZ-LPEV was much bigger than that of LPEV, confirming the coating of MZ with LPEV. These findings highlighted the importance of LPEV coating onto the MZ nanocomposite, which not only stabilized the nanocomposite but also potentiated its antibacterial activity (discussed in the latter section). In separate experiments, zeta potential measurements (Table 1) were performed to characterize the physical difference between MZ and MZ-LPEV. The zeta potential values of MZ, LPEV, and MZ-LPEV were −43.7, −19.9, and −21.5 mV, respectively. This indicated a similarity between LPEV with MZ-LPEV in terms of zeta potential, in addition to confirming the coating of MZ with LPEV. Overall, NTA and zeta potential analyses proved the formation of the LPEV-coated MZ nanocomposite (MZ-LPEV).

Table 1. Characterization of MZ, LPEV, and MZ-LPEV. Hydrodynamic size (Mean diameter, nm) from NTA analysis and zeta potential values were shown. Data are presented as mean ± standard deviation ($p < 0.05$).

Sample	Size (nm)	Zeta Potential (mV)
MZ	Not measured	−43.7 ± 0.4
LPEV	160.4 ± 13.1	−19.93 ± 0.35
MZ-LPEV	465.2 ± 12.4	−21.5 ± 2.8

3.3. *Evaluation of Anti-S. aureus Activity of MZ-Lactobacillus-Derived EVs*

Lactobacillus species exhibit anti-*S. aureus* activity [32,33]. In addition, EVs derived from *Lactobacillus* species could be used as natural anti-bacterial materials [21]. However, we could not find any clear ZOI for *Lactobacillus*-derived EVs against the *S. aureus* ATCC 25923 strain. This suggested that *Lactobacillus*-derived EVs could be used to achieve a synergistic effect with MZ against *S. aureus*.

To verify this notion, MZ-*Lactobacillus* EV nanocomposites (MZ-LPEV, MZ-LMEV, MZ-LFEV, and MZ-LAEV) were prepared, and their MIC values against *S. aureus* were determined (Table 2). Subsequently, the bactericidal activity of MZ, LPEV, and MZ-LPEV from corresponding MIC plates was assessed. MZ and MZ-LPEV exhibited MICs of 10 and 2.5 $\mu g \cdot mL^{-1}$, respectively; however, LPEV itself did not exhibit antibacterial efficacy against *S. aureus* up to 100 $\mu g \cdot mL^{-1}$ (Figure S1). Compared to the MIC of ZO NPs against *S. aureus* (50 $\mu g \cdot mL^{-1}$) (Table 2; Figure S2), the MIC of the MZ nanocomposite was 10 $\mu g \cdot mL^{-1}$ (Figures S1 and S2), indicating that functionalization of ZO NPs via PEGylated MoS_2 enhanced their bactericidal activity against *S. aureus* 5-fold. Next, the MICs of MZ-*Lactobacillus*-derived EV nanocomposites against *S. aureus* were determined. Only MZ cloaked with LPEV (MZ-LPEV) enhanced the anti-*S. aureus* activity of MZ 4-fold, thereby decreasing the MIC to 2.5 $\mu g \cdot mL^{-1}$ (Table 2; Figures S1 and S2). The MIC of MZ-LAEV and MZ-LMEV was 100 $\mu g \cdot mL^{-1}$, while that of MZ-LFEV was 50 $\mu g \cdot mL^{-1}$, antagonizing the MZ activity ~5–10 fold (Table 2; Figure S2). The result itself shows that the ZO NP, with MIC of 50 $\mu g \cdot mL^{-1}$, is an effective antibacterial agent against *S. aureus*. Additionally, the MoS_2 and LPEV together potentiated ZO NPs activity against *S. aureus* 20-fold, with LPEV promoting antibacterial specificity. The excellent antibacterial activity and high specificity of the LPEV-coated MZ nanocomposite were attributed to the enhanced uptake of the MZ-LPEV nanocomposite by *S. aureus* cells. However, it is also possible that the mixture of MZ with LPEV, rather than the MZ-LPEV single nanocomposite, could exhibit synergistic activity against *S. aureus*. To verify this notion, checkerboard assays with LPEV and MZ nanocomposite were performed, thus revealing no synergy between LPEV and MZ against *S. aureus* without any change in the MIC of MZ (10 $\mu g \cdot mL^{-1}$) (Figure S3). Overall, our results show that the LPEV coating of MZ as a combined nanocomposite conferred potent and selective synergistic activity to the inherent antibacterial properties of ZO and MoS_2.

Table 2. MIC values of ZO NP, MZ, and *Lactobacillus* strain EV-coated MZ against *S. aureus* (ATCC 25923) [1].

Sample	MIC ($\mu g \cdot mL^{-1}$)
ZO NP	50
MZ	10
MZ-LPEV	2.5
MZ-LMEV	100
MZ-LFEV	50
MZ-LAEV	100

[1] Data shown here are representative of the triplicate experiments. Abbreviations: MIC, Minimum inhibitory concentration; ZO, Zinc Oxide; NP, Nanoparticle; MZ, PEGylated MoS_2-ZO NP; LPEV, *Lactobacillus paracasei*-derived extracellular vesicle; MZ-LPEV, LPEV-cloaked MZ; LMEV, *Lactobacillus plantarum*-derived extracellular vesicle; MZ-LMEV, LMEV-cloaked MZ; LFEV, *Lactobacillus fructosus*-derived extracellular vesicle; MZ-LFEV, LFEV-cloaked MZ; LAEV, *Lactobacillus acidophilus*-derived extracellular vesicle; MZ-LAEV, LAEV-cloaked MZ.

3.4. Species Selectivity of MZ-LPEV

The selective antibacterial activity of MZ, LPEV, and MZ-LPEV nanocomposites was evaluated by determining MICs against different standard Gram-positive strains dwelling with *S. aureus* (*S. epidermidis* and *S. saprophyticus*; Figure S4) as well as Gram-negative bacterial strains (*A. baumannii, E. coli*, and *P. aeruginosa*; Figure S5). As shown in Figures S4 and S5, MZ-LPEV was not synergistically active against the bacterial strains except *S. aureus* (ATCC 25923). This indicated that MZ-LPEV is a potential and selective antibacterial agent against *S. aureus*. More interestingly, the MIC of MZ-LPEV against *S. aureus* was 4-fold higher compared to that of other MZ nanocomposites with EVs derived from other *Lactobacillus* strains (Table 2), indicating that LPEV potentiates both the activity and selectivity of the MZ nanocomposite against *S. aureus*. Taken together, MZ-LPEV could have the potential as a nanoplatform against *S. aureus*.

3.5. Plausible Antibacterial Mechanism

Disruption of the bacterial cell membrane and ROS generation are well-known and widely established antibacterial mechanisms of nanomaterials [35,39]. Therefore, the morphological changes (Figure 4) of bacterial cells (*S. aureus*) treated with MZ, LPEV, and MZ-LPEV were evaluated to confirm the antibacterial mechanism of action at play. The ROS production ability (Figure 5) of samples was also assessed to further verify the antibacterial mechanism of MZ-LPEV.

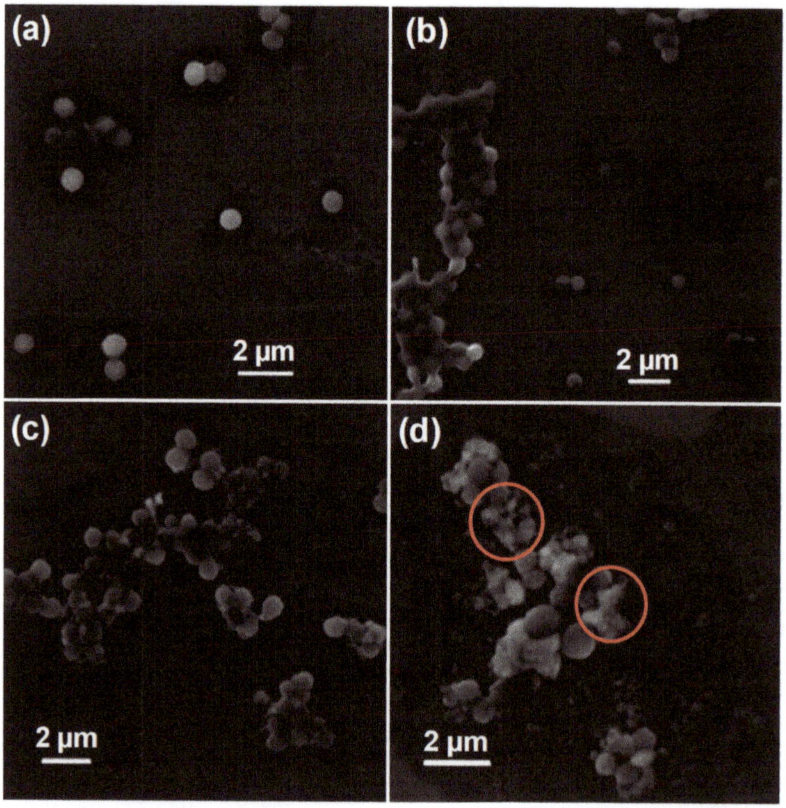

Figure 4. Scanning electron microscopy images of *S. aureus* after various treatments. (**a**) Untreated, (**b**) LPEV-treated, (**c**) MZ-treated, and (**d**) MZ-LPEV-treated. The red circles indicate morphological changes in bacterial cells.

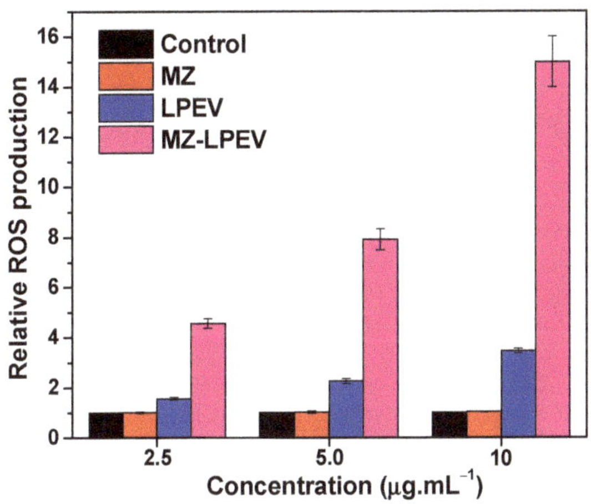

Figure 5. Relative ROS production. Fluorescence intensities at 520 nm were measured for *S. aureus* (ATCC 25923) cells treated with MZ, LPEV, and MZ-LPEV, respectively, and a relative ratio to the control sample is shown. Bacterial cell suspension in PBS without treatment was used as a control. MARS Data Analysis software (ver. 3.02 R2; BMG Labtech GmbH, Ortenber, Germany) was used for data processing and averaged values of relative ROS production from triplicate experiments are shown ($p < 0.05$).

3.5.1. Morphological Characterization of Bacteria

SEM was utilized to assess the morphological changes of *S. aureus* (Figure 4) under treatment with nanomaterials and LPEV. As expected, the untreated *S. aureus* (Figure 4a) bacterial cells displayed a smooth surface without disruption. When bacterial cells were treated with LPEV, the bacterial cell surface was smooth as in the control condition; a population of grouped cells was also detected (Figure 4b), suggesting that the LPEV itself does not exert antibacterial effects and might promote attachment between cells. However, bacterial cells under treatment with the MZ nanocomposite exhibited membrane disruption, as shown in Figure 4c. The phenotype was more pronounced under treatment with MZ-LPEV (Figure 4d). The observed cell membrane disruption can be attributed to ZO NPs [35], the MoS_2 nanosheet [40], and LPEV attaching to the bacterial cell surface. Hence, this result confirmed that the synergistic antibacterial activity of the MZ-LPEV nanocomposite against *S. aureus* is mediated via bacterial membrane disruption.

3.5.2. ROS Production

ROS production via nanomaterials damages various intracellular components of bacteria (DNA, proteins, or other functional cellular components), resulting in cell death [50]. To determine whether MZ-LPEV increases ROS production against *S. aureus*, ROS production of the MZ-LPEV nanocomposite was measured at a fluorescence intensity of 520 nm and then compared to that of the MZ nanocomposite and LPEV at multiple concentrations (Figure 5). As shown in Figure 5, ROS production via the MZ nanocomposite against *S. aureus* cells did not change at all tested concentrations. Thus, the MZ nanocomposite itself had no ROS production capacity. Meanwhile, ROS production by LPEV was 1.6 to 3.4 times higher than the control and showed a concentration-dependent increase. More interestingly, ROS production by the MZ-LPEV nanocomposite at 2.5 $\mu g \cdot mL^{-1}$ (MIC) was 4.5 times greater than that of the control sample and similar to that achieved by LPEV at 10 $\mu g \cdot mL^{-1}$. ROS production by MZ-LPEV was concentration-dependent and ~3 times greater at 10 $\mu g \cdot mL^{-1}$ when compared to the MIC. This higher ROS production from MZ-LPEV can be attributed to the formation of nanocomposite and the synergistic capability of nanocomposite in terms of antibacterial properties [51,52]. This indicated that

MZ nanocomposite coated with LPEV (MZ-LPEV) exhibited strong synergistic activity when compared to individual samples. The 4-fold increase of synergistic antibacterial activity observed for the MZ-LPEV nanocomposite (Table 1) relative to individual mixtures (Figure S3) could therefore be attributed to enhanced ROS production.

3.6. *In Vitro Cytotoxicity of Materials*

One of the key criteria for nanocomposite application is biocompatibility. To evaluate biocompatibility, WST-1 assays (Figure 6) were performed to determine the cytotoxic effects of MZ and MZ-LPEV nanocomposite at varying concentrations on HEK293 cells, for which the penetration ability and cellular interactions of ZO NPs have been well defined [53]. As shown in Figure 6, the cell viability under MZ treatment was ~25% greater when compared to that under ZO NPs at 10 $\mu g \cdot mL^{-1}$, which is 4-times the MIC (2.5 $\mu g \cdot mL^{-1}$) and thus indicative of greater biocompatibility. However, the feature was not retained at 25 $\mu g \cdot mL^{-1}$, and >90% of cells were non-viable. Meanwhile, cells treated with MZ-LPEV remained viable at 10 $\mu g \cdot mL^{-1}$ and even 25 $\mu g \cdot mL^{-1}$. Therefore, LPEV, as part of the MZ-LPEV nanocomposite, helps alleviate the toxicity of ZO NPs and the MZ nanocomposite. Taken together, our newly developed MZ-LPEV nanocomposite is a potent and biocompatible antibacterial nanoplatform against *S. aureus*.

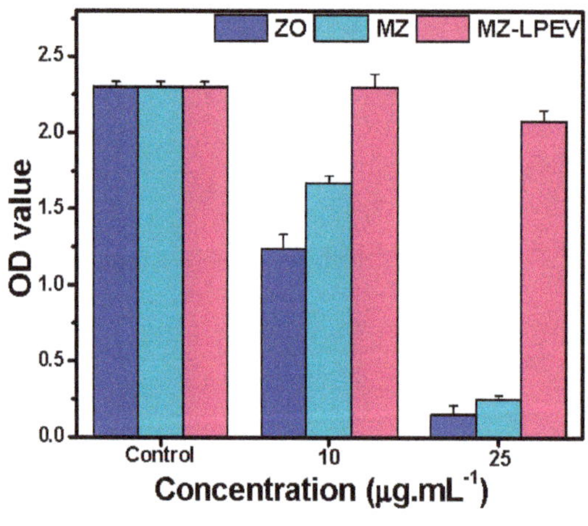

Figure 6. Viability (WST assay) of the human embryonic kidney (HEK 293) cells treated with ZO, MZ, and MZ-LPEV at various concentrations for 48 h. Averaged values from triplicate experiments are shown ($p < 0.05$).

4. Conclusions

In summary, we successfully prepared a nanocomposite comprising PEG-modified-MoS_2/ZO NPs cloaked with *L. paracasei*-derived EVs (MZ-LPEV), which we then characterized as a selective and biocompatible antibacterial platform against hazardous *S. aureus* species. This nanocomposite exhibited superb synergistic activity by utilizing the advantages of both the functionalized MZ and LPEV, which resulted in enhanced ROS production and membrane disruption. Overall, our study demonstrated the specific usage of *L. paracasei*-derived EVs for selective targeting by the modified 2D antibacterial nanocomposite. Therefore, LPEV clocked with multiple 2D antibacterial nanocomposites represents a unique platform for the nanoantibiotic remediation of *S. aureus* infection and transmission across environmental matrices. Since different types of 2D nanocomposites would have distinct selectivity, our new strategy holds promise for the treatment of different bacterial infections that are harmful to the environment.

Supplementary Materials: The following supporting information can be downloaded at: https://www.mdpi.com/article/10.3390/pharmaceutics14112273/s1, Figure S1: Bactericidal activity of nanocomposites; Figure S2: Antibacterial activity of nanomaterials and LPEV; Figure S3: Evaluation of synergistic activity between MZ and LPEV; Figure S4: Antibacterial activity of nanocomposites and MZ-LPEV against Gram-positive bacteria; Figure S5: Antibacterial activity of nanocomposites and MZ-LPEV against Gram-negative bacteria.

Author Contributions: A.N.: Conceptualization, investigation, methodology, validation, and writing-original draft. H.C.: Investigation, methodology, and validation. K.-s.K.: Conceptualization, supervision, resources, and writing—review & editing. All authors have read and agreed to the published version of the manuscript.

Funding: This research was funded by a National Research Foundation of Korea (NRF) grant funded by the Korean government (MSIT) (grant number NRF-2021R1A2C1007413).

Institutional Review Board Statement: Not applicable.

Informed Consent Statement: Not applicable.

Data Availability Statement: Not applicable.

Acknowledgments: We would like to thank the Korean Collection for Type Cultures (KCTC) for providing bacterial strains.

Conflicts of Interest: The authors declare no conflict of interest.

References

1. Kavanaugh, J.S.; Horswill, A.R. Impact of environmental cues on *Staphylococcal* quorum sensing and biofilm development. *J. Biol. Chem.* **2016**, *291*, 12556–12564. [CrossRef] [PubMed]
2. Denissen, J.; Reyneke, B.; Waso-Reyneke, M.; Havenga, B.; Barnard, T.; Khan, S.; Khan, W. Prevalence of ESKAPE pathogens in the environment: Antibiotic resistance status, community-acquired infection and risk to human health. *Int. J. Hyg. Environ. Health* **2022**, *244*, 114006. [CrossRef] [PubMed]
3. Kozajda, A.; Jezak, K.; Kapsa, A. Airborne *Staphylococcus aureus* in different environments-a review. *Environ. Sci. Pollut. Res.* **2019**, *26*, 34741–34753. [CrossRef] [PubMed]
4. Wertheim, H.F.; Melles, D.C.; Vos, M.C.; van Leeuwen, W.; van Belkum, A.; Verbrugh, H.A.; Nouwen, J.L. The role of nasal carriage in *Staphylococcus aureus* infections. *Lancet Infect. Dis.* **2005**, *5*, 751–762. [CrossRef]
5. Zhu, F.; Zhuang, H.; Ji, S.; Xu, E.; Di, L.; Wang, Z.; Jiang, S.; Wang, H.; Sun, L.; Shen, P.; et al. Household transmission of community-associated methicillin-resistant *Staphylococcus aureus*. *Front. Public Health* **2021**, *9*, 658638. [CrossRef]
6. Lee, A.S.; de Lencastre, H.; Garau, J.; Kluytmans, J.; Malhotra-Kumar, S.; Peschel, A.; Harbarth, S. Methicillin-resistant *Staphylococcus aureus*. *Nat. Rev. Dis. Primers* **2018**, *4*, 18033. [CrossRef]
7. DeLeo, F.R.; Chambers, H.F. Reemergence of antibiotic-resistant *Staphylococcus aureus* in the genomics era. *J. Clin. Investig.* **2009**, *119*, 2464–2474. [CrossRef] [PubMed]
8. Matai, I.; Sachdev, A.; Dubey, P.; Kumar, S.U.; Bhushan, B.; Gopinath, P. Antibacterial activity and mechanism of Ag-ZnO nanocomposite on *S. aureus* and GFP-expressing antibiotic resistant *E. coli*. *Colloids Surf. B Biointerfaces* **2014**, *115*, 359–367. [CrossRef]
9. Naskar, A.; Kim, K.-S. Nanomaterials as delivery vehicles and components of new strategies to combat bacterial infections: Advantages and limitations. *Microorganisms* **2019**, *7*, 356. [CrossRef]
10. Ganguly, P.; Breen, A.; Pillai, S.C. Toxicity of nanomaterials: Exposure, pathways, assessment, and recent advances. *ACS Biomater. Sci. Eng.* **2018**, *4*, 2237–2275. [CrossRef]
11. Naskar, A.; Cho, H.; Lee, S.; Kim, K.-S. Biomimetic nanoparticles coated with bacterial outer membrane vesicles as a new-generation platform for biomedical applications. *Pharmaceutics* **2021**, *13*, 1887. [CrossRef] [PubMed]
12. Malhotra, S.; Dumoga, S.; Singh, N. Red blood cells membrane-derived nanoparticles: Applications and key challenges in their clinical translation. *Wiley Interdiscip. Rev. Nanomed.* **2022**, *14*, e1776. [CrossRef] [PubMed]
13. Wang, D.; Wang, S.; Zhou, Z.; Bai, D.; Zhang, Q.; Ai, X.; Gao, W.; Zhang, L. White blood cell membrane-coated nanoparticles: Recent development and medical applications. *Adv. Healthc. Mater.* **2022**, *11*, e2101349. [CrossRef] [PubMed]
14. Han, H.; Bártolo, R.; Li, J.; Shahbazi, M.A.; Santos, H.A. Biomimetic platelet membrane-coated nanoparticles for targeted therapy. *Eur. J. Pharm. Biopharm.* **2022**, *172*, 1–15. [CrossRef]
15. Harris, J.C.; Scully, M.A.; Day, E.S. Cancer cell membrane-coated nanoparticles for cancer management. *Cancers* **2019**, *11*, 1836. [CrossRef]
16. Guerrero-Mandujano, A.; Hernández-Cortez, C.; Ibarra, J.A.; Castro-Escarpulli, G. The outer membrane vesicles: Secretion system type zero. *Traffic* **2017**, *18*, 425–432. [CrossRef]

17. Wang, X.; Koffi, P.F.; English, O.F.; Lee, J.C. *Staphylococcus aureus* extracellular vesicles: A story of toxicity and the stress of 2020. *Toxins* **2021**, *13*, 75. [CrossRef] [PubMed]
18. Schrempf, H.; Merling, P. Extracellular *Streptomyces lividans* vesicles: Composition, biogenesis and antimicrobial activity. *Microb. Biotechnol.* **2015**, *8*, 644–658. [CrossRef] [PubMed]
19. Woo, J.H.; Kim, S.; Lee, T.; Lee, J.C.; Shin, J.H. Production of membrane vesicles in *Listeria monocytogenes* cultured with or without sub-inhibitory concentrations of antibiotics and their innate immune responses *in vitro*. *Genes* **2021**, *12*, 415. [CrossRef]
20. Brown, L.; Kessler, A.; Cabezas-Sanchez, P.; Luque-Garcia, J.L.; Casadevall, A. Extracellular vesicles produced by the Gram-positive bacterium *Bacillus subtilis* are disrupted by the lipopeptide surfactin. *Mol. Microbiol.* **2014**, *93*, 183–198. [CrossRef]
21. Lee, B.H.; Wu, S.C.; Shen, T.L.; Hsu, Y.Y.; Chen, C.H.; Hsu, W.H. The applications of *Lactobacillus plantarum*-derived extracellular vesicles as a novel natural antibacterial agent for improving quality and safety in tuna fish. *Food Chem.* **2021**, *340*, 128104. [CrossRef] [PubMed]
22. Grande, R.; Celia, C.; Mincione, G.; Stringaro, A.; Di Marzio, L.; Colone, M.; Di Marcantonio, M.C.; Savino, L.; Puca, V.; Santoliquido, R.; et al. Detection and physicochemical characterization of membrane vesicles (MVs) of *Lactobacillus reuteri* DSM 17938. *Front. Microbiol.* **2017**, *8*, 1040. [CrossRef] [PubMed]
23. Shi, Y.; Meng, L.; Zhang, C.; Zhang, F.; Fang, Y. Extracellular vesicles of *Lacticaseibacillus paracasei* PC-H1 induce colorectal cancer cells apoptosis via PDK1/AKT/Bcl-2 signaling pathway. *Microbiol. Res.* **2021**, *255*, 126921. [CrossRef]
24. Elsharkasy, O.M.; Nordin, J.Z.; Hagey, D.W.; de Jong, O.G.; Schiffelers, R.M.; Andaloussi, S.E.; Vader, P. Extracellular vesicles as drug delivery systems: Why and how? *Adv. Drug Deliv. Rev.* **2020**, *159*, 332–343. [CrossRef]
25. Gao, F.; Xu, L.; Yang, B.; Fan, F.; Yang, L. Kill the real with the fake: Eliminate intracellular *Staphylococcus aureus* using nanoparticle coated with its extracellular vesicle membrane as active-targeting drug carrier. *ACS Infect. Dis.* **2019**, *5*, 218–227. [CrossRef]
26. Wu, S.; Huang, Y.; Yan, J.; Li, Y.; Wang, J.; Yang, Y.Y.; Yuan, P.; Ding, X. Bacterial outer membrane-coated mesoporous silica nanoparticles for targeted delivery of antibiotic rifampicin against gram-negative bacterial infection in vivo. *Adv. Funct. Mater.* **2021**, *31*, 2103442. [CrossRef]
27. Ortiz, A. Not all extracellular vesicles were created equal: Clinical implications. *Ann Transl. Med.* **2017**, *5*, 111. [CrossRef]
28. Qin, Y.; Long, L.; Huang, Q. Extracellular vesicles in toxicological studies: Key roles in communication between environmental stress and adverse outcomes. *J. Appl. Toxicol.* **2020**, *40*, 1166–1182. [CrossRef]
29. Dean, S.N.; Leary, D.H.; Sullivan, C.J.; Oh, E.; Walper, S.A. Isolation and characterization of *Lactobacillus*-derived membrane vesicles. *Sci. Rep.* **2019**, *9*, 877. [CrossRef]
30. Bhogoju, S.; Nahashon, S. Recent advances in probiotic application in animal health and nutrition: A review. *Agriculture* **2022**, *12*, 304. [CrossRef]
31. Di Cerbo, A.; Palmieri, B.; Aponte, M.; Morales-Medina, J.C.; Iannitti, T. Mechanisms and therapeutic effectiveness of *lactobacilli*. *J. Clin. Pathol.* **2016**, *69*, 187–203. [CrossRef] [PubMed]
32. Kang, M.S.; Lim, H.S.; Oh, J.S.; Lim, Y.J.; Wuertz-Kozak, K.; Harro, J.M.; Shirtliff, M.E.; Achermann, Y. Antimicrobial activity of *Lactobacillus salivarius* and *Lactobacillus fermentum* against *Staphylococcus aureus*. *Pathog. Dis.* **2017**, *75*, ftx009. [CrossRef] [PubMed]
33. Shaaban, M.; Abd El-Rahman, O.A.; Al-Qaidi, B.; Ashour, H.M. Antimicrobial and antibiofilm activities of probiotic *Lactobacilli* on antibiotic-resistant *Proteus mirabilis*. *Microorganisms* **2020**, *8*, 960. [CrossRef] [PubMed]
34. Guerrero Correa, M.; Martínez, F.B.; Vidal, C.P.; Streitt, C.; Escrig, J.; de Dicastillo, C.L. Antimicrobial metal-based nanoparticles: A review on their synthesis, types and antimicrobial action. *Beilstein J. Nanotechnol.* **2020**, *11*, 1450–1469. [CrossRef] [PubMed]
35. Cho, H.; Naskar, A.; Lee, S.; Kim, S.; Kim, K.-S. A new surface charge neutralizing nano-adjuvant to potentiate polymyxins in killing Mcr-1 mediated drug-resistant *Escherichia coli*. *Pharmaceutics* **2021**, *13*, 250. [CrossRef] [PubMed]
36. Vandebriel, R.J.; De Jong, W.H. A review of mammalian toxicity of ZnO nanoparticles. *Nanotechnol. Sci. Appl.* **2012**, *5*, 61–71. [CrossRef]
37. Naskar, A.; Bera, S.; Bhattacharya, R.; Saha, P.; Roy, S.S.; Sen, T.; Jana, S. Synthesis, characterization and antibacterial activity of Ag incorporated ZnO–graphene nanocomposites. *RSC Adv.* **2016**, *6*, 88751–88761. [CrossRef]
38. Naskar, A.; Khan, H.; Sarkar, R.; Kumar, S.; Halder, D.; Jana, S. Anti-biofilm activity and food packaging application of room temperature solution process based polyethylene glycol capped Ag-ZnO-graphene nanocomposite. *Mater. Sci. Eng. C Mater. Biol. Appl.* **2018**, *91*, 743–753. [CrossRef]
39. Naskar, A.; Cho, H.; Kim, K.-S. Black phosphorus-based CuS nanoplatform: Near-infrared-responsive and reactive oxygen species-generating agent against environmental bacterial pathogens. *J. Environ. Chem. Eng.* **2022**, *10*, 108226. [CrossRef]
40. Zhao, Y.; Jia, Y.; Xu, J.; Han, L.; He, F.; Jiang, X. The antibacterial activities of MoS_2 nanosheets towards multi-drug resistant bacteria. *Chem. Commun.* **2021**, *57*, 2998–3001. [CrossRef]
41. Zhao, X.; Chen, M.; Wang, H.; Xia, L.; Guo, M.; Jiang, S.; Wang, Q.; Li, X.; Yang, X. Synergistic antibacterial activity of streptomycin sulfate loaded PEG-MoS_2/rGO nanoflakes assisted with near-infrared. *Mater. Sci. Eng. C Mater. Biol. Appl.* **2020**, *116*, 111221. [CrossRef] [PubMed]
42. Naskar, A.; Lee, S.; Lee, Y.; Kim, S.; Kim, K.-S. A new nano-platform of erythromycin combined with Ag nano-particle ZnO nano-structure against methicillin-resistant *Staphylococcus aureus*. *Pharmaceutics* **2020**, *12*, 841. [CrossRef]
43. Kim, T.I.; Kwon, B.; Yoon, J.; Park, I.J.; Bang, G.S.; Park, Y.; Seo, Y.S.; Choi, S.Y. Antibacterial activities of graphene oxide–molybdenum disulfide nanocomposite films. *ACS Appl. Mater. Interfaces* **2017**, *9*, 7908–7917. [CrossRef]

44. Kim, T.; Bak, G.; Lee, J.; Kim, K.-S. Systematic analysis of the role of bacterial Hfq-interacting sRNAs in the response to antibiotics. *J. Antimicrob. Chemother.* **2015**, *70*, 1659–1668. [CrossRef] [PubMed]
45. Naskar, A.; Lee, S.; Kim, K.-S. Antibacterial potential of Ni-doped zinc oxide nanostructure: Comparatively more effective against Gram-negative bacteria including multi-drug resistant strains. *RSC Adv.* **2020**, *10*, 1232–1242. [CrossRef]
46. Comfort, N.; Cai, K.; Bloomquist, T.R.; Strait, M.D.; Ferrante, A.W., Jr.; Baccarelli, A.A. Nanoparticle tracking analysis for the quantification and size determination of extracellular vesicles. *J. Vis. Exp.* **2021**, *169*, e62447. [CrossRef] [PubMed]
47. Qi, Y.; Wang, N.; Xu, Q.; Li, H.; Zhou, P.; Lu, X.; Zhao, G. A green route to fabricate MoS_2 nanosheets in water-ethanol-CO_2. *Chem. Commun.* **2015**, *51*, 6726–6729. [CrossRef] [PubMed]
48. Li, B.; Jiang, L.; Li, X.; Ran, P.; Zuo, P.; Wang, A.; Qu, L.; Zhao, Y.; Cheng, Z.; Lu, Y. Preparation of monolayer MoS_2 quantum dots using temporally shaped femtosecond laser ablation of bulk MoS_2 targets in water. *Sci. Rep.* **2017**, *7*, 11182. [CrossRef]
49. Filipe, V.; Hawe, A.; Jiskoot, W. Critical evaluation of nanoparticle tracking analysis (NTA) by NanoSight for the measurement of nanoparticles and protein aggregates. *Pharm. Res.* **2010**, *27*, 796–810. [CrossRef]
50. Wen, T.; Liu, J.; He, W.; Yang, A. Nanomaterials and Reactive Oxygen Species (ROS). In *Nanotechnology in Regenerative Medicine and Drug Delivery Therapy*; Xu, H., Gu, N., Eds.; Springer: Singapore, 2020.
51. Bidkar, A.P.; Sanpui, P.; Ghosh, S.S. Red blood cell-membrane-coated Poly(Lactic-*co*-glycolic Acid) nanoparticles for enhanced chemo- and hypoxia-activated therapy. *ACS Appl. Bio Mater.* **2019**, *2*, 4077–4086. [CrossRef]
52. Su, J.; Sun, H.; Meng, Q.; Zhang, P.; Yin, Q.; Li, Y. Enhanced blood suspensibility and laser-activated tumor-specific drug release of theranostic mesoporous silica nanoparticles by functionalizing with erythrocyte membranes. *Theranostics* **2017**, *7*, 523–537. [CrossRef] [PubMed]
53. Reshma, V.G.; Mohanan, P.V. Cellular interactions of zinc oxide nanoparticles with human embryonic kidney (HEK 293) cells. *Colloids Surf. B Biointerfaces* **2017**, *157*, 182–190.

pharmaceutics

MDPI

Article

Synthesis and Characterization of Quercetin–Iron Complex Nanoparticles for Overcoming Drug Resistance

Lucas Prestianni [1], Eric R. Espinal [2], Sarah F. Hathcock [2], Nadine Vollmuth [2], Pixiang Wang [3], Robert A. Holler [4], Shaoyang Liu [3], Brandon J. Kim [2,5,6,7,*] and Yuping Bao [1,6,7,*]

1 Chemical and Biological Engineering, The University of Alabama, Tuscaloosa, AL 35487, USA
2 Department of Biological Sciences, The University of Alabama, Tuscaloosa, AL 35487, USA
3 Department of Chemistry and Physics, Center for Materials and Manufacturing Sciences, Troy University, Troy, AL 36082, USA
4 Alabama Analytical Research Center, The University of Alabama, Tuscaloosa, AL 35487, USA
5 Department of Microbiology, Heersink School of Medicine, The University of Alabama at Birmingham, Birmingham, AL 35487, USA
6 Center for Convergent Biosciences and Medicine, The University of Alabama, Tuscaloosa, AL 35487, USA
7 Alabama Life Research Institute, The University of Alabama, Tuscaloosa, AL 35487, USA
* Correspondence: bjkim4@ua.edu (B.J.K.); ybao@eng.ua.edu (Y.B.)

Abstract: Quercetin, one of the major natural flavonoids, has demonstrated great pharmacological potential as an antioxidant and in overcoming drug resistance. However, its low aqueous solubility and poor stability limit its potential applications. Previous studies suggest that the formation of quercetin-metal complexes could increase quercetin stability and biological activity. In this paper, we systematically investigated the formation of quercetin-iron complex nanoparticles by varying the ligand-to-metal ratios with the goal of increasing the aqueous solubility and stability of quercetin. It was found that quercetin-iron complex nanoparticles could be reproducibly synthesized with several ligand-to-iron ratios at room temperature. The UV-Vis spectra of the nanoparticles indicated that nanoparticle formation greatly increased the stability and solubility of quercetin. Compared to free quercetin, the quercetin-iron complex nanoparticles exhibited enhanced antioxidant activities and elongated effects. Our preliminary cellular evaluation suggests that these nanoparticles had minimal cytotoxicity and could effectively block the efflux pump of cells, indicating their potential for cancer treatment.

Keywords: iron complex; quercetin; drug resistance; flavonoids; efflux pump

1. Introduction

Cancer remains a leading cause of death globally, and chemotherapy is still the most common treatment [1,2]. Unfortunately, tumor cells tend to develop resistance to multiple anticancer drugs, which greatly affects clinical outcomes [3]. Several mechanisms of drug resistance have been reported, such as drug efflux by overexpressed transporters (e.g., P-glycoprotein—P-gp), inhibition of the PI3K/AKT pathway, and activated cell growth factors [3]. Among these explored mechanisms of drug resistance, P-gp overexpression in cancer cells has been well accepted. This results in the exclusion of drugs from tumor cells, which prevents drug accumulation inside cancer cells [4–6]. Strategies have been developed to overcome drug resistance [7], such as inhibiting drug efflux transporters, structural alternation of drug molecules, gene delivery, etc. [8]. As natural antioxidants, flavonoids have attracted much attention for reversing multidrug resistance (MDR) to chemotherapeutics for cancer [7,9]. It is believed that flavonoids are involved in several regulatory processes, such as the regulation of drug efflux transporters, critical enzymes, oxidative stress, and cell cycles [7,10]. In particular, it has been shown that complexation with metal ions enhances the biological activities of flavonoids [11,12].

As one of the major naturally occurring flavonoids, quercetin (Q) has been extensively studied for cancer therapy [13–16]. For example, Q molecules have demonstrated activity in overcoming drug resistance, inducing cell apoptosis, and modulating tumor microenvironments in several cancer types [13–16]. Much evidence suggests that Q molecules are able to inhibit the efflux effects of several ATP-binding cassette (ABC) transporters, such as *ABCB1* (P-gp) [16,17], *ABCC1*, and *ABCC2* (MDR proteins 1 and 2) [11]. However, Q's clinical applications in cancer therapy are greatly hindered by its extremely low aqueous solubility, poor stability from oxidation, and rapid enzymatic degradation, which lead to limited bioavailability [18,19]. To overcome these limitations, many efforts have been made to alter Q properties for enhanced biological activity [20], improved solubility [21], and improved bioavailability by forming protein complexes [22]. Additionally, the encapsulation of Q molecules inside nanocarriers has been explored for enhanced circulation time, increased bioavailability, and tumor targeting [23]. Particularly, complexation of Q with various metallic ions has exhibited enhanced biological activity, such as stronger antioxidant activity of Q metal complexes compared to free Q, [24,25], enhanced inhibitory effects on tumor cell growth, and increased bioavailability compared with free Q [26,27]. In addition, Q has multiple metal binding sites and can coordinate with various metallic ions to form complexes [24,28,29], such as cobalt, zinc, ruthenium, and iron. Compared to other complexes, iron (Fe) coordination has drawn special attention due to the demonstrated potential of Q-Fe complexes as MRI contrast agents [30]. Q-Fe complexes also exhibit the best antioxidant and antiacetylcholinesterase activities as promising agents for Alzheimer's disease [24]. Therefore, the Q-Fe complex is explored in our study. Compared to Q-metal complex molecules, the formation of nanostructures based on Q-metal complexes led to additional benefits, such as nanoparticles for effective delivery [30], thin films and capsules for surface coating [31], and nanocomposites [32]. In our study, we aim at creating Q-Fe complex nanoparticles.

Here, we systematically investigated the feasibility of synthesizing Q-Fe complex nanoparticles (QFeNPs) under different conditions. In particular, the effects of Q-Fe ratios on NP formation, aqueous solubility, and stability were studied. Q molecules have distinct UV-Vis absorption bands, which were used to monitor the complex and QFeNP formation, study the stability, and quantify the solubility. The NP formation was also examined by transmission electron microscopy (TEM) for size and morphology, while the coordination between Q and Fe^{3+} was studied with Fourier-transform infrared spectroscopy (FTIR). Finally, we performed a preliminary evaluation of the inhibitory effects of these NPs on P-gp, which is expressed in human brain endothelial cells.

2. Materials and Methods

2.1. Chemicals

The majority of the chemicals were purchased from VWR, including quercetin dihydrate (97%, VWR, Aurora, OH, USA), iron (III) chloride anhydrous ($FeCl_3$, 98%, VWR, Aurora, OH, USA), 2, 2-Bis (hydroxymethyl)-2, 2′, 2″-nitrilotriethanol (Bistris, ultra-pure, VWR, Ohio, USA), tris(hydroxymethyl)aminomethane (Tris, ultra-pure, VWR, Aurora, OH, USA), 10× phosphate-buffered saline (PBS) solution (VWR, Aurora, OH, USA), and ethanol (70%, VWR, Aurora, OH, USA). The following chemicals were purchased from other vendors as indicated, including sodium chloride (NaCl, 99%, Acros, Waltham, NJ, USA), methanol (99.8%, low acetone, Alfa Aesar, Haverhill, MA, USA), ultra-pure (4-(2-hydroxyethyl)-1-piperazineethanesulfonic acid) (HEPES) sodium salt (BDH, Radnor, PA, USA), and 1,1-Diphenyl-2-picrylhydrazyl free radical (DPPH, 97%, TCI, JP).

2.2. Synthesis of QFeNPs

A quantity of 5 mL of a 10 mM Q dihydrate methanol solution was mixed with 5 mL of a $FeCl_3$ water solution of different molarities (50, 40, 30, 20, 10, 5, 3.3, 2.5, and 2 mM) to achieve Q-Fe ratios of 5:1, 4:1, 3:1, 1:1, 1:2, 1:3, 1:4, and 1:5. The reaction solutions were stirred at room temperature for 2 h. For temperature effects, experiments were performed with a Q-Fe ratio of 1:5, and the reaction solutions were stirred at room temperature at 37 °C and 60 °C. Then, the samples were processed for characterization and analysis. For TEM examination of NP formation and NP morphology, TEM samples were prepared by dropping 100 µL of an as-synthesized solution onto TEM grids. For UV-Vis spectrum collection, each as-synthesized solution (50 µL) was brought up to 5 mL with DI water and was then measured by a UV-Vis spectrometer. For solubility, stability, and activity tests, the reaction solutions were dialyzed in G2 Floatilizers for 4 h in sterilized DI water to remove methanol before freeze-drying. The dried powders were used for different analyses.

2.3. *Stability of QFeNPs*

The stability of QFeNPs was studied by monitoring their time-dependent UV-Vis spectra for up to two weeks at three different conditions: as-synthesized NPs in a 50/50 methanol/water solution, NPs stored in powder form after freeze-drying, and NPs in various buffers. For as-synthesized NPs, at day 1, day 7, and day 14, each 50 µL of the original NP solution was diluted into 5 mL of DI water and a UV-Vis spectrum was collected. For NP powders at the intervals of day 1, day 7, and day 14, 5 mg of QFeNPs for each ratio were dissolved into 1 mL of DI water and underwent 10 s of sonication. After further diluting to approximately 0.05 mg/mL with DI water, UV-Vis spectra were collected. For NPs in various buffers, ~5 mg of freeze-dried powders for each NP-forming ratio were dissolved into 1 mL of DI water, 150 mM of NaCl, 10 mM of Bis Tris, 10 mM of Tris, 10 mM of HEPES, and 1 × PBS under sonication. Then, 50 µL of the top solution at day 1, day 7, and day 14 were diluted into 5 mL of the respective buffer, and the UV-Vis spectra were collected.

2.4. *Solubility of QFeNPs*

The solubility of QFeNPs with clear and stable NP formations at Q-Fe ratios of 1:3, 1:4, and 1:5 was estimated. Specifically, standard curves of QFeNPs with Q-Fe ratios of 1:3, 1:4, and 1:5 were created using the UV-Vis absorbance at 293 nm, which was used to quantify the concentration of NPs at each ratio in different solutions. Approximately 5 mg of freeze-dried NP powders were dispersed into 1 mL of 1 × PBS, 10 mM of Bis Tris, 10 mM of Tris, 10 mM of HEPES, 150 mM of NaCl, or DI water, and each underwent sonication to create saturated NP solutions. Then, the UV-Vis spectra were collected on 50× diluted top supernatants after 24 h. The standard curves for each ratio were generated as follows: QFeNPs DI water solutions (~1 mg/mL) were created and then diluted to create concentrations within a range of 0.05 mg/mL and 0.005 m/mL, which were analyzed using a VWR V 3100PC UV-Vis spectrophotometer.

2.5. *DPPH Antioxidant Activity*

The antioxidant activity of the QFeNPs was measured using a DPPH antioxidant assay [33] and compared with free Q. Q and QFeNPs were dissolved in a water/methanol (50/50 *v/v*) mixture at various concentrations of 100, 75, 50, 25, and 10 µM. Then, 3 mL of a 0.1 mM DPPH solution was added to 1 mL of the sample solution while mixing. After 40 min, the absorbance of the solution was measured at 517 nm (A_s). A quantity of 3 mL of DPPH (0.1 mM) was mixed with 1 mL of methanol and water and used as a control (A_0). The absorbance of representative samples (100 µM) at 517 nm was also measured as a function of time, such as free Q and QFeNPs with a Q-Fe ratio of 1:5 and 2:1. The absorbance was recorded immediately after mixing and in 5 min increments for 30 min, after which absorbance was recorded at 1, 2, 4, and 6 h after mixing. The experiments were performed in triplicate, and the inhibition percentage of DPPH was then calculated using the following equation:

$$\text{Inhibition } (\%) = 100 \times (A_0 - A_s)/A_0$$

2.6. Characterization

The morphology of QFeNPs was examined using a Hitachi H-7650 TEM (Hitachi, Ibaraki, Japan). The UV-Vis absorption spectra were collected in a range of 200–900 nm using 1 cm quartz cells on a VWR V 3100PC UV-Vis spectrophotometer. The FTIR spectra were recorded for powder samples in the range of 400–4000 cm^{-1} on an Agilent Cary 630 FTIR spectrometer (Agilent, Boulder, CO, USA). Freeze-drying was performed in a SP VirTis Benchtop Pro BTP-8ZL0VW freeze dryer (SP, Warminster, PA, USA). The heat-treated NP powder was analyzed by X-ray diffraction (XRD) on a Rigaku Miniflex with a Cu source at 30 kV and 15 mA. Thermogravimetric analyses (TGA) were performed on QFeNPs powders from freeze-drying using a TGA-550 (TA Instruments, New Castle, DE, USA) with a platinum-HT sample pan. Specifically, ~5 mg QFeNPs powder was placed into a platinum-HT sample pan, and the temperature was raised from room temperature to 800 °C at a heating rate of 10 °C/min. The measurements were carried out in a nitrogen environment with a gas flow of 60 mL/min for sample purge and 40 mL/min for balance purge.

2.7. P-gp Expression and Blocking Assay

Prior to studying the inhibition of QFeNPs on P-gp activity, we first evaluated the P-gp expression by immunostaining two types of cells: MDA-MB231br, a variant of triple-negative highly metastatic breast cancer cell lines, and human induced pluripotent stem-cell-derived brain-like endothelial cells (iBECs) [34–37]. Briefly, cells were fixed for 15 min with ice-cold methanol and blocked with 10% FBS in 1 × PBS for one hour at room temperature. P-gp antibody (Thermo Fisher Scientific, Waltham, MA, USA) was diluted 1:25 into a blocking solution, and cells were then stained overnight at 4 °C. After 24 h, the cells were washed three times with 1 × PBS, and a secondary antibody, Alexa-Fluor 488 mouse (Thermo Fisher Scientific, Waltham, MA, USA), diluted 1:200 in blocking solution, was added and incubated for one hour at room temperature, protected from the light. After incubation, the cells were washed twice with 1 × PBS, incubated with DAPI diluted at a ratio of 1:5000 in 1 × PBS for 15 min at room temperature in the dark, washed once more with 1× PBS, and then imaged on a TI2 Nikon microscope.

The effectiveness of QFeNPs on inhibiting P-gp activity was measured in iBECs using a fluorescent substrate Rhodamine 123 (R123) accumulation assay [38]. Cyclosporin A (CsA), a known P-gp inhibitor, was used as a positive control, while cells without treatment served as a negative control. The inhibition activity of three representative samples was tested, including free Q and QFeNPs with Q-Fe ratios of 2:1 and 1:5. All three samples were diluted to 100 μM and 50 μM in EC growth media without basic fibroblast growth factor (bFGF) or retinoic acid. Cells were incubated with the diluted samples for 2 h at 37 °C with 5% CO_2. Then, cells were incubated with R123 (10 μM) with or without inhibitor and QFeNPs for 2 h at 37 °C with 5% CO_2. Cells were then washed twice with PBS and lysed with 200 μL of RIPA buffer on a rocker for 10 min at room temperature, protected from light. The fluorescent intensity of R123 was measured on a Molecular Devices ID3 plate reader.

3. Results and Discussion

The objective of this study is to create QFeNPs with controlled sizes reproducibly and to increase Q's aqueous solubility and stability in order to generate potential anti-drug resistance agents for cancer therapy. Prior to NP synthesis, we first investigated the pH-dependent structural stability of free Q using UV-Vis spectrometry and FTIR. Subsequently, the Fe^{3+} and Q complexation were studied by varying the Q-Fe ratios. For reactions with successful NP formation, we investigated the stability and aqueous solubility of QFeNPs. Finally, the inhibitory effects of QFeNPs were preliminarily tested on P-gp using iPSC-derived BECs in cell culture. Q was chosen as a coordination ligand for complex formation because of its proven anti-drug resistance activity and multiple binding sites [32]. The multiple binding sites allow adjusting the ratio of metal ions and further crosslinking for NP formation. The use of iron as the coordination metal ion is due to the potential of Fe complexes as MRI contrast agents [30]. Specifically, we studied the effects of temperature and Q-Fe ratios on NP formation with the goal of increasing Q's aqueous solubility and stability.

3.1. Stability of Free Quercetin

As one of the major naturally occurring flavonoids, Q is known to have anti-drug resistance and anti-inflammatory activity, which is mainly attributed to its chemical structure [39]. Q has multiple metal binding sites [40], which allows adjusting Q-metal ion ratios for NP formation through crosslinking. Metal ions can coordinate through the catechol and carbonyl groups at the C4 position, assisted by hydroxyl groups at the C3 or C5 positions (Figure 1A), yielding catechol-like, maltol-like, and acetylacetone-like coordination interactions [40]. The functional groups have different pKa's, leading to pH dependent stability and coordination behaviors. Although Q has five different pKas associated with its hydroxyl groups (-C4′-OH: 6.41, -C7-OH: 7.81, C3-OH: 10.19, C3′-OH: 11.53, and C5-OH: 12.91), Q methanol solutions at different pHs only exhibited two typical absorption peaks (Figure 1B). Without any pH adjustment, two typical absorbance bands were observed at 254 and 365 nm, which were consistent with reported studies with assigned B-ring cinnamoyl bands and A-ring benzoyl bands [30,41,42].

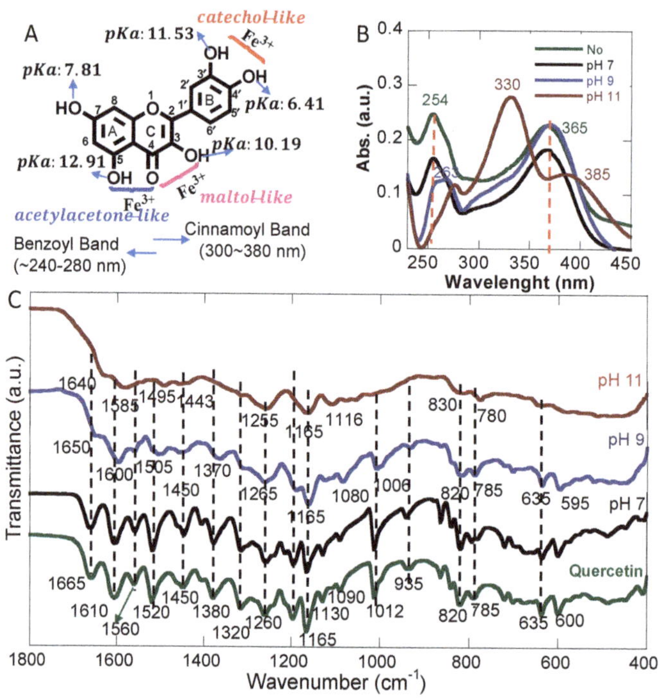

Figure 1. (**A**) Structure of quercetin with typical pKa values of hydroxyl groups and metal coordination sites along with typical absorbance, (**B**) UV-Vis absorption spectra of Q solution at different pHs compared with no pH adjustment, and (**C**) FTIR spectra of Q at different pHs compared with no pH adjustment.

After adjusting the solution pH to 7 with 100 mM of NaOH, no changes in absorption were observed after 2 h at room temperature. Increasing the pH to 9, evident shifts were observed for both peaks (254 → 263 nm and 365 → 370 nm), likely due to deprotonation of some hydroxyl groups. In addition, a peak shoulder appeared around 300 nm, indicating some Q degradation. However, after pH was increased to 11, further shifts and decreases in intensities of the bands at 254 nm and 365 nm were observed. In addition, a major absorption band at 330 nm appeared, suggesting a significant structural change in Q. It has been previously reported that Q experiences rapid degradation at higher pH in solution, and the absorption band at 330 nm was mainly from degradation products, such as 2-(3,4-dihydroxyphenyl)-2-oxoacetic acid, as reported previously [43]. These degradation products showed three distinct bands at 274, 330, and 385 nm, with the 330 nm band being the most pronounced one [43].

The structural change of Q was also studied by comparing the alteration of functional groups based on the FTIR spectra of Q freeze-dried powders at different pHs. Similar to UV-Vis analysis, the FTIR spectra of free Q without pH adjustment and at pH 7 were identical. However, evident changes could be seen for pH 9 and pH 11 samples. The -OH stretching band around 3400 cm^{-1} showed significant broadening at higher pH, suggesting a structure change and the formation of likely carboxylic group-containing degradation products (Figure S1). Aromatic out-of-plane C-H bending vibrations at 820 and 785 cm^{-1} were not affected at pH 9 but broadened at pH 11, indicating ring-related changes. The bands at 600 and 635 cm^{-1} were likely associated with C-OH bending and ring stretching within ring C, which were not altered at pH 9 but completely disappeared at pH 11. Ring C breakdown is a direct indicator of Q degradation (Figure S2). In fact, previous studies have reported that the C3-OH position within ring C is considered the weakest point of Q and is susceptible to degradation [43]. The FTIR information of metal coordination site functional groups is mainly in the range of 1000–1800 cm^{-1}, which is presented in Figure 1C. For Q powder prepared at pH 7, the FTIR spectra were identical and were consistent with previous studies with several characteristic peaks, including the band at 1665 cm^{-1} associated with the –C=O stretching at the C4 position and the C=C aromatic ring stretching bands at 1610, 1560, and 1520 cm^{-1} [44,45]. Increasing the pH caused Q degradation to start with the rearrangement and subsequent breakdown of ring C, leading to different single-ring degradation products (Figure S2). Briefly, the band at 1012 cm^{-1} could be attributed to C-CO-C stretching and bending in ketone at C4. This band did not change much at pH 9, suggesting the structural integrity of Q. However, this band completely disappeared at pH 11, indicating ring C breakdown and degradation of Q. Similarly, the 1200 cm^{-1} band refers to the C-O stretching in the aryl ether ring, which disappeared in the degradation products, consistent with the reported degradation products lacking the C-O ring [43]. The band at 1165 cm^{-1} could be assigned to the C-O stretching in phenol, which still existed in all degradation products, so the peaks were evident for all pHs tested. The stretching related to =C-O-H of the phenolic group was also observed at 1320 and 1380 cm^{-1} (OH in-plane bending). Both peaks broadened at pH 9, suggesting deprotonation. However, at pH 11, the peaks disappeared, indicating structural change. The aromatic ring stretching at 1260 cm^{-1} was not changed drastically at three different pHs because aromatic rings were also present in degraded products. Therefore, both UV-Vis and FTIR spectra suggest that Q molecules were relatively stable in methanol with no pH adjustment and at pH 7, but experienced degradation at pH 9 and pH 11. Therefore, all further studies were performed with Q in methanol without pH adjustment to minimize Q degradation.

3.2. *Synthesis of QFeNPs*

3.2.1. Temperature Effects

Previous studies suggest that higher temperatures promote Q degradation [46]. Prior to the study on the effects of different parameters on NP formation, we first tested the effects of reaction temperature on NP formation using a Q-Fe ratio of 1:5 and an excess amount of Fe for cross-linking. Three reaction temperatures were chosen: 25 °C, 37 °C, and 60 °C, to represent typical storage, application, and elevated temperatures. The Q-Fe interaction was mainly studied by UV-Vis spectroscopy. The morphology and size distribution were examined by TEM. NPs were formed at all three temperatures without much difference in morphologies, except for a slightly smaller size at a higher temperature (Figure 2). The UV-Vis spectra of QFeNPs prepared at different temperatures were almost identical, with a single peak around 293 nm, indicating similar coordination behaviors of Q and Fe. Comparing to previously reported molecular absorption of the Q-Fe complex with multiple peaks [26,47], QFeNPs only exhibited a single peak at 293 nm. The typical peaks of free Q at 254 and 365 nm were not observed, suggesting interactions of iron ions with both rings within the Q molecules. The higher absorbance of the sample made at 60 °C was likely due to the significant evaporation of methanol during the reaction. Even though NP formation was observed at all temperatures, all further reactions were performed at 25 °C to minimize Q degradation with increasing temperature.

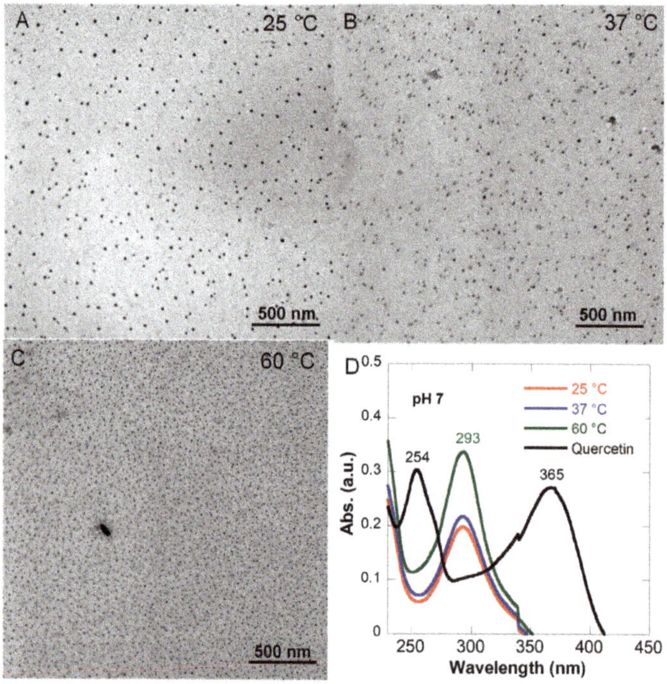

Figure 2. TEM images of QFeNPs prepared with a Q-Fe ratio of 1:5 at different temperatures: (**A**) 25 °C, (**B**) 37 °C, and (**C**) 60 °C, and (**D**) UV-Vis spectra of QFeNPs compared with free Q.

3.2.2. Q-Fe Ratio Effects

As illustrated in Figure 1A, a Q molecule has three iron coordination sites: catechol-like coordination on the B ring through catechol groups; maltol-like coordination through the hydroxyl group at C3 and the keto group on C4; and acetylacetone-like coordination through the C5-hydroxy- and C4-keto groups on the C ring. However, due to complex stability and steric hindrance when multiple molecules coordinate to a metal ion, the optimal ratio of Q to Fe for NP formation is difficult to predict. Therefore, the ratio effects on NP formation, aqueous solubility, and stability were investigated by varying the Q-Fe ratios from 5:1 to 1:5. The NP formation was monitored by examining the morphology of the products with TEM. The free Q methanol solution was light yellow, while the $FeCl_3$ water solution was orange-brown. Upon mixing at room temperature, the reaction solution color changed to greenish-black, indicating a fast coordination process. After 2 h, the reactions were stopped, and the reaction solutions at different ratios exhibited variation in not only color but also translucency levels. Sample solutions with Q-Fe ratios of 5:1, 4:1, and 3:1 were completely turbid, while samples with Q-Fe ratios of 1:2–1:5 were translucent. However, samples with Q-Fe ratios of 2:1 and 1:1 were somewhere in between (Figure 3A). Further TEM analysis suggests a direct correlation between the formed products and their solution appearance. For example, with Q-Fe ratios of 5:1, 4:1, and 3:1, no NPs were formed; instead, large organic-like aggregate bundles were observed (Figure S4). With increasing Fe^{3+} amounts, NP formation was observed, and large aggregate bundles were barely seen at the 1:1 ratio. However, a dark TEM background was observed for samples with Q-Fe ratios of 1:2 and 1:1, suggesting that many of the Q molecules may exist as molecular Q-Fe complexes. Further decreasing the Q-Fe ratio, NPs were readily formed, as shown in Figure 3B,C. NPs with relatively uniform sizes around 6 nm were formed except for the 1:5 ratio, where a larger particle population around 10 nm was observed.

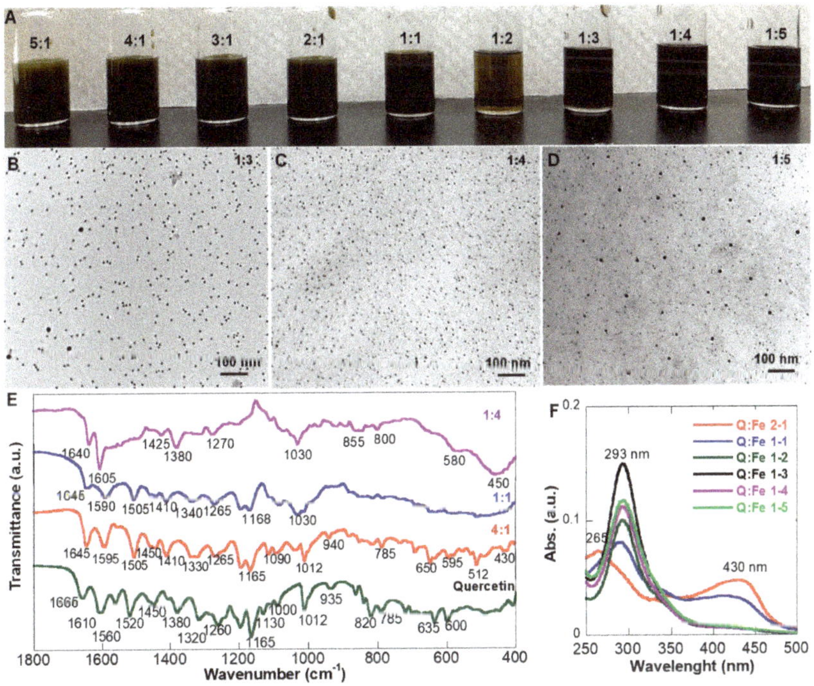

Figure 3. Ratio effect on NP formation: (**A**) photos of the reaction solutions at different ratios with different turbid levels; (**B–D**) representative TEM images of samples with NP formation at Q-Fe ratios of 1:3, 1:4, and 1:5; (**E**) FTIR spectra of representative samples with/or without NP formation; and (**F**) UV-Vis spectra of samples with NP formation at different ratios.

Based on the TEM observation, FTIR spectra were presented on selective samples representing the three types of products (bundles without NPs—4:1, some NP formation—1:1, and NPs—1:4) and compared with free Q (Figure 3E). The 4:1 ratio sample showed very similar IR bands to free Q, with a small band of Fe-O at 430 cm^{-1} and a visible decrease of the –C=O stretching band around 1560 cm^{-1}, indicating some binding involvement of the –C=O group. The hydroxyl C-OH in-plane (1320 cm^{-1}) and out-of-plane (785 cm^{-1}) bending was clearly seen. In contrast, in the spectrum of the 1:4 ratio sample, the Fe-O band around 450 cm^{-1} was significant, and the –C=O stretching band around 1560 cm^{-1} was barely seen. Keto -C=O in-plane (1012 cm^{-1}) and out-of-plane (820 cm^{-1}) bands were shifted and broadened. Hydroxyl CO-H bending (1165 cm^{-1}) became a broad shoulder. For the 1:1 ratio sample, the C=O in-plane (1012 cm^{-1}) and out-of-plane (820 cm^{-1}) bands were shifted and broadened, but the C=O stretching band around 1560 cm^{-1} was well reserved. The hydroxyl CO-H bending (1165 cm^{-1}) was still clearly seen, suggesting Fe^{3+} ions were primarily interacting through the –C=O functional group. Hydroxyl C-OH in-plane (600 cm^{-1}) and out-of-plane (785 cm^{-1}) bending involved in the coordination was significantly altered at high iron concentrations. Previous studies on the Fe (II)–Q complex suggest Fe-O stretching occurs at ~630 cm^{-1} [26], which was absent in the FTIR spectra of free Q and QFeNPs. Therefore, the Fe^{3+} was not reduced. The spectral information suggests that coordination of metals occurred with the carbonyl group and OH linked to the C-3 carbon of Q.

Like the FTIR spectra, the UV-Vis spectra also depended on the Q-Fe ratios (Figure 3F). For samples with clear NP formation, such as Q-Fe ratios of 1:3, 1:4, and 1:5, only one major 293 nm absorption band was observed. In contrast, for 2:1 and 1:1 samples with a significant amount of molecular Q-Fe complex, two distinct peaks (at 265 and 430 nm) were observed related to a ligand-metal charge transfer, as reported by other studies [26,30]. For samples with evident NP formation, the absorption peaks of free quercetin at 254 and 365 nm disappeared. Instead, the UV-Vis spectra of QFeNPs exhibited a single peak around 293 nm, regardless of the reaction ratios of Q-Fe. However, the 2:1 ratio sample showed clear band shifts from free quercetin (254→265 nm and 365→430 nm) with a shoulder close to 290 nm. This observation is consistent with most previous studies in that the 2:1 Q:metal ratio provides the most favorable conditions for complex formation. The 420 nm peak also indicates the chemical reaction of iron (III) at the hydroxychromone site of Q, according to a previous report [47]. Our results are very different from a previous report using Q at pH 11 for NP formation as an MRI contrast agent [30]. Our pH-dependent stability assessment of free Q suggests that Q would be completely degraded at pH 11 and that the products would no longer be Q-Fe complex nanoparticles. Interestingly, after freeze-drying, QFeNP samples with all NP-forming ratios (2:1, 1:1, 1:2, 1:3, 1:4, and 1:5) only exhibited a single peak at 293 nm, indicating that the freeze-dried powder mainly contained QFeNPs (Figure S4A). The absorption peak around 430 nm from the as-synthesized samples with Q-Fe ratios of 2:1 and 1:1 disappeared. To understand whether the samples changed or the Q-Fe complex with absorption at 430 nm was removed during dialysis, several sample processes were conducted: samples before and after dialysis, samples with vacuum drying without dialysis, and water solutions of freeze-dried and vacuum-dried powders, as shown in Figure S4B,C. The presence of a Q-Fe complex absorbance for samples without dialysis suggests that the dialysis step removed the molecular complex.

3.3. Stability of NPs

We hypothesized that NP formation would increase the stability of free Q molecules because the Fe coordination at the weak site of the molecule is prone to degradation. Here, we investigated the stability of QFeNPs by monitoring the time dependent UV-Vis spectra of NPs at three conditions: as-synthesized NPs in a 50/50 methanol/water solution, NPs stored in powder form after freeze-drying, and NPs in various buffers. Special attention was given to the appearance of degradation products with absorptions around 330 nm, additional peak formation, and peak intensity changes at 293 nm. Our goal was to understand the effects of the relative Q-Fe ratios on NP stability. If the absorbance peak around 293 nm remained unchanged in terms of peak position and intensity, the NPs would be considered stable. Alternatively, if the absorbance of the NP solution changed greatly with additional absorption peaks, it would be attributed to Q degradation.

Figure 4A shows the UV-Vis spectra of as-synthesized samples in 50/50 methanol/water solutions after two weeks. We observed that NP formation samples only showed relative intensity changes compared to Figure 3F. The absorption at 293 nm of 2:1 and 1:1 ratio samples became evident, and the 254 nm peak completely disappeared. In addition, the 430 nm peak is slightly redshifted with increased intensity. No peaks indicating degradation of the free Q peak were observed for all samples. Therefore, the NP formation did increase the stability of free Q. Once QFeNPs were formed and freeze-dried, they were very stable in powder form. Figure 4B shows the UV-Vis spectra of freeze-dried QFeNPs redispersed in DI water, where the peak position was not changed after two weeks. However, once the QFeNPs were dispersed in different buffers, a variation in stability was observed depending on the Q-Fe ratios. Figure 4C shows the representative UV-Vis spectra of QFeNPs with a Q-Fe ratio of 1:4, where the NPs were stable in all six tested conditions but had the lowest solubility in the Bis-Tris buffer. In contrast, the samples with a Q-Fe ratio of 2:1 showed clear degradation after two weeks in PBS, Bis Tris, and HEPES, with a degradation peak around 330 nm (Figure 4D). This observation could be attributed to a competing interaction with Fe^{3+} in the Q-Fe complex.

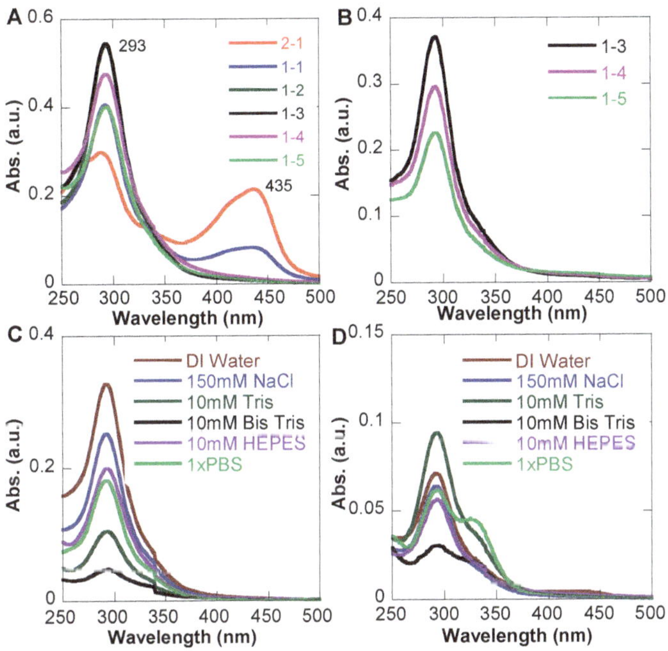

Figure 4. UV-Vis spectra of QFeNPs at various conditions after two weeks: (**A**) as-synthesized NPs at various ratios in 50/50 methanol/water; (**B**) NP powders with Q-Fe ratios of 1:3, 1:4, and 1:5 after freeze-drying; (**C**) QFeNPs with a Q-Fe ratio of 1:4 in different solutions; and (**D**) QFeNPs with a Q-Fe ratio of 2:1 in different solutions.

3.4. Solubility of NPs

Another goal of NP formation was to increase Q solubility in aqueous solutions. Most commercial vendors classify free Q as insoluble in aqueous solution. A few studies suggest that free Q in water has a solubility of 2–4 µg/mL, which does not reach the therapeutic threshold suggested by in vitro and in vivo studies in the order of tens micromolar [48,49]. Metal complex formation has clearly demonstrated increased biological activity, but no clear solubility information can be found. Our stability studies of QFeNPs also showed different absorption intensities, suggesting a solubility variation in different solutions. Here, we quantified the solubility of QFeNPs with clear and stable NP formation at Q-Fe ratios of 1:3, 1:4, and 1:5 in various solutions. Specifically, standard curves of QFeNPs at Q-Fe ratios of 1:3, 1:4, and 1:5 were created using the UV-Vis absorbance at 293 nm, which was used to quantify the concentration of NPs at each ratio. The table in Figure 5A presents the average solubility of QFeNPs from three tests by creating a saturated solution (5 mg/mL) and measuring the top absorbance after 24 h. DI water and 150 mM salt conditions exhibited a higher solubility compared to Bis-Tris and PBS. Tris and HEPES fell in between. The solubility of QFeNPs at all ratios was increased compared to free Q.

A

Buffer	Q-Fe (1:5) (mg/mL)	Q-Fe (1:4) (mg/mL)	Q-Fe (1:3) (mg/mL)
DI Water	1.07	1.65	1.45
150 mM NaCl	1.17	1.44	1.95
10 mM Tris	0.85	1.41	1.87
10 mM Bis Tris	0.73	0.69	0.82
10 mM HEPES	0.91	1.03	1.06
1xPBS	0.87	0.78	0.80

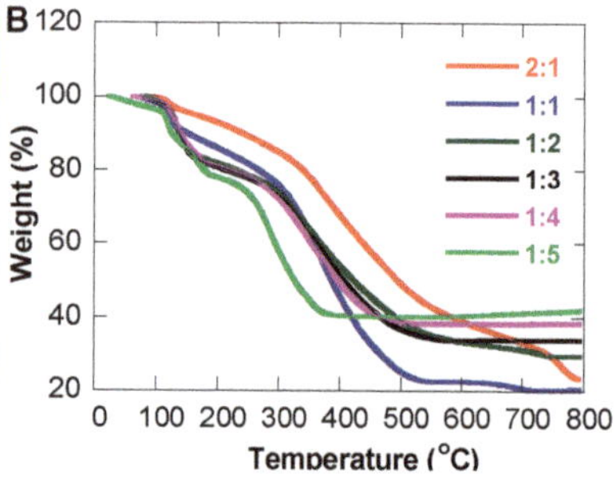

Figure 5. (**A**) Solubility of QFeNPs with Q-Fe ratios of 1:5, 1:4, and 1:3 in various solutions; and (**B**) TGA plots of QFeNPs powders with all Q-Fe ratios after freeze-drying.

In order to understand the Q-Fe ratio-dependent behaviors, TGA experiments were performed on freeze-dried QFeNPs in a nitrogen atmosphere in the temperature range from room temperature to 800 °C at a heating rate of 10 °C/min. As expected, NPs with different Q-Fe ratios exhibited distinct weight loss onsets and different decomposition behaviors, as shown in Figure 5B. No weight loss was observed for all samples below 100 °C, suggesting a lack of surface-adsorbed water molecules. The weight losses below 200 °C were mainly from complex or Fe-bound water molecules [26,50]. Depending on the Q-Fe ratios, the bound water molecules varied, and the onsets of Q decomposition were also different, with the 1:5 ratio sample being the lowest at around 250 °C until a stable weight was reached. When the weight reached a plateau, Q decomposition was complete, and iron formed inorganic compounds. X-ray diffraction analysis of QFeNP powders after heating up to 450 °C for 4 h suggests a hematite iron oxide (Fe_2O_3) phase (Figure S5), where the Fe content (70%) and O weight percentage (30%) were used to estimate the Q-Fe ratios within QFeNPs. The detailed information is presented in Table 1. For samples with a Q-Fe ratio of 2:1, the H2O-Q-Fe ratio could not be obtained because the sample continued to decompose beyond 800 °C, a similar degradation behavior to free Q molecules [24]. With increasing Fe content to 1:1 and 1:2 ratios, the sample decomposition showed two weight loss windows: a window in the range of 300–500 °C likely associated with the Q-Fe complex and another higher temperature window starting at 700 °C from the complete decomposition of free Q. For higher Fe contents, the Q decomposition only had one window with a lower stated temperature at higher Fe contents, suggesting that the Fe coordination decreased the decomposition temperature of the complex with Q-Fe ratios of 1:3, 1:4, and 1:5 which correspond to inorganic compound formation around 575, 500, and 400 °C, respectively. The calculated ratio of H2O-Q-Fe for all the samples suggests that the bound water molecules kept increasing when the Q-Fe ratios were greater than 1:1, but the Fe coordination only became saturated for the 1:5 Q-Fe ratio. Our TGA analysis (Table 1) suggests an increase in water coordination with NP formation, which could be correlated with the stability and solubility of QFeNPs.

Table 1. TGA analysis of nanoparticles with different Q-Fe ratios.

Sample	2:1	1:1		1:2		1:3		1:4		1:5	
Dehydration (°C/%)	112–131 4%	110–131 13%		118–149 20%		120–155 20%		116–160 20%		113–124 10%	159–181 10%
Q Decomposition (°C/%)	-	312–463 64%	653–715 2%	299–491 49%	702–747 3%	302–471 46%		290–442 54%		258–345 38%	
Inorganics (°C/%)	N/A	>750 °C	6% O 15% Fe	>750 °C	8% O 20% Fe	>575 °C	10% O 24% Fe	>500 °C	11% O 26% Fe	>400 °C	13% O 28% Fe
H_2O:Q:Fe	-	3:1:1.1		5.5:1:1.8		6:1:2.3		6.2:1:2.6		6.6:1:3	

3.5. Antioxidant Activity of QFeNPs

Free Q and Q-metal complexes are known to have antioxidant activities [24,25]. To study whether NP formation affects the antioxidant activity, the DPPH assay [33] was performed on QFeNPs with various Q-Fe ratios at 25, 50, and 100 μM, and the inhibition (%) was calculated and compared with free Q (Figure 6). DPPH exists in a stable free radical form at room temperature and has a strong absorbance at 517 nm. In the presence of an antioxidant molecule, DPPH will be reduced to a colorless form. Thus, the DPPH assay provides an easy way to assess the antioxidant activity of compounds by monitoring DPPH inhibition [33]. Here, we observed DPPH inhibition for QFeNPs with all ratios at three concentrations (Figure 6A). In general, the percentage of DPPH inhibition increased with increasing NP concentrations. However, compared to free Q controls, QFeNPs at lower concentrations (25 and 50 μM) showed greater antioxidant activity. However, at 100 μM, free Q exhibited higher antioxidant activity. Previous studies on Q-metal complexes with 2:1 Q-metal ratios suggest that the antioxidant activity of the complex might be metal ion dependent, similar to the lower antioxidant activities for Sb (II) and Tb (III) Q complexes [50,51] and the higher antioxidant activities for Co (II) and Pb (II) Q complexes [52–54]. The key difference of our samples from reported studies is the NP formation. We hypothesize that the NP formation could potentially affect the release rate of free Q molecules and consequently elongate the time of action. Therefore, time-dependent DPPH inhibition was performed on representative samples at 100 μM, such as QFeNPs with Q-Fe ratios of 2:1 and 1:5, compared with free Q controls for up to 6 h (Figure 6B). Within the first 30 min, the inhibition was measured every 5 min, then the inhibition was measured at 1, 2, 4, and 6 h. After around 25 min, free Q reached maximum DPPH inhibition, while the QFeNPs showed continuous inhibition and did not reach maximum inhibition after 6 h. This observation confirmed our hypothesis that NP formation can increase the release time of free Q.

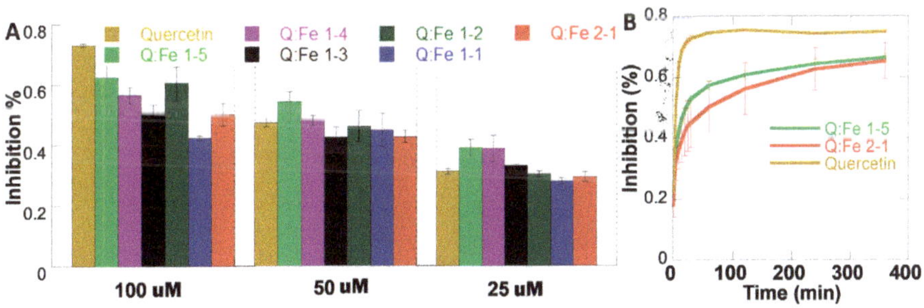

Figure 6. DPPH assay: (**A**) inhibition (%) of DPPH by free Q and QFeNPs with various Q-Fe ratios after 40 min at 100 μM, 50 μM, and 25 μM; and (**B**) time-dependent inhibition (%) of DPPH by free Q and QFeNPs with Q-Fe ratios of 2:1 and 1:5 at 100 μM.

3.6. Inhibitory Activity of QFeNPs on P-Glycoprotein Function

P-gp is an ABC membrane MDR transporter that acts as a drug efflux pump and is encoded by the gene *ABCB1* [6]. This membrane protein is known to be overexpressed in various cancer cells [6]. For example, the triple-negative and highly metastatic breast cancer cell line MDA-MB-231, after developing drug resistance, showed a much higher level of P-gp expression [55,56]. In the human body, various tissues and organs related to drug pharmacokinetics also physiologically express P-gp, such as the intestine, liver, kidney, and brain endothelial cells of the blood–brain barrier [57]. Therefore, P-gp is directly involved in the regulation of drug intestinal absorption, brain tissue penetration, and liver and renal accumulation and serves as an important factor of the drug pharmacokinetics [57]. Previous studies have shown that BECs not only have functional P-gp expression but are also able to pump out a wide range of molecules [58,59]. The functional expression of

MDR transporters in BECs was also reported [60]. First, we evaluated P-gp expression through immunostaining on two types of cells: MDA-MB231br, a variant of MDA-MB 231, and iPSC-derived BECs (iBECs), as shown in Figure 7. Cells were labeled with the anti-P-gp antibody, followed by the Alexa-488-labeled secondary antibody. Cells without the P-gp antibody treatment were used as a comparison. Significant green fluorescence was observed for P-gp antibody-labeled iBECs (Figure 7A) compared to control cells (Figure 7B), suggesting a high level of expression of P-gp in iBECs. In contrast, green fluorescence was also observed for the P-gp antibody-labeled MDA-MB-231br cells (Figure 7C) compared to the control cells (Figure 7D). However, the fluorescence levels were significantly lower than those of iBECs. This is consistent with the literature reports that only the selected resistant breast cancer cells exhibit significantly higher P-gp expression, in contrast to the original cell lines [56,57]. We have also performed viability assays on these two types of cells: MDA-Mb-23br and iBECs, to study the cytotoxicity of QFeNPs (Figure S6). Here, cells were treated with representative QFeNPs at Q-Fe ratios of 2:1 and 1:5 at 50 and/or 100 μM. Cell viability was presented as the percentage of live cells using untreated cells as a control. We did not observe a significant alteration in cell viability for both cell types. Cell viability was slightly altered in some cases, such as cells treated with 50 and 100 μM QFeNPs with Q-Fe ratios of 2:1 (Figure S6A), but statistical analyses showed that the variation was not drastic in iBECs. The viability of iBECs was similar for all treatments (Figure S6B).

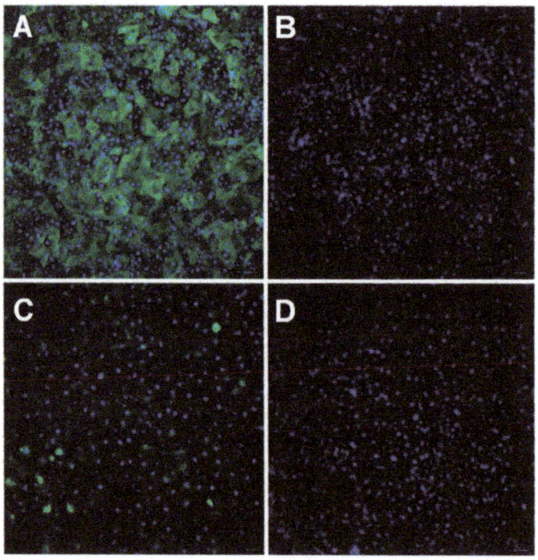

Figure 7. The immunostaining of P-gp on (**A**) iBECs labeled with P-gp antibody Alexa-488 tagged secondary antibody; (**B**) iBECs labeled only with Alexa-488 tagged secondary antibody; (**C**) MDA-Mb-231 Br labeled with P-gp antibody Alexa-488 tagged secondary antibody; and (**D**) MDA-Mb-231 Br labeled only with Alexa-488 tagged secondary antibody. Cells were observed using a 20× objective. Cell nuclei were stained with DAPI blue.

Because of the higher expression levels of P-gp in iBECs, as shown, iBECs were chosen as a model system to investigate the use of QFeNPs to modulate the function of P-gp in BECs. We tested three representative samples: free Q, samples with a Q-Fe ratio of 2:1, which formed stable complex molecules, and samples with a Q-Fe ratio of 1:5, which formed QFeNPs. The P-gp function was measured using a fluorescent substrate R123 accumulation assay [33]. The accumulation of the substrate inside the cells is an indication of the blockage of the P-gp efflux pump. We observed a trend toward increased R123 accumulation with higher concentrations of all QFeNPs (Figure 8). The R123 accumulation inside cells treated with 100 μM QFeNPs with a Q-Fe ratio of 1:5 showed statistically significant but higher R123 accumulation. Even though further detailed investigation is needed, our preliminary results suggest the contribution and effectiveness of QFeNPs in regulating P-gp function in BECs.

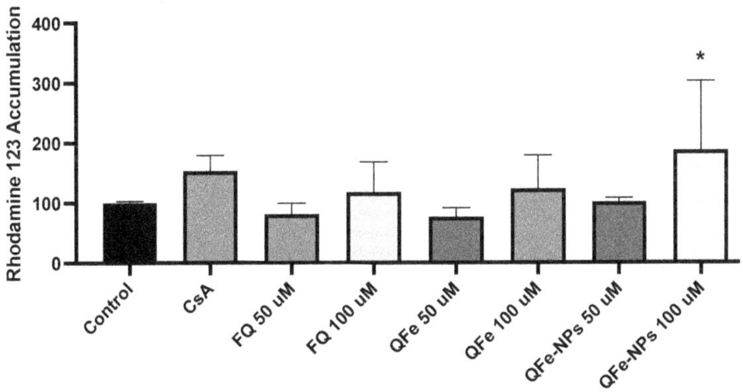

Figure 8. Rhodamine 123 accumulation inside BECs treated with free quercetin (FQ), the QFe complex with a 2:1 Q-Fe ratio, or QFeNPs with a 1:5 Q-Fe ratio at 50 μM and 100 μM along with CsA, as a positive control, and cells without treatment as a negative control. Data are presented as mean values from two independent iPSC-derived BEC differentiations conducted in triplicate ($n = 6$). Error bars represent SD. An ANOVA was used to determine significance compared to the control. * $p < 0.05$.

4. Conclusions

In conclusion, QFeNPs have been successfully synthesized with several Q-Fe ratios. The Q-Fe ratios directly affected NP formation, but UV-Vis absorbance and TGA analysis suggest that only a 1:5 Q-Fe ratio achieved full coordination of all three binding sites of Q. The QFeNPs at all Q-Fe ratios exhibited increased stability and aqueous solubility when compared to free Q. For example, QFeNPs with Q-Fe ratios of 1:3, 1:4, and 1:5 showed increased solubility (>1 mg/mL) in DI water and 150 mL of NaCl. Stability monitoring using UV-Vis spectroscopy suggests that close to full coordination of Q-Fe (1:3) made NPs more stable in buffers. For example, QFeNPs showed clear degradation in PBS and tris buffer, likely because buffer molecules (e.g., phosphate and amine groups) could interact with Fe, leading to Fe dissociation from the QFeNPs. The cellular viability tests indicated that these NPs had minimal cytotoxicity. Our preliminary cellular testing suggests that the Q-Fe nanoparticles could effectively inhibit the P-gp efflux pump in cells with high levels of P-gp expression. Therefore, these NPs have great potential for overcoming several pharmacokinetic limitations of free Q and opening possibilities for multiple purposes and different applications. The proposed NPs are based on dietary natural products for overcoming MDR in cancer treatment and have great potential for cancer prevention with less safety concern and better public acceptance. This system can be used in combination with multiple drugs to reduce side effects and increase overall efficacy and safety. Our future studies will focus on QFeNP's effectiveness in overcoming drug resistance in different drug-resistant cell lines and further understanding the anti-cancer mechanisms of natural products that can help prevent and manage many types of cancer.

Supplementary Materials: The following supporting information can be downloaded at: https://www.mdpi.com/article/10.3390/pharmaceutics15041041/s1, Figure S1: FTIR spectra of free quercetin at different PHs in the range of 2000–4000 cm^{-1}; Figure S2: Quercetin degradation process and major degradation products; Figure S3: TEM images of products formed at different Q-Fe ratios; Figure S4: UV-Vis spectra of samples with Q-Fe ratios of 2:1 and 1:2 at different processing conditions; Figure S5: XRD spectra of QFeNPs powder heated at 450 °C under argon for 2 h; Figure S6: Cell viability.

Author Contributions: Conceptualization, Y.B. and L.P.; methodology, Y.B. and L.P.; validation, L.P., S.L. and B.J.K.; formal analysis, Y.B., L.P., S.F.H., N.V. and B.J.K.; investigation, L.P., E.R.E., P.W. and R.A.H.; data curation, writing—original draft preparation, Y.B. and L.P.; writing—review and S.F.H., N.V. and B.J.K.; editing, Y.B. and L.P.; visualization, Y.B. and L.P.; supervision, Y.B.; project administration, Y.B.; funding acquisition, Y.B. All authors have read and agreed to the published version of the manuscript.

Funding: This work was supported in part by NSF-CBET 1915873 and the Breast Cancer Research Foundation of Alabama. L.P. was supported by the U.S. Department of Education as a GAANN Fellow (P200A210069).

Institutional Review Board Statement: Not applicable.

Informed Consent Statement: Not applicable.

Data Availability Statement: Not applicable.

Acknowledgments: This work was supported in part by NSF-CBET 1915873 and the Breast Cancer Research Foundation of Alabama. Y.B. acknowledges the University of Alabama Department of Biological Sciences for the use of TEM.

Conflicts of Interest: The authors declare no conflict of interest.

References

1. Schirrmacher, V. From chemotherapy to biological therapy: A review of novel concepts to reduce the side effects of systemic cancer treatment (Review). *Int. J. Oncol.* **2019**, *54*, 407–419. [CrossRef] [PubMed]
2. Bidram, E.; Esmaeili, Y.; Ranji-Burachaloo, H.; Al-Zaubai, N.; Zarrabi, A.; Stewart, A.; Dunstan, D.E. A concise review on cancer treatment methods and delivery systems. *J. Drug Deliv. Sci. Technol.* **2019**, *54*, 101350. [CrossRef]
3. Bukowski, K.; Kciuk, M.; Kontek, R. Mechanisms of multidrug resistance in cancer chemotherapy. *Int. J. Mol. Sci.* **2020**, *21*, 3233. [CrossRef] [PubMed]
4. Seelig, A. P-glycoprotein: One mechanism, many tasks and the consequences for pharmacotherapy of cancers. *Front. Oncol.* **2020**, *10*, 576559. [CrossRef] [PubMed]
5. Robinson, K.; Tiriveedhi, V. Perplexing Role of P-Glycoprotein in Tumor Microenvironment. *Front. Oncol.* **2020**, *10*, 265. [CrossRef] [PubMed]
6. Karthika, C.; Sureshkumar, R.; Zehravi, M.; Akter, R.; Ali, F.; Ramproshad, S.; Mondal, B.; Tagde, P.; Ahmed, Z.; Khan, F.S.; et al. Multidrug resistance of cancer cells and the vital role of P-glycoprotein. *Life* **2022**, *12*, 897. [CrossRef]
7. Ye, Q.; Liu, K.; Shen, Q.; Li, Q.; Hao, J.; Han, F.; Jiang, R.-W. Reversal of multidrug resistance in cancer by multi-functional flavonoids. *Front. Oncol.* **2019**, *9*, 487. [CrossRef]
8. Saraswathy, M.; Gong, S. Different strategies to overcome multidrug resistance in cancer. *Biotechnol. Adv.* **2013**, *31*, 1397–1407. [CrossRef]
9. To, K.K.; Cho, W.C. Flavonoids overcome drug resistance to cancer chemotherapy by epigenetically modulating multiple mechanisms. *Curr. Cancer Drug Targets* **2021**, *21*, 289–305. [CrossRef]
10. Liskova, A.; Samec, M.; Koklesova, L.; Brockmueller, A.; Zhai, K.; Abdellatif, B.; Siddiqui, M.; Biringer, K.; Kudela, E.; Pec, M.; et al. Flavonoids as an effective sensitizer for anti-cancer therapy: Insights into multi-faceted mechanisms and applicability towards individualized patient profiles. *EPMA J.* **2021**, *12*, 155–176. [CrossRef]
11. Khater, M.; Ravishankar, D.; Greco, F.; Osborn, H.M. Metal complexes of flavonoids: Their synthesis, characterization and enhanced antioxidant and anticancer activities. *Futur. Med. Chem.* **2019**, *11*, 2845–2867. [CrossRef] [PubMed]
12. Dong, H.; Yang, X.; He, J.; Cai, S.; Xiao, K.; Zhu, L. Enhanced antioxidant activity, antibacterial activity and hypoglycemic effect of luteolin by complexation with manganese (ii) and its inhibition kinetics on xanthine oxidase. *RSC Adv.* **2017**, *7*, 53385–53395. [CrossRef]
13. Maruszewska, A.; Tarasiuk, J. Quercetin triggers induction of apoptotic and lysosomal death of sensitive and multidrug resistant leukaemia HL60 cells. *Nutr. Cancer* **2020**, *73*, 484–501. [CrossRef]
14. Singh, A.; Patel, S.K.; Kumar, P.; Das, K.C.; Verma, D.; Sharma, R.; Tripathi, T.; Giri, R.; Martins, N.; Garg, N. Quercetin acts as a P-gp modulator via impeding signal transduction from nucleotide-binding domain to transmembrane domain. *J. Biomol. Struct. Dyn.* **2020**, *40*, 4507–4515. [CrossRef] [PubMed]
15. Zhou, Y.; Zhang, J.; Wang, K.; Han, W.; Wang, X.; Gao, M.; Wang, Z.; Sun, Y.; Yan, H.; Zhang, H.; et al. Quercetin overcomes colon cancer cells resistance to chemotherapy by inhibiting solute carrier family 1, member 5 transporter. *Eur. J. Pharmacol.* **2020**, *881*, 173185. [CrossRef] [PubMed]

16. Chen, Z.; Huang, C.; Ma, T.; Jiang, L.; Tang, L.; Shi, T.; Zhang, S.; Zhang, L.; Zhu, P.; Li, J.; et al. Reversal effect of quercetin on multidrug resistance via FZD7/β-catenin pathway in hepatocellular carcinoma cells. *Phytomedicine* **2018**, *43*, 37–45. [CrossRef] [PubMed]
17. Fang, H.; Zohaib, B.; Li, G.; Wang, L. Effect of quercetin on P-glycoprotein expression and efflux function in liver and jejunum of rat. *Acta Vet. Et Zootech. Sin.* **2018**, *49*, 422–431.
18. Cai, X.; Fang, Z.; Dou, J.; Yu, A.; Zhai, G. Bioavailability of quercetin: Problems and promises. *Curr. Med. Chem.* **2013**, *20*, 2572–2582. [CrossRef]
19. Pinheiro, R.G.R.; Pinheiro, M.; Neves, A.R. Nanotechnology Innovations to Enhance the Therapeutic Efficacy of Quercetin. *Nanomaterials* **2021**, *11*, 2658. [CrossRef]
20. Massi, A.; Bortolini, O.; Ragno, D.; Bernardi, T.; Sacchetti, G.; Tacchini, M.; De Risi, C. Research Progress in the Modification of Quercetin Leading to Anticancer Agents. *Molecules* **2017**, *22*, 1270. [CrossRef]
21. Mulholland, P.J.; Ferry, D.R.; Anderson, D.; Hussain, S.A.; Young, A.M.; Cook, J.E.; Hodgkin, E.; Seymour, L.W.; Kerr, D.J. Pre-clinical and clinical study of QC12, a water-soluble, pro-drug of quercetin. *Ann. Oncol.* **2001**, *12*, 245–248. [CrossRef] [PubMed]
22. Yuan, Z.-P.; Chen, L.-J.; Fan, L.-Y.; Tang, M.-H.; Yang, G.-L.; Yang, H.-S.; Du, X.-B.; Wang, G.-Q.; Yao, W.-X.; Zhao, Q.-M.; et al. Liposomal quercetin efficiently suppresses growth of solid tumors in murine models. *Clin. Cancer Res.* **2006**, *12*, 3193–3199. [CrossRef]
23. Zang, X.; Cheng, M.; Zhang, X.; Chen, X. Quercetin nanoformulations: A promising strategy for tumor therapy. *Food Funct.* **2021**, *12*, 6664–6681. [CrossRef]
24. da Silva, W.M.B.; Pinheiro, S.D.O.; Alves, D.R.; de Menezes, J.E.S.A.; Magalhães, F.E.A.; Silva, F.C.O.; Silva, J.; Marinho, E.S.; de Morais, S.M. Synthesis of quercetin-metal complexes, in vitro and in silico anticholinesterase and antioxidant evaluation, and in vivo toxicological and anxiolitic activities. *Neurotox. Res.* **2019**, *37*, 893–903. [CrossRef] [PubMed]
25. Ravichandran, R.; Rajendran, M.; Devapiriam, D. Antioxidant study of quercetin and their metal complex and determination of stability constant by spectrophotometry method. *Food Chem.* **2014**, *146*, 472–478. [CrossRef]
26. Raza, A.; Xu, X.; Xia, L.; Xia, C.; Tang, J.; Ouyang, Z. Quercetin-iron complex: Synthesis, characterization, antioxidant, DNA binding, DNA cleavage, and antibacterial activity studies. *J. Fluoresc.* **2016**, *26*, 2023–2031. [CrossRef] [PubMed]
27. Xu, D.; Hu, M.-J.; Wang, Y.-Q.; Cui, Y.-L. Antioxidant activities of quercetin and its complexes for medicinal application. *Molecules* **2019**, *24*, 1123. [CrossRef]
28. Shastrala, K.; Kalam, S.; Damerakonda, K.; Sheshagiri, S.B.B.; Kumar, H.; Guda, R.; Kasula, M.; Bedada, S.K. Synthesis, characterization, and pharmacological evaluation of some metal complexes of quercetin as P-gp inhibitors. *Futur. J. Pharm. Sci.* **2021**, *7*, 99. [CrossRef]
29. Liu, Y.; Guo, M. Studies on transition metal-quercetin complexes using electrospray ionization tandem mass spectrometry. *Molecules* **2015**, *20*, 8583–8594. [CrossRef]
30. Papan, P.; Kantapan, J.; Sangthong, P.; Meepowpan, P.; Dechsupa, N. Iron (III)-quercetin complex: Synthesis, physicochemical characterization, and mri cell tracking toward potential applications in regenerative medicine. *Contrast Media Mol. Imaging* **2020**, *2020*, 1–22. [CrossRef]
31. Bertleff-Zieschang, N.; Rahim, A.; Ju, Y.; Braunger, J.A.; Suma, T.; Dai, Y.; Pan, S.; Cavalieri, F.; Caruso, F. Biofunctional metal–phenolic films from dietary flavonoids. *Chem. Commun.* **2017**, *53*, 1068–1071. [CrossRef]
32. Parhi, B.; Bharatiya, D.; Swain, S.K. Application of quercetin flavonoid based hybrid nanocomposites: A review. *Saudi Pharm. J.* **2020**, *28*, 1719–1732. [CrossRef]
33. Huang, D.; Ou, B.; Prior, R.L. The Chemistry behind antioxidant capacity assays. *J. Agric. Food Chem.* **2005**, *53*, 1841–1856. [CrossRef]
34. Lippmann, E.S.; Azarin, S.M.; Kay, J.E.; Nessler, R.A.; Wilson, H.K.; Al-Ahmad, A.; Palecek, S.P.; Shusta, E.V. Derivation of blood-brain barrier endothelial cells from human pluripotent stem cells. *Nat. Biotechnol.* **2012**, *30*, 783–791. [CrossRef]
35. Stebbins, M.J.; Wilson, H.K.; Canfield, S.G.; Qian, T.; Palecek, S.P.; Shusta, E.V. Differentiation and characterization of human pluripotent stem cell-derived brain microvascular endothelial cells. *Methods* **2015**, *101*, 93–102. [CrossRef] [PubMed]
36. Endres, L.M.; Schubert-Unkmeir, A.; Kim, B.J. Neisseria meningitidis infection of induced pluripotent stem-cell derived brain endothelial cells. *J. Vis. Exp.* **2020**, *161*, e61400. [CrossRef]
37. Espinal, E.R.; Sharp, S.; Kim, B.J. Induced pluripotent stem cell (iPSC)-derived endothelial cells to study bacteri-al-brain endothelial cell interactions. *Methods Mol. Biol.* **2022**, *2492*, 73–101.
38. Forster, S.; Thumser, A.E.; Hood, S.R.; Plant, N. Characterization of Rhodamine-123 as a tracer dye for use in in vitro drug transport assays. *PLoS ONE* **2012**, *7*, e33253. [CrossRef] [PubMed]
39. Leopoldini, M.; Russo, N.; Toscano, M. The molecular basis of working mechanism of natural polyphenolic antioxidants. *Food Chem.* **2011**, *125*, 288–306. [CrossRef]
40. Kasprzak, M.M.; Erxleben, A.; Ochocki, J. Properties and applications of flavonoid metal complexes. *RSC Adv.* **2015**, *5*, 45853–45877. [CrossRef]
41. Lee, Y.-H.; Tuyet, P.-T. Synthesis and biological evaluation of quercetin–zinc (II) complex for anti-cancer and anti-metastasis of human bladder cancer cells. *Vitr. Cell. Dev. Biol.-Anim.* **2019**, *55*, 395–404. [CrossRef] [PubMed]

42. de Castilho, T.S.; Matias, T.B.; Nicolini, K.P.; Nicolini, J. Study of interaction between metal ions and quercetin. *Food Sci. Hum. Wellness* **2018**, *7*, 215–219. [CrossRef]
43. Ramešová, S.; Sokolová, R.; Degano, I.; Bulíčková, J.; Zabka, J.; Gál, M. On the stability of the bioactive flavonoids quercetin and luteolin under oxygen-free conditions. *Anal. Bioanal. Chem.* **2012**, *402*, 975–982. [CrossRef]
44. Porto, I.C.C.M.; Nascimento, T.G.; Oliveira, J.M.S.; Freitas, P.H.; Haimeur, A.; França, R. Use of polyphenols as a strategy to prevent bond degradation in the dentin-resin interface. *Eur. J. Oral Sci.* **2018**, *126*, 146–158. [CrossRef] [PubMed]
45. Baranović, G.; Šegota, S. Infrared spectroscopy of flavones and flavonols. Reexamination of the hydroxyl and carbonyl vibrations in relation to the interactions of flavonoids with membrane lipids. Spectrochim. *Acta Part A Mol. Biomol. Spectrosc.* **2018**, *192*, 473–486. [CrossRef]
46. Qiao, L.; Sun, Y.; Chen, R.; Fu, Y.; Zhang, W.; Li, X.; Chen, J.; Shen, Y.; Ye, X. Sonochemical effects on 14 flavonoids common in citrus: Relation to stability. *PLoS ONE* **2014**, *9*, e87766. [CrossRef]
47. Ryan, P.; Hynes, M.J. The kinetics and mechanisms of the reactions of iron(III) with quercetin and morin. *J. Inorg. Biochem.* **2008**, *102*, 127–136. [CrossRef]
48. Salehi, B.; Machin, L.; Monzote, L.; Sharifi-Rad, J.; Ezzat, S.M.; Salem, M.A.; Merghany, R.M.; El Mahdy, N.M.; Kılıç, C.S.; Sytar, O.; et al. Therapeutic potential of quercetin: New insights and perspectives for human health. *ACS Omega* **2020**, *5*, 11849–11872. [CrossRef]
49. Tang, S.-M.; Deng, X.-T.; Zhou, J.; Li, Q.-P.; Ge, X.-X.; Miao, L. Pharmacological basis and new insights of quercetin action in respect to its anti-cancer effects. *Biomed. Pharmacother.* **2020**, *121*, 109604. [CrossRef]
50. Kalinowska, M.; Świderski, G.; Matejczyk, M.; Lewandowski, W. Spectroscopic, thermogravimetric and biological studies of Na(I), Ni(II) and Zn(II) complexes of quercetin. *J. Therm. Anal. Calorim.* **2016**, *126*, 141–148. [CrossRef]
51. Tong, L.; Zhang, J.; Liu, Q.; Zhai, G. Sb(IIII)-quercetin complex: Synthesis, characterization and antioxidant activity. *Life Sci. J.* **2016**, *13*, 127–133.
52. Cherrak, S.A.; Mokhtari-Soulimane, N.; Berroukeche, F.; Bensenane, B.; Cherbonnel, A.; Merzouk, H.; Elhabiri, M. In vitro antioxidant versus metal ion chelating properties of flavonoids: A structure-activity investigation. *PLoS ONE* **2016**, *11*, e0165575. [CrossRef] [PubMed]
53. Kalinowska, M.; Lewandowska, H.; Pruszyński, M.; Świderski, G.; Gołębiewska, E.; Gryko, K.; Braun, J.; Borkowska, M.; Konieczna, M.; Lewandowski, W. Co(II) complex of quercetin–spectral, anti-/pro-oxidant and cytotoxic activity in HaCaT cell lines. *Appl. Sci.* **2021**, *11*, 9244. [CrossRef]
54. Dolatabadi, J.E.N.; Mokhtarzadeh, A.; Ghareghoran, S.M.; Dehghan, G. Synthesis, Characterization and antioxidant property of quercetin-Tb(III) complex. *Adv. Pharm. Bull.* **2013**, *4*, 101–104. [CrossRef]
55. Mutoh, K.; Tsukahara, S.; Mitsuhashi, J.; Katayama, K.; Sugimoto, Y. Estrogen-mediated post transcriptional down-regulation of P-glycoprotein in MDR1-transduced human breast cancer cells. *Cancer Sci.* **2006**, *97*, 1198–1204. [CrossRef]
56. Bao, L.; Hazari, S.; Mehra, S.; Kaushal, D.; Moroz, K.; Dash, S. Increased Expression of P-Glycoprotein and Doxorubicin Chemoresistance of Metastatic Breast Cancer Is Regulated by miR-298. *Am. J. Pathol.* **2012**, *180*, 2490–2503. [CrossRef]
57. Staud, F.; Ceckova, M.; Micuda, S.; Pavek, P. Expression and function of p-glycoprotein in normal tissues: Effect on pharmacokinetics. *Methods Mol. Biol.* **2010**, *596*, 199–222. [PubMed]
58. Tsuji, A.; Terasaki, T.; Takabatake, Y.; Tenda, Y.; Tamai, I.; Yamashima, T.; Moritani, S.; Tsuruo, T.; Yamashita, J. P-glycoprotein as the drug efflux pump in primary cultured bovine brain capillary endothelial cells. *Life Sci.* **1992**, *51*, 1427–1437. [CrossRef] [PubMed]
59. Löscher, W.; Potschka, H. Blood-brain barrier active efflux transporters: ATP-binding cassette gene family. *NeuroRx* **2005**, *2*, 86–98. [CrossRef]
60. Lye, P.; Bloise, E.; Imperio, G.E.; Chitayat, D.; Matthews, S.G. Functional expression of multidrug-resistance (MDR) trans-porters in developing human fetal brain endothelial cells. *Cells* **2022**, *11*, 2259. [CrossRef]

pharmaceutics

MDPI

Article

Eluxadoline-Loaded Eudragit Nanoparticles for Irritable Bowel Syndrome with Diarrhea: Formulation, Optimization Using Box–Behnken Design, and Anti-Diarrheal Activity

Md. Khalid Anwer [1,*], Mohammed Muqtader Ahmed [1], Mohammed F. Aldawsari [1], Muzaffar Iqbal [2,3], Gamal A. Soliman [4,5] and Ibrahim A. Aljuffali [6]

1 Department of Pharmaceutics, College of Pharmacy, Prince Sattam Bin Abdulaziz University, Al-Kharj 11942, Saudi Arabia
2 Department of Pharmaceutical Chemistry, College of Pharmacy, King Saud University, Riyadh 11451, Saudi Arabia
3 Bioavailability Laboratory, College of Pharmacy, King Saud University, Riyadh 11451, Saudi Arabia
4 Department of Pharmacology and Toxicology, College of Pharmacy, Prince Sattam Bin Abdulaziz University, Al-Kharj 11942, Saudi Arabia
5 Department of Pharmacology, College of Veterinary Medicine, Cairo University, Giza 12613, Egypt
6 Department of Pharmaceutics, College of Pharmacy, King Saud University, Riyadh 11451, Saudi Arabia
* Correspondence: m.anwer@psau.edu.sa

Abstract: Eluxadoline (ELD), a recently approved drug, exhibits potential therapeutic effects in the management and treatment of IBS-D. However, its applications have been limited due to poor aqueous solubility, leading to a low dissolution rate and oral bioavailability. The current study's goals are to prepare ELD-loaded eudragit (EG) nanoparticles (ENPs) and to investigate the anti-diarrheal activity on rats. The prepared ELD-loaded EG-NPs (ENP1-ENP14) were optimized with the help of Box–Behnken Design Expert software. The developed formulation (ENP2) was optimized based on the particle size (286 ± 3.67 nm), PDI (0.263 ± 0.01), and zeta potential (31.8 ± 3.18 mV). The optimized formulation (ENP2) exhibited a sustained release behavior with maximum drug release and followed the Higuchi model. The chronic restraint stress (CRS) was successfully used to develop the IBS-D rat model, which led to increased defecation frequency. The in vivo studies revealed a significant reduction in defecation frequency and disease activity index by ENP2 compared with pure ELD. Thus, the results demonstrated that the developed eudragit-based polymeric nanoparticles can act as a potential approach for the effective delivery of eluxadoline through oral administration for irritable bowel syndrome diarrhea treatment.

Keywords: eluxadoline; eudragit; optimization; dissolution; defecation frequency; disease activity index

1. Introduction

Irritable bowel syndrome (IBS) is one of the common types of gastrointestinal disorders, having a global incidence of 11–15% [1,2]. The most common symptoms of IBS include systematic pain in the abdominal region related to the alterations in the frequency of stools and are categorized depending upon the major stool patterns: IBS-diarrhea (IBS-D), IBS-constipation, both mixed, or uncategorized. Amongst all these, the most common category is IBS, which comprises nearly 45–50% of all cases of IBS [3]. Studies have reported limited therapeutic strategies for the effective management of IBS-D. Conventional therapeutic strategies involve anti-diarrheals and modifications in the diet, as well as lifestyle, of the patient. A negative impact is observed in the quality of life of the patients due to IBS-D, surpassing the quality-of-life deteriorations observed in asthmatic, gastrointestinal reflux diseases [4,5], and even IBS constipation [6]. Numerous comorbid circumstances have been related with IBS, such as fibromyalgia, migraine headaches, interstitial cystitis, major depression, anxiety, and others [7]. IBS-D executes a considerable financial burden on society and financiers due to augmented healthcare uses [8–10].

Loperamide (LPM) is one of the most used therapeutics for the effective management of IBS-D. LPM is a peripherally acting m-opioid receptor (m-OR) agonist that pharmacologically reduces the gut motility and enhances fluid re-absorption [11,12]. However, LPM is not directed for long-term usage and does not regulate abdominal pain or swelling [13–15]. Thus, there is substantial necessity for new and effective therapies with promising safety profiles exhibiting potential effects of long-term reprieve from symptoms of IBS-D patients.

Eluxadoline (ELD) is local-acting and exhibits diverse pharmacological effects, including m-OR and kappa opioid receptor agonists and delta opioid receptor antagonists. It exerts negligible oral bioavailability yet is officially approved by the United States Food and Drug Administration for IBS-D treatment [16]. Due to its collective pharmacological properties, ELD (Figure 1) significantly decreases the gut motility and reduces the probabilities of drug-induced constipation issues. Studies, including the animal models, have demonstrated that the combinatorial dosage of a d-opioid receptor antagonist and an l-opioid receptor agonist significantly improves its effects on intuitive sensations, while reduces the possibility of constipation [17,18]. These exclusive properties differentiate ELD from peripherally acting m-OR agonists such as LPR [18]. ELD is commercially available in tablet dosage form (75 and 100 mg) for treating IBS-D, but other dosage forms, including capsules and liquid systems for pediatric usage, are commercially unavailable [19].

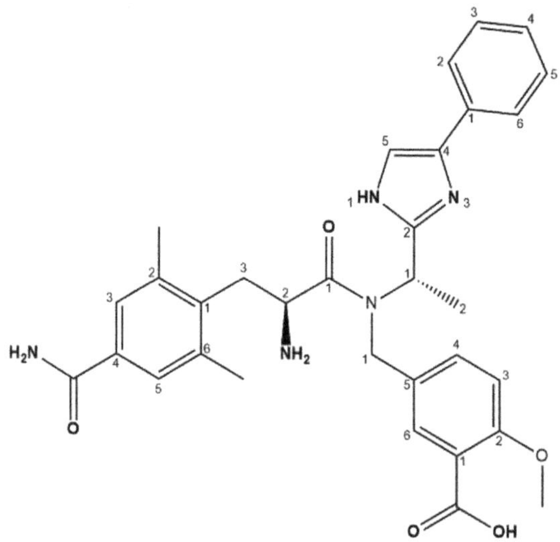

Figure 1. Chemical structure of eluxadoline.

More importantly, ELD shows poor bioavailability, primarily due to poor aqueous solubility, restricted absorption, and first-pass metabolism, and thus its frequent use is limited [20]. Thus, a novel and targeted therapeutic strategy is necessary to improve the solubility, permeability, and oral bioavailability of ELD, with reduced or negligible toxicity profiles, for the effective management of IBS-D. Nanotechnology-derived therapeutic strategies, including polymeric nanocarriers, lipid-based nanoparticles, metallic nanoparticles, and others have shown immense potential for delivering therapeutics to targeted disease sites with controlled release behavior, particularly for delivering drugs with low oral bioavailability [21].

Polymeric nanocarrier systems have shown immense potential and have attracted significant interest over recent years owing to their diverse characteristics [22,23]. Several drugs have been successfully delivered using the nanoencapsulation of drugs, which has been shown to increase solubility, protect against toxicity, increase pharmacological activity and stability, provide sustained release, provide physical protection, and protect against chemical degradation [23–26]. Amongst various polymers, eudragit is one of the most used polymers for the fabrication of drug-loaded polymeric systems. Eudragit exhibits protective effects against the environmental moisture, masks the smells/flavors, and also shows versatility, subsequently due to the choice of a precise type as per the required delivery system, i.e., sustained, immediate, or controlled. Moreover, it is also well-defined as a pH-sensitive polymer due to its solubilizing abilities at varying pH values [27,28].

The aim of the current study was to enhance the oral bioavailability of ELD through loading into eudragit nanoparticles and to investigate the ability of ELD-loaded EG-NPs' (ENPs) effective treatment of IBS-D. The optimization of developed formulations was performed using Box–Behnken Design Expert software, considering independent variables such as weight of eudragit polymer, PVA (%w/v), and sonication time and dependent variables such as particle size, polydispersity index, and zeta potential. The optimized ELD-loaded EG-NPs (ENP2) were finally evaluated for different pharmaceutical attributes and their ability to improve the oral efficacy against irritable bowel syndrome with diarrhea.

2. Materials and Methods

2.1. Materials

Eluxadoline (ELD) was procured from Mesochem Technology Co., Ltd., Beijing, China. The poly (vinyl alcohol) and eudragit RS100 were purchased from Sigma-Aldrich (St. Louis, MO, USA). Analytical grade chemicals and reagents were employed throughout the experiment.

2.2. Box–Behnken Design (BBD) Optimization

A Box–Behnken response surface approach experimental design (Design-Expert® Software Version 13) was used to optimize the eluxadoline-loaded eudragit nanoparticles (ENPs) (3 factors, 3 levels). The independent variables selected were: the weight of the eudragit polymer (X1), %w/v, PVA (X2), and sonication time (X3), with their high, medium, and low levels for the preparation of 14 formulations, as shown in Table 1. Particle size (Y1), polydispersity index (Y2), and zeta potential (Y3) were the responses that were examined. Additionally, 3D response surface graphs were plotted to show how the specified factors affected the responses that were measured.

Table 1. Variables for the development of formulations.

Independent Variables	Levels		
	Low (−1)	Medium (0)	High (+1)
X1 = Eudragit (mg)	100	200	300
X2 = PVA (%w/v)	0.1	0.3	0.5
X3 = Sonication time (min.)	3	6	9
Responses	**Target to**		
Y1 = Size (nm)	Minimum size		
Y2 = PDI	Minimum PDI		
Y3 = Zeta potential	Maximum zeta potential		

2.3. Preparation of Eluxodoline-Loaded Eudragit Nanoparticles (ENPs)

ELD-loaded EG-NPs (ENPs) were prepared by the emulsion solvent diffusion method, using different proportions of EG (polymer) and PVA (stabilizer). The disperse phase consisted of ELD and EG in 5 mL of dichloromethane, which was further added in the PVA aqueous phase (10 mL) using a probe sonicator (ultrasonic processor, Fisher scientific, Waltham, MA, USA) at 65% W with 5 s on/off for 3 to 9 min. Thereafter, continuous stirring took place for 24 h at 1000 rpm using a magnetic stirrer. The prepared nanoparticles were collected by filtration and freeze dried (Millirock Technology, Kingston, NY, USA) and finally packed for further evaluations in a sealed vial.

2.4. Measurement of Particle Size, PDI, and Zeta Potential

The average particle size and PDI of all the developed formulations (ENP1-ENP14) were estimated using a Malvern zetasizer (ZEN-3600, Malvern Instruments Ltd., Worcestershire, WR14 1XZ, UK) at 25 ± 2 °C. The colloidal suspension of ENPs was diluted with deionized water (200 times) with a refractive index of 1.33 and a dielectric constant of 78.5; an angle of angle of measurement was set at 90° to incident laser light, ultrasonicated for 10 min, then the diluted sample (1.5 mL) was kept in the sample holder of the instrument in a disposable plastic cuvette, after which the particle size and PDI were measured three times. The zeta potential (ZP) of ENPs was measured following the same procedure, except using a glass electrode cuvette in the place of the glass cuvette [29]. The data were analyzed using a software DTS V–4.1 (Malvern, UK) equipped with the system; the measurements were performed in triplicate.

2.5. Drug Encapsulation

The drug encapsulation (%DE) in ELD-loaded EG-NPs (ENP2) was determined indirectly by estimating the supernatant after centrifugation at 15,000 rpm for 10 min. The drug in the filtrate was then quantified using the HPLC technique [30]. The ratio between the amount of drug encapsulated in the nanoparticles and the amount added to prepare NPs was used to calculate the %DE. The experiment was carried out three times.

$$\%\text{DE} = \frac{\text{ELD added in NPs} - \text{ELD in supernatant}}{\text{ELD added in NPs}}$$

2.6. DSC Analysis

DSC spectra of pure ELD, optimized ELD-loaded EG NPs (ENP2), eudragit (EG), and PVA were taken by a DSC thermal analyzer using Scinco N650 (made in Korea, Scinco, Seoul, South Korea). The sample (5 mg) was cramped into a hemispherical aluminum pan and placed beside a reference (empty pan) in the sample holder, supplied with nitrogen (20 mL/min), and heated at a rate of 20 °C in the temperature range of 50–300 °C.

2.7. FTIR Studies

FTIR studies assisted in estimating the probability of the interaction of the drug with the excipients. Initially, a blank sample of potassium bromide (KBr) was run to eliminate the background errors. Further, pure ELD, EG, PVA, and the optimized formulation (ENP2) were mixed separately with KBr, physically compressed to form a transparent film, and analyzed within a wavelength range of 4000–400 cm^{-1} (Jasco 4600 Mid-IR FTIR spectrometer, Jasco, Tokyo, Japan).

2.8. In Vitro Drug Release Studies

In vitro drug release studies were performed to analyze the drug release behavior and the release mechanism of the optimized formulation. The analysis of pure ELD and the optimized formulation (ENP2) were determined using the dialysis membrane method. The pure ELD and ENP2 (5 mL) were loaded into the dialysis bag (Spectra/Por® Standard RC Tubing, MWCO 12 KDa) and tied at both ends. Then, the bags were dipped into a beaker containing a dissolution medium of pH 1.2 and pH 6.8 (200 mL), maintained at a temperature of 37 ± 2 °C, and kept under stirring at 100 rpm. At pre-estimated time intervals, 0.5 mL aliquots were withdrawn from each beaker and the sink condition was maintained by adding fresh media [31]. Furthermore, the aliquots were analyzed for drug content by the HPLC method and the percent drug release was calculated and plotted against the time. [30]. All the studies were performed in triplicate (n = 3). Additionally, the drug release mechanism of ELD from the optimized formulation at pH (1.2 and 6.8) was estimated by fitting the drug release results into different mathematical modeling, including zero order, first order, Higuchi, and Korsmeyer–Peppas kinetics models [32,33].

2.9. SEM Studies

The surface morphology of optimized NPs (ENP2) was visualized using SEM (Zeiss EVO LS10, Cambridge, UK) by using the gold sputter method. The imaging was performed after the sample was coated with gold and put in a stub.

2.10. Effect on Irritable Bowel Syndrome in Rats

2.10.1. Animals

A total of 30 Wistar albino male rats weighing between 110 and 120 g were obtained from the lab animal unit, College of Pharmacy, University of Prince Sattam bin Abdulaziz. The animals were maintained in ventilated cages (Rat IVC Blue Line, Techniplast, Buguggiate VA, Italy) in controlled environmental conditions (25 ± 1 °C and 12 h/12 h light/dark cycle). All rats were fed a standard rat pellet and water ad libitum.

2.10.2. Induction of Irritable Bowel Syndrome (IBS) Model

In this study, the IBS rat model was induced by chronic restraint stress (CRS) as described by Lu et al. [34]. All rats were randomly divided into two groups (24 rats in the model group and 6 rats in the control group) after 7 days of adaptation. The rats in the model group were subjected to CRS using an elastic bandage to restrict the movement of the upper body and forelimbs and then anesthetized with ether. Their fore shoulders, upper forelimbs, and thoracic trunk were wrapped in elastic bandage for 2 h each day for 14 days to produce a steady and consistent amount of stimulation to restrict but not prevent movement. The control animals were anesthetized with ether but not restrained.

Grouping and Administration

The rats were divided into five groups (n = 6) as follows:

1. Normal control group (NC): normal rats received saline (1 mL/kg).
2. IBS control group (IBS-C): CRS rats received saline (1 mL/kg).
3. Reference group (REF): CRS rats received loperamide (LRD) at 10 mg/kg.
4. Pure drug group (ELD-std): CRS rats received (20 mg/kg).
5. Formulation group (ENP2): CRS rats received (20 mg/kg).

Treatments were administered orally, started 6 h after IBS induction, and continued for 14 consecutive days. Body weights were recorded daily.

2.10.3. Evaluation of Fecal Parameters

After 14 days of treatment, stool frequency and the wet weight of fecal pellets were recorded per rat over 12 h. The stool frequency of each rat was measured at 2 h intervals for 12 h (e.g., 0–2 h, 2–4 h, 4–6 h, etc.). The wet fecal pellets were weighed, desiccated in an oven (50 °C, 6 h), and weighed again (dry weight in mg). The ratio of the wet to dry weights was calculated and used as a marker of fecal water content according to the following equation:

$$\text{Water content}(\%) = \frac{\text{wet weight} - \text{dry weight}}{\text{wet weight}} \times 100$$

2.10.4. Disease Activity Index (DAI)

According to Murthy et al. [35], the disease activity index (DAI) was calculated as follows: total score (body weight loss + stool consistency + rectal hemorrhage)/3. Scores were given based on the percentage of weight loss (none = 0; 1–5% = 1; 5–10% = 2; 10–15% = 3; >15% = 4), stool consistency (normal = 0; pasty stool that does not stick to the anus = 1; pasty stool that does not stick to the anus = 2; pasty stool that stuck to the anus = 3; watery stool = 4), and rectal bleeding (hemoccult (-) = 0; hemoccult (±) = 1; hemoccult (+) = 2; hemoccult (++) = 3; obvious blood in stool = 4).

2.11. Statistical Analysis

The mean and standard error (SEM) of the mean were used to express the results. One-way analysis of variance (ANOVA) was used to assess the statistical variances among the various treatment groups and the post hoc Tukey's test was used to confirm the results. Statistics were deemed significant at $p < 0.05$. The GraphPad Prism application (version 4) was used to perform statistical analysis (GraphPad Software, San Diego, CA, USA).

3. Results

3.1. Box–Behnken Design (BBD) Optimization

By using the Box–Behnken Design (BBD), the current study improved the development of eluxadoline-loaded eudragit nanoparticles (ENPs) using the emulsion solvent diffusion method with varying proportions of eudragit (polymer) and polyvinyl alcohol (stabilizer). The particle size, PDI, and zeta potential (ZP) of the developed ENPs were examined as dependent factors in order to achieve the optimized formulation by BBD; these characteristics are shown in Table 2. The equation in terms of coded factors can be used to make predictions regarding the response for the given levels of each factor. The coded equation is useful for identifying the relative impact of the factors by comparing the factor coefficients [36]. The quadratic model was used to examine all dependent variables and 3D surface plots of the results were produced. The statistical analysis of the quadratic model discovered significant p-values, indicating a best fit for chosen responses (Table 3).

Table 2. Developed formulations and observed responses.

Formulae (ENPs)	Eudragit (mg)	PVA (%*w*/*v*)	Sonication Time (min.)	Particle Size (nm)	PDI	ZP (mV)
ENP1	300	0.3	3	523 ± 5.43	0.321 ± 0.05	36.1 ± 1.23
ENP2	200	0.5	9	286 ± 3.67	0.263 ± 0.01	31.8 ± 3.18
ENP3	300	0.1	6	534 ± 8.24	0.321 ± 0.06	33.6 ± 4.60
ENP4	300	0.5	6	421 ± 6.55	0.276 ± 0.02	34.4 ± 2.94
ENP5	200	0.3	6	327 ± 4.83	0.176 ± 0.09	30.2 ± 3.21
ENP6	100	0.1	6	531 ± 6.51	0.31 ± 0.02	20.7 ± 5.27
ENP7	200	0.3	6	327 ± 2.36	0.176 ± 0.09	35.2 ± 3.21
ENP8	200	0.5	3	563 ± 4.57	0.286 ± 0.12	34.8 ± 4.44
ENP9	100	0.3	3	575 ± 9.41	0.267 ± 0.11	18.8 ± 3.84
ENP10	300	0.3	9	348 ± 5.25	0.273 ± 0.03	34.1 ± 3.21
ENP11	200	0.1	3	634 ± 3.69	0.312 ± 0.12	25.6 ± 6.52
ENP12	100	0.5	6	541 ± 8.37	0.298 ± 0.16	21.7 ± 6.31
ENP13	100	0.3	9	349 ± 6.95	0.269 ± 0.06	22.3 ± 5.48
ENP14	200	0.1	9	441 ± 8.89	0.297 ± 0.07	32.3 ± 2.63

Table 3. ANOVA data of the quadratic models.

Responses (Y)	R^2	Adjusted R^2	Predicted R^2	Adequate Precision	SD	%CV	*p* Value
Y1	0.9857	0.9673	0.7708	18.90	20.70	4.70	Significant
Y2	0.9983	0.9734	0.8135	21.61	0.0093	3.61	Significant
Y3	0.9439	0.8719	0.6793	10.89	2.00	6.78	Significant

3.1.1. The Effect of Independent Variables on Response Particle Size (Y1)

The selected independent factors affected the size of developed ENPs; the average size of several batches of formulations ranged from 286 to 634 nm, as shown in Table 2. The mathematical relationship between independent variables and particle size of developed ENPs is seen in the following polynomial Equation (1), that can be used to determine how factors and particle size are correlated using the coded equation.

$$Y1 = +327.00 - 21.25\,A - 41.12\,B - 108.88C - 30.75\,AB + 12.75\,AC - 21.00\,BC + 73.75\,A^2 + 106.00\,B^2 + 48.00\,C^2 \quad (1)$$

According to response Y1, the above equation reflects the quantitative effects of independent variables (A, B, and C) and their interactions in terms of AB, AC, and BC. In this case A, B, C, AB, A^2, B^2, and C^2 are significant ($p < 0.05$) model terms. The model's model F-value of 53.51 ($p < 0.05$) proved that it was significant. A negative impact is indicated by the minus sign of the coefficient (A, B, and C), showing that the particle size decreased with the decrease in the concentration of EG, PVA, and sonication time. The predicted R^2 of 0.7708 is in reasonable agreement with the adjusted R^2 of 0.9673, i.e., the difference is less than 0.2 (Table 1). Adequate precision measures the signal to noise ratio. A ratio greater than 4 is desirable. The adequate precision of 18.90 indicates an adequate signal. This model can be used to navigate the design space.

With the use of a 3D-response surface graph, interaction patterns were examined. It is clear from the 3D-response surface graph in Figure 2 that the concentrations of PVA and sonication time had a substantial impact on the particle size of ENPs. The particle size decreased with the increase in PVA concentration and sonication time.

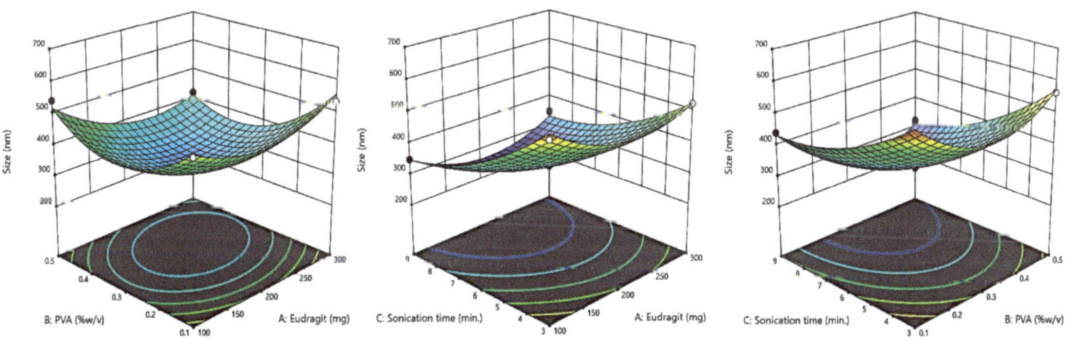

Figure 2. A 3D plot showing the effect of independent variables on particle size.

3.1.2. The Effect of Independent Variables on Response PDI (Y2)

Table 2 lists the influence of independent variables on the PDI of various formulations. The experimental setup demonstrated that the quadratic model was the one that suited the data the best. The model was clearly fitted, as evidenced by the F-value of 65.96. The predicted R^2 of 0.8135 was in reasonable agreement with the adjusted R^2 of 0.9734, i.e., the difference was less than 0.2. Adequate precision measures the signal to noise ratio. A ratio greater than 4 is desirable. The ratio of 21.612 indicated an adequate signal. This model can be used to navigate the design space. Figure 3 shows graphs of the 3D actual and expected values of PDI, illustrating how the independent factors affected the PDI and showing how closely the two variables were related.

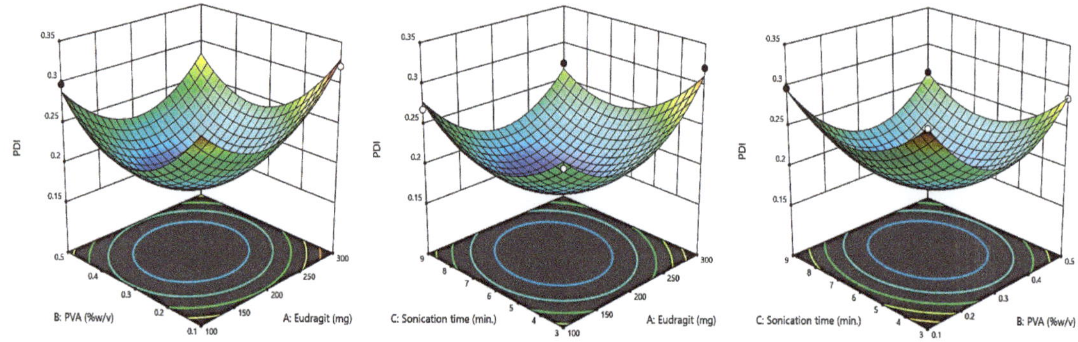

Figure 3. A 3D plot showing the effect of independent variables on PDI.

$$Y2 = +0.1760 + 0.0059\,A - 0.0146\,B - 0.0105\,C - 0.0083\,AB - 0.0020\,AC + 0.0591\,A^2 + 0.0661\,B^2 + 0.0474\,C^2 \quad (2)$$

3.1.3. The Effect of Independent Variables on Response ZP (Y3)

The surface charges of the ENP formulations with ELD loading ranged from 18.8 ± 3.84 to 36.1 ± 1.23 (Table 2). The presence of freely ionized amino groups, which are required for electrostatic repulsion between particles to generate stable nano-dispersions, was shown by the positive charge on the surface of the NPs. The mathematical representation of the measured response, Y3, as a polynomial equation is listed below. The stability of the developed formulations, where the nanoparticles have a tendency to de-aggregate rather than assemble, was significantly impacted by these high zeta potential values. The model F-value of 19.69 implied the model is significant. There was only a 0.04% chance that an F-value this large could occur due to noise. Figure 4 shows graphs of the 3D actual and expected values of zeta potential, illustrating how the independent factors affected the zeta potential.

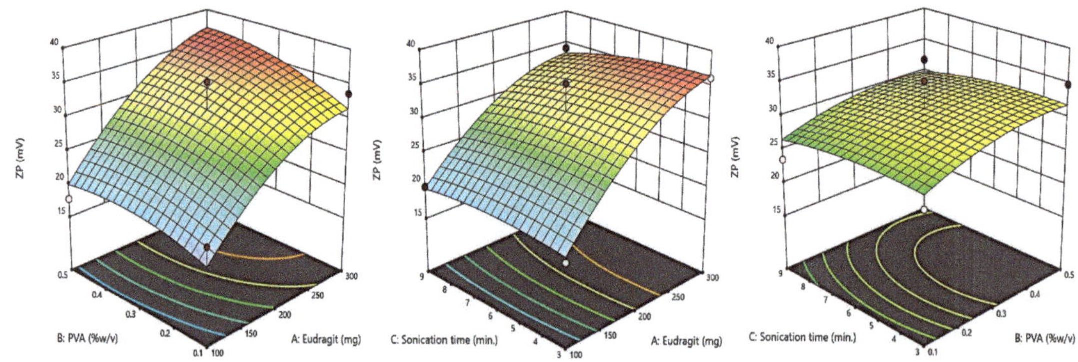

Figure 4. A 3D plot showing the effect of independent variables on zeta potential.

$$Y3 = +31.20 + 6.84\,A + 1.31\,B + 0.6500\,C - 0.0500\,AB - 1.38\,AC - 2.42\,BC - 3.45\,A^2 - 0.1500\,B^2 + 0.0750\,C^2 \quad (3)$$

For the analysis of particle size, PDI, and zeta potential, the obtained data suggested a quadratic model, which is shown in Table 3. The difference between adjusted and predicted R^2 values for the investigated responses were less than 0.2, indicating a reasonable degree of agreement in the study design [37]. The particle size, PDI, and ZP of developed ENPs measured in the range of 286 to 634 nm, 0.263 to 0.321, and 18.8 to 36.1 mV, respectively (Table 2).

3.2. Selection of Optimized Formulation

The ideal composition for the development of the optimized ELD-loaded EG-NP (ENP2) was identified by imposing constraints on the particle size, PDI, and ZP (Table 2); expert design software suggested an optimized composition with overall desirability 1.000. The software suggested an optimized formulation (ENP2) having a composition of eudragit (200 mg), PVA (0.5%, *w*/*v*), and sonication time (9 min.) The optimized formulation (ENP2) exhibited the particle size (286 ± 3.67 nm), PDI (0.263 ± 0.01) (Figure 5), and ZP (31.8 ± 3.18 mV) (Table 2).

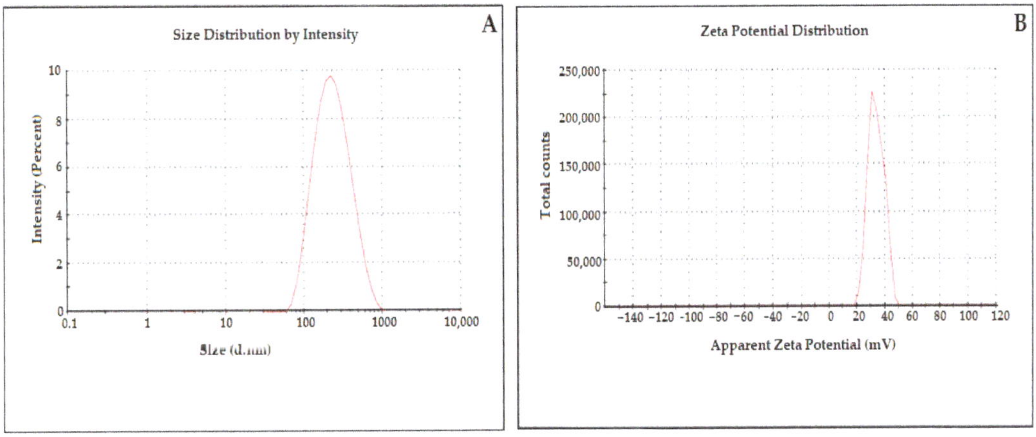

Figure 5. Particle size (**A**) and zeta potential (**B**) of optimized formulation (ENP2).

3.3. Measurement of Particle Size, PDI, and Zeta Potential

Polymeric NPs must have a small particle size, low PDI, and high ZP values for the effective biodistribution of a drug [38]. The prepared ELD-loaded EG-NPs (ENP1-ENP14) were found to have a mean particle size in the range of 286–634 nm, PDI values between 0.176 and 0.321, and ZP between 18.8 and 36.1 mV. Based on particle characterization, ELD-loaded EG-NPs (ENP2) were optimized with particle size (286 ± 3.67 nm), PDI (0.263 ± 0.01) (Figure 5), and ZP (37.7 ± 3.18) (Table 2). The homogeneity of the particles in a nanocarrier system is shown by the PDI. Therefore, a good nanocarrier system should have a low PDI to deliver the drug and to increase oral bioavailability. The particles were considered extremely homogeneous, with a PDI value of 0.3 [39,40]. High zeta potential values were determined for each formulation, demonstrating the produced NPs having high stability. The ammonium quaternary groups of the eudragit, as was previously mentioned, caused the surface of the NPs to be positively charged [41,42]. The positively charged nanocarrier was typically advantageous due to its interactions with the negatively charged mucosal membrane. The drug that was encapsulated showed the prolonged residence time due to electrostatic interaction with the mucosal membrane in the small intestine [43].

3.4. Drug Encapsulation

The stability of the polymer matrix and the way the drug interacts with it both have a role in drug entrapment. The %DE of ELD-loaded EG-NPs (ENP2) showed 82.35 ± 4.1%.

3.5. DSC Analysis

The DSC spectra of pure ELD, EG, PVA, and optimized ELD-loaded EG NPs (ENP2) were analyzed; the results are shown in Figure 6. The DSC spectra of ELD showed characteristic endothermic peaks at 118, 158, and 183 °C, as reported in the literature [42]. The DSC spectra of eudragit RS100 exhibited two endothermic peaks at 60 °C and 195 °C, related to water loss and melting temperature, respectively [44,45]. The DSC spectra of PVA showed melting endotherm at 221 °C [46]. The ELD peak completely disappeared from the spectra of the optimized ELD-loaded EG NPs (ENP2), probably due to encapsulation and stabilization of the drug by the polymer. The successful entrapment of ELD within the EG polymer was evidenced by the DSC studies.

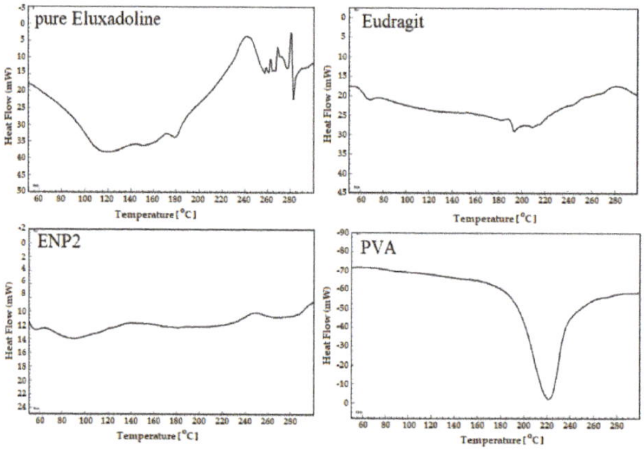

Figure 6. Comparative DSC spectra of pure ELD, eudragit, PVA, and optimized formulation (ENP2).

3.6. FTIR Studies

A comparative FTIR spectra of pure ELD, EG, PVA, and optimized ELD-loaded EG NPs (ENP2) were studied for the identification of the encapsulated drug inside NPs (Figure 7). The pure ELD showed prominent functional group peaks at 3117 cm^{-1} (-NH- str), 3117 cm^{-1} (-NH-), 1696 cm^{-1} (-COOH), 1658 cm^{-1} (-RCONH2-), and 1429 cm^{-1} (-C=C-), which confirmed the purity of the drug [47]. The peaks at 3532 cm^{-1} and 3239 cm^{-1} (CH aliphatic stretching) were visible in the spectra of eudragit RS100 [48]. The characteristic absorption bands of ELD diminished or disappeared in the fingerprint region of the drug, which indicated that the drug encapsulated inside the eudragit polymer, and the appearance of new peaks in the ENP2 corresponding eudragit and PVA confirmed successful entrapment.

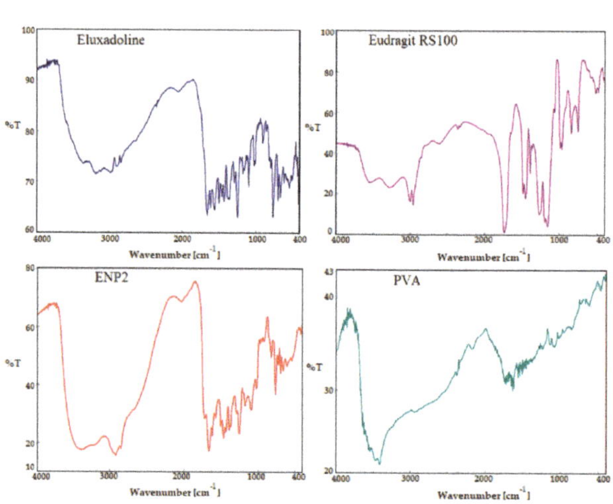

Figure 7. Comparative FTIR spectra of pure ELD, eudragit, PVA, and optimized formulation (ENP2).

3.7. In Vitro Drug Release Studies

Figures 8 and 9, display the ELD release profiles at different pH levels. There was no drug adsorbed to the surface of the ENP2, as evidenced by the lack of burst releases of ELD in the beginning of the release profiles at pH 1.2 (Figure 8). However, at pH 6.8, a burst release could be seen at 2 h in the studies (Figure 9). The release profile of ELD from ENP2 at pH 1.2 exhibited a slow release in comparison with pure ELD, probably due to eudragit RS100 protection from the acidic environment. Over a 24 h period, the release of ELD from ENP2 in PBS (pH 6.8) was roughly 99% compared with less than 40% of pure ELD. These findings suggest that ELD was enclosed in eudragit RS100 polymeric nanoparticles and shielded from the stomach's highly acidic environment. This indicates that the majority of ELD was released once the ENP2 reached the small intestine [49]. This nano-size of ENP2 enhanced drug release was due to the availability of a greater surface area (Figure 5). The release kinetics equations were used to study the ELD release pattern from ENP2 at two pHs (1.2 and 6.8). Applying the kinetic models, it was observed that the Higuchi model could adequately describe the release of ELD from ENP2 at both pHs (Table 3). The Higuchi model had the highest coefficient of correlation values among the applied release models (R2 = 0.8855 and 0.9680 at pH 1.2 and pH 6.8), as shown in Table 4. The best fit correlations were found by the Higuchi model based on the diffusion controlled release of the drug at both pHs [50].

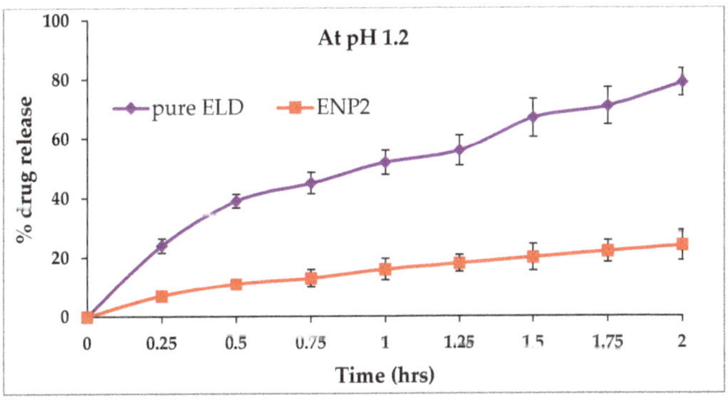

Figure 8. In vitro release profile of pure ELD and optimized formulation (ENP2) at pH 1.2.

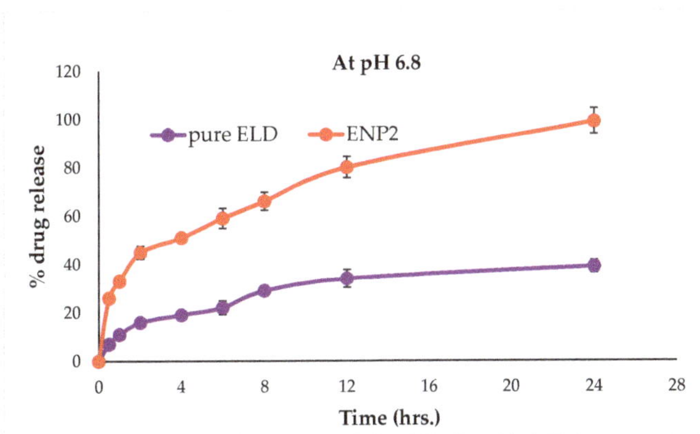

Figure 9. In vitro release profile of pure ELD and optimized formulation (ENP2) at pH 6.8.

Table 4. Release kinetic models of EPN2.

Models	Equations	R^2 (At pH 1.2)	R^2 (At pH 6.8)
Zero order	$Q = kt + b$	0.6303	0.7943
First order	$In(100 - Q) = -kt + b$	0.6653	0.9550
Korsmeyer–Peppas	$Q_t/Q = k^n$	0.4626	0.3776
Higuchi	$Q = kt^{0.5} + b$	0.8855	0.9680

3.8. SEM Studies

The SEM images of the optimized formulation (ENP2) demonstrated the smooth and spherical structure of particles (Figure 10). The particles were aggregated or stuck to each other, probably due to the PVA used in the formulation.

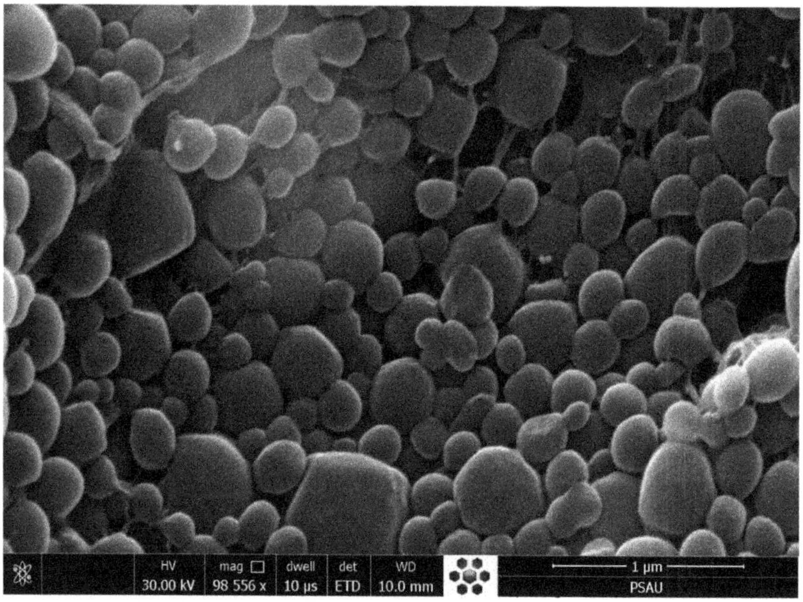

Figure 10. SEM images of optimized formulation (ENP2).

3.9. Assessment of Chronic Restraint Stress-Induced Irritable Bowel Syndrome

There were no observable behavioral or activity changes in the rats during the experiment and no illness or deaths from the therapy took place. According to Figure 11, IBS-C-induced rats had considerably more bowel movements than normal rats ($p < 0.05$) and ENP2 dramatically decreased IBD-S rats' bowel movements ($p < 0.05$). The body weight of rats in the ENP2-treated group was significantly higher ($p < 0.05$) than the ELD-std model group rats. Physical stool hardness reflects physical stool consistency, since it closely correlates with physical stool water content. A significant decrease in fecal water content in the ENP2 (45.47 ± 1.19%) -treated rats was observed compared with the ELD-std (53.36 ± 1.81%) and IBS-C (65.13 ± 2.29%) model group rats (Tables 5 and 6). This finding suggests that chronic restraint stress (CRS) caused the stress models' stools to include more water and to develop diarrhea. The formulation (ENP2) also exhibited reduced body weight, stool consistency, and bleeding scores in comparison with the ELD-std and control (IBS-C) groups ($p < 0.05$) (Figure 12). Thus, low scores of DAI of the formulation (ENP2) indicated a reduction in the severity of irritable-induced diarrhea. This improvement might be due to nano-sized particles and hence enhanced bioavailability. The results demonstrated that the formulation (ENP2) ameliorated IBS-D better than the pure ELD.

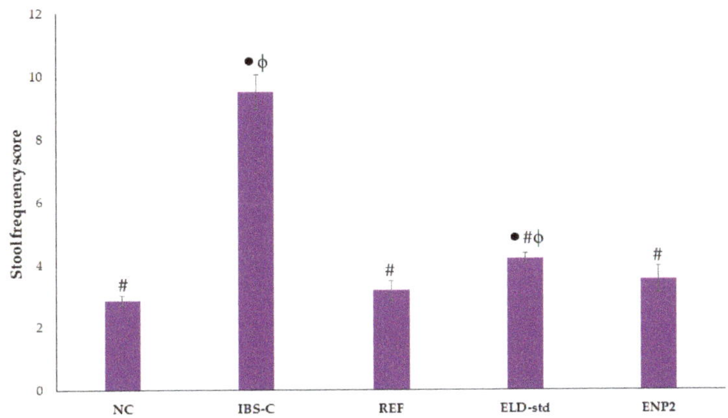

Figure 11. Effects of ELD-std and ENP2 on stool frequency in chronic restraint stress-induced IBS rats. Values are expressed as mean ± S.E.M., n = 6 rats/group. • indicates significant difference versus normal control (NC) group at $p < 0.05$. # indicates significant difference versus IBS control (IBS-C) group at $p < 0.05$. ϕ indicates significant difference versus reference (REF) group at $p < 0.05$.

Table 5. Effects of ELD-std and formulation (ENP2) on body weight of IBD-S rats.

Groups	Body Weight		
	Day 0	**Day 14**	**% wt Change**
NC	116.33 ± 0.88	127.33 ± 2.23 #	9.42 ± 1.10 #
IBS-C	115.00 ± 0.93	111.33 ± 1.43 •	−3.19 ± 1.02 •
REF	116.33 ± 0.80	124.00 ± 3.07 #	6.59 ± 2.48 #
ELD-Std	115.67 ± 1.09	120.67 ± 1.71 •#	4.39 ± 2.00 •#
ENP2	115.83 ± 0.87	122.17 ± 3.59 #	5.44 ± 2.78 #

• indicates significant difference versus normal control (NC) group at $p < 0.05$. # indicates significant difference versus IBS control (IBS-C) group at $p < 0.05$.

Table 6. Effects of ELD-std and formulation (ENP2) on fecal weight and the percentage of water fecal content of IBD-S rats.

Groups	Fecal Weight (mg/h)		Fecal Water Content (%)
	Wet Weight	**Dry Weight**	
NC	314.50 ± 19.35 #	193.17 ± 19.69	39.25 ± 2.89 #
IBS-C	414.17 ± 16.03 •	146.00 ± 14.77	65.13 ± 2.29 •
REF	318.67 ± 13.37 #	184.50 ± 19.57	42.40 ± 4.59 #
ELD-Std	364.83 ± 9.20 •#ϕ	169.83 ± 6.50	53.36 ± 1.81 •#ϕ
ENP2	327.17 ± 16.51 #	177.83 ± 7.81	45.47 ± 1.19 #

Values are expressed as mean ± S.E.M., n = 6 rats/group. • indicates significant difference versus normal control (NC) group at $p < 0.05$. # indicates significant difference versus IBS control (IBS-C) group at $p < 0.05$. ϕ indicates significant difference versus reference (REF) group at $p < 0.05$.

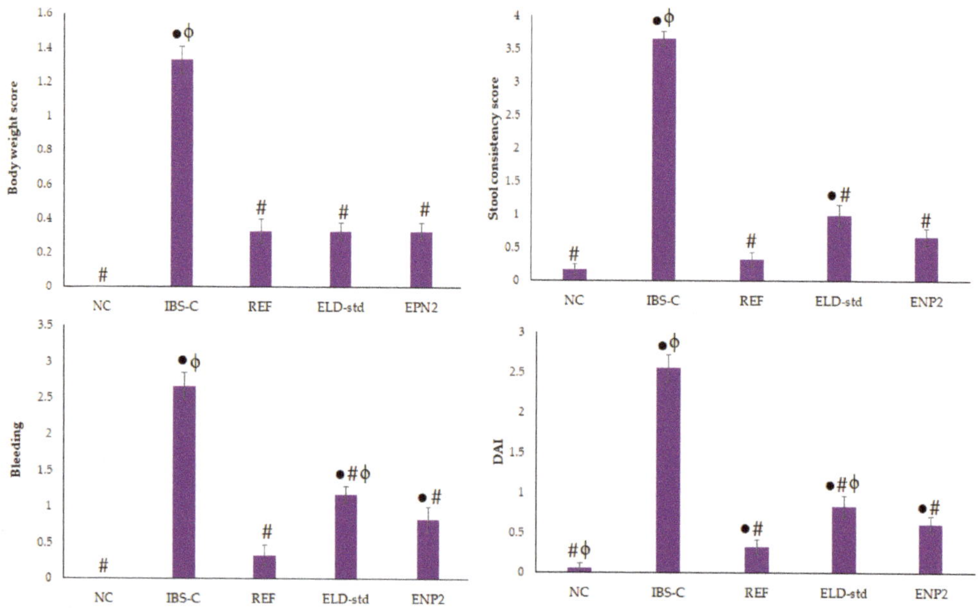

Figure 12. Effects of ELD-std and ENP2 on body weight, stool consistency, bleeding, and DAI scores in chronic restraint stress-induced IBS rats. Values are expressed as mean ± S.E.M., n = 6 rats/group. • indicates significant difference versus normal control (NC) group at $p < 0.05$. # indicates significant difference versus IBS control (IBS-C) group at $p < 0.05$. ϕ indicates significant difference versus reference (REF) group at $p < 0.05$.

4. Conclusions

In this research work, ELD-loaded EG-NPs (ENP1-ENP14) were prepared using an eudragit polymer and PVA and formulations were optimized using a Box–Behnken Design software. The optimized ELD-loaded EG-NPs (ENP2) exhibited particle size, PDI, ZP, and drug entrapment 286 ± 3.67 nm, 0.263 ± 0.01, 31.8 ± 3.18 mV, and 82.35 ± 4.1%., respectively. The ENP2 exhibited enhanced and prolonged drug release at pH 6.8 due to the acidic protection of the drug by the eudragit RS100 polymer. The assessment of chronic restraint stress-induced irritable bowel syndrome revealed that ENP2 exhibited reduced body weight, stool consistency, and bleeding scores in comparison with the ELD-std and control (IBS-C) group ($p < 0.05$) and low scores of DAI of the formulation (ENP2) indicated a reduction in the severity of irritable-induced diarrhea. The formulation (ENP2) could be considered an effective treatment of IBS-D and other GIT-allied conditions. This novel drug delivery system needs to be further evaluated to ascertain its effectiveness and safety in in vivo experimental models before going on to the clinical stage.

Author Contributions: Conceptualization, M.K.A. and M.M.A.; methodology, M.K.A. and G.A.S.; validation, M.I. and G.A.S.; formal analysis, G.A.S.; investigation, M.M.A. and M.K.A. resources, M.F.A.; writing—original draft preparation, M.K.A. and M.M.A.; writing—review and editing, I.A.A.; supervision, M.K.A.; project administration, M.K.A.; funding acquisition, M.K.A. All authors have read and agreed to the published version of the manuscript.

Funding: This research was funded by Deputyship for Research and Innovation, Ministry of Education in Saudi Arabia, grant number IF/PSAU-2022/03/22663.

Institutional Review Board Statement: This study was conducted after approval from the Research Ethics Committee, Prince Sattam Bin Abdulaziz University (Approval number: BERC 003-03-21; dated: March 2021).

Informed Consent Statement: Not applicable.

Data Availability Statement: The data presented in this study are available on request from the corresponding author.

Acknowledgments: The authors extend their appreciation to the Deputyship for Research and Innovation, Ministry of Education in Saudi Arabia, for funding the research work.

Conflicts of Interest: The authors declare no conflict of interest.

References

1. Chey, W.D.; Kurlander, J.; Eswaran, S. Irritable bowel syndrome: A clinical review. *JAMA* **2015**, *313*, 949–958. [CrossRef] [PubMed]
2. Longstreth, G.F.; Thompson, W.G.; Chey, W.D.; Houghton, L.A.; Mearin, F.; Spiller, R.C. Functional bowel disorders. *Gastroenterology* **2006**, *130*, 1480–1491. [CrossRef]
3. Lovell, R.M.; Ford, A.C. Global prevalence of and risk factors for irritable bowel syndrome: A meta-analysis. *Clin. Gastroenterol. Hepatol.* **2012**, *10*, 712–721.e714. [CrossRef] [PubMed]
4. Buono, J.L.; Carson, R.T.; Flores, N.M. Health-related quality of life, work productivity, and indirect costs among patients with irritable bowel syndrome with diarrhea. *Health Qual. Life Outcomes* **2017**, *15*, 35. [CrossRef] [PubMed]
5. ten Berg, M.J.; Goettsch, W.G.; van den Boom, G.; Smout, A.J.; Herings, R.M. Quality of life of patients with irritable bowel syndrome is low compared to others with chronic diseases. *Eur. J. Gastroenterol. Hepatol.* **2006**, *18*, 475–481. [CrossRef]
6. Singh, P.; Staller, K.; Barshop, K.; Dai, E.; Newman, J.; Yoon, S.; Castel, S.; Kuo, B. Patients with irritable bowel syndrome-diarrhea have lower disease-specific quality of life than irritable bowel syndrome-constipation. *World J. Gastroenterol.* **2015**, *21*, 8103–8109. [CrossRef]
7. Lackner, J.M.; Ma, C.X.; Keefer, L.; Brenner, D.M.; Gudleski, G.D.; Satchidanand, N.; Firth, R.; Sitrin, M.D.; Katz, L.; Krasner, S.S.; et al. Type, rather than number, of mental and physical comorbidities increases the severity of symptoms in patients with irritable bowel syndrome. *Clin. Gastroenterol. Hepatol.* **2013**, *11*, 1147–1157. [CrossRef]
8. Buono, J.L.; Mathur, K.; Averitt, A.J.; Andrae, D.A. Economic Burden of Irritable Bowel Syndrome with Diarrhea: Retrospective Analysis of a U.S. Commercially Insured Population. *J. Manag. Care Spec. Pharm.* **2017**, *23*, 453–460. [CrossRef]
9. Canavan, C.; West, J.; Card, T. Review article: The economic impact of the irritable bowel syndrome. *Aliment. Pharmacol. Ther.* **2014**, *40*, 1023–1034. [CrossRef]
10. Tornblom, H.; Goosey, R.; Wiseman, G.; Baker, S.; Emmanuel, A. Understanding symptom burden and attitudes to irritable bowel syndrome with diarrhoea: Results from patient and healthcare professional surveys. *United Eur. Gastroenterol. J.* **2018**, *6*, 1417–1427. [CrossRef]
11. Ruppin, H. Review: Loperamide—A potent antidiarrhoeal drug with actions along the alimentary tract. *Aliment. Pharmacol. Ther.* **1987**, *1*, 179–190. [CrossRef] [PubMed]
12. Sayuk, G.S.; Wolf, R.; Chang, L. Comparison of Symptoms, Healthcare Utilization, and Treatment in Diagnosed and Undiagnosed Individuals with Diarrhea-Predominant Irritable Bowel Syndrome. *Am. J. Gastroenterol.* **2017**, *112*, 892–899. [CrossRef] [PubMed]
13. Efskind, P.S.; Bernklev, T.; Vatn, M.H. A double-blind placebo-controlled trial with loperamide in irritable bowel syndrome. *Scand. J. Gastroenterol.* **1996**, *31*, 463–468. [CrossRef] [PubMed]
14. Talley, N. Pharmacologic therapy for the irritable bowel syndrome. *Am. J. Gastroenterol.* **2003**, *98*, 750–758. [CrossRef]
15. Talley, N.J. Evaluation of drug treatment in irritable bowel syndrome. *Br. J. Clin. Pharm.* **2003**, *56*, 362–369. [CrossRef]
16. US Food Drug Administration. VIBERZI (eluxadoline) Tablets for Oral Use, C.I.V. Available online: https://www.accessdata.fda.gov/drugsatfda_docs/label/2018/206940s003lbl.pdf (accessed on 24 October 2015).
17. Ananthan, S. Opioid ligands with mixed mu/delta opioid receptor interactions: An emerging approach to novel analgesics. *AAPS J.* **2006**, *8*, E118–E125. [CrossRef]
18. Wade, P.R.; Palmer, J.M.; McKenney, S.; Kenigs, V.; Chevalier, K.; Moore, B.A.; Mabus, J.R.; Saunders, P.R.; Wallace, N.H.; Schneider, C.R.; et al. Modulation of gastrointestinal function by MuDelta, a mixed micro opioid receptor agonist/micro opioid receptor antagonist. *Br. J. Pharm.* **2012**, *167*, 1111–1125. [CrossRef]
19. Özdener, A.E.; Rivkin, A. Eluxadoline in the treatment of diarrhea-predominant irritable bowel syndrome. *Drug Des. Dev. Ther.* **2017**, *11*, 2827–2840. [CrossRef]
20. Anwer, M.K.; Ahmed, M.M.; Aldawsari, M.F.; Alshahrani, S.; Fatima, F.; Ansari, M.N.; Rehman, N.U.; Al-Shdefat, R.I. Eluxadoline Loaded Solid Lipid Nanoparticles for Improved Colon Targeting in Rat Model of Ulcerative Colitis. *Pharmaceutics* **2020**, *13*, 255. [CrossRef]
21. Das, S.S.; Bharadwaj, P.; Bilal, M.; Barani, M.; Rahdar, A.; Taboada, P.; Bungau, S.; Kyzas, G.Z. Stimuli-Responsive Polymeric Nanocarriers for Drug Delivery, Imaging, and Theragnosis. *Polymers* **2020**, *12*, 1397. [CrossRef]
22. Cano, A.; Sanchez-Lopez, E.; Ettcheto, M.; Lopez-Machado, A.; Espina, M.; Souto, E.B.; Galindo, R.; Camins, A.; Garcia, M.L.; Turowski, P. Current advances in the development of novel polymeric nanoparticles for the treatment of neurodegenerative diseases. *Nanomedicine* **2020**, *15*, 1239–1261. [CrossRef] [PubMed]
23. Soppimath, K.S.; Aminabhavi, T.M.; Kulkarni, A.R.; Rudzinski, W.E. Biodegradable polymeric nanoparticles as drug delivery devices. *J. Control. Release* **2001**, *70*, 1–20. [CrossRef] [PubMed]

24. Sivasankarapillai, V.S.; Das, S.S.; Sabir, F.; Sundaramahalingam, M.A.; Colmenares, J.C.; Prasannakumar, S.; Rajan, M.; Rahdar, A.; Kyzas, G.Z. Progress in natural polymer engineered biomaterials for transdermal drug delivery systems. *Mater. Today Chem.* **2021**, *19*, 100382. [CrossRef]
25. Qazvini, N.T.; Zinatloo, S. Synthesis and characterization of gelatin nanoparticles using CDI/NHS as a non-toxic cross-linking system. *J. Mater. Sci. Mater. Med.* **2011**, *22*, 63–69. [CrossRef]
26. Zinatloo-Ajabshir, Z.; Zinatloo-Ajabshir, S. Preparation and Characterization of Curcumin Niosomal Nanoparticles via a Simple and Eco-friendly Route. *J. Nanostruct.* **2019**, *9*, 784–790. [CrossRef]
27. Júlia, A.; Dalcin, F.; Ferreira Ourique, A.; Gomes, P. Cationic Nanocapsules Containing Eudragit RS100®and Its Potential for Application in Nanomedicine. *Discip. Sci. Nat. Tecnol.* **2017**, *18*, 545–566.
28. Sonje, A.; Chandra, A. Comprehensive Review on Eudragit Polymers. *Int. Res. J. Pharm.* **2013**, *4*, 71–74. [CrossRef]
29. Almutairy, B.K.; Alshetaili, A.; Alali, A.S.; Ahmed, M.M.; Anwer, M.K.; Aboudzadeh, M.A. Design of Olmesartan Me-doxomil-Loaded Nanosponges for Hypertension and Lung Cancer Treatments. *Polymers* **2021**, *13*, 2272. [CrossRef]
30. Prasad, P.U.; Kumar RA, S. A novel validated RP-HPLC-DAD method for the estimation of Eluxadoline in bulk and pharmaceutical dosage form. *Res. J. Pharm. Technol.* **2015**, *8*, 1469–1476. [CrossRef]
31. Alali, A.S.; Kalam, M.A.; Ahmed, M.M.; Aboudzadeh, M.A.; Alhudaithi, S.S.; Anwer, M.K.; Fatima, F.; Iqbal, M. Nanocrystallization Improves the Solubilization and Cytotoxic Effect of a Poly (ADP-Ribose)-Polymerase-I Inhibitor. *Polymers* **2022**, *14*, 4827. [CrossRef]
32. Ritger, P.L.; Peppas, N.A. A simple equation for description of solute release II. Fickian and anomalous release from swellable devices. *J. Control. Release* **1987**, *5*, 37–42. [CrossRef]
33. Gigliobianco, M.R.; Casadidio, C.; Censi, R.; Di Martino, P. Nanocrystals of Poorly Soluble Drugs: Drug Bioavailability and Physicochemical Stability. *Pharmaceutics* **2018**, *10*, 134. [CrossRef] [PubMed]
34. Lu, Y.; Huang, J.; Zhang, Y.; Huang, Z.; Yan, W.; Zhou, T.; Wang, Z.; Liao, L.; Cao, H.; Tan, B. Therapeutic Effects of Berberine Hydrochloride on Stress-Induced Diarrhea-Predominant Irritable Bowel Syndrome Rats by Inhibiting Neurotransmission in Colonic Smooth Muscle. *Front. Pharmacol.* **2021**, *12*, 596686. [CrossRef] [PubMed]
35. Murthy, S.N.; Cooper, H.S.; Shim, H.; Shah, R.S.; Ibrahim, S.A.; Sedergran, D.J. Treatment of dextran sulfate sodium-induced murine colitis by intracolonic cyclosporin. *Dig. Dis. Sci.* **1993**, *38*, 1722–1734. [CrossRef] [PubMed]
36. Mujtaba, M.A.; Alotaibi, N.M.; Alshehri, S.M.; Yusuf, M.; Anwer, M.K.; Rahman, M.A.; Parveen, A. Novel Therapeutic Approach in PEGylated Chitosan Nanoparticles of Apigenin for the Treatment of Cancer via Oral Nanomedicine. *Polymers* **2022**, *14*, 4344. [CrossRef] [PubMed]
37. Abla, K.K.; Mneimneh, A.T.; Allam, A.N.; Mehanna, M.M. Application of Box-Behnken Design in the Preparation, Optimization, and In-Vivo Pharmacokinetic Evaluation of Oral Tadalafil-Loaded Niosomal Film. *Pharmaceutics* **2023**, *15*, 173. [CrossRef] [PubMed]
38. Bhattacharya, S.; Mondal, L.; Mukherjee, B.; Dutta, L.; Ehsan, I.; Debnath, M.C.; Gaonkar, R.H.; Pal, M.M.; Majumdar, S. Apigenin loaded nanoparticle delayed development of hepatocellular carcinoma in rats. *Nanomedicine* **2018**, *14*, 1905–1917. [CrossRef]
39. Imam, S.S.; Gilani, S.J.; Bin Jumah, M.N.; Rizwanullah, M.; Zafar, A.; Ahmed, M.M.; Alshehri, S. Harnessing Lipid Polymer Hybrid Nanoparticles for Enhanced Oral Bioavailability of Thymoquinone: In Vitro and In Vivo Assessments. *Polymers* **2022**, *14*, 3705. [CrossRef]
40. Anwer, M.K.; Mohammad, M.; Ezzeldin, E.; Fatima, F.; Alalaiwe, A.; Iqbal, M. Preparation of sustained release apremilast-loaded PLGA nanoparticles: In vitro characterization and in vivo pharmacokinetic study in rats. *Int. J. Nanomed.* **2019**, *14*, 1587–1595. [CrossRef]
41. Froiio, F.; Ginot, L.; Paolino, D.; Lebaz, N.; Bentaher, A.; Fessi, H.; Elaissari, A. Essential Oils-Loaded Polymer Particles: Preparation, Characterization and Antimicrobial Property. *Polymers* **2019**, *11*, 1017. [CrossRef]
42. Sharma, U.K.; Verma, A.; Prajapati, S.K.; Pandey, H.; Pandey, A.C. In vitro, in vivo and pharmacokinetic assessment of amikacin sulphate laden polymeric nanoparticles meant for controlled ocular drug delivery. *Appl. Nanosci.* **2015**, *5*, 143–155. [CrossRef]
43. Zhu, Y.; Gu, Z.; Liao, Y.; Li, S.; Xue, Y.; Firempong, M.A.; Xu, Y.; Yu, J.; Smyth, H.D.; Xu, X. Improved intestinal absorption and oral bioavailability of astaxanthin using poly (ethylene glycol)-graft-chitosan nanoparticles: Preparation, in vitro evaluation and pharmacokinetics in rats. *J. Sci. Food Agric.* **2022**, *102*, 1002–1011. [CrossRef]
44. Barreca, G.; Ventimiglia, G.; Masciocchi, N. Eluxadoline Crystalline Forms and Process of Their Preparation. EP3573958A1, 26 January 2018. Available online: https://patentscope.wipo.int/search/en/detail.jsf?docId=WO2018138274 (accessed on 5 February 2023).
45. Ceballos, A.; Cirri, M.; Maestrelli, F.; Corti, G.; Mura, P. Influence of formulation and process variables on in vitro release of theophylline from directly-compressed Eudragit matrix tablets. *Farmaco* **2005**, *60*, 913–918. [CrossRef] [PubMed]
46. Zhu, J.; Li, Q.; Che, Y.; Liu, X.; Dong, C.; Chen, X.; Wang, C. Effect of Na_2CO_3 on the Microstructure and Macroscopic Properties and Mechanism Analysis of PVA/CMC Composite Film. *Polymers* **2020**, *12*, 453. [CrossRef] [PubMed]
47. Anwer, M.K.; Al-Shdefat, R.; Ezzeldin, E.; Alshahrani, S.M.; Alshetaili, A.S.; Iqbal, M. Preparation, Evaluation and Bioavailability Studies of Eudragit Coated PLGA Nanoparticles for Sustained Release of Eluxadoline for the Treatment of Irritable Bowel Syndrome. *Front. Pharmacol.* **2017**, *8*, 844. [CrossRef] [PubMed]
48. Alhamhoom, Y.; Ravi, G.; Osmani, R.A.M.; Hani, U.; Prakash, G.M. Formulation, Characterization, and Evaluation of Eudragit-Coated Saxagliptin Nanoparticles Using 3 Factorial Design Modules. *Molecules* **2022**, *27*, 7510. [CrossRef] [PubMed]

49. Wei, L.; Yang, Y.; Shi, K.; Wu, J.; Zhao, W.; Mo, J. Preparation and Characterization of Loperamide-Loaded Dynasan 114 Solid Lipid Nanoparticles for Increased Oral Absorption in the Treatment of Diarrhea. *Front. Pharmacol.* **2016**, *7*, 332. [CrossRef]
50. Siepmann, J.; Siepmann, F. Modeling of diffusion controlled drug delivery. *J. Contrl. Rel.* **2012**, *161*, 351–362. [CrossRef]

pharmaceutics

MDPI

Article

Gold-Polypyrrole-Loaded Eosin in Photo-Mediated Treatment of Hidradenitis Suppurativa: In Vivo Trans-Epidermal Permeation Study and Clinical Case Report

Abdullah I. El-Kholy [1], Maha Fadel [1,*], Maha Nasr [2], Ibrahim El-Sherbiny [3], Abeer Tawfik [4], Yasser O. Mosaad [5] and Doaa Abdel Fadeel [1]

[1] Department of Medical Applications of Laser, Pharmaceutical Nano-Technology Unit, National Institute of Laser Enhanced Sciences (NILES), Cairo University, Giza 12613, Egypt
[2] Department of Pharmaceutics and Industrial Pharmacy, Faculty of Pharmacy, Ain Shams University, Cairo 11566, Egypt
[3] Nanomaterials Lab, Center for Materials Science, Zewail City of Science and Technology, 6th October City, Giza 12578, Egypt
[4] Department of Medical Applications of Laser, Dermatology Unit, National Institute of Laser Enhanced Sciences (NILES), Cairo University, Giza 12613, Egypt
[5] Department of Pharmacy Practice and Clinical Pharmacy, Faculty of Pharmaceutical Sciences and Pharmaceutical Industries, Future University, Cairo 11835, Egypt
* Correspondence: mahafmali@niles.cu.edu.eg; Tel.: +20-1001649550

Abstract: This study reports a new protocol for the management of Hidradenitis Suppurativa (HS), depending on the synergistic photodynamic and photothermal effect of eosin yellow-gold-polypyrrole hybrid nanoparticles (E-G-Ppy NPs). E-G-Ppy NPs and gold-polypyrrole NPs (G-Ppy NPs) were synthesized, characterized, and formulated in topical hydrogels. Then, in vivo trans-epidermal permeation study, under both dark and white light-irradiation conditions, was done on albino mice. The E-G-Ppy hydrogel was then applied on a twenty-four years old female with recurrent axillary HS lesions pretreated with fractional CO_2 laser. Thereafter, the treated lesions were irradiated sequentially, using an IPL system, in the visible (~550 nm) and NIR band (630–1100 nm) to activate the synthesized nanoparticles. Results showed that, upon application to mice skin, E-G-Ppy exhibited good tolerance and safety under dark conditions and induced degenerative changes into dermal layers after white-light activation, reflecting deep penetration. Photo-activation of E-G-Ppy hydrogel to a severe Hidradenitis Suppurativa case showed an improvement of 80% of the lesions according to average HS-LASI scores after 4 sessions with no recurrence during a follow-up period of six months. In summary, the dual photodynamic/photothermal activation of E-G-Ppy NPs can represent a promising modality for management of HS. Further expanded clinical studies may be needed.

Keywords: polypyrrole; gold; eosin yellow; photodynamic; photothermal; Hidradenitis Suppurativa

1. Introduction

Hidradenitis Suppurativa (HS), is an inflammatory recurrent dermatosis affecting different areas of the skin. It is characterized by the presence of thick scarring, oozing abscesses, and painful nodules in different areas such as armpits, buttocks, groin, or below the breast [1,2]. Causes of HS are not well established, but potentially thought to be mainly related to apocrine glands problems. Yet, HS may also be related to other factors such as hair follicle structural anomalies, obesity, and smoking, among others [3]. HS is commonly treated by oral/topical antibiotics, oral/topical isotretinoin, anti-inflammatory drugs, or surgery [4]. Photodynamic therapy (PDT) was studied as a promising new technique for the treatment of HS; with encouraging results obtained [5,6]. PDT depends on the activation of a photosensitive compound (a photosensitizer; PS) by light of an appropriate wavelength in the presence of oxygen. The activated PS returned to its ground state liberating free radicals and/or reactive oxygen species that cause tissue destruction [7,8]. Previous studies reported the use of PSs as 5-aminolevulinic acid (ALA) [2], and methylene blue [4,6] for PDT treatment of HS. The main drawbacks were the low penetration of the PS, which can be overcome by the proper choice of a delivery system [4]. In a previous work, highly dispersible, ultra-nanonized, and highly stable polypyrrole-coated gold nanoparticles (G-Ppy NPs) were synthesized and showed promising photothermal effects. In that method of synthesis, chloroauric acid was used as an oxidizing agent to induce the oxidative polymerization of pyrrole into polypyrrole, resulting in the formation of gold-conjugated polypyrrole with highly enhanced pharmaceutical properties in comparison to polypyrrole synthesized via the conventional methods [9]. Later, we conjugated two hydrophilic PSs; eosin yellow (E) and rose bengal (RB) with the synthesized nanoparticles and studied their combined photothermal and photodynamic effect in vitro using HeG2 as a model for cancerous cell lines [10]. Eosin yellow is a water-soluble dye that we used successfully as a photosensitizer in topical PDT of recalcitrant plantar warts [11] and onychomycosis [12]. The goal of this work is to report our experience with a new protocol in a case report for HS management that depends on the combined synergistic photodynamic and photothermal effect of the synthesized (E-G-Ppy NPs). The synthesized nanoparticles were formulated as a topical hydrogel and evaluated in vivo for trans-epidermal permeation (on albino mice skin) before application on a patient with HS (clinical case report).

2. Materials and Methods

2.1. Materials

Eosin yellow sodium salt, chloroauric acid ($HAuCl_4$), and pyrrole were purchased from Sigma-Aldrich Corp. (St. Louis, MO, USA). Sodium-carboxymethylcellulose (Na-CMC) was purchased from Normest Company for scientific development, Egypt. All other reagents and solvents were of analytical grade.

2.2. Synthesis of Free and Eosin-Conjugated Gold-Polypyrrole Nanoparticles (G-Ppy and E-G-Ppy)

Gold-polypyrrole nanoparticles loaded with eosin were synthesized as described in a previous paper [10]. Briefly, aqueous pyrrole solution (25 mM) was mixed with an aqueous eosin solution (0.5 mM). A solution of 1 mL $HAuCl_4$ (10 mM) was added to 20 mL of the pre-prepared pyrrole-eosin solution, under stirring for 4–5 min, followed by centrifugation at 10,000 rpm to separate any byproducts and unreacted pyrrole. The precipitated nanoparticles were re-dispersed in 20 mL double distilled water and left as a stock colloidal solution. G-Ppy NPs (free of E) were also synthesized in the same molar ratio ($HAuCl_4$: Pyrrole at MR: 1:50, respectively) for comparison, according to the procedure previously described by Fadel et al. [9].

2.3. Characterization of G-Ppy NPs and E-G-Ppy NPs

Morphological characteristics of the synthesized G-Ppy NPs and E-G-Ppy NPs were examined by transmission electron microscope TEM (JEOL Ltd., Tokyo, Japan). Zetasizer (Malvern Ltd., Malvern, UK) was used for particle size and zeta potential measurements. A double-beam spectrophotometer (Rayleigh UV-2601, Beijing, China) was used to study the UV–visible-NIR absorption spectra of eosin yellow and the synthesized nanoparticles.

2.4. Topical Hydrogel Preparations of E, G-Ppy NPs, and E-G-Ppy NPs

Free E, free G-Ppy NPs, and E-G-Ppy NPs were all formulated in a 3% carboxymethylcellulose (CMC) hydrogel base as described by Fadel et al. [13]. The concentration of E in free E hydrogel and E-G-Ppy hydrogel was 0.03455% w/w and the concentrations of G-Ppy in G-Ppy hydrogel and E-G-Ppy hydrogel were equivalent. The produced hydrogels were visually examined for appearance and uniformity. The pH values of the produced hydrogels were determined using a digital pH meter (HANNA, RI, USA). Samples from different areas of the free E and E-G-Ppy NPs hydrogels were taken, diluted with distilled water, and measured colorimetrically at 515 nm for the study of hydrogel uniformity and the actual E concentration.

2.5. In Vivo Evaluation of Trans-Epidermal Permeation Following the Application of G-Ppy NPs and E-G-Ppy NP Hydrogels

Trans-epidermal permeation was studied by tracking the histological changes in skin layers after the application of hydrogels in dark and after irradiation of the animal's skin. This experiment was carried out following the same protocol as described by Fadel et al. [13] on male *Mus musculus* albino mice, applying the regulations of Cairo University Institutional Animal Care and Use Committee (CUIACUC); with the approval number (CU-I-F-83-20). All of the animals' dorsal skin hair was shaved, and the animals were divided into different groups and treated as listed in Table 1.

Table 1. Topical treatment and light irradiation of different animal groups for trans-epidermal permeation study.

Groups (2 Animals per Group)	Topical Treatment *	Light Condition **
Control	-	-
Group 1	G-Ppy hydrogel	Dark
		Light
Group 2	Free E hydrogel	Dark
		Light
Group 3	E-G-Ppy hydrogel	Dark
		Light

NB: * Gel was applied for 15 min to a shaved dorsal skin (1 cm^2 area). ** Animals irradiation was carried out by white light source (Photon scientific, Cairo, Egypt) for 20 min (fluence of 90 mW/cm^2).

Animal behavior was observed during the irradiation time, and animals that suffered from distress signs or pain were administered isoflurane inhalation of low doses. After the experiment, each animal was kept in a separate clean plastic cage for 24 h. Afterwards, the animals were anesthetized and executed. For histopathological examination, the treated skin areas were separated and fixed in 10% neutral buffered formalin for 72 h. They were then processed and 4μm thick tissue skin sections were stained with hematoxylin and eosin and examined by a light microscope (Leica Microsystems GmbH, Wetzlar, Germany).

2.6. Clinical Case Study

This case study was carried out at the National Institute of Laser Enhanced Sciences (NILES) clinic, Cairo University, Egypt. Approval number of the board of the research ethics committee of the Institute obtained is (CU-NILES/25/21). The study protocol conformed to the guidelines of the Declaration of Helsinki. We affirm that the patient was provided informed consent for publication of images illustrating the clinical improvement. The study was conducted on a twenty-four-year-old female who presented with recurrent lesions of HS at the axilla on one side for 2 years. The recurrence of the lesions appeared after oral medicines such as isotretinoin and topical clarithromycin. Dermatological examination showed hemispheric nodules with a diameter of 0.3–2 cm that were distributed at and around her axilla. Some of the abscesses became ulcerated with noticed local haphalgesia. The patient's main complaint was recurrent infection, oozing, and a disfiguring scar. The lesions were of grade 4 according to Hurley classification.

2.7. Treatment Protocol

Pretreatment with Fractional CO_2 Laser before hydrogel application was applied to increase trans-epidermal delivery of E-G-Ppy NPs through the patient's thick skin. The lesions were subjected to one pass of fractional CO_2 Laser (Bison, Italy). Fractional CO_2

Laser parameters were as follows; scanning area 3 ~ 20 mm, fluence: 7.5 mJ/cm^2, pulse duration: 500 µsec, and dot density: 0.8. Then, 1 g ± 0.2 of E-G-Ppy NPs hydrogel was spread on the lesions as a thin film and applied for 15 min. The lesions were then irradiated, sequentially, using an IPL system (EPI-C PLUS; Espansione Group, Bologna, Italy) using a 550 nm filter and 630–1100 nm wide-band filter, respectively, with 2.5 × 4.5 cm spot area, 20 ms pulse duration, and fluence of 25 J/cm^2. Sessions were carried out every 2 weeks over a period of 8 weeks. The elimination of the lesions was the treatment endpoint. Photographs were taken before treatment, as a baseline, and after treatment. Treatment efficacy assessment was recorded using the modified Hidradenitis Suppurativa Lesion, Area and Severity Index (HS-LASI) [14] by three independent blinded dermatologists to the intervention protocol. A follow-up period of 6 months was carried out to report any recurrent lesions or side effects.

3. Results

3.1. Preparation and Characterization of G-Ppy NPs and E-G-Ppy NPs

It was clear from the UV–vis-NIR spectra that conjugation of E to G-Ppy has changed the spectroscopic properties of the E-G-Ppy NPs with an increase in the absorption peak and the appearance of new peaks in the NIR region (Figure 1). TEM imaging revealed the morphologies of both types of nanoparticles which resemble those pre-reported by El-Kholy et al. [10] (Figure 2). The zeta potential of G-Ppy was 45 ± 5.9 mV with an average diameter of 55 ± 6.4 nm and the zeta potential of E-G-Ppy was −33 mV with an average diameter of 33 ± 5.63 nm. Both zeta potential values revealed a good colloidal stability [15].

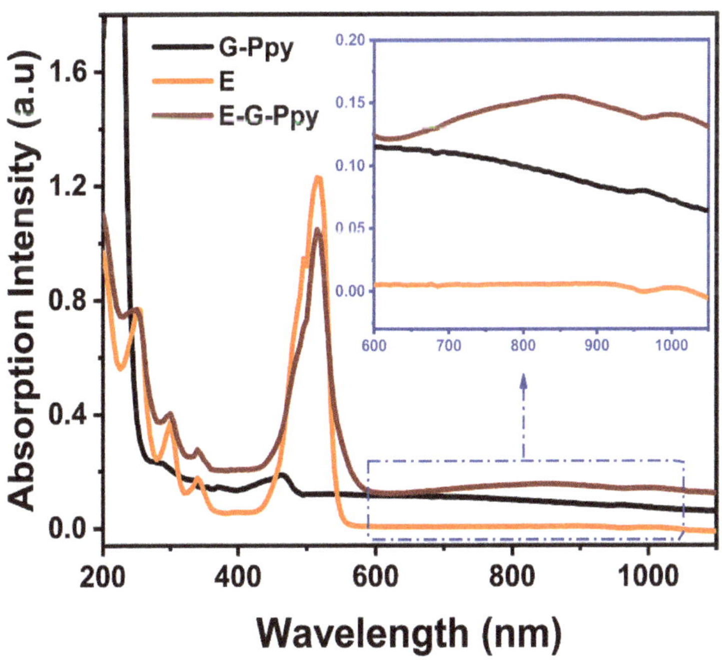

Figure 1. UV–vis-NIR spectra of E, G-Ppy, and E-G-Ppy.

The prepared hydrogels were clear in color and homogeneous. Hydrogels' pH values ranged from 6.7 to 6.9 ± 0.5, which are close to skin pH. Therefore, no irritation was expected upon use [16]. The different examined samples were found to retain around 95.3–97.7% of the initially incorporated E, showing acceptable homogeneity and uniformity.

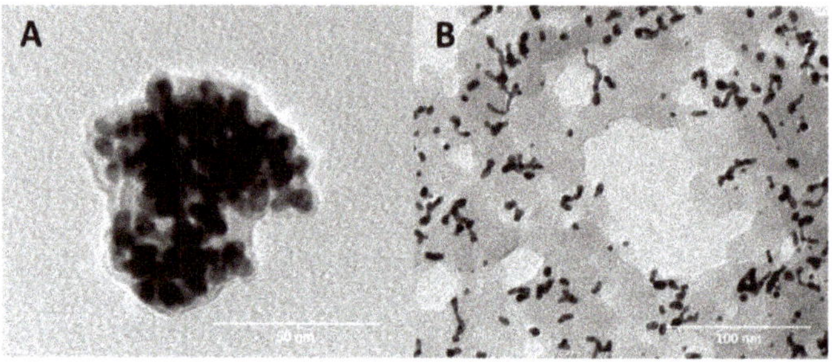

Figure 2. TEM imaging of (**A**) free G-Ppy and (**B**) E-G-Ppy. Preparation and characterization of E, G-Ppy NPs, and E-G-Ppy NPs hydrogels.

3.2. In Vivo Evaluation of Trans-Epidermal Permeation Following the Application of E, G-Ppy NPs and E-G-Ppy NP Hydrogels

The histopathological changes in the skin samples of the studied groups are shown in Figure 3 and summarized in Table 2.

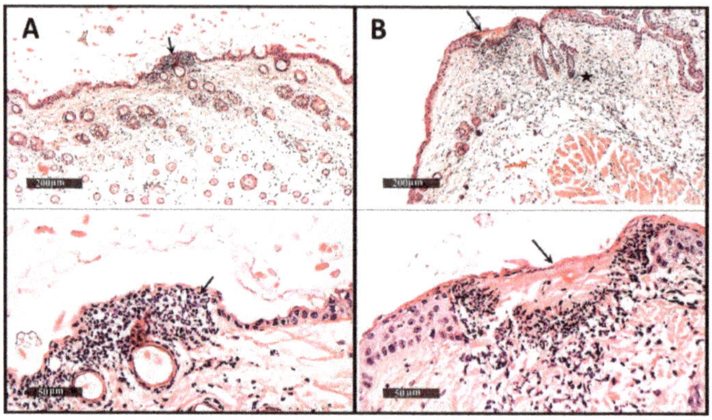

Figure 3. (**A**) Transverse sections of the dorsal mice skin stained (H&E) taken from group 2 (Free E under irradiation): showing the epidermal degenerative changes (black arrows) and (**B**) Transverse sections of the dorsal mice skin stained (H&E) taken from group 3 (E-G-Ppy under irradiation) showing the epidermal degenerative changes (black arrows), ulceration and inflammatory cells in dermal regions (black stars), and the congestive blood vessels (red arrows).

Table 2. Histopathological changes due to trans-epidermal permeation before and after light irradiation of different animal groups.

Group	Epidermal Degenerative Changes	Dermal Ulceration	Inflammatory Cells Infiltrate	Congested Subcutaneous Blood Vessels
Control	-	-	-	-
Group 1-Dark (G-Ppy)	-	-	-	-
Group 1(G-Ppy)-Light	-	-	-	-
Group 2-Dark (free E)	+	-	+	-
Group 2-Light (Free E)	++	-	++	-
Group 3-Dark (E-G-Ppy)	+	-	+	+
Group 3-Light (E-G-Ppy)	+	++	+++	+

Coding system: (-): nil, (+): mild (less than 25% of examined sections), (++): moderate (26–50% of examined sections). (+++): severe (>50% of examined sections).

3.3. Clinical Outcome

The E-G-Ppy hydrogel was used for the photo-induced treatment of HS. As stated by the patient, there was a marked improvement as the oozing stopped after 2 sessions and the scars were improved. According to average HS-LASI scores reported by blinded dermatologists, an improvement of 80% of the lesion was achieved (Figure 4) after 4 sessions. The patient did not report pain, erythema, or hyperpigmentation during treatment. No side effects or recurrence of lesions were reported during the 6 months of the follow-up period.

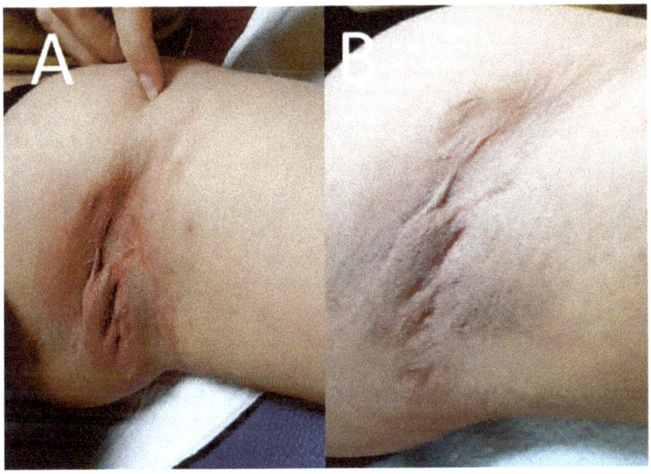

Figure 4. HS lesion (**A**) before treatment showed inflamed oozing hemispheric nodules, and (**B**) after treatment showed improvement to nodules with disappearance of oozing and inflammation.

4. Discussion

In a previous work, we synthesized polypyrrole-coated gold nanoparticles (G-Ppy NPs) by oxidative polymerization of pyrrole mediated by gold ions [9]. The use of polypyrrole as a delivery system has many advantages as it is a conductive biodegradable polymer that can absorb light in the near-infrared (NIR) region, thus producing a photothermal effect [17]. The produced gold-coated polypyrrole differs from conventionally-synthesized polypyrrole in being highly water dispersible which, in turn, makes it suitable for use in pharmaceutical formulations. Besides, the photothermal activity of the synthesized G-Ppy NPs was found to surpass that of polypyrrole synthesized by the chemical conventional method, under the same conditions [9]. Later, we conjugated eosin to the prepared nanoparticles in a one-step method giving eosin-loaded gold-polypyrrole nanoparticles (E-G-Ppy NPs) with high loading efficiency, higher photocytotoxicity, and lower dark cytotoxicity (in comparison to those of either free E or G-Ppy NPs alone); using the HepG2 cell line as a model for cancer cells [10]. In the current study, we extended the work to go deeply into the applications of the synthesized E-G-Ppy NPs. So, we formulated the synthesized E-G-Ppy NPs, as well as free E and G-Ppy NPs, in the form of topical hydrogels and studied their trans-epidermal permeation through skin layers by in vivo investigation of their photo-induced effects on mice skin. Then, we used E-G-Ppy clinically as a dual photodynamic/photothermal treatment in the management of HS. Results revealed that E loaded within G-Ppy penetrated to deep layers and exhibited a pronounced photo-destructive effect that extended to the dermis and the subcutaneous regions if compared to free E and free G-Ppy NPs (Figures 2 and 3, respectively). This can be attributed to the synergism between the photodynamic effect of E and the photothermal effect of G-Ppy NPs, because IPL was applied using two wavelength bands; the first in the visible light (~550 nm; activates E) and the second in a wide band of the NIR region (630–1100 nm; activates polypyrrole). As revealed from UV–Visible-NIR spectra, conjugation of E to G-Ppy NPs led to an increase in the absorption in the NIR region, thus enhancing the G-Ppy NPs' photothermal effect. Additionally, polypyrrole allows more efficient delivery of eosin into deeper layers due to its polymeric nature, giving more efficiency. In fact, IPL has been used previously to activate 5-aminolevulinic acid (ALA) [18] and methylene blue [4] for PDT treatment of HS. However, in our study, the incubation time was shorter (the hydrogel was applied for only 15 min) which is more convenient for the patient and the improvement was pronounced after four sessions only. The scars of HS were characterized by thick skin. That is why the fractional CO_2 laser was used prior to the PDT session to assist the trans-epidermal E delivery as it facilitates the penetration and distribution of the hydrogel [18]. Fractional CO_2 causes ablation of the epidermal layer. The ablative holes may extend to deeper layers generating micro-channels through which the topically applied formula can penetrate and accumulate in deep skin layers [19].

5. Conclusions

Eosin-gold-polypyrrole hybrid nanoparticles exhibited good tolerance and safety under dark conditions. Gold-polypyrrole, as a delivery system, proved high efficacy in loading capacity, skin-penetration, and photothermal effect. The latter was concluded from the enhanced photo-mediated effect of gold-polypyrrole-loaded eosin, compared to its free form. Light-activation of topically applied eosin-gold-polypyrrole induced observed damages and degenerative changes through skin layers reflecting deep penetration, as tested on albino mice skin. Clinical application of eosin-gold-polypyrrole hydrogel, after pretreatment with fractional CO_2 laser, resulted in accelerated improvement of the lesions, proving its combined photodynamic/photothermal effects. In summary, the dual photo-activation of eosin-gold-polypyrrole nanoparticles, after pretreatment with fractional CO_2 laser, can represent a promising modality for the management of Hidradenitis Suppurativa.

Author Contributions: All authors contributed to the study conception and design. Material preparation, data collection and analysis were performed by M.F., D.A.F., M.N., I.E.-S., A.I.E.-K., A.T. and Y.O.M. The first draft of the manuscript was written by D.A.F., A.I.E.-K., M.F., A.T., M.N., I.E.-S. and Y.O.M. All authors commented on previous versions of the manuscript. All authors have read and agreed to the published version of the manuscript.

Funding: This research received no external funding.

Institutional Review Board Statement: The clinical study was conducted in accordance with the Declaration of Helsinki, and approved by the board of the research ethics committee of the National Institute of Laser Enhanced sciences with the approval number (CU-NILES/25/21). The animal study protocol was approved by the Cairo University Institutional Animal Care and Use Committee (CUIACUC); with the approval number (CU-I-F-83-20).

Informed Consent Statement: Informed consent was obtained from all subjects involved in the study.

Data Availability Statement: The datasets generated during and/or analyzed during the current study are available from the corresponding author on reasonable request.

Acknowledgments: This work is supported by a Cairo University project 2016 entitled: Nanosystems in topical photodynamic therapy and photodynamic diagnosis: preparation, characterization and clinical evaluation.

Conflicts of Interest: The authors declare no conflict of interest.

References

1. Mordon, S.J. Treating hidradenitis suppurativa with photodynamic therapy. *Cosmet. Laser Ther.* **2018**, *20*, 223–228. [CrossRef] [PubMed]
2. Valladares, M.J.S.; Salvado, N.E.; Prieto, M.A.R. Treatment of hidradenitis suppurativa with intralesional photodynamic therapy with 5-aminolevulinic acid and 630 nm laser beam. *J. Dermatol. Sci.* **2017**, *85*, 241–246. [CrossRef] [PubMed]
3. Paus, L.R.; Kurzen, H.; Kurokawa, I.; Jemec, G.B.E.; Emtestam, L.; Sellheyer, K.; Giamarellos-Bourboulis, E.J.; Nagy, I.; Bechara, F.G.; Sartorius, K.; et al. What causes hidradenitis suppurativa? *Exp. Dermatol.* **2008**, *17*, 455–456. [CrossRef]
4. Fadel, M.A.; Tawfik, A.A. New topical photodynamic therapy for treatment of hidradenitis suppurativa using methylene blue niosomal gel: A single-blind, randomized, comparative study. *Clin. Exp. Dermatol.* **2015**, *40*, 116–122. [CrossRef] [PubMed]

5. Zhou, Z.-W.; Chen, X.-D.; Wu, X.-Y. 5-ALA PDT successfully treats facial hidradenitis suppurativa-induced severe hypertrophic scar. *Photodiagn. Photodyn. Ther.* **2019**, *28*, 343–345. [CrossRef] [PubMed]
6. Agut-Busquet, E.; Romaní, J.; Gilaberte, Y.; García-Malinis, A.; Ribera-Pibernat, M.; Luelmo, J. Photodynamic therapy with intralesional methylene blue and a 635 nm light-emitting diode lamp in hidradenitis suppurativa: A retrospective follow-up study in 7 patients and a review of the literature. *Photochem. Photobiol. Sci.* **2016**, *15*, 1020–1028. [CrossRef] [PubMed]
7. Maha, F.; Kawser, K.; Nevien, S.; Doaa, A.; Ghada, Y.; Nasr, M. Nanovesicular photodynamic clinical treatment of resistant plantar warts. *Curr. Drug Deliv.* **2020**, *17*, 396–405.
8. Juarranz, Á.; Jaén, P.; Sanz-Rodríguez, F.; Cuevas, J.; González, S. Photodynamic therapy of cancer. Basic principles and applications. *Clin. Transl. Oncol.* **2008**, *10*, 148–154. [CrossRef] [PubMed]
9. Fadel, M.; Fadeel, D.A.; Ibrahim, M.; Hathout, R.M.; El-Kholy, A.I. One-step synthesis of polypyrrole-coated gold nanoparticles for use as a photothermally active nano-system. *Int. J. Nanomed.* **2020**, *15*, 2605–2615. [CrossRef] [PubMed]
10. El-Kholy, A.I.; Fadeel, D.A.; Nasr, M.; El-Sherbiny, I.; Fadel, M. (Rose Bengal)/(Eosin Yellow)-Gold-Polypyrrole Hybrids: A Design for Dual Photo-Active Nano-System with Ultra-High Loading Capacity. *Drug Des. Dev. Ther.* **2021**, *15*, 5011–5023. [CrossRef] [PubMed]
11. Ibrahim, N.A.; Fadeel, D.A.A.; Sadek, A.; Fadel, M.; Tawfik, A. Intralesional vitamin D3 versus new topical photodynamic therapy in recalcitrant palmoplanter warts Randomized comparative controlled study. *Photodiagn. Photodyn. Ther.* **2020**, *32*, 101979. [CrossRef] [PubMed]
12. Shamali, N.; Preuß, A.; Saltsman, I.; Mahammed, A.; Gross, Z.; Däschlein, G.; Röder, B. In vitro photodynamic inactivation (PDI) of pathogenic germs inducing onychomycosis. *Photodiagn. Photodyn. Ther.* **2018**, *24*, 358–365. [CrossRef] [PubMed]
13. Fadel, M.; Fadeel, D.A.; Tawfik, A.; El-Kholy, A.I.; Mosaad, Y.O. Rose Bengal-gold-polypyrrole nanoparticles as a photothermal/photodynamic dual treatment of recalcitrant plantar warts: Animal and clinical study. *J. Drug Deliv. Sci. Technol.* **2022**, *69*, 103095. [CrossRef]
14. Sartorius, K.; Emtestam, L.; Jemec, G.B.E.; Lapins, J. Objective scoring of hidradenitis suppurativa reflecting the role of tobacco smoking and obesity. *Br. J. Dermatol.* **2009**, *161*, 831–839. [CrossRef] [PubMed]
15. Fadel, M.; Kassab, K.; Youssef, T.; El-Kholy, A.I. One-step synthesis of phyto-polymer coated gold nanospheres as a delivery system to enhance resveratrol cytotoxicity. *Drug Dev. Ind. Pharm.* **2019**, *45*, 937–945. [CrossRef] [PubMed]
16. Abdulbaqi, I.M.; Darwis, Y.; Assi, R.A.; Khan, N.A.K. Transethosomal gels as carriers for the transdermal delivery of colchicine: Statistical optimization, characterization, and ex vivo evaluation. *Drug Des. Dev. Ther.* **2018**, *12*, 795–813. [CrossRef] [PubMed]
17. Shi, G.; Rouabhia, M.; Wang, Z.; Dao, L.H.; Zhang, Z. A novel electrically conductive and biodegradable composite made of polypyrrole nanoparticles and polylactide. *Biomaterials* **2004**, *25*, 2477–2488. [CrossRef] [PubMed]
18. Alexiades, M. Randomized, controlled trial of fractional carbon dioxide laser resurfacing followed by ultrashort incubation aminolevulinic acid blue light photodynamic therapy for actinic keratosis. *Dermatol. Surg.* **2017**, *43*, 1053–1064. [CrossRef] [PubMed]
19. Ma, G.; Wu, P.; Lin, X.; Chen, H.; Hu, X.; Jin, Y.; Qiu, Y. Fractional carbon dioxide laser–assisted drug delivery of topical timolol solution for the treatment of deep infantile hemangioma: A pilot study. *Pediatr. Dermatol.* **2014**, *31*, 286–291. [CrossRef] [PubMed]

pharmaceutics

MDPI

Article

Response of the Endogenous Antioxidant Defense System Induced in RAW 264.7 Macrophages upon Exposure to Dextran-Coated Iron Oxide Nanoparticles

Mihaela Balas [1], Simona Liliana Iconaru [2,*], Anca Dinischiotu [1], Nicolas Buton [3] and Daniela Predoi [2,*]

[1] Department of Biochemistry and Molecular Biology, Faculty of Biology, University of Bucharest, 91-95 Splaiul Independentei, 050095 Bucharest, Romania

[2] HORIBA Jobin Yvon S.A.S., 6-18, Rue du Canal, CEDEX, 91165 Longjumeau, France

[3] National Institute of Materials Physics, 405A Atomistilor Street, 077125 Magurele, Romania

* Correspondence: simonaiconaru@gmail.com (S.L.I.); dpredoi@gmail.com (D.P.)

Abstract: Presently, iron oxide nanoparticles are the only ones approved for clinical use as contrast agents in magnetic resonance imaging (MRI). Even though there is a high demand for these types of nanoparticles both for clinical use as well as for research, there are difficulties in obtaining stable nanoparticles with reproducible properties. In this context, in this study, we report the obtaining by an adapted coprecipitation method of dextran-coated maghemite nanoparticles (γ-Fe_2O_3 NPs). The morphology and structure of the dextran-coated maghemite nanoparticles (γ-Fe_2O_3 NPs) were determined using scanning electron microscopy (SEM) and transmission electron microscopy (TEM). The TEM and SEM micrographs highlighted the obtaining of particles of nanometric size and spherical shape morphology. Furthermore, the high-resolution transmission electron microscopy (HRTEM), as well as selected area diffraction (SAED), revealed that the obtained samples presented the structure of cubic maghemite. In this study, we also explored the effects of the co-precipitation synthesized dextran-coated maghemite nanoparticles (γ-Fe_2O_3 NPs) on the redox status of macrophages. For cytotoxicity evaluation of these NPs, murine macrophages (RAW 264.7 cell line) were exposed to different concentrations of dextran-coated maghemite nanoparticles (γ-Fe_2O_3 NPs) corresponding to 0–500 µg Fe^{3+}/mL and incubated for 24, 48, and 72 h. Intracellular iron uptake, changes in the oxidative stress parameters (reactive oxygen species production and malondialdehyde level), and the activity of antioxidant enzymes, as well as GSH concentration in cells, were evaluated after incubation with a lower (50 µg Fe^{3+}/mL) and higher (500 µg Fe^{3+}/mL) dose of NPs. The results indicated a significant decrease in RAW 264.7 cell viability after 72 h in the presence of NPs at concentrations above 25 µg Fe^{3+}/mL. An important accumulation of NPs, dependent on dose and exposure time, was detected in macrophages, but it induced only a limited raise in the oxidative status. We showed here that the antioxidant capacity of RAW 264.7 macrophages was efficient in counteracting dextran-coated maghemite nanoparticles (γ-Fe_2O_3 NPs) toxicity even at higher doses.

Keywords: iron oxide nanoparticles; dextran; RAW 264.7 macrophages; oxidative stress; antioxidant enzyme activity

1. Introduction

In the last decades, iron oxide nanoparticles (IONPs) have been extensively researched and used in the biomedical field as contrast agents, as carriers of biomolecules for drug delivery to specific organs and tissues, for gene therapy or as iron supplements for the treatment of patients suffering from anemia [1–5]. Over the years, researchers have made considerable efforts toward the elaboration of IONPs with improved physicochemical and surface properties [6–10]. In order to be considered for use in biomedical applications, the IONPs need to meet a series of criteria and, most of all, to be able to have excellent biocompatibility properties and to exhibit good biodistribution and pharmacokinetics properties [11–13]. It has been reported that the pharmacokinetic and biodistribution behavior of the IONPs is strongly correlated with the surface properties and physicochemical properties of the nanoparticles [14]. In this context, many attempts were made in order to improve the surface chemistry of IONPs and usually, those attempts involved the coating and/or functionalization of IONPs with different polymers, such as dextran, chitosan, starch and dextrin [3,15,16]. Amongst these, some have been successfully transferred to clinical trials [17], and some have even been approved for use by the U.S. Food and Drug Administration (FDA) [18] as contrast agents for MRI. One of the most successful polymers used in the functionalization of IONPs has been dextran, mainly due to its own excellent biological properties [19]. Dextran is used in the medical field as an antithrombotic because it has the ability to reduce blood viscosity [20]. Therefore, in this context, dextran-coated magnetic nanoparticles have been intensively studied over the years for their potential biomedical applications [21,22]. Even though there have been drawbacks with the iron oxide nanoparticles developed and approved for use over the years, there are still continuous worldwide efforts made for the optimizations of a synthesis route that will allow the obtaining of IONPs with reproducible properties and enhanced biological effects for biomedical applications. Therefore, in the last years, due to the tremendous efforts made by the scientific community, some iron oxide nanoparticles were approved by the FDA for clinical use, Feraheme® was approved in the treatment of iron deficiency, and Combidex® (U.S.) and Sinerem® (Europe) were also approved to be used as magnetic resonance imaging (MRI) agents. In addition, Nanotherm® (MagForce) was approved for being used in cancer treatment, and Lumirem® was given approval to be used as an imaging agent for the oral gastrointestinal tract [23–27]. The biological effects of IONPs are dependent on various factors, including size, surface characteristics, dose, solubility, and cell type [28–30]. The interaction of NPs with biological components (e.g., serum proteins) is another important factor that modulates their bioreactivity and toxic effects on cells [31].

Upon intravenous administration, IONPs are opsonized (adsorption of plasma proteins on the NP's surface) in the bloodstream before being phagocytized by macrophages and accumulated in the reticuloendothelial (RES) organs. This process promotes the accumulation of NPs in tissues, especially in tumor ones, due to the enhanced permeability and retention (EPR) effect [32]. Despite coating with plasma proteins, NPs may be cleared through opsonin-independent mechanisms by macrophages residing in the liver and spleen. Previously it was shown that either dextran or exposed IONPs could be directly recognized by macrophages [33]. Multiple alterations caused by exposure of macrophages to IONPs were previously reported [34,35]; however, the specific mechanisms of protective cellular response induced in the presence of various IONPs in macrophages are not clear.

The effects induced by these NPs on macrophage activation are a concern in terms of nanomaterial imaging, therapeutic efficacy, or systemic nanotoxicity. Excessive alterations drive macrophages to cell death, which has been associated with the development of several inflammatory diseases. Macrophages are equipped with a complex network of protective mechanisms against oxidative bursts (rapid release of ROS against pathogens) to survive during the inflammatory process [36]. How these mechanisms help macrophages to fight against oxidative stress induced by IONPs is an intriguing matter to reveal.

A deeper understanding of the interactions between NPs and macrophages is of great importance for researchers and clinicians as it can be directed toward generating biocompatible nanomaterials with specific surface characteristics fitting the biological environment.

In this context, we aimed to characterize the properties of newly synthesized dextran-coated maghemite nanoparticles (γ-Fe_2O_3 NPs) and to study the biological implications of their interaction with macrophages. Our focus was on cellular redox modulation after exposure to NPs, including oxidative stress induction and the activity of the endogenous antioxidant defense system.

2. Materials and Methods

2.1. Sample Preparation

The dextran-coated maghemite nanoparticles (γ-Fe_2O_3 NPs) suspension was synthesized by the adapted coprecipitation method in agreement with anterior studies [37–41].

2.2. Physicochemical Characterization

Information regarding the morphology and structure of dextran-coated maghemite nanoparticles (γ-Fe_2O_3 NPs) were determined using transmission electron microscopy. The TEM studies were carried out using a CM20 (Philips FEI, Eindhoven, The Netherlands) transmission electron microscope (TEM) equipped with a Lab6 instrument.

Furthermore, the morphology of the dextran-coated maghemite nanoparticles (γ-Fe_2O_3 NPs) was investigated using the scanning electron microscopy technique with the aid of an FEI Quanta Inspect microscope. Furthermore, the SEM micrographs were used to determine the particle size distribution of the nanoparticles.

The mean hydrodynamic diameter and zeta potential of dextran-coated maghemite nanoparticles (γ-Fe_2O_3 NPs) suspension were determined by dynamic light scattering (DLS) using a ZetaSizer Nano ZS (Malvern Instruments Limited, UK). All measurements were effectuated 3 times at 25 °C.

The changes of residual mass of dextran, dextran-coated γ-Fe_2O_3 NPs and γ-Fe_2O_3 NPs with temperature were analyzed by TG analysis using a Perkin Elmer instrument. The thermogravimetric data were obtained from a thermogravimetric analyzer (TGA) performed under a dry nitrogen atmosphere from 30 to 1000 °C. The heating rate was 10 °C /min.

2.3. Biological Assays

2.3.1. Cell Culture and Treatment

The macrophage RAW 264.7 cell line was purchased from American Type Culture Collection (ATCC, TIB-71, Manassas, VA, USA). The cells were grown in high-glucose Dulbecco Modified Eagle Medium (DMEM), supplemented with 10% fetal bovine serum (10270-106, origin South America, Gibco, Life Technologies, Carlsbad, CA, USA) and 1% antibiotic-antimycotic solution (A5955, Sigma, St. Louis, MO, US, USA) and maintained at 37 °C in a humidified atmosphere (95%) with 5% CO_2. For treatment, the cells were seeded at a density of 5×10^4 cells/mL and allowed to adhere for 24 h. Then, cells were exposed to different concentrations of dextran-coated γ-Fe_2O_3 NPs corresponding to 5, 10, 25, 50, 100, 250, and 500 µg Fe^{3+}/mL and incubated for 24, 48, and 72 h. Untreated RAW 264.7 cells were used as control.

2.3.2. MTT Assay

The cell viability was assessed using the colorimetric MTT (3-(4,5-dimethylthiazol-2-yl)-2,5-diphenyltetrazolium bromide) test relying on the reduction of the yellow MTT tetrazolium salt to purple formazan crystals in metabolically active cells. RAW 264.7 cells were seeded in a 24-well plate at a density of 5×10^4 cells/mL/well. After treatment, the medium from each well was removed, and a volume of 250 µL 1 mg/mL MTT solution was added. After 2 h of incubation, the formazan crystals were dissolved in 250 µL 2-propanol solution. The absorbance was measured at 595 nm using a Tecan multi-plate reader (TecanGENios, Grödic, Germany).

2.3.3. Quantification of Intracellular Iron Content

The level of intracellular iron was measured as previously described [42]. After treatment with NPs, cells were trypsinized, washed with phosphate-buffered saline (PBS), centrifuged and counted. The cell pellet was digested in 5 N HCl for 24 h at 37 °C and then centrifuged at 2000× *g* rpm for 10 min. A volume of 50 µL of supernatant was mixed with 50 µL 1% ammonium persulfate solution (to convert the Fe^{2+} to Fe^{3+} ions) and 100 µL of 0.5 M potassium thiocyanate and shaken for 5 min in order to develop the red colored iron-thiocyanate. The formed complexes were spectrophotometrically detected at 450 nm. A standard curve with $FeCl_3 \bullet 6H_2O$ ranging from 0–250 µg Fe^{3+}/mL was used to quantify the intracellular iron. The total amount of iron was related to the cell number.

2.3.4. Measurement of ROS Production

The level of reactive oxygen species (ROS) generated in RAW 264.7 cells was estimated using the dye 2′,7′-dichlorodihydrofluorescein diacetate (H_2DCF-DA; D6883, Sigma-Aldrich, St. Louis, MO, USA). Only two NPs concentrations, selected after cell viability evaluation, were investigated: 50 and 500 µg/mL. After treatment with NPs, the cells seeded in a 6-well plate were washed with PBS and incubated at 37 °C in the dark with a volume of 1.5 mL of 10 µM H_2DCFDA solution for 30 min. Then, the cells were trypsinized, centrifuged and resuspended in 2 mL of PBS solution. The fluorescence of dichlorofluorescein (DCF) was spectrofluorimetrically recorded at 488 nm ex./515 nm em wavelength. The RFU values were related to the cell number in each sample.

2.3.5. Preparation of Cell Lysate

RAW 264.7 cells were seeded in 75 cm^2 culture flasks at a density of 2 × 10^6 cells/flask. After treatment with NPs, the cell suspensions were centrifuged for 5 min at 1500× *g* rpm, and the cellular pellets were washed and resuspended in PBS. Cell lysis was obtained through ultrasonication 3 times for 30 s each, on ice, using a UP50H ultrasonicator (80% amplitude, 1 cycle) from Hielscher Ultrasound Technology (Teltow, Germany). The total extract was centrifuged at 3000× *g* rpm for 10 min at 4 °C, and the supernatants were collected. The protein concentration in each sample was measured using the Bradford method and a calibration curve of bovine serum albumin (BSA) ranging from 0 to 1.5 mg/mL protein.

2.3.6. Detection of Lipid Peroxidation Products

The level of malondialdehyde (MDA) in RAW 264.7 cells was assessed as an indicator of lipid peroxidation via the thiobarbituric acid reaction, according to Dinischiotu et al. [43]. Briefly, a volume of 200 µL from cell lysate was mixed with 700 µL 0.1 N HCl and incubated for 20 min at room temperature. After adding 900 µL of 0.025 M thiobarbituric acid (TBA), the samples were incubated for another 65 min at 37 °C. Finally, a volume of 400 µL of PBS was added. The fluorescence of MDA (RFU) was recorded using a 520 nm/549 nm (excitation/emission) filter. A calibration curve with 1,1,3,3-tetramethoxy propane in the range of 0.05–5 µM was used to calculate the MDA concentration in each sample. The results are expressed as nmoles of MDA/mg protein.

2.3.7. Quantification of Reduced Glutathione (GSH) Concentration

The intracellular GSH content was estimated in RAW 264.7 cells using the Glutathione Assay Kit (CS0260, Sigma-Aldrich, St. Louis, MO, USA). Thus, cell lysates were precipitated with 5-sulfosalicylic acid (1:1) and centrifugated at 10,000× *g* rpm for 10 min at 4 °C. A volume of 10 µL from the supernatant was mixed with 150 µL Assay buffer containing 5,50-dithiobis(2-nitrobenzoic acid) and incubated for 10 min at room temperature. The 5-thio-2-nitrobenozoic acid (TNB) formed was measured spectrophotometrically at 405 nm. A calibration curve of GSH (3.125–50 µM) was similarly prepared. The GSH levels were expressed as nmoles of GSH/mg protein.

2.3.8. Measurement of Antioxidant Enzymatic Activity

i. Superoxide dismutase (SOD, EC 1.15.1.1) activity was measured according to the method of Paoletti et al. [44], which is based on NADPH oxidation by the superoxide anions. Superoxide anions were generated from oxygen molecules by the addition of triethanolamine: diethanolamine (100 mM) buffer pH 7.4, containing $MnCl_2$-EDTA (100 mM /50 mM) and 2-mercaptoethanol (100 mM) to each sample of cell lysate. After the addition of 7.5 mM NADPH solution, the decrease of absorbance was followed at 340 nm for 10 min at 37 °C. A sample-free control was run in parallel. SOD activity was calculated in terms of U/mg of protein, where one unit (U) of activity was defined as the amount of enzyme required to inhibit the rate of NADPH oxidation of the control by 50%.

ii. Catalase (CAT, EC 1.11.1.6) activity was assessed by monitoring the disappearance of H_2O_2 at 240 nm, according to the Aebi method [45]. The cell lysate was mixed with 0.059 M H_2O_2 and 0.1 M K_2HPO_4/KH_2PO_4 buffer, pH 7.1, and the reaction kinetics was recorded spectrophotometrically for 1 min. CAT activity was calculated in terms of U/mg protein, where 1 U was the amount of enzyme that catalyzed the conversion of one μmole H_2O_2 in 1 min.

iii. Glutathione peroxidase (GPX, EC 1.11.1.9) activity was assessed by the Beutler method [46] from cell lysate, using 7 mM tert-butyl hydroperoxide and 2 mM NADPH as substrates. The conversion of NADPH to $NADP^+$ was followed by recording the changes in absorption intensity at 340 nm for 5 min. One unit was defined as the amount of enzyme that catalyzes the conversion of 1 μmole of NADPH per minute. The activity was calculated as U/mg protein, using a molar extinction coefficient (ε_{NADPH}) of $6.22 \times 10^3\ M^{-1}cm^{-1}$.

2.4. Statistical Analysis

Data were obtained from 3 independent experiments and expressed in terms of mean ± standard deviation. The results from each sample were represented on graphs as percentages from the control (100%). Statistical analysis was performed through GraphPad Prism version 8.0.2 (GraphPad Software, Inc., San Diego, CA, USA) using two-way ANOVA variance with the Geisser-Greenhouse correction followed by Sidak's multiple comparison test. Values of * $p < 0.05$, ** $p < 0.01$, and *** $p < 0.001$ were considered statistically significant (each sample vs. control).

3. Results and Discussion

Nanoparticles in general, and maghemite nanoparticles in particular, due to their adaptability, represent a promising platform that could improve therapeutic delivery and controlled release in the area of different affected organs. The size of the particles and their stability are two very important parameters that characterize the behavior of nanoparticles. Thus, studies that contribute to the understanding of these nanometric suspensions are very important.

The morphology and structure of the prepared dextran-coated maghemite nanoparticles (γ-Fe_2O_3 NPs) were investigated by TEM (Figure 1a–d). The large bright field TEM image (Figure 1a) revealed that the dextran-coated iron oxide nanoparticles have a uniform particle distribution of nanometric sizes and spherical shapes. Moreover, the particle size distribution was also determined by measuring the mean diameter, D, of approximately 500 particles.

The average grain size distribution obtained from the TEM image is depicted in Figure 1b, and it was emphasized that the particle size distribution was approximately 12.4 nm. Furthermore, the high-resolution TEM image, presented in Figure 1c, revealed the existence of regular fringes in the nanoparticle having a distance of 2.51 Å, which is characteristic of the (311) interplanar distance of the cubic maghemite. The clear lattice fringe observed in the HRTEM image highlighted the obtaining of nanoparticles with a crystalline nature. The SAED patterns obtained for the dextran-coated iron oxide nanoparticles were indexed to be of cubic maghemite, γ-Fe_2O_3, and the obtained rings were attributed to the (220), (311), (400), (422), (511) and (440) planes, respectively in agreement with existing reported data [47,48].

Furthermore, additional information about the morphology of the dextran-coated maghemite nanoparticles (γ-Fe_2O_3 NPs) was also gathered using scanning electron microscopy. The results obtained from the SEM studies are depicted in Figure 2a–c. The SEM micrograph presented in Figure 2a, as well as the inset of the high magnification SEM image (Figure 2b), confirmed the data obtained from the TEM studies and revealed the obtaining of particles having nanometric sizes and spherical shapes. In addition, the SEM micrograph also depicted the uniformity a homogeneity of the particles. More than that, the particle size distribution obtained using the SEM micrograph determined the grain size distribution at 13.1 nm, which is consistent with the one obtained from the TEM image.

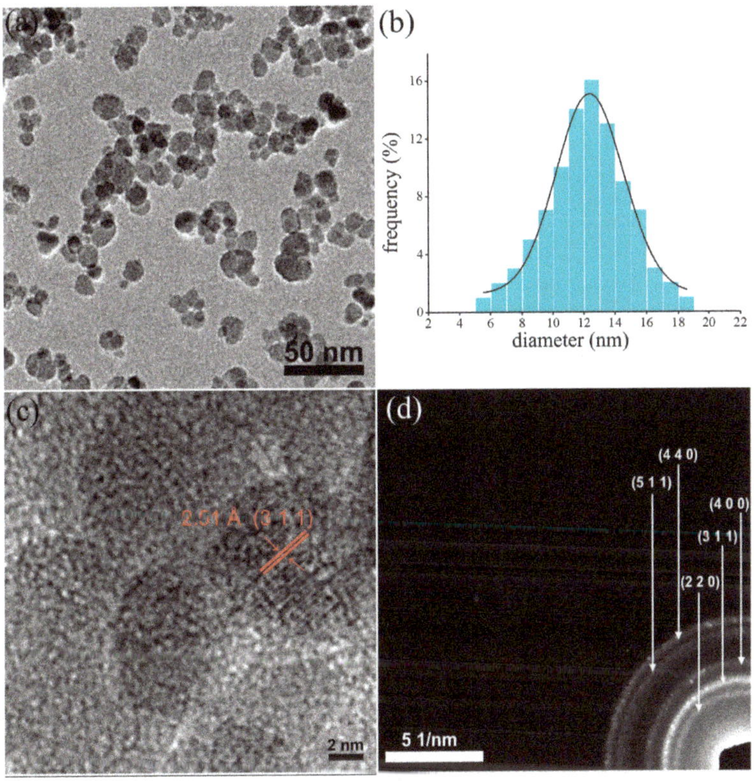

Figure 1. TEM image (**a**), particle size distributions obtained from large area TEM image (**b**), high-resolution TEM (HRTEM) image (**c**) and selected area electron diffraction (SAED) (**d**) of dextran-coated maghemite nanoparticles (γ-Fe_2O_3 NPs).

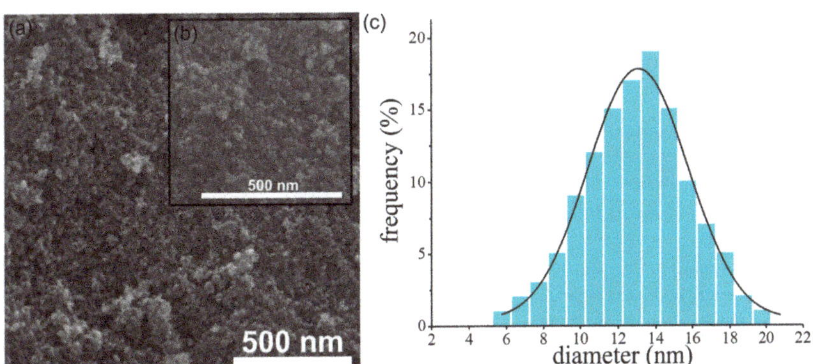

Figure 2. SEM image (**a**), inset of high magnification SEM image (**b**) and particle size distributions obtained from SEM image (**c**) of dextran-coated maghemite nanoparticles (γ-Fe_2O_3 NPs).

The stabilization of maghemite nanoparticles by the adsorption of a layer of dextran around the particles is very important in biological and medical applications. The formation of the dispersant layer (adlayer, in our case, dextran) was very important for the stabilization of maghemite suspensions. It is known that the thin layers on the surface of the particles lead to the agglomeration of the particles. For this purpose, DLS studies were carried out to determine the hydrodynamic diameter of maghemite nanoparticles covered with dextran in suspension. The zeta potential was also determined for the studied suspensions.

Figure 3 shows the distribution based on volume (a) and the distribution based on numbers (b). Both the distribution based on volume and the one based on numbers clearly show that the suspension of maghemite nanoparticles covered with dextran does not present aggregates. As can be seen from the volume size distribution, the analyzed sample is composed of approximately 45.4 nm particles (Figure 3a). The number distribution presented in Figure 3b was monomodal, with an average peak at 38 nm. Figure 3c revealed the intensity particle size distribution obtained for maghemite nanoparticles coated with dextran in suspension. The graph shows a monomodal distribution with a distinct peak at 45.7 nm without indicating the presence of aggregates in the studied sample. The ratio D_H/D_{TEM} representing the hydrodynamic diameter (D_H) calculated from DLS studies and the nanoparticle diameter calculated by TEM (D_{TEM}) was 3.7 nm. On the other hand, the ratio D_H/D_{SEM} representing the hydrodynamic diameter (D_H) calculated from DLS studies and the nanoparticle diameter calculated by SEM (D_{SEM}) was 3.5 nm. Both the D_H/D_{TEM} ratio and the D_H/D_{SEM} ratio show that the dextran present on the surface of the maghemite nanoparticles results in an increase in the size of the obtained sample. This result is in full agreement with previous studies [49–52]. The dispersion stability of dextran-coated maghemite suspension was measured through the absolute value of zeta potential. According to previous studies [53], it can be said that a nanofluid has a colloidal dispersion stability if the absolute zeta potential is greater than 30 mV. The colloidal stability of dextran-coated maghemite suspension using zeta potential was presented in Figure 3d. The zeta potential measured for dextran-coated maghemite suspension was −38.4 mV. Since the measured value is higher than 30 mV, it can be said that the dextran-coated maghemite suspension is at good colloidal stability condition.

The numerical value of the polydispersity index (PDI) of the γ-Fe_2O_3 NPs was 0.165. In agreement with previous studies [54,55], the PDI is a representation of the population size distribution in a sample. Moreover, previous studies [56] have demonstrated that values lower than or equal to 0.2 are considered to be accepted in practice for nanoscale materials containing polymers. Moreover, PDI values between 0.0 and 0.5 highlight the fact that the analyzed sample is uniform in relation to the particle size [57]. The DLS and zeta potential studies showed that the dextran layer on the surface of the maghemite nanoparticles has a fairly significant thickness, which led to very good stability, as could be seen from the zeta potential analysis.

Furthermore, the stability of the dextran-coated γ-Fe_2O_3 NPs was also investigated visually. Images of dextran-coated γ-Fe_2O_3 NPs suspensions kept at room temperature in glass vials over different periods of time are depicted in Figure 4a–i. The images were taken after 1 day, 3 days and 7 days. As can be observed from the images presented in Figure 4, the suspensions were stable over time, and there was no sign of precipitation or deposition of the nanoparticles at the bottom of the vials. Moreover, Figure 4a depicts the image of the dextran-coated γ-Fe_2O_3 NPs suspensions obtained from the synthesis without dilution. The images of the vials taken after 1 day, 3 days, and 7 days emphasized that the obtained suspension is stable and there were no signs of particle agglomeration or particle deposition in the investigated time interval. Furthermore, the diluted dextran-coated γ-Fe_2O_3 NPs suspensions used in the biological assays were also studied, and their images after 1 day, 3 days and 7 days are depicted in Figure 4d–i. The results were in agreement with previous studies and determined that the obtained suspensions were stable in time.

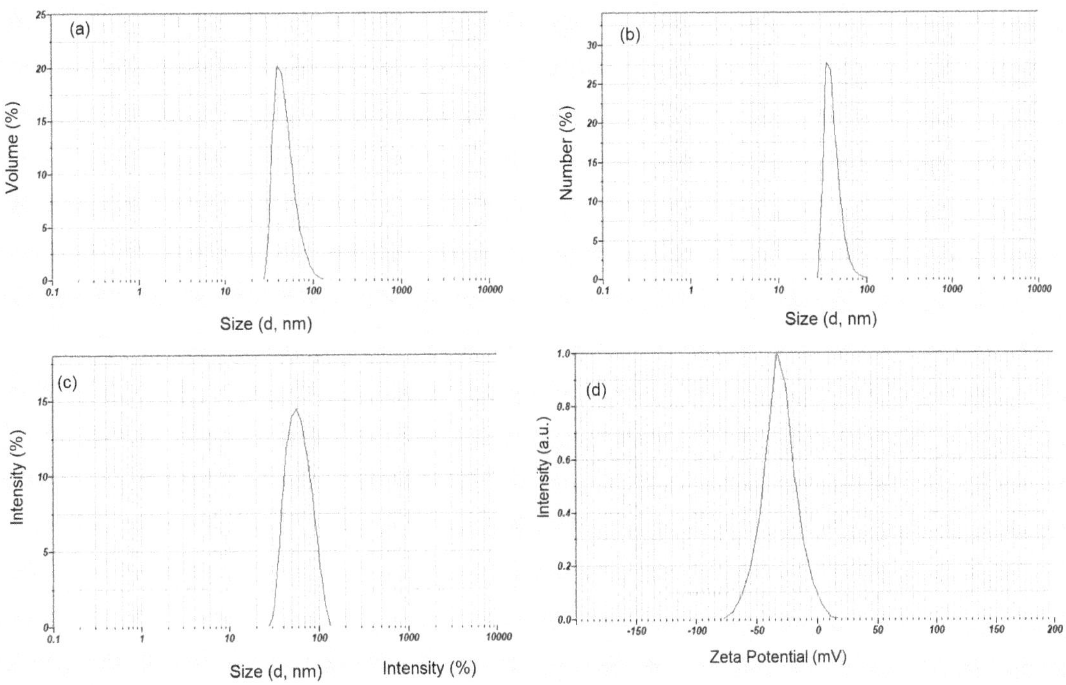

Figure 3. Volume size distribution (**a**), particle size by number distribution (**b**), intensity size distribution (**c**) and zeta potential (**d**) for maghemite nanoparticles coated with dextran in suspension.

The TGA curves of dextran (a), dextran-coated γ-Fe_2O_3 NPs (b) and γ-Fe_2O_3 NPs (c) in the temperature range of 30−1000 °C are presented in Figure 5. For all the samples, we observed an initial small weight loss (between 30–150 °C). This small weight loss was due to the amount of water physically absorbed from their surface and the dehydroxylation of hydroxyl groups on the surface. This behavior was in accordance with the other previous results [58,59]. As can be seen in Figure 5, the decomposition of dextran takes place in a single step in the temperature range of 180–750 °C. The thermal decomposition of γ-Fe_2O_3 NPs takes place in two stages. The first stage of dextran degradation takes place with a mass loss in the range of 150–400 °C. The second stage of dextran degradation takes place in the range of 400–700 °C. After 700 °C, we have no more mass loss, which shows that the dextran has been completely decomposed, and what remains are only maghemite nanoparticles.

The obtained results were in good agreement with previous studies [60–62]. According to previous studies [63], the percentage of dextran molecules attached to the surface of γ-Fe_2O_3 NPs can be simply calculated by measuring the difference in residual weight between uncoated γ-Fe_2O_3 NPs and dextran-coated γ-Fe_2O_3 NPs. This result reveals that the coating efficiency of the γ-Fe_2O_3 NPs was about 52.13 %. The TGA results are in agreement with the results obtained from DLS and zeta potential studies. Moreover, our results obtained from TGA analysis are in agreement with previous studies [63] that obtained a dextran-coating efficiency of magnetite nanoparticles of approximately 50.12% and 53.89%, respectively.

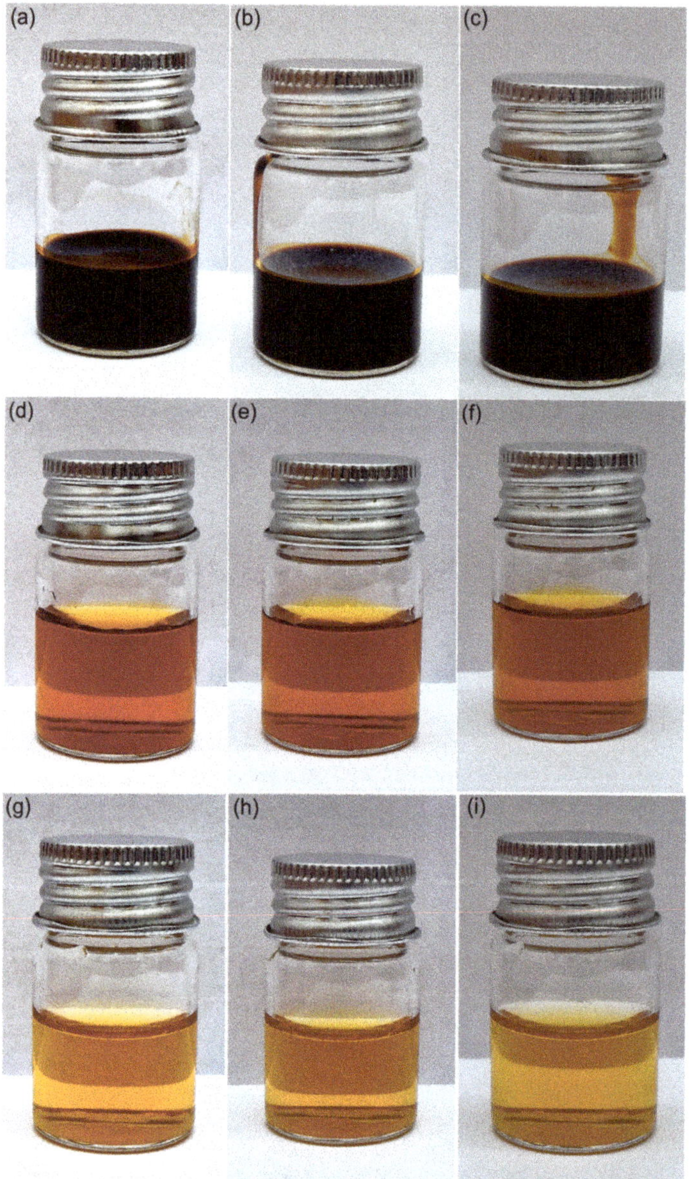

Figure 4. Visual appearance of prepared dextran-coated γ-Fe_2O_3 NPs (**a–c**), dextran-coated γ-Fe_2O_3 NPs with 500 µg Fe^{3+}/mL (**d–f**) and dextran-coated γ-Fe_2O_3 NPs with 50 µg Fe^{3+}/mL (**g–i**) observed after 1 day (**a**,**d**,**g**), 3 days (**b**,**e**,**h**) and 7 days (**c**,**f**,**i**).

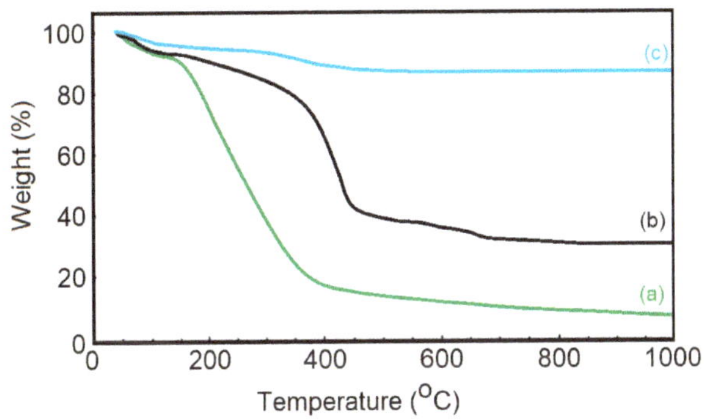

Figure 5. TGA curves of dextran (**a**), dextran-coated ɤ-Fe_2O_3 NPs (**b**) and ɤ-Fe_2O_3 NPs (**c**).

The cell viability of RAW 264.7 murine cells exposed to dextran-coated maghemite nanoparticles (ɤ-Fe_2O_3 NPs) in a concentration range of 5–500 µg Fe^{3+}/mL varied in a dose and time-dependent manner (Figure 6). For doses below 250 µg Fe^{3+}/mL, no significant decrease of viability, compared to control, was noticed after 24 and 48 h from treatment except for the dose of 100 µg Fe^{3+}/mL at 24 h. For the same exposure intervals, the dose of 500 µg Fe^{3+}/mL induced a significant reduction of cellular viability by 35% and 38%, respectively, compared to control cells. After 72 h of treatment, all doses above 25 µg Fe^{3+}/mL caused a significant decrease in this parameter. Two doses of NPs of 50 and 500 µg Fe^{3+}/mL have been chosen for the following determinations.

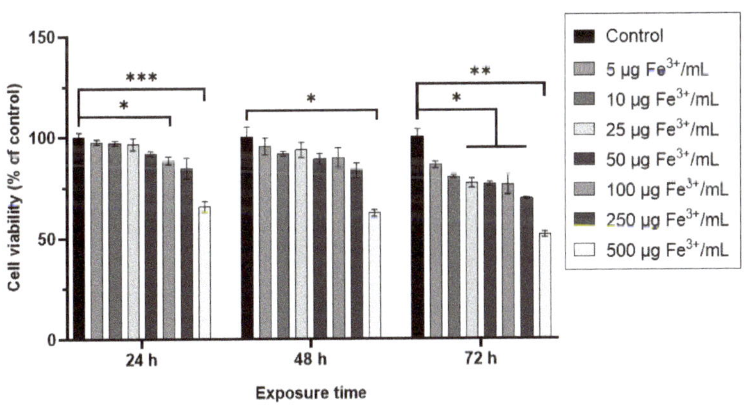

Figure 6. Cell viability of RAW 264.7 cells after 24, 48, and 72 h exposure to different doses of dextran-coated ɤ-Fe_2O_3 NPs (corresponding to 5–500 µg Fe^{3+}/mL). Data (n = 3) are expressed as relative values (%) related to control ± SD. The results were considered statistically significant at * $p < 0.05$, ** $p < 0.01$ and *** $p < 0.001$ (sample vs. control).

The internalization of NPs was quantified by measuring the level of iron in the treated RAW 264.7 cells with NPs corresponding to doses of 50 µg Fe^{3+}/mL and 500 µg Fe^{3+}/mL, respectively (Figure 7a). The intracellular concentration of Fe^{3+} increased in time, depending on the applied dose. The lower dose determined a significant increase of Fe^{3+} concentration by about 42%, 101%, and 132% after 24 h, 48 h, and 72 h, respectively, whereas the higher one generated a significant raise of the intracellular Fe^{3+} level by about 383%, 721%, and 997% respectively, compared to control cells. According to Figure 7b, the production of ROS in RAW 264.7 murine cells exposed to NPs increased in a concentration and time-dependent manner up to 48 h of exposure, followed by a slight decrease after 72 h.

The dose of 50 μg/mL determined a significant raise of ROS levels by about 17%, 75%, and 57% after 24 h, 48 h, and 72 h, respectively, whereas the higher dose generated a significant increase of these by 104%, 185% and 130% after the same intervals of exposure, compared to control cells. Malondialdehyde (MDA) is an end-product of the oxidative degradation of polyunsaturated fatty acids (PUFA) and is an indicator of cellular oxidative stress. In the RAW 264.7 murine cells exposed for 24 h to both doses of NPs, the MDA concentrations increased significantly by 56% (lower dose) and 212% (higher dose) in comparison with control cells (Figure 7c). The treatment of RAW 264.7 cells with a dose of 50 μg Fe^{3+}/mL for 48 h and 72 h generated insignificant increases in MDA levels by 7% and 25%, respectively, compared to the control. Instead, exposure to NPs corresponding to 500 μg Fe^{3+}/mL determined significant raises of MDA concentrations by 82% and 48% after 48 h and 72 h, respectively, relative to the control.

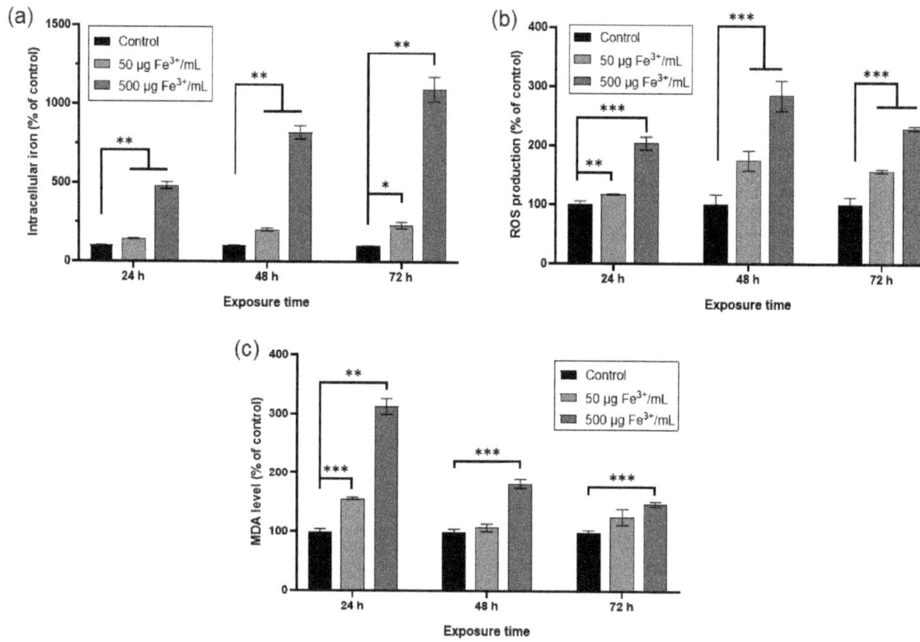

Figure 7. Cellular iron uptake and levels of oxidative stress parameters in RAW 264.7 cells after 24, 48, and 72 h exposure to two doses of dextran-coated γ-Fe_2O_3 NPs corresponding to 50 and 500 μg Fe^{3+}/mL. (**a**) intracellular iron content quantified by iron-thiocyanate reaction; (**b**) level of reactive oxygen species detected by H_2DCF-DA assay; (**c**) level of malondialdehyde estimated by TBA reaction. Data (n = 3) are expressed as relative values (%) related to control ± SD. The results were considered statistically significant at * $p < 0.05$, ** $p < 0.01$ and *** $p < 0.001$ (sample vs. control).

The cellular antioxidant defense system is formed by non-enzymatic and enzymatic molecules. Reduced glutathione (γ-glutamyl-cysteinyl-glycine) is a tripeptide that represents the main non-enzymatic molecule. The exposure of RAW 264.7 cells to NPs corresponding to 50 μg Fe^{3+}/mL determined a significant increase of GSH level by 148% after 24 h related to the control (Figure 8a). At longer periods of treatment, this increase was by about 81% and 63% after 48 h and 72 h, respectively, compared to the control. Even if this increase is diminished in a time-dependent manner, the level of this non-enzymatic antioxidant remains higher in comparison with the control. In the case of treatment with the higher dose, the level of GSH decreased by 66% and 42% after 24 h and 48 h, respectively, and increased by 44% after 72 h, although at this time point, the result was not statistically significant.

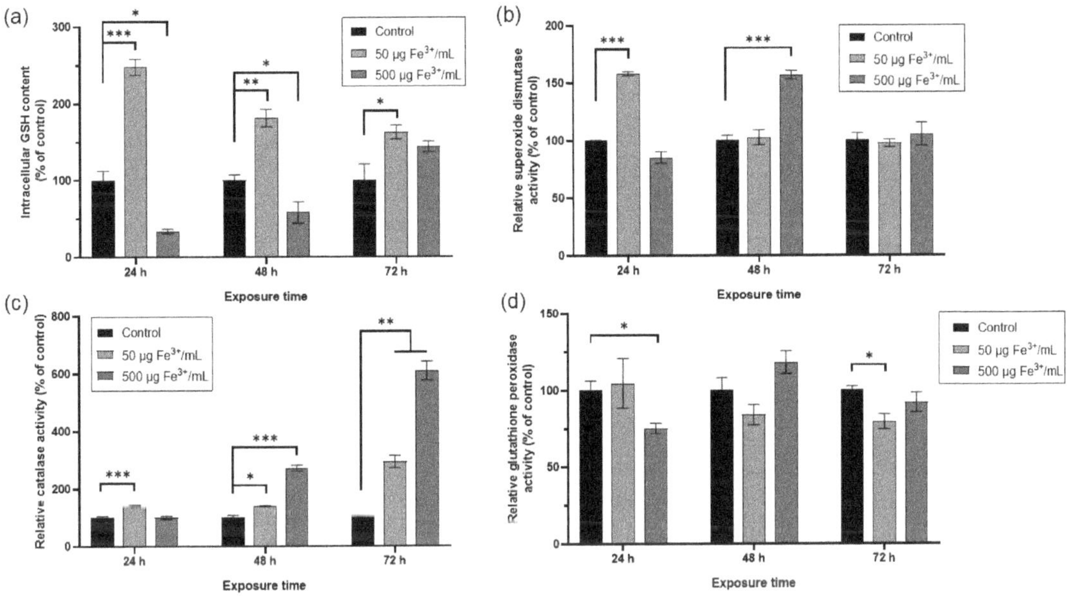

Figure 8. Antioxidant response of RAW 264.7 cells after 24, 48, and 72 h exposure to two doses of dextran-coated γ-Fe_2O_3 NPs corresponding to 50 and 500 µg Fe^{3+}/mL. (**a**) level of intracellular GSH concentration; (**b**) enzymatic activity of SOD; (**c**) enzymatic activity of CAT; (**d**) enzymatic activity of GPX. Data ($n = 3$) are expressed as relative values (%) related to control ± SD. The results were considered statistically significant at * $p < 0.05$, ** $p < 0.01$ and *** $p < 0.001$ (sample vs. control).

Antioxidant enzymes such as superoxide dismutase (SOD), catalase (CAT), and glutathione peroxidase (GPX) work together to counteract the toxic ROS produced in cells.

The specific activity of SOD (Figure 8b) increased in the cells exposed to NPs corresponding to 50 µg Fe^{3+}/mL by 58% after 24 h and returned to the control level after 48 h and 72 h. However, post-treatment with NPs corresponding to 500 µg Fe^{3+}/mL, this enzymatic activity decreased by 15% after 24 h, increased significantly by 57% after 48 h and returned to the control level after 72 h.

The specific activity of CAT (Figure 8c) increased significantly by about 40% after 24 h and 48 h of exposure to NPs corresponding to 50 µg Fe^{3+}/mL. After 72 h, this enzymatic activity raised significantly by 193% compared to the control. The treatment of RAW 264.7 cells with NPs corresponding to 500 µg Fe^{3+} /mL determined no significant change in the specific activity of CAT after 24 h and a significant increase by 171% and 510%, respectively, after 48 h and 72 h.

The specific activity of GPX (Figure 8d) in the RAW 264.7 cells exposed to NPs corresponding to 50 µg Fe^{3+}/mL decreased significantly only after 72 h, by 20% related to control. High dose administration significantly inhibited the specific activity of GPX by 25% only after 24 h, then after 48 h, only a slight activation by 18% was noticed, and after 72 h, the level returned to normal.

The RAW 246.7 murine macrophage cell line is used to screen natural and engineered products to predict their potential effect in vivo [64]. Macrophage responses to different NPs are influenced by dose, size, composition, and surface properties and uptake these by endocytosis or phagocytosis, undergoing polarization [65].

In the presence of serum-containing culture media, NPs' surfaces form protein coronae that confer properties involved in their interaction with cells. Previously, it was shown that the uptake of NPs by macrophages was directly related to the amounts of proteins adsorbed on the NPs' surface [66]. Also, studies in vivo revealed that dextran-coated supermagnetic iron (SPIO) NPs presented on their surface, mannan-binding lectins bound to the dextran coating, and histidine-rich glycoprotein and kininogen bound to the iron oxide part. Also, secondary binders such as complement lectin and contact clotting factors were identified [33].

In our study, the uptake of NPs containing protein corona is highlighted by the increase of Fe^{3+} ions concentration in the treated RAW 246.7 cells, these ions being released from the maghemite core. There is a significant probability that Fe^{3+} ions to be complexed by low molecular weight compounds such as citrate, nucleotides, and glycosaminoglycans. These Fe^{3+}-chelates could be reduced to Fe^{2+} by NAD(P)H-dependent flavoenzymes, lipoyl dehydrogenase being probably the dominant catalyst within cells [67]. As a result, the level of Fe^{2+} probably increased, and the Fenton reaction occurred, generating hydroxyl radicals (HO•) and hydroxide ions (OH−).

On the other hand, due to the interaction of NPs with RAW 246.7 cells, NADPH oxidase could be activated, producing superoxide anions ($O_2^{\bullet -}$), as was proved in the case of other types of NPs [68]. Metabolism of iron occurs predominately in mitochondria, and its overload can also affect mitochondrial function because this transition metal is involved in ROS production, which can diminish the expression of mitochondrial-encoded respiratory chain subunits [69]. Superoxide passage by simple diffusion inside cells is highly unfavorable [70], but this anion can use anion channels of membranes to enter cells [71]. Superoxide can also react with H_2O_2 in the Haber-Weiss reaction, catalyzed by iron [72], also generating hydroxyl radicals (HO•).

ROS can attack PUFA and generate MDA, which is an end-product of lipid peroxidation. These considerations are supported by the same pattern of cellular Fe^{3+} and ROS levels up to 48 h of exposure. The highest level of MDA was registered after 24 h, being correlated with ROS concentration. Later on, MDA concentrations decreased in a time-dependent manner, probably due to the activation of the non-enzymatic and enzymatic antioxidant systems.

Alternatively, superoxide can be dismutated in the reaction catalyzed by SOD, generating H_2O_2 and molecular oxygen [73]. In mammalian cells, there are 2 types of SOD: Cu/Zn-SOD, present mainly in the cytosol, and mitochondrial MnSOD. The lower dose (50 µg Fe^{3+}/mL) of NPs determined an increase in the total SOD activity after 24 h of exposure, followed by a decrease to the control level after 48 h and 72 h, respectively. Probably, this decrease occurred due to the significant level of H_2O_2 generated, which could inhibit Cu/Zn-SOD [74]. Also, the exposure to the higher dose (500 µg Fe^{3+}/mL) of NPs slightly diminished the total SOD after 24 h, probably due to the same reason. Instead, the increase of total SOD after 24 h in cells exposed to the lower dose we assumed it might be a consequence of the Mn-SOD activation. As shown in a previous study [75], Mn-SOD activity could be induced in macrophages as a mechanism for the acquirement of oxidative stress resistance through the participation of PARP1 in the regulation of Mn-SOD gene expression. Mn-SOD is possible to respond to an endogenous redox imbalance that involves superoxide leakage as a result of disruption of mitochondria functions in iron-overloaded cells. However, how much Mn-SOD contributes to the strongly elevated level of total SOD after 24 h is unclear and needs to be further investigated. Possibly, after 48 h, the incorporation of iron instead of Mn into Mn-SOD switched its activity to a prooxidant peroxidase that utilizes H_2O_2 for the oxidation of other molecules [76]. Previously, it was also proved that the accumulation of iron decreased the expression and activity of Mn-SOD [77]. In our opinion, after 48 h, the high concentration of Fe^{2+} generated an increase in Mn-SOD activity due to the two-ion switch. After 72 h, possibly the accumulation of Fe^{2+} decreased the expression and activity of Mn-SOD.

CAT catalyzes the reaction of decomposition of H_2O_2, a product of the reaction catalyzed by SOD, in water and molecular oxygen. CAT is a porphyrin-containing tetramer that is located mainly in peroxisomes [78]. The variation of CAT-specific activity in time can be correlated with that of total SOD in the case of treatment with the lower dose. In the case of the higher dose, the significant increase of CAT-specific activity after 48 h could be correlated with the high total SOD activity. Possibly, the high quantity of H_2O_2 generated after the switch of Mn with iron ions was involved in the up-regulation of Mn-SOD and CAT gene transcription [79].

The level of H_2O_2 produced in cells can be controlled not only by CAT activity but also by GPX. This latter enzyme catalyzes H_2O_2 decomposition in the presence of GSH to form water and oxidized glutathione (GSSG). The Michaelis constant for H_2O_2 is 50 times higher for CAT compared to that of GPX [80]. GPX is the first enzyme that is activated under high levels of ROS, playing an important role as a first line of defense against oxidative stress [81]. However, taking into account the high level of CAT activity, we could consider that the quantity of H_2O_2 generated was removed by CAT action.

GPX also catalyzes the reaction between GSH and lipid peroxides, playing a role in the detoxification of these molecules. After exposure to the lower dose, GPX-specific activity was not changed after 24 h and decreased after the other time intervals, suggesting that this enzyme was not involved in the removal of MDA. Taking into account the pattern of GSH variation corresponding to this dose, probably this tripeptide was a substrate for glutathione-S-transferase (GST), which could be implicated in MDA removal [82]. At the same time, in the case of treatment of RAW 246.7 cells with the higher dose of NPs, GPX was not efficient in MDA detoxification.

In the present study, at a lower dose (50 μg Fe^{3+}/mL), the GSH level decreased after 24 h and increased in a time-dependent manner up to 72 h when it became higher than the control level. The higher dose (500 μg Fe^{3+}/mL) increased the GSH level by 150% after 24 h exposure and decreased later on, remaining higher than the control level at all time intervals. Previous studies revealed that dextran-coated maghemite nanoparticles (γ-Fe_2O_3 NPs) modulate the GSH level in a cell-type-dependent manner [47,83].

Our results highlight the need to evaluate in-depth the interactions between IONPs and cells to take full advantage of the intrinsic properties of these NPs in biological systems.

4. Conclusions

The present study was focused on the response of the endogenous antioxidant defense system induced in RAW 264.7 macrophages upon exposure to dextran-coated maghemite nanoparticles (γ-Fe_2O_3 NPs). The dextran-coated maghemite nanoparticles (γ-Fe_2O_3 NPs) were obtained using an adapted coprecipitation method. The morphology of the dextran-coated maghemite nanoparticles (γ-Fe_2O_3 NPs) was investigated by TEM and SEM studies. The SEM and TEM micrographs highlighted that the particles were well-dispersed, presenting a nanometric size distribution and spherical shape. The particle size distributions determined from TEM and SEM micrographs were 12.4 nm and 13.1 nm. Moreover, the HRTEM studies revealed clear lattice fringes, which suggested a good crystallinity of the samples. In addition, the SAED patterns obtained for the dextran-coated iron oxide nanoparticles were indexed to be of cubic maghemite, γ-Fe_2O_3. As observed in the DLS studies, the dextran layer on the surface of the maghemite particles is large enough to ensure the very good stability of these nanoparticles. Therefore, maghemite nanoparticles functionalized with dextran could be successfully applied in different biological and medical fields.

RAW 246.7 cells efficiently counteracted the oxidative stress induced by the exposure to these NPs. This statement is supported by the increased GSH level and the diminished MDA content in the RAW 246.7 cells after the maximum exposure time.

The results obtained in this study emphasized that dextran-coated maghemite nanoparticles (γ-Fe_2O_3 NPs) obtained by an adapted coprecipitation method could be used in the medical and pharmaceutical fields due to their physicochemical and biological properties.

Author Contributions: Conceptualization, D.P. and A.D.; methodology, D.P. and A.D.; software, M.B., D.P. and S.L.I.; validation, D.P., A.D., M.B., S.L.I. and N.B.; formal analysis, D.P.; investigation, M.B. and S.L.I. resources, D.P., A.D. and N.B.; data curation, D.P., A.D., M.B., S.L.I. and N.B.; writing—original draft preparation, D.P., A.D., M.B. and S.L.I.; writing—review and editing, D.P., A.D., M.B. and S.L.I.; visualization, D.P., A.D., M.B., S.L.I. and N.B.; supervision, D.P., A.D., M.B., S.L.I. and N.B.; project administration, D.P.; funding acquisition, D.P. All authors have read and agreed to the published version of the manuscript.

Funding: This research received no external funding.

Institutional Review Board Statement: Not applicable.

Informed Consent Statement: Not applicable.

Data Availability Statement: Data is available on demand from the corresponding authors.

Conflicts of Interest: The authors declare no conflict of interest.

References

1. Edge, D.; Shortt, C.M.; Gobbo, O.L.; Teughels, S.; Prina-Mello, A.; Volkov, Y.; MacEneaney, P.; Radomski, M.W.; Markos, F. Pharmacokinetics and bio-distribution of novel super paramagnetic iron oxide nanoparticles (SPIONs) in the anaesthetized pig. *Clin. Exp. Pharmacol. Physiol.* **2016**, *43*, 319–326. [CrossRef] [PubMed]
2. Kievit, F.M.; Veiseh, O.; Bhattarai, N.; Fang, C.; Gunn, J.W.; Lee, D.; Ellenbogen, R.G.; Olson, J.M.; Zhang, M. PEI-PEG-Chitosan Copolymer Coated Iron Oxide Nanoparticles for Safe Gene Delivery: Synthesis, complexation, and transfection. *Adv. Funct. Mater.* **2009**, *19*, 2244–2251. [CrossRef] [PubMed]
3. Arami, H.; Stephen, Z.; Veiseh, O.; Zhang, M. Chitosan-Coated Iron Oxide Nanoparticles for Molecular Imaging and Drug Delivery. *Adv. Polym. Sci.* **2011**, *243*, 163–184.
4. Berman, S.M.C.; Walczak, P.; Bulte, J.W.M. Tracking stem cells using magnetic nanoparticles. *Nanomed. Nanobiotechnol.* **2011**, *3*, 343–355. [CrossRef]
5. Lu, M.; Cohen, M.H.; Rieves, D.; Pazdur, R. FDA report: Ferumoxytol for intravenous iron therapy in adult patients with chronic kidney disease. *Am. J. Hematol.* **2010**, *85*, 315–319. [CrossRef] [PubMed]
6. Kicheeva, A.G.; Sushko, E.S.; Bondarenko, L.S.; Kydralieva, K.A.; Pankratov, D.A.; Tropskaya, N.S.; Dzeranov, A.A.; Dzhardimalieva, G.I.; Zarrelli, M.; Kudryasheva, N.S. Functionalized Magnetite Nanoparticles: Characterization, Bioeffects, and Role of Reactive Oxygen Species in Unicellular and Enzymatic Systems. *Int. J. Mol. Sci.* **2023**, *24*, 1133. [CrossRef] [PubMed]
7. Laurent, S.; Forge, D.; Port, M.; Roch, A.; Robic, C.; Elst, L.V.; Muller, R.N. Magnetic iron oxide nanoparticles: Synthesis, stabilization, vectorization, physicochemical characterizations, and biological applications. *Chem. Rev.* **2008**, *108*, 2064–2110. [CrossRef]
8. Hao, R.; Xing, R.; Xu, Z.; Hou, Y.; Gao, S.; Sun, S. Synthesis, functionalization, and biomedical applications of multifunctional magnetic nanoparticles. *Adv. Mater.* **2010**, *22*, 2729–2742. [CrossRef]
9. Xie, J.; Liu, G.; Eden, H.S.; Ai, H.; Chen, X. Surface-engineered magnetic nanoparticle platforms for cancer imaging and therapy. *Acc. Chem. Res.* **2011**, *44*, 883–892. [CrossRef]
10. Bondarenko, L.S.; Kovel, E.S.; Kydralieva, K.A.; Dzhardimalieva, G.I.; Illés, E.; Tombácz, E.; Kicheeva, A.G.; Kudryasheva, N.S. Effects of Modified Magnetite Nanoparticles on Bacterial Cells and Enzyme Reactions. *Nanomaterials* **2020**, *10*, 1499. [CrossRef]
11. Naahidi, S.; Jafari, M.; Edalat, F.; Raymond, K.; Khademhosseini, A.; Chen, P. Biocompatibility of Engineered Nanoparticles for Drug Delivery. *J. Control. Release* **2013**, *166*, 182–194. [CrossRef]
12. Gamucci, O.; Bertero, A.; Gagliardi, M.; Bardi, G. Biomedical Nanoparticles: Overview of Their Surface Immune-Compatibility. *Coatings* **2014**, *4*, 139–159. [CrossRef]
13. Ghosh, S.; Ghosh, I.; Chakrabarti, M.; Mukherjee, A. Genotoxicity and biocompatibility of superparamagnetic iron oxide nanoparticles: Influence of surface modification on biodistribution, retention, DNA damage and oxidative stress. *Food Chem. Toxicol.* **2020**, *136*, 110989. [CrossRef] [PubMed]
14. Kievit, F.M.; Zhang, M.Q. Surface Engineering of Iron Oxide Nanoparticles for Targeted Cancer Therapy. *Acc. Chem. Res.* **2011**, *44*, 853–862. [CrossRef] [PubMed]
15. Tassa, C.; Shaw, S.Y.; Weissleder, R. Dextran-coated Iron Oxide Nanoparticles: A Versatile Platform for Targeted Molecular Imaging, Molecular Diagnostics, and Therapy. *Acc. Chem. Res.* **2011**, *44*, 842–852. [CrossRef]
16. Cole, A.J.; David, A.E.; Wang, J.X.; Galban, C.J.; Hill, H.L.; Yang, V.C. Polyethylene Glycol Modified, Cross-Linked Starch-Coated Iron Oxide Nanoparticles for Enhanced Magnetic Tumor Targeting. *Biomaterials* **2011**, *32*, 2183–2193. [CrossRef]
17. Auerbach, M.; Pappadakis, J.A.; Bahrain, H.; Auerbach, S.A.; Ballard, H.; Dahl, N.V. Safety and Efficacy of Rapidly Administered (One Hour) One Gram of Low Molecular Weight Iron Dextran (INFeD) for the Treatment of Iron Deficient Anemia. *Am. J. Hematol.* **2011**, *86*, 860–862. [CrossRef] [PubMed]

18. Ros, P.R.; Freeny, P.C.; Harms, S.E.; Seltzer, S.E.; Davis, P.L.; Chan, T.W.; Stillman, A.E.; Muroff, L.R.; Runge, V.M.; Nissenbaum, M.A. Hepatic MR Imaging With Ferumoxides: A Multicenter Clinical Trial of the Safety and Efficacy in the Detection of Focal Hepatic Lesions. *Radiology* **1995**, *196*, 481–488. [CrossRef]
19. Peng, M.; Li, H.; Luo, Z.; Kong, J.; Wan, J.; Zheng, Z.; Zhang, Q.; Niu, H.; Vermorken, A.; Van de Ven, W.; et al. Dextran-coated superparamagnetic nanoparticles as potential cancer drug carriers in vivo. *Nanoscale* **2015**, *7*, 11155–11162. [CrossRef]
20. Lewis, S.L. *Medical Surgical Nursing*, 8th ed.; Mosby: St. Louis, MI, USA, 2010; ISBN 978-0323079150.
21. Turrina, C.; Milani, D.; Klassen, A.; Rojas-González, D.M.; Cookman, J.; Opel, M.; Sartori, B.; Mela, P.; Berensmeier, S.; Schwaminger, S.P. Carboxymethyl-Dextran-Coated Superparamagnetic Iron Oxide Nanoparticles for Drug Delivery: Influence of the Coating Thickness on the Particle Properties. *Int. J. Mol. Sci.* **2022**, *23*, 14743. [CrossRef]
22. Weissleder, R.; Bogdanov, A.; Neuwelt, E.A.; Papisov, M. Long-circulating iron oxides for MR imaging. *Adv. Drug Deliv. Rev.* **1995**, *16*, 321–334. [CrossRef]
23. Huang, Y.; Hsu, J.C.; Koo, H.; Cormode, D.P. Repurposing ferumoxytol: Diagnostic and therapeutic applications of an FDA-approved nanoparticle. *Theranostics* **2022**, *12*, 796–816. [CrossRef] [PubMed]
24. Sakamoto, J.H.; van de Ven, A.L.; Godin, B.; Blanco, E.; Serda, R.E.; Grattoni, A.; Ziemys, A.; Bouamrani, A.; Hu, T.; Ranganathan, S.I.; et al. Enabling individualized therapy through nanotechnology. *Pharmacol Res.* **2010**, *62*, 57–89. [CrossRef] [PubMed]
25. Iv, M.; Telischak, N.; Feng, D.; Holdsworth, S.J.; Yeom, K.W.; Daldrup-Link, H.E. Clinical applications of iron oxide nanoparticles for magnetic resonance imaging of brain tumors. *Nanomedicine* **2015**, *10*, 993–1018. [CrossRef] [PubMed]
26. Gerb, J.; Strauss, W.; Derman, R.; Short, V.; Mendelson, B.; Bahrain, H. Ferumoxytol for the treatment of iron deficiency and iron-deficiency anemia of pregnancy. *Ther. Adv. Hematol.* **2021**, *12*, 20406207211018042. [CrossRef]
27. Blumenstein, I.; Shanbhag, S.; Langguth, P.; Kalra, P.A.; Zoller, H.; Lim, W. Newer formulations of intravenous iron: A review of their chemistry and key safety aspects-Hypersensitivity, hypophosphatemia, and cardiovascular safety. *Expert Opin Drug Saf.* **2021**, *20*, 757–769. [CrossRef]
28. Feng, Q.; Liu, Y.; Huang, J.; Chen, K.; Huang, J.; Xiao, K. Uptake, distribution, clearance, and toxicity of iron oxide nanoparticles with different sizes and coatings. *Sci. Rep.* **2018**, *8*, 2082. [CrossRef]
29. Patil, R.M.; Thorat, N.D.; Shete, P.B.; Bedge, P.A.; Gavde, S.; Joshi, M.G., Bohara, R.A. Comprehensive cytotoxicity studies of superparamagnetic iron oxide nanoparticles. *Biochem. Biophys. Rep.* **2018**, *13*, 63–72. [CrossRef]
30. Vakili-Ghartavol, R.; Momtazi-Borojeni, A.A.; Vakili-Ghartavol, Z.; Aiyelabegan, H.T.; Jaafari, M.R.; Rezayat, S.M.; Arbabi Bidgoli, S. Toxicity assessment of superparamagnetic iron oxide nanoparticles in different tissues. *Artif. Cells. Nanomed. Biotechnol.* **2020**, *48*, 443–451. [CrossRef]
31. Saptarshi, S.R.; Duschl, A., Lopata, A.L. Interaction of nanoparticles with proteins: Relation to bio-reactivity of the nanoparticle. *J. Nanobiotechnol.* **2013**, *11*, 26. [CrossRef]
32. Colino, C.I.; Lanao, J.M.; Gutierrez-Millan, C. Targeting of Hepatic Macrophages by Therapeutic Nanoparticles. *Front. Immunol.* **2020**, *11*, 218. [CrossRef]
33. Simberg, D.; Park, J.-H.; Karmali, P.P.; Zhang, W.-M.; Merkulov, S.; McCrae, K.; Bhatia, S.N.; Sailor, M.; Ruoslahti, E. Differential proteomics analysis of the surface heterogeneity of dextran iron oxide nanoparticles and the implications for their in vivo clearance. *Biomaterials* **2009**, *30*, 3926–3933. [CrossRef]
34. Rojas, J.M.; Sanz-Ortega, L.; Mulens-Arias, V.; Gutiérrez, L.; Pérez-Yagüe, S.; Barber, D.F. Superparamagnetic iron oxide nanoparticle uptake alters M2 macrophage phenotype, iron metabolism, migration and invasion. *Nanomed. Nanotechnol. Biol. Med.* **2016**, *12*, 1127–1138. [CrossRef]
35. Mulens-Arias, V.; Rojas, J.M.; Barber, D.F. The Intrinsic Biological Identities of Iron Oxide Nanoparticles and Their Coatings: Unexplored Territory for Combinatorial Therapies. *Nanomaterials* **2020**, *10*, 837. [CrossRef]
36. Virág, L.; Jaén, R.I.; Regdon, Z.; Boscá, L.; Prieto, P. Self-defense of macrophages against oxidative injury: Fighting for their own survival. *Redox Biol.* **2019**, *26*, 101261. [CrossRef] [PubMed]
37. Predoi, D. A Study on iron oxide nanoparticles coated with dextrin obtained by coprecipitation. *Dig. J. Nanomater. Biostruct.* **2007**, *2*, 169–173.
38. Ciobanu, C.S.; Iconaru, S.L.; Gyorgy, E.; Radu, M.; Costache, M.; Dinischiotu, A.; Le Coustumer, P.; Lafdi, K.; Predoi, D. Biomedical properties and preparation of iron oxide-dextran nanostructures by MAPLE technique. *Chem. Cent. J.* **2012**, *6*, 17. [CrossRef]
39. Butoi, B.; Ciobanu, C.S.; Iconaru, S.L.; Negrilă, C.C.; Badea, M.A.; Balas, M.; Dinischiotu, A.; Predoi, G.; Bita, B.; Groza, A.; et al. Iron-Oxide-Nanoparticles-Doped Polyaniline Composite Thin Films. *Polymers* **2022**, *14*, 1821. [CrossRef] [PubMed]
40. Prodan, A.M.; Iconaru, S.L.; Chifiriuc, C.M.; Bleotu, C.; Ciobanu, C.S.; Motelica-Heino, M.; Sizaret, S.; Predoi, D. Magnetic Properties and Biological Activity Evaluation of Iron Oxide Nanoparticles. *J. Nanomater.* **2013**, *2013*, 893970. [CrossRef]
41. Iconaru, S.L.; Prodan, A.M.; Motelica-Heino, M.; Sizaret, S.; Predoi, D. Synthesis and characterization of polysaccharide-maghemite composite nanoparticles and their antibacterial properties. *Nanoscale Res. Lett.* **2012**, *7*, 576–584. [CrossRef]
42. Radu, M.; Dinu, D.; Sima, C.; Burlacu, R.; Hermenean, A.; Ardelean, A.; Dinischiotu, A. Magnetite nanoparticles induced adaptive mechanisms counteract cell death in human pulmonary fibroblasts. *Toxicol. In Vitro* **2015**, *29*, 1492–1502. [CrossRef]
43. Dinischiotu, A.; Stanca, L.; Gradinaru, D.; Petrache, S.N.; Radu, M.; Serban, A.I. Lipid peroxidation due to in vitro and in vivo exposure of biological samples to nanoparticles. *Oxid. Stress Nanotechnol.* **2013**, *1028*, 155–164.
44. Paoletti, F.; Aldinucci, D.; Mocali, A.; Caparrini, A. A sensitive spectrophotometric method for the determination of superoxide dismutase activity in tissue extracts. *Anal. Biochem.* **1986**, *154*, 538–541. [CrossRef]

45. Aebi, H. Catalase in vitro. In *Methods of Enzymatic Analysis*; Bergmayer, H.U., Ed.; FRG: Weinheim, Germany, 1984; pp. 673–684.
46. Beutler, E. Red cell metabolism. In *A Manual of Biochemical Methods*; Grune, S., Ed.; Elsevier: New York, NY, USA, 1971; pp. 71–73.
47. Balas, M.; Ciobanu, C.S.; Burtea, C.; Stan, M.S.; Bezirtzoglou, E.; Predoi, D.; Dinischiotu, A. Synthesis, Characterization, and Toxicity Evaluation of Dextran-Coated Iron Oxide Nanoparticles. *Metals* **2017**, *7*, 63. [CrossRef]
48. Predoi, S.-A.; Iconaru, S.L.; Predoi, D. In Vitro and In Vivo Biological Assays of Dextran Coated Iron Oxide Aqueous Magnetic Fluids. *Pharmaceutics* **2023**, *15*, 177. [CrossRef] [PubMed]
49. Nikitin, M.P.; Orlov, A.V.; Znoyko, S.L.; Bragina, V.A.; Gorshkov, B.G.; Ksenevich, T.I.; Cherkasov, V.R.; Nikitin, P.I. Multiplex biosensing with highly sensitive magnetic nanoparticle quantification method. *J. Magn. Magn. Mater.* **2018**, *459*, 260–264. [CrossRef]
50. Ryu, J.-H.; Jiwpanich, S.; Chacko, R.; Bickerton, S.; Thayumanavan, S. Surface-Functionalizable Polymer Nano-gels with Facile Hydrophobic Guest Encapsulation Capabilities. *J. Am. Chem. Soc.* **2010**, *132*, 8246–8247. [CrossRef]
51. Ryu, J.-H.; Chacko, R.T.; Jiwpanich, S.; Bickerton, S.; Babu, R.P.; Thayumanavan, S. Self-Cross-Linked Polymer Nanogels: A Versatile Nanoscopic Drug Delivery Platform. *J. Am. Chem. Soc.* **2010**, *132*, 17227–17235. [CrossRef] [PubMed]
52. Aktan, B.; Chambre, L.; Sanyal, R.; Sanyal, A. "Clickable" Nanogels via Thermally Driven Self-Assembly of Polymers: Facile Access to Targeted Imaging Platforms using Thiol– Maleimide Conjugation. *Biomacromolecules* **2017**, *18*, 490–497. [CrossRef]
53. Suganthi, K.S.; Rajan, K.S. Temperature induced changes in ZnO-water nanofluid: Zeta potential, size distribution and viscosity profiles. *Int. J. Heat Mass Transf.* **2012**, *55*, 7969–7980. [CrossRef]
54. Nobbmann, U.L. Polydispersity–What Does It Mean for DLS and Chromatography. 2014. Available online: http://www.materials-talks.com/blog/2014/10/23/polydispersity-what-does-it-mean-for-dls-and-chromatography/ (accessed on 14 March 2018).
55. Bera, B. Nanoporous silicon prepared by vapor phase strain etch and sacrificial technique. In Proceedings of the International Conference on Microelectronic Circuit and System (Micro), Kolkata, India, 11–12 July 2015; pp. 42–45.
56. Clarke, S. Development of Hierarchical Magnetic Nanocomposite Materials for Biomedical Applications. Ph.D. Thesis, Dublin City University, Northside, Dublin, 2013.
57. Worldwide, M.I. *Dynamic Light Scattering, Common Terms Defined*; Inform White Paper; Malvern Instruments Limited: Malvern, UK, 2011; pp. 1–6.
58. Saraswathy, A.; Nazeer, S.S.; Nimi, N.; Arumugam, S.; Shenoy, S.J.; Jayasree, R.S. Synthesis and characterization of dextran stabilized superparamagnetic iron oxide nano-particles for in vivo MR imaging of liver fibrosis. *Carbohydr. Polym.* **2014**, *101*, 760–768. [CrossRef] [PubMed]
59. Carp, O.; Patron, L.; Culita, D.; Budrugeac, P.; Feder, M.; Diamandescu, L. Thermal analysis of two types of dextran-coated magnetite. *J. Therm. Anal. Calorim.* **2010**, *101*, 181–187. [CrossRef]
60. Can, H.K.; Kavlak, S.; ParviziKhosroshahi, S.; Güune, A. Preparation, characterization and dynamical mechanical properties ofdextran-coated iron oxide nanoparticles (DIONPs). *Artif. Cells Nanomed. Biotechnol.* **2018**, *46*, 421–431. [CrossRef] [PubMed]
61. Easo, S.L.; Mohanan, P.V. Dextran stabilized iron oxide nanoparticles:synthesis, characterization and in vitro studies. *Carbohydr Polym.* **2013**, *92*, 726–732. [CrossRef] [PubMed]
62. Bautista, M.C.; Miguel-Bomati, O.; Morales, M.P.; Serna, C.J. Veintemillas-Verdaguer, S. Surface characterization of dextran-coated iron oxide nanoparticles prepared bylaser pyrolysis and coprecipitation. *J. Magn. Magn. Mater.* **2005**, *293*, 20–27. [CrossRef]
63. Shaterabadi, Z.; Nabiyouni, G.; Soleymani, M. High impact of in situ dextran coating on biocompatibility, stability and magnetic properties of iron oxide nanoparticles. *Mater. Sci. Eng. C* **2017**, *75*, 947–956. [CrossRef] [PubMed]
64. Merly, L.; Smith, S.L. Murine RAW264.7 cell line as an immune target: Are we missing something? *Immunopharm Immunotox* **2017**, *39*, 55–58. [CrossRef] [PubMed]
65. Reichell, D.; Tripathi, M.; Perez, J.M. Biological Effects of Nanoparticles on Macrophage Polarization in the Tumor Microenvironment. *Nanotheranostics* **2019**, *3*, 66–88. [CrossRef]
66. Saha, K.; Rahimi, M.; Yazdani, M.; Kim, S.T.; Moyano, D.F.; Hou, S.; Das, R.; Mout, R.; Rezaee, F.; Mahmoudi, M.; et al. Regulation of Macrophage Recognition through the Interplay of Nanoparticle Surface Functionality and Protein Corona. *ACS Nano* **2016**, *10*, 4421–4430. [CrossRef]
67. Petrat, F.; Paluch, S.; Dogruöz, E.; Dörfler, P.; Kirch, M.; Korth, H.-G.; Sustmann, R.; de Groot, H. Reduction of Fe (III) Ions Complexed to Physiological Ligands by Lipoyl Dehydrogenase and Other Flavoenzymes Iin Vitro. *J. Biol. Chem.* **2003**, *278*, 46403–46413. [CrossRef]
68. Masoud, R.; Bizouarn, T.; Trepout, S.; Wien, F.; Baciou, L.; Marco, S.; Houée Levin, C. Titanium Dioxide Nanoparticles Increase Superoxide Anion Production by Acting on NADPH Oxidase. *PLoS ONE* **2015**, *10*, e0144829. [CrossRef]
69. Paul, B.T.; Manz, D.H.; Torti, F.M.; Torti, S.V. Mitochondria and Iron: Current Question. *Expert. Rev. Hematol.* **2017**, *10*, 65–79. [CrossRef]
70. Möller, M.N.; Cuevasanta, E.; Orrico, F.; Lopez, A.C.; Thomson, L.; Denicola, A. Diffusion and Transport of Reactive Species Across Cell Membrane. In *Bioactive Lipids in Health and Disease*; Trostchansky, A., Rubbo, H., Eds.; (AEMB, 1127); Springer: Berlin/Heidelberg, Germany, 2019; pp. 3–19.
71. Lynch, R.E.; Fridovich, I. Permeation of the erythrocyte stroma by superoxide radical. *J. Biol. Chem.* **1978**, *253*, 4697–4699. [CrossRef]
72. Kehrer, J.P. The Haber-Weiss reaction and mechanisms of toxicity. *Toxicology* **2000**, *149*, 43–50. [CrossRef] [PubMed]

73. Wang, Y.; Branicky, R.; Noë, A.; Hekimi, S. Superoxide dismutases: Dual roles in controlling ROS damage and regulating ROS signaling. *J. Cell. Biol.* **2018**, *217*, 1915–1928. [CrossRef]
74. Gottfredsen, R.H.; Larsen, U.G.; Enghild, J.J.; Petersen, S.V. Hydrogen peroxide induce modifications of human extracellular superoxide dismutase that results in enzyme inhibition. *Redox Biol.* **2013**, *1*, 24–31. [CrossRef]
75. Tokarz, P.; Płoszaj, T.; Regdon, Z.; Virag, L.; Robaszkiewicz, A. PARP1-LSD1 functional interplay controls transcription of SOD2 that protects human pro-inflammatory macrophages from death under an oxidative condition. *Free Radic. Biol. Med.* **2019**, *131*, 218–224. [CrossRef]
76. Ganini, D.; Santos, J.H.; Bonini, M.G.; Mason, R.P. Switch of Mitochondrial Superoxide Dismutase into a Prooxidant Peroxidase in Manganese-Deficient Cells and Mice. *Cell. Chem. Biol.* **2018**, *25*, 413–425. [CrossRef] [PubMed]
77. Holley, A.K.; Bakthavatchalu, V.; Velez-Roman, J.M.; Clair, D.K. Manganese Superoxide Dismutase: Guardian of the Powerhouse. *Int. J. Molec. Sci.* **2011**, *12*, 7114–7162. [CrossRef] [PubMed]
78. Aguilar, T.A.F.; Hernández Navarro, B.C.; Pérez, J.A.M. Endogenous Antioxidants: A Review of their Role in Oxidative Stress. In *A Master Regulator of Oxidative Stress-The Transcription Factor Nrf2*; Morales-Gonzalez, J.A., Morales-Gonzalez, A., Madrigal-Santillan, E.O., Eds.; IntechOpen: London, UK, 2016.
79. Röhrdanz, E.; Schmuck, G.; Ohler, S.; Kahl, R. The influence of oxidative stress on catalase and Mn SOD gene transcription in astrocytes. *Brain. Res.* **2001**, *900*, 128–136. [CrossRef]
80. Makino, N.; Mochizuki, Y.; Bannai, S.; Sugita, Y. Kinetic studies on the removal of extracellular hydrogen peroxide by cultured fibroblasts. *J. Biol. Chem.* **1994**, *269*, 1020–1025. [CrossRef] [PubMed]
81. Halliwell, B.; Gutteridge, J.M.C. *Free Radicals in Biology and Medicine*, 5th ed.; Oxford University Press: Oxford, UK, 2015; p. 753.
82. Singhal, S.S.; Singh, S.P.; Singhal, P.; Horne, D.; Singhal, J.; Awathi, S. Antioxidant role of glutathione-S-transferase: 4-Hydroxynonenal, a key molecule in stress-mediated signals. *Tox. Appl. Pharm.* **2015**, *289*, 361–370. [CrossRef] [PubMed]
83. Easo, S.L.; Mohanan, P.V. Toxicological evaluation of dextran stabilized iron oxide nanoparticles in human peripheral blood lymphocytes. *Biointerfases* **2016**, *16*, 058601. [CrossRef] [PubMed]

pharmaceutics

MDPI

Article

A Single Infusion of Polyethylene Glycol-Coated Superparamagnetic Magnetite Nanoparticles Alters Differently the Expressions of Genes Involved in Iron Metabolism in the Liver and Heart of Rats

Michal Kluknavsky [1,†], Andrea Micurova [1,†], Martin Skratek [2], Peter Balis [1], Monika Okuliarova [3], Jan Manka [2] and Iveta Bernatova [1,*]

[1] Centre of Experimental Medicine, Slovak Academy of Sciences, Institute of Normal and Pathological Physiology, 813 71 Bratislava, Slovakia
[2] Institute of Measurement Science, Slovak Academy of Sciences, 841 04 Bratislava, Slovakia
[3] Department of Animal Physiology and Ethology, Faculty of Natural Sciences, Comenius University, 842 15 Bratislava, Slovakia
* Correspondence: iveta.bernatova@savba.sk
† These authors contributed equally to this work.

Abstract: This study investigated genotype- and tissue-related differences in the biodistribution of superparamagnetic magnetite (Fe_3O_4) nanoparticles (IONs) into the heart and liver of normotensive Wistar Kyoto (WKY) and spontaneously hypertensive (SHR) rats after a single i.v. infusion of polyethylene glycol-coated IONs (~30 nm, 1mg Fe/kg) 100 min post-infusion. The effects of IONs on the expression of selected genes involved in the regulation of iron metabolism, including *Nos*, *Sod* and *Gpx4*, and their possible regulation by nuclear factor (erythroid-derived 2)-like 2 (NRF2, encoded by *Nfe2l2*) and iron-regulatory protein (encoded by *Irp1*) were investigated. In addition, superoxide and nitric oxide (NO) production were determined. Results showed reduced ION incorporations into tissues of SHR compared to WKY and in the hearts compared to the livers. IONs reduced plasma corticosterone levels and NO production in the livers of SHR. Elevated superoxide production was found only in ION-treated WKY. Results also showed differences in the regulation of iron metabolism on the gene level in the heart and liver. In the hearts, gene expressions of *Nos2*, *Nos3*, *Sod1*, *Sod2*, *Fpn*, *Tf*, *Dmt1* and *Fth1* correlated with *Irp1* but not with *Nfe2l2*, suggesting that their expression is regulated by mainly iron content. In the livers, expressions of *Nos2*, *Nos3*, *Sod2*, *Gpx4*, and *Dmt1* correlated with *Nfe2l2* but not with *Irp1*, suggesting a predominant effect of oxidative stress and/or NO.

Keywords: iron oxide nanoparticles; blood pressure; iron metabolism; oxidative stress; nitric oxide; magnetometry; NRF2

1. Introduction

In organisms, iron absorption, storage and usage are highly regulated. Briefly, the main regulator of systemic iron homeostasis is hepcidin (HEPC, encoded by the *Hamp* gene)—a hormone primarily secreted by hepatocytes and, to a lesser extent, also in the heart [1] and other tissues, in response to iron loading. Hepcidin binds to ferroportin (FPN, encoded by the *Fpn1* gene), the iron exporter on the cell surface. This initiates FPN internalization and degradation resulting in a reduced efflux of iron from the enterocytes, macrophages and other peripheral cells into the circulation [2,3]. In circulation, iron is transported via the circulating transporter transferrin (TF, encoded by the *Tf* gene). After TF binding to transferrin receptor-1 (TFR1, encoded by the *Tfr1* gene) on the peripheral cells, transferrin-bound iron enters the cells in which iron accomplishes its biological functions. Non-transferrin-bound iron enters the cells via the divalent metal transporter (DMT1, encoded by the *Dmt1* gene) [4]. Intracellular iron metabolism is regulated predominantly through the iron-regulatory protein (IRP1 encoded by the *Irp1* gene) that binds to iron-responsive elements in specific mRNAs [5]. While iron absorption is highly regulated, the organism has no active mechanism to excrete the redundant iron; however, iron can be deposited in ferritin (FTH, encoded by the *Fth1* and *Ftl* genes) cores [6]. The absence of active excretion mechanisms can thus result in the cellular accumulation of iron and/or free iron can occur in circulation, while both can be cytotoxic.

Disorders in iron metabolism were found in many diseased states. Epidemiological studies provide evidence that elevated iron stores are a risk factor for developing cardiovascular and metabolic abnormalities [7]. On the other hand, low iron concentration was found in heart failure [8]. In addition, Seravalle et al. have shown that hepatic iron overload correlated positively with muscle sympathetic nerve activity in hypertensive patients, suggesting that hepatic iron overload may participate in increased cardiovascular risk [9]. There is also crosstalk between the liver and heart: liver dysfunction may induce cardiac disorders and vice versa [10], thus iron-overload-induced hepatic disorders may have a negative impact on the cardiovascular system.

Nowadays, iron oxide nanoparticles (IONs) are widely used in various areas, such as the cosmetic industry, biomedical research, medicine and others. In medicine and biomedical research, IONs can be used as contrast agents to improve magnetic resonance imaging, for cell labelling, targeted drug delivery, vascular tissue repair or for cancer treatment with hyperthermia [11]. Pharmacokinetics and biodistribution of IONs and other metal nanoparticles [12,13] and blood half-lives of IONs coated with different types of molecules in mammal models were reviewed previously [14]. The pharmacokinetics and half-life of IONs depend on various factors, such as size, shape and surface chemistries, and IONs can enter cells via phagocytosis and pinocytosis [14,15]. Under certain conditions (low pH in lysosomes, instability of ION coating or in the case of interactions with other substances), the ION coating may become unstable and the iron can be released. Free iron can cause oxidative stress due to the production of reactive oxygen species (ROS) in the superoxide-driven Fenton reaction, which consequently leads to peroxide radical formation, lipid oxidation and, in case of reduced glutathione peroxidase 4 (GPX4, encoded by the *Gpx4* gene) activity, iron-dependent cell death called ferroptosis [16,17]. On the other hand, following the elevation of ROS levels, cytoprotective pathways are activated, which are mediated via transcription nuclear factor (erythroid-derived 2)-like 2 (NRF2, encoded by the *Nfe2l2* gene) [18]. The *Nfe2l2* gene is constitutively expressed in all cell types, thus ensuring their prompt response to oxidative, inflammatory and metabolic stresses. Under normal conditions, the NRF2 protein has a rapid turnover with a half-life of about 20–30 min [19]. NRF2 translocation into the nucleus is elevated in the presence of elevated ROS as well as nitric oxide (NO) [20,21] and it induces the transcription of genes involved in antioxidant defence [22].

Another role of NRF2 is the iron-independent regulation of genes involved in iron metabolism, such as *Fth1*, *Ftl*, *Fpn1*, heme oxygenase 1 and others [18]. In addition, recent studies found that NRF2 indirectly controls the release of HEPC [23,24]. In conditions of oxidative stress, peroxisome proliferator-activated receptor gamma (PPARγ, encoded by *Pparg* gene) also plays an important regulatory role, which directly modulates the expression of superoxide dismutases (SOD1 and SOD2, encoded by the *Sod1* and *Sod2* genes), catalase [25] and inducible and endothelial NO synthases (NOS2 and NOS3, encoded by the *Nos2* and *Nos3* genes, respectively) [26,27]. A recent study also showed that i.v. administration of amino-modified IONs led to significantly increased *Hamp* mRNA in mice with non-alcoholic fatty liver disease [28]. In another study, TF saturation and TFR1 serum levels were increased along with increased *Hamp* expression and HEPC serum levels [29]. These findings support the hypothesis of changes in hepatic iron metabolism following the administration of IONs. In addition, the administration of IONs was also shown to interfere with the gene expression of NRF2 and nuclear receptor PPARγ [30,31].

In recent studies, we have shown that elevated BP was associated with alterations in the distribution of IONs compared to rats with normal blood pressure [13,32]. However, little is known about differences in iron metabolism and the incorporation of IONs into the heart and liver in hypertensive rats and whether and how IONs affect the expression of genes involved in iron metabolism, antioxidant defence and NO production in these organs after a single i.v. infusion, a condition that is relevant if IONs are used for diagnostic or therapeutic purposes in patients with various BP levels.

Thus, this study investigated the influence of a single intravenous infusion of IONs in the liver and the heart in normotensive Wistar Kyoto (WKY) and spontaneously hypertensive rats (SHR). We focused on genotype- and tissue-related differences in the biodistribution of IONs, superoxide and NO productions, gene expressions of the selected genes involved in iron metabolism as well as in genes involved in NO production and maintenance of redox balance in the liver and heart. We hypothesized that chronic elevation of blood pressure (hypertension) significantly alters the biodistribution of IONs and thus alters the expression of the above-mentioned genes, with more pronounced alterations in the liver than in the heart.

2. Materials and Methods

2.1. Animals and Treatment

In our study, 12–16 weeks old normotensive WKY and SHR male rats were used. They were fed with pelleted diet 1320, variant P (Altromin 1314, variant P; Altromin Spezialfutter, Lage, Germany), with reduced phytoestrogen content and defined iron content (192.51 mg/kg of diet). Rats had free access to food and water. The rats were held in standard conditions (humidity 45–65%; temperature 20–22 °C) with a regular rotation of light and darkness (12/12 h). Before the experiment, all of the rats had implanted catheters in the carotid artery for blood pressure (BP) and heart rate (HR) measurements and a catheter in the jugular vein for infusion of nanoparticles dispersed in physiological saline solution or saline alone (in the control rats). The rats were cannulated under anaesthesia (2.5–3% isoflurane) by the procedure described previously [33] one day before the experiment. The rats were divided into 2 groups in each genotype: control groups to which saline alone was administered (Cont, n = 6–7) and ION treated group (ION, n = 6–7) to which a dispersion of IONs in saline was administered.

Commercially available superparamagnetic PEG-coated IONs were purchased from Merck (previously Sigma-Aldrich) Bratislava, Slovakia (cat. No. 747408, PubChem SID 329765832, accessed on 18 March 2021). Coated IONs were chosen because bare IONs were shown to be toxic due to their ability to induce haemolysis, DNA breakdown and oxidative stress [34,35]. PEG was chosen as a suitable coating as it is a hydrophilic, biocompatible and neutral polymer that enhances the dispersion of IONs in aqueous media. Furthermore, PEGylation of nanoparticles has been demonstrated to reduce immunogenicity, liver uptake, hemotoxic effects and haemolysis, as well as increase the blood circulation time of nanoparticles in vivo [36–38]. IONs concentration was 1 mg Fe/mL and they were dispersed in water. The manufacturer declared the size of IONs confirmed by the transmission electron microscope was 28–32 nm, the zeta potential was −12 mV, the polydispersity index was 0.1 and the hydrodynamic size was approximately 45 nm. The exact properties of IONs used in this study were described previously [39]. IONs were autoclaved at 121 °C for 30 min and dispersed in sterile saline to reach a final dose of 1 mg of Fe/kg of body weight and administered in 10 min-lasting infusions into the jugular vein of rats. At the end of the experiment, i.e., 100 min after the IONs (or saline to control rats) administration, a small amount of blood was collected from the carotid artery catheter into ethylenediaminetetraacetic acid-coated test tubes to prepare plasma for determination of plasma corticosterone. Rats were then decapitated unconsciously after short exposure to CO_2, and trunk blood was collected into heparinized test tubes for determination of plasma iron concentration. Then the hearts and livers were dissected for further analyses.

2.2. Blood Pressure and Heart Rate Determination

Before the experiment, the conscious rats were placed into a plastic box 27 × 14 × 9 cm in size, which allowed free movement. BP and HR were recorded with a sampling rate of 1 kHz via a catheter inserted into the carotid artery using the BP-recording device PowerLab system (ADInstruments, Bella Vista, Australia). BP and HR were recorded during the entire experiment, basal mean arterial pressure (MAP) and HR were calculated as the average values of a 200 sec segment between 16 and 20 min of the recording (about 10 min before IONs application) and end MAP and HR were calculated as the average values of a 200 sec segment between 138 and 142 min of the experiment (100 min after ION application) [32].

2.3. Determination of Plasma Corticosterone and Iron Concentrations

After collection, blood was centrifuged at 4 °C, 850× *g* for 10 min and plasma was kept at −80 °C until further analysis. Plasma corticosterone was determined in plasma samples using the Corticosterone Rat/Mouse ^{125}I radioimmunoassay kit (DRG Instruments GmBH, Germany) according to the manufacturer's instructions. All samples were measured in a single assay with the intra-assay variation coefficient of 4%. The assay sensitivity was 6.3 ng/mL [32].

Iron concentrations were determined in blood plasma from heparinized trunk blood in the accredited laboratory of Laboklin s.r.o. (Bratislava, Slovakia) using the standard laboratory methods [40].

2.4. Determinations of NOS Activity and Superoxide Production

Total nitric oxide synthase (NOS) activity was determined in the 20% of tissue homogenates (*w:v*) of the liver and left heart ventricle (LHV) as described previously [32]. Briefly, tissues were collected into ice-cold buffer (0.05 mol/L Tris–HCl, pH 7.4, containing 1% protease inhibitor cocktail, homogenized 4 °C and centrifuged (4 °C, 10 min, 3000× *g*). After centrifugation, NO synthase activity was determined in the supernatants by the conversion of [^{3}H]-L-arginine to [^{3}H]-L-citrulline. NO synthase activity was expressed as pkat per gram of protein. The protein concentration was determined using the Lowry method [41].

Superoxide production was determined in approximately 15 mg tissue of the liver and LHV by determination of lucigenin-enhanced chemiluminescence as described previously [42,43]. The results were expressed as cpm/mg of tissue.

2.5. Determination of the Relative Content of Biogenic Iron and ION-Originated Iron Content in Plasma, Liver and Heart

To determine the relative content of biogenic iron and iron-containing compounds in the liver and LHV samples, we used a Quantum Design MPMS-XL 7AC (SQUID) magnetometer with a reciprocating sample operation option with a sensitivity of 10^{-11} Am^2. The advantage of this method is its ability to determine all the iron forms in a small sample of biological material with high sensitivity [44–46]. It also allows us to distinguish biogenic iron from that originated from IONs based on their different magnetic properties [39].

Samples of the liver and LHV were dissected using ceramic scissors and forceps, frozen immediately in liquid nitrogen and kept at −80 °C until further analysis. Before the analysis, the tissues were defrosted and cut using the cylindrical shaped instrument to obtain repeatedly the same shape of all samples with d = ~4.5 mm as described previously [39]. These were vacuum dried and inserted into a plastic measuring straw. For the determination of the relative content of biogenic iron, the magnetic characteristics of the samples were measured in the form of isothermal hysteresis curves at a temperature of 2 K (−271.15 °C) and at a magnetic field up to 7 T once the saturation magnetization (M_S) was reached. M_S is the parameter for determining the relative amount of magnetic compounds in the biological samples, of which iron is a dominant component [44,45,47]. Results are expressed as *Ms* (memu/g of dried weight). For determination of magnetic characteristics of ION-originated iron in tissues, samples were prepared as described above, but the magnetic characteristics were measured at temperature 300 K (26.85 °C) in a magnetic field up to 1 T. ION-originated iron content was calculated as described previously [32,39] and expressed as μg of iron per g of dried weight of the tissue. The magnetic properties of the tissues and iron contents were determined in 5–6 rats per group.

2.6. Determination of Gene Expression

The relative mRNA expression of *Nfe2l2*, *Pparg*, inducible NOS (*Nos2*), endothelial NOS (*Nos3*), superoxide dismutase 1 (*Sod1*), superoxide dismutase 2 (*Sod2*), glutathione peroxidase 4 (*Gpx4*), *Hamp*, *Fth1*, *Fpn1*, *Tf*, *Tfr1*, *Dmt1*, *Irp1* and β-actin (*Actb*, as housekeeping gene) were determined by using a two-step reverse transcription quantitative polymerase chain reaction (RT-qPCR).

The total RNA of the tissue samples was isolated by using the PureZOL™ RNA Isolation Reagent (Bio-Rad, Hercules, CA, USA) according to the manufacturer's protocols. The amount of total isolated RNA was spectrophotometrically quantified at 260/280 nm and 260/230 nm by using a NanoDrop spectrophotometer (Thermo Scientific, Waltham, MA, USA). In the next step, the isolated RNA was reverse transcribed into cDNA by using Eppendorf Mastercycler (Eppendorf AG, Elbmarsch, Germany) and the reaction mixture of iScript™ cDNA Synthesis Kit (Bio-Rad, Hercules, CA, USA) according to the manufacturer's instructions. Gene amplification by using qPCR was performed on a CFX96 Real-Time PCR detection system (Bio–Rad, Hercules, CA, USA). SsoAdvanced Universal SYBR Green Supermix (Bio-Rad, Hercules, CA, USA) was used for gene amplification.

The PCR mixture contained 1.5 μL of five-fold diluted template cDNA, 10 μL SsoAdvanced mix, 1.5 μL of both forward and reverse primers (Metabion, Germany, 4 μmol/L) and 5.5 μL of nuclease-free water (Sigma–Aldrich, Germany) in a final volume of 20 μL. The thermal cycling conditions were as follows: (1) 50 °C for 1 min, (2) 95 °C for 30 sec, (3) 39 cycles consisting of (a) 95 °C for 10 sec, (b) annealing temperature (depending on the selected primer (see Table 1) for 30 sec and (4) melt curve analysis. Determination of melt curves for amplicon analyses was constructed at 59–95 °C, 5 sec/1 °C. Samples were measured using Bio–Rad CFX Manager software (version 2.0). Expression of studied genes was expressed as the ratio of gene expression with respect to β-actin levels (*Actb*). Gene-specific primers were designed using the PubMed database (Gene) and program (Primer-BLAST). The following pairs of primer sequences, melting temperatures, accession number and amplicon size of studied genes are described in Table 1. The plates with samples were measured with CFX96 Touch™ Real Time-PCR Detection System (Bio-Rad, Hercules, CA, USA); the program started with heating up the plate to 50 °C (2 min), then increasing the temperature to 95 °C (30 s). The program continued with 39 cycles repeating the steps of denaturation (95 °C, 10 s) and annealing (30 s). The fluorescent dye SYBR Green (Bio-Rad, Hercules, CA, USA) was used for the detection of PCR products. The signal intensity during amplification was detected with Bio-Rad CFX Manager software. The gene expression is presented as the ratio of gene expression to *Actb*.

Table 1. Primer pairs used to amplify selected genes.

Gene	Primer Pairs	Tm (°C)	Amp (bp)
Nos3 (NM_021838.2)	Forward: GAT CCC CCG GAG AAT GGA GA Reverse: TCG GAT TTT GTA ACT CTT GTG CT	60	105
Nos2 (NM_012611.3)	Forward: AAA CGC TAC ACT TCC AAC GC Reverse: TGC TGA GAG CTT TGT TGA GGT C	59	91
Nfe2l2 (NM_031789.2)	Forward: TGC CAT TAG TCA GTC GCT CTC Reverse: ACC GTG CCT TCA GTG TGC	60	102
Pparg (NM_013124.3)	Forward: CTC ACA ATG CCA TCA GG TTT GG Reverse: GCT GGT CGA TAT CAC TGG AGA T	59	84

Table 1. *Cont.*

Gene	Primer Pairs	Tm (°C)	Amp (bp)
Sod1 (NM_017050.1)	Forward: CTG AAG GCG AGC ATG GGT TC Reverse: TCC AAC ATG CCT CTC TTC ATC C	60	131
Sod2 (NM_017051.2)	Forward: GCT GGC CAA GGG AGA TGT TAC Reverse: TGC TGT GAT TGT ATG GCC CC	60	83
Gpx4 (NM_001368043.1)	Forward: TAA GTA CAG GGG TTG CGT GTG Reverse: CAA GGG AAG GCC AGG ATT CG	60	135
Dmt1 (Slc11a2) (NM_013173.2)	Forward: CTA CTT GGG TTG GCA GTG TTT G Reverse: ATC TTC GCT CAG CAG GAC TTT	60	94
Tf (NM_001013110.1)	Forward: GCT CCG AAC AAC AGA GAG GG Reverse: AGC AGT GTT CTT TCC GTT CGT	60	126
Tfr1 (NM_022712.1)	Forward: GCT ATG AGG AAC CAG ACC GC Reverse: CAC TGG ACT TCG CAA CAC CA	58	78
Fth1 (NM_012848.2)	Forward: ACG TCT ATC TGT CCA TGT CTT GTT Reverse: GAA GAT TCG TCC ACC TCG CT	60	149
Fpn1 (Slc40a1) (NM_133315.2)	Forward: GAC CTC ACC TAA AGA TAC TGA GCC Reverse: GAA GGG TTC TGC GAT CTG GG	59	130
Irp1 (Aco1) (NM_017321.1)	Forward: ACC TCA AAA CCA GCC TGT CT Reverse: ACC ACG TCA AAC CCT AAC TGG	59	100
Hamp (Hepc) (NM_053469.1)	Forward: CTA TCT CCG GCA ACA GAC GAG Reverse: TGT CTC GCT TCC TTC GCT TC	60	110
Actb (NM_031144.3)	Forward: CTC TGT GTG GAT TGG TGG CT Reverse: CGC AGC TCA GTA ACA GTC CG	59	139

Abbreviations: *Nos3*, endothelial nitric oxide synthase; *Nos2*, inducible nitric oxide synthase; *Nfe2l2*, nuclear factor (erythroid-derived 2)-like 2; *Pparg*, peroxisome proliferator-activated receptor gamma; *Sod1*, superoxide dismutase 1; *Sod2*, superoxide dismutase 2; *Gpx4*, glutathione peroxidase 4; *Dmt1*, divalent metal transporter; *Tf*, transferrin; *Tfr1*, transferrin receptor; *Fth1*, ferritin heavy chain 1; *Fpn*, ferroportin; *Irp1* (*Aco1*), iron-regulatory protein 1 or aconitase 1; *Hamp*, hepcidin; *Actb*, β-actin; Tm, metlting temperature; Amp, amplicon; bp, base pare of DNA.

3. Results

3.1. MAP, HR and Plasma Corticosterone Levels

The basal MAP of WKY and SHR rats were 130 ± 4 and 178 ± 3 mmHg, respectively (genotype: $F_{(1,21)} = 136.2$, $p < 0.0001$). The MAP at the end of the experiment (i.e., 100 min post-infusion) did not change significantly in any group of rats (Figure 1a).

The basal HR of WKY and SHR rats were 327 ± 7 and 370 ± 11 bpm, respectively ($F_{(1,21)} = 27.8.2$, $p < 0.0001$). There was a significant interaction of genotype and time for HR ($F_{(1,21)} = 6.6$, $p < 0.02$) with a significantly lower final (i.e., 100 min post-infusion) HR in WKY rats compared to their basal levels (Figure 1b), which was not seen in SHR.

There were no significant differences in plasma corticosterone levels between genotypes ($F_{(1,20)} = 3.6$, $p = 0.07$). Interaction of genotype and treatment ($F_{(1,20)} = 7.3$, $p < 0.02$) revealed a significant decrease of plasma corticosterone in ION-treated SHR (SHR_{ION}) vs. control SHR (SHR_{Cont}) and ION-treated WKY (WKY_{ION}, Figure 1c). Determination of total iron content in plasma of rats revealed a significant effect of treatment ($F_{(1,20)} = 5.6$, $p < 0.03$), with higher levels in ION-treated rats vs. controls (Figure 1d).

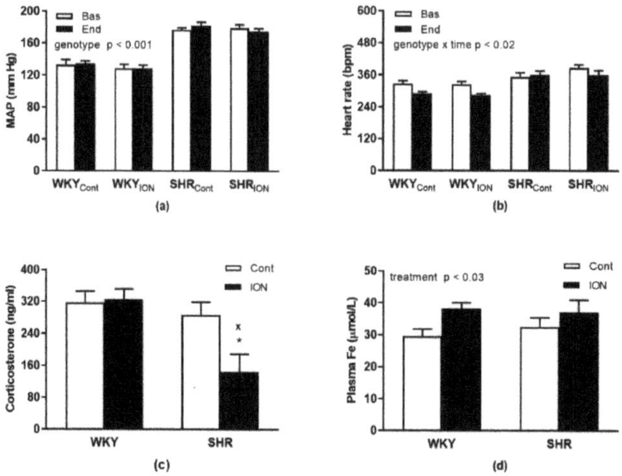

Figure 1. Mean arterial blood pressure (**a**), heart rate (**b**), plasma corticosterone (**c**) and plasma iron levels (**d**). The results are the mean ± SEM. * $p < 0.01$ vs. control SHR, ^{x} $p < 0.03$ vs. ION-treated WKY group. Abbreviations: MAP, mean arterial blood pressure; Bas, basal levels; End, levels determined 100 min post-infusion; SHR, spontaneously hypertensive rats; WKY, Wistar-Kyoto rats; Cont, control group; ION, iron oxide nanoparticle-treated group.

3.2. Nitric Oxide Synthase Activities and Superoxide Productions

Regarding NOS activity, two-way ANOVA revealed significant interaction of genotype and treatment in the liver ($F_{(1,21)} = 5.5$, $p < 0.03$) with significantly lower values of NOS activity in ION-treated SHR vs. control SHR (Figure 2a). No changes in NOS activities were found in the LHV (Figure 2b).

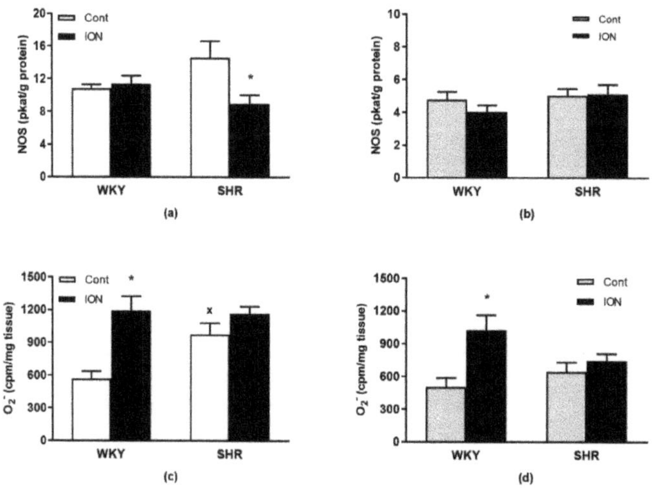

Figure 2. Nitric oxide synthase activity in the liver (**a**) and left heart ventricle (**b**). Superoxide production in the liver (**c**) and left heart ventricle (**d**). The results are the mean ± SEM, * $p < 0.04$ vs. the control group of the same genotype, ^{x} $p < 0.05$ vs. control WKY, n = 6/group. Abbreviations: NOS, nitric oxide synthase; cpm, counts/min; for other abbreviations see the legend to Figure 1.

For superoxide productions, there were significant interactions of genotype and treatment in both the liver ($F_{(1,20)} = 4.9, p < 0.04$) and the LHV ($F_{(1,20)} = 4.7, p < 0.05$) with significantly higher levels found in ION-treated WKY compared to control WKY (Figure 2c,d). Higher superoxide production was found in the liver of control SHR vs. control WKY (Figure 2c). However, no changes in superoxide productions were found in ION-treated SHR vs. control SHR in both the liver and LHV (Figure 2c,d).

3.3. Relative Contents of Biogenic Iron and ION-Originated Iron

Saturation magnetization *Ms* (relative parameter of biogenic iron content) of the liver of control SHR was significantly higher than in WKY ($p < 0.001$, Figure 3a). In contrast, the saturation magnetization of the LHV of SHR was reduced compared to WKY ($p < 0.001$, Figure 3b). ION-originated Fe content was significantly lower in the liver ($p < 0.02$) and the decreasing tendency was also in the LHV ($p = 0.06$, n = 10) of SHR compared to that in the respective WKY value (Figure 3c,d).

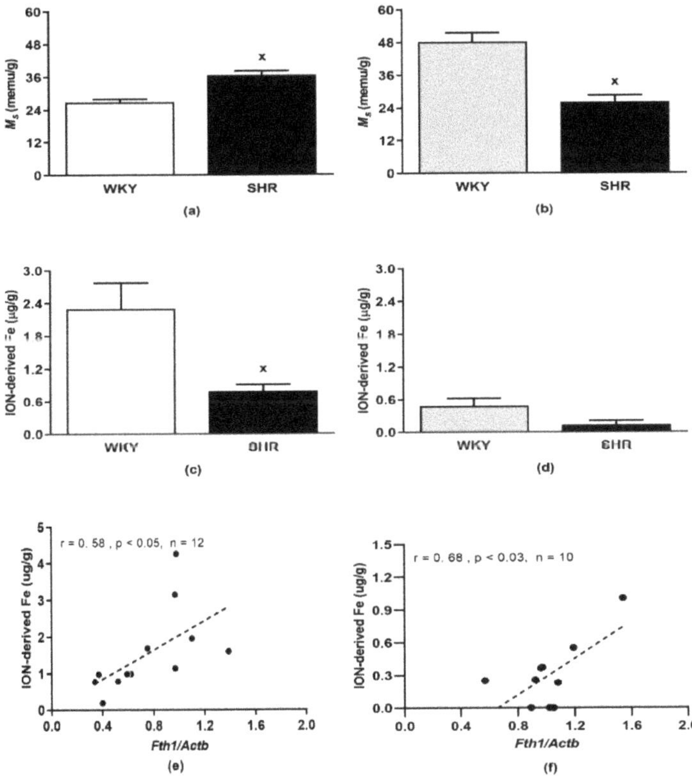

Figure 3. Saturation magnetization in the liver (**a**) and left heart ventricle (**b**). Iron oxide nanoparticle-originated iron content in the liver (**c**) and left heart ventricle (**d**). Pearson correlations between ION-originated iron and *Fth1* gene expressions in the liver (**e**) and left heart ventricle (**f**). The results are the mean ± SEM, ^{x} $p < 0.04$ vs. the WKY group, n = 5–6/group. Abbreviations: *Ms*, saturation magnetization; ION, iron oxide nanoparticles; *Fth1*, ferritin gene; *Actb*, β-actin gene. For other abbreviations see the legend to Figure 1.

In the liver and LHV of ION-treated rats, the amount of ION-originated iron correlated positively with the *Fth1*: r = 0.58, $p < 0.05$ in the liver (Figure 3e) and r = 0.68, $p < 0.03$ in LHV (Figure 3f).

3.4. Expression of Genes Involved in Iron Metabolism, Antioxidant Defence and Nitric Oxide Production

Relative mRNA expressions of *Nfe2l2*, *Pparg*, *Nos2* and *Nos3* in the liver and LHV are shown in Figure 4. There were significant main effects of genotype for *Nfe2l2* ($F_{(1,20)} = 4.59$, $p < 0.05$, Figure 4a) and *Pparg* ($F_{(1,20)} = 16.23$, $p < 0.001$, Figure 4b) in the liver and for *Nos3* ($F_{(1,20)} = 17.96$, $p < 0.001$, Figure 4h) in the LHV, with higher levels found in SHR. A significant effect of ION treatment was found only for *Pparg* ($F_{(1,20)} = 4.59$, $p < 0.05$) in the LHV with lower levels in ION-treated rats compared to controls (Figure 4f).

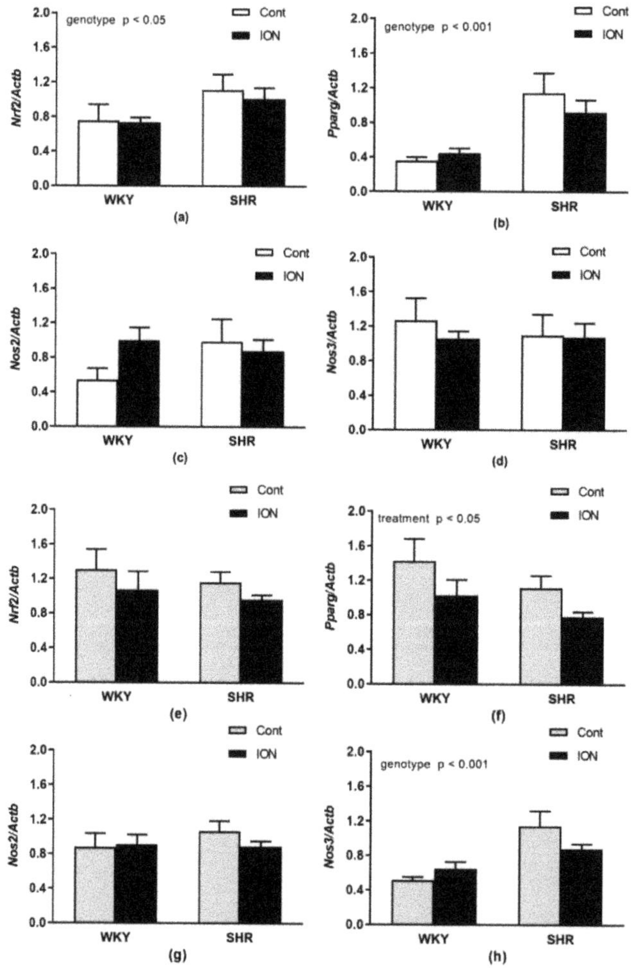

Figure 4. Relative mRNA expressions of nuclear transcription factor *Nfe2l2* (**a**,**e**), *Pparg* (**b**,**f**) and genes involved in nitric oxide production *Nos2* (**c**,**g**) and *Nos3* (**d**,**h**) in the liver (**a**–**d**) and left heart ventricle (**e**–**h**). The values represent the mean ± SEM. See Results section for detailed results of 2-way ANOVA analysis. Abbreviations: *Nfe2l2*, nuclear factor (erythroid-derived 2)-like 2; *Pparg*, peroxisome proliferator-activated receptor gamma; *Nos2*, inducible nitric oxide synthase; *Nos3*, endothelial nitric oxide synthase. Other abbreviations are the same as in Figure 1.

Relative mRNA expressions of genes encoding antioxidant enzymes *Sod1*, *Sod2* and *Gpx4* in the liver and LHV are shown in Figure 5. In the liver, there were significant interactions of genotype and treatment for *Sod1* ($F_{(1,20)} = 15.37$, $p < 0.001$, Figure 5a) and *Sod2* ($F_{(1,20)} = 28.55$, $p < 0.0001$, Figure 5b). In the LHV, significant interactions of genotype and treatment were found only for *Sod1* ($F_{(1,20)} = 7.20$, $p < 0.02$, Figure 5d); no effects were found for *Sod2* (Figure 5e). The mRNA expressions of *Gpx4* were unchanged in the liver (Figure 5c), but in the LHV, significant effects of genotype ($F_{(1,20)} = 14.71$, $p < 0.01$) and treatment $F_{(1,20)} = 5.7$, $p < 0.03$, Figure 5f) were found, with lower levels in SHR vs. WKY and for ION-treated rats vs. controls.

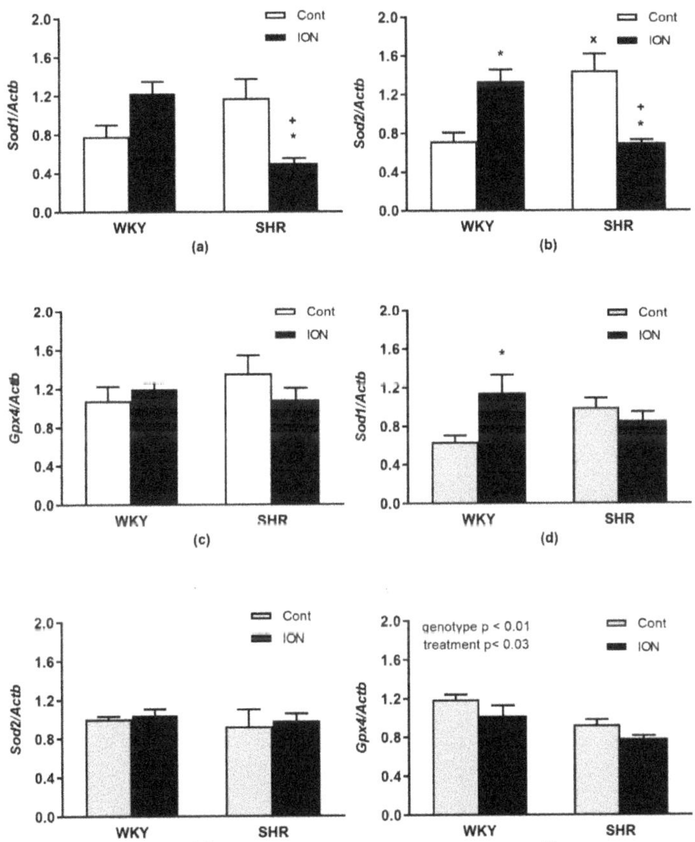

Figure 5. Gene expressions of selected enzymes involved in antioxidant defence *Sod1* (**a**,**d**), *Sod2* (**b**,**e**) and *Gpx4* (**c**,**f**) in the liver (**a**–**c**) and left heart ventricle (**d**–**f**). The values represent the mean ± SEM. * $p < 0.03$ vs. the control group of the same genotype, $^{+}$ $p < 0.02$ vs. ION-treated WKY group, $^{\times}$ $p < 0.01$ vs. WKY control group, n = 6/group. See Results section for detailed results of 2-way ANOVA analysis. Abbreviations: *Sod1*, superoxide dismutase 1; *Sod2*, superoxide dismutase 2; *Gpx4*, glutathione peroxidase 4. Other abbreviations are the same as in the Figure 1.

In Figure 6, relative mRNA expressions of genes involved in iron metabolism regulation or iron carrying and storage are depicted. A significant effect of ION treatment was found only for *Hamp* ($F_{(1,20)} = 6.74$, $p < 0.02$) in the liver with higher levels in ION-treated rats compared to controls (Figure 6a). Significant interactions of genotype and treatment in the liver were found only for *Fth1* ($F_{(1,20)} = 9.06$, $p < 0.01$, Figure 6d); there was a significant decrease in *Fth1* mRNA in ION-treated SHR vs. control SHR. In the LHV, there was a significant reduction in *Tf* gene expression in SHR vs. WKY (effect of genotype, $F_{(1,20)} = 4.58$, $p < 0.05$, Figure 6g). No differences were found in the gene expression of *Irp1* and *Tf* in the liver (Figure 6b,c) and in the *Hamp*, *Irp1* and *Fth1* in the LHV (Figure 6e,f,h). In the liver, *Hamp* gene expression correlated positively with plasma iron levels (r = 0.58, $p < 0.006$, n = 21), which was not found in the LHV.

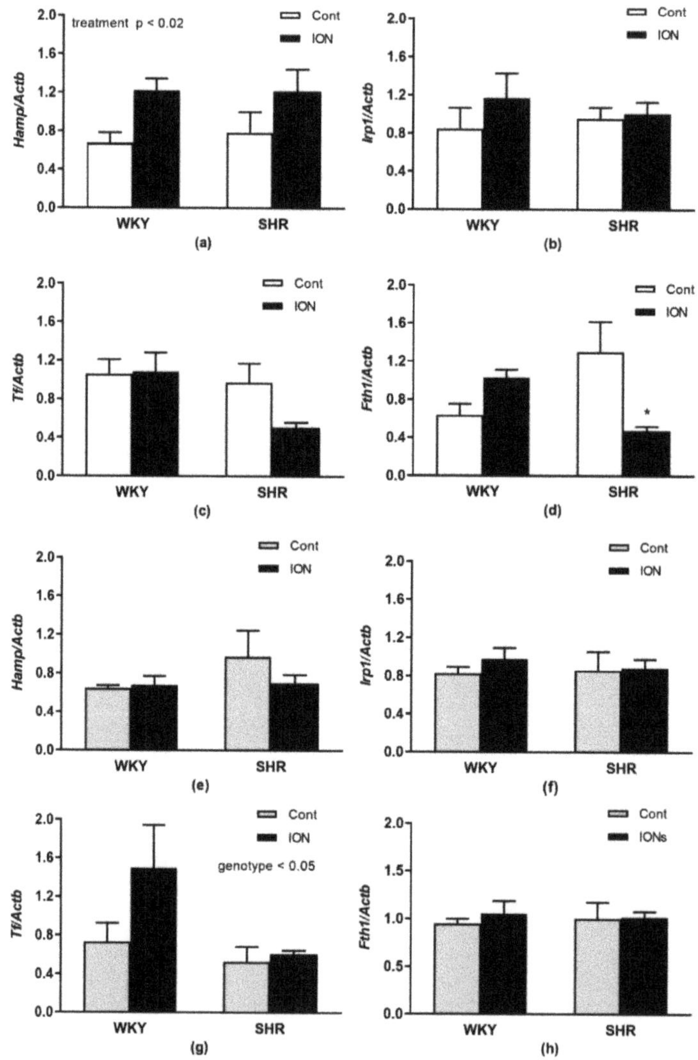

Figure 6. Gene expressions of selected genes associated with iron metabolism regulation or iron carrying and storage in the liver (**a**–**d**) and left heart ventricle (**e**–**h**). The values represent the mean ± SEM. * $p < 0.03$ vs. the control group of the same genotype, n = 6/group. See Results section for detailed results of 2-way ANOVA analysis. Abbreviations: *Hamp*, hepcidin; *Irp1*, iron regulatory protein 1; *Fth1*, ferritin heavy chain 1; *Tf*, transferrin. Other abbreviations are the same as in Figure 1.

In Figure 7, relative mRNA expressions of genes involved in iron transport are depicted. No genotype and/or treatment-related changes in *Tfr1*, *Dmt1* and *Fpn1* gene expressions were found in the liver (Figure 7 a–c). In the LHV, a significant effect of genotype ($F_{(1,20)} = 30.02$, $p < 0.0001$), treatment ($F_{(1,20)} = 15.27$, $p < 0.001$) and interactions of genotype and treatment were found for *Tfr1* ($F_{(1,20)} = 757$, $p < 0.02$, Figure 7d). A significant effect of treatment was found in the LHV for *Dmt1* ($F_{(1,20)} = 5.03$, $p < 0.04$, Figure 7e). No changes were found in the gene expression of *Fpn1* in the LHV (Figure 7f). The correlations among the genes are in the Supplementary Table S1.

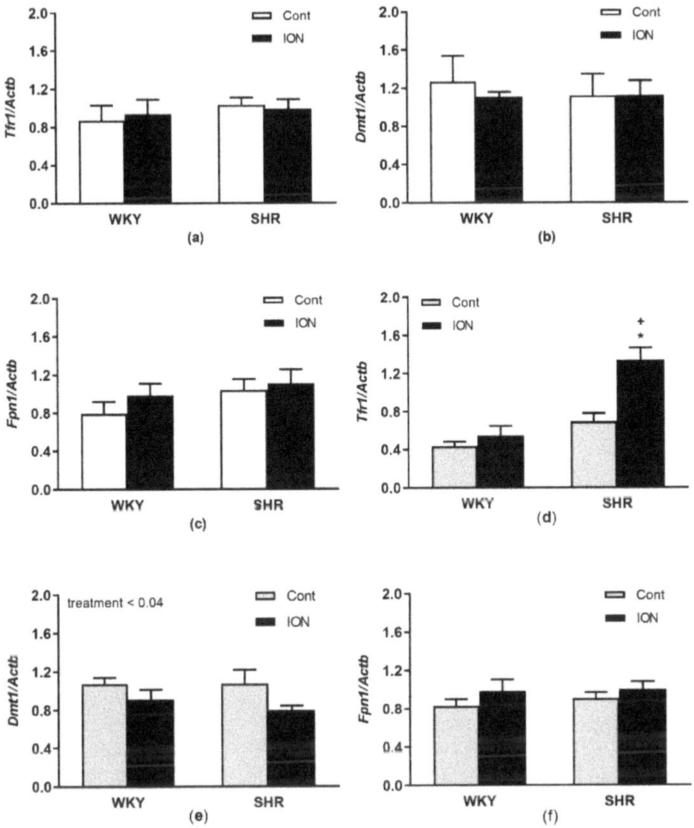

Figure 7. Gene expressions of selected genes associated with iron transport in the liver (**a**–**c**) and left heart ventricle (**d**–**f**). The values represent the mean ± SEM. * $p < 0.03$ vs. the control group of the same genotype, $^{+}$ $p < 0.02$ vs. ION-treated WKY group, n = 6/group. See Results section for detailed results of 2-way ANOVA analysis. Abbreviations: *Tfr1*, transferrin receptor 1; *Dmt1*, divalent metal transporter 1; *Fpn 1*, ferroportin 1. Other abbreviations are the same as in Figure 1.

4. Discussion

Superparamagnetic iron oxide nanoparticles of γ-Fe_2O_3 (maghemite) and Fe_3O_4 (magnetite) can be used in various biomedical applications. The advantage of such NPs lies in the possibility to use them for targeted drug delivery in the presence of the magnetic field. However, it is also very important to know the pharmacokinetics of the NPs and their effect on the living organism because iron is an essential biogenic element. In our previous studies, we confirmed the superparamagnetism of IONs used in this study [39] as well as their presence in different tissues depending on the blood pressure [13,32,39,40].

The main findings of this study are that ION-originated iron was found in the livers and hearts of normotensive and hypertensive rats, but considerably less in the tissues of hypertensive SHR than normotensive WKY. ION-originated iron content found in the hearts was roughly around 20% of that determined in the liver of the given genotype. In addition, our study showed considerable tissue differences in the expression of genes involved in iron metabolism, as well as in *Sod* and *Nos* expression, in the livers and hearts. Regarding genotype differences, we found that elevated ION content in the tissues of WKY led to elevated superoxide production, which was not seen in SHR. Lower ION content in the tissues of SHR was associated with reduced plasma corticosterone, reduced total NOS activity in the liver as well as with reduced liver expressions of *Sod1*, *Sod2* and *Fth1*. On the other hand, in WKY, *Sod2* was elevated in the liver and *Sod1* in the heart in ION-treated rats. Despite these genotype- and tissue-related differences, positive correlations were found between plasma iron concentration and hepatic *Hamp* expression as well as between ION-originated iron content and *Fth1* gene expressions in both tissues investigated, suggesting the considerable influence of ION-derived iron on intracellular iron metabolism in these tissues when all rats were taken into account.

Previously we showed that hypertension (i.e., chronic high BP) was associated with an increased incorporation of IONs into the liver and vascular wall of SHR when determined 24 h after the second ION infusion at the dose of 2 mg Fe/kg/day [13]. On the other hand, an acute stress-induced increase in BP in WKY rats treated with a single infusion of IONs (1 mg Fe/kg) led to a decrease in ION-derived iron in circulation and in the liver when determined 100 min post-ION infusion [32]. Those studies showed that high BP, either chronic or acute, is an important factor affecting ION deposition in the liver. In this study, we focused on the heart and liver after a single ION infusion in normotensive and hypertensive rats, which is relevant to the situation of patients with various levels of BP.

We found that a single ION infusion in rest conditions did not induce significant changes in BP and HR in SHR despite an ION-induced decrease in NO production in the liver of SHR (vs. control SHR) and elevated superoxide production in both tissues investigated in WKY. Unchanged BP after ION administration suggests that mild changes in the above-mentioned parameters as well as the increase in overall hepatic iron content due to the incorporation of ION-derived iron had no effect on BP regulation in any rat strain. This finding corresponds with the results of Seravalle et al., who also found no changes in BP in hypertensive patients with hepatic iron overload compared to hypertensive individuals [9]. Surprisingly, we found a significant decrease in corticosterone levels after ION infusion in SHR, suggesting that IONs can interfere with hypothalamic–pituitary–adrenal axis function, specifically under conditions of hypertension, though the exact mechanisms need to be further studied. In the present study, we did not determine iron content in the adrenal glands, but there are reports in humans showing enhanced acute accumulation of iron nanoparticles within the adrenals that was comparable to that in the tissues of the reticuloendothelial system, such as the liver and spleen [48]. In spite of missing data in hypertensive patients, our study demonstrates that the adrenals of hypertensive individuals may display increased sensitivity to ION administration.

Our study also revealed that plasma iron concentrations were elevated in both rat genotypes after ION infusion. However, plasma iron levels do not reflect ION-originated iron content in the tissues. Using SQUID magnetometry, we found elevated M_S, an indirect but very sensitive parameter, reflecting total iron content [39] in the liver of control SHR compared to control WKY. Despite that the liver is considered a rich source of iron in the organism, high levels of iron are also in the heart, in which iron metabolism has to be regulated very precisely to prevent cardiac dysfunction [49]. In addition, SQUID magnetometry allows us to determine the amount of ION-originated iron, which is not possible to distinguish from biogenic iron present in the tissues by biochemical or histological methods [39]. We found that, in conditions of this study, the content of ION-originated iron was lower in the hearts than in the livers and also in tissues of ION-treated SHR compared to the ION-treated WKY. In fact, in three of five hearts of ION-treated SHR we did not find ION-originated iron. However, in both tissues, positive correlations were found between ION-originated iron and *Fth1* gene expressions, suggesting the significant influence of ION-originated iron on innate iron metabolism.

This effect was also confirmed by elevated *Hamp* expression in the liver of ION-treated rats and by a positive correlation between plasma iron and *Hamp* gene expression in the liver. It is known that the hepatic release of hepcidin is regulated predominantly by intrahepatic iron concentration [50]. However, hepcidin can also be synthesized in smaller amounts by the other tissues, including the heart [51] in which it participates in the regulation of local iron levels [52]. Recent studies show that hepcidin has an irreplaceable role in regulating iron homeostasis in the heart; hepcidin deficiency results in cardiac dysfunction, left ventricular hypertrophy and apoptosis [53]. In our study, no changes in cardiac *Hamp* expression were found, suggesting that the heart functions should not be considerably altered by ION-originated iron after a single low-dose ION infusion. However, IONs and/or iron released after nanoparticle disintegration can enter redox processes and induce oxidative stress [54,55]. Here we found elevated superoxide production only in the tissues of WKY, which is in agreement with the higher ION-originated iron content found in the tissues of WKY. In addition, *Sod2* was elevated in the liver and *Sod1* in the heart of WKY, while both *Sod1* and *Sod2* were significantly reduced in the liver of ION-treated SHR vs. control SHR. Despite our expectation, no corresponding changes (regarding *Sod* expressions) were found in the expression of the *Nfe2l2* gene in both tissues investigated. On the other hand, we found positive correlations between *Nfe2l2* and *Nos2, Nos3, Dmt1, Gpx4, Sod2* and *Pparg* in the liver. No such correlations with *Nfe2l2* were found in the heart, except for that with *Pparg*, which correlated positively with *Nfe2l2* in both tissues investigated. This study also showed two interesting relations among the gene expressions in the liver and heart when all rats were taken into account. Firstly, Of the 24 correlations found among the genes investigated in this study in the liver, only 1 was negative. In the heart, of the 39 correlations found among the genes investigated, 17 were negative and 22 were positive. Secondly, all correlations with *Dmt1* or *Fth1* were positive in the liver and only two genes (*Fpn1* and *Tfr1*) correlated positively with *Irp1*. In contrast, in the heart, all genes which correlated positively with *Fth1* or *Irp1*, correlated negatively with *Dmt1*. These findings suggest considerable differences in the expression of genes involved in iron metabolism in the liver and heart. Since the optimal iron concentration in the heart is critical for normal cardiac function [49], we assume that the sensitivity of cardiomyocytes to iron is higher compared to that in the liver. Rapid, but not necessarily big, changes in the expression of various genes and corresponding proteins can maintain optimal intracellular iron concentrations in the heart, specifically under oxidative and/or nitrosative stress, as both ROS and NO participate in the regulation of iron metabolism [56,57]. In the heart, we also found a negative correlation between the *Fth1* and *Dmt1* genes, supposedly under the control of *Irp1*, which suggests the finely tuned regulation of intracellular iron concentration. In addition, opposite correlations of the *Fth1* and *Dmt1* genes with other genes mentioned in the supplementary Table S1, especially with *Nos* and *Sod* genes, can result in the increase in antioxidant defence and reduction of NO production. NO, in addition to its role in cardiovascular functions [58,59], has an important role in iron metabolism by modulation of cytosolic aconitase (ACO1)/IRP1 function [60]. In conditions of low levels of intracellular iron, the apo form of ACO1 has the function of IRP1, while at high iron levels, its holo form containing the $[4Fe\text{-}4S]^{2+}$ cluster possesses ACO1 enzymatic activity [61]. NO can promote the release of iron from the Fe-S centres of ACO1 and thus induce the IRP1 function of this bifunctional protein [61]. High levels of IRP1 protein support an increase of *Fth1* mRNA translation resulting in elevated iron storage capacity in ferritin cores. In addition, high levels of IRP1 decrease *Dmt1* and *Tfr1* mRNA stability, which leads to a reduced influx of iron into the cell [62]. Surprisingly, in this study, there were no correlations with the *Nfel2l* and *Pparg* genes and other genes investigated in the heart, which is in contrast to the liver. In the liver, the antioxidant genes (*Sod2, Gpx4*) and *Nos2* and *Nos3* genes correlated positively with *Nfel2l*, in agreement with previous findings of elevated NRF2 translocation into the nucleus in the presence of ROS and NO [20,21]. Interestingly, none of the genes investigated in the liver correlated with hepatic *Hamp* and only two genes (*Fpn1, Tfr1*) correlated with *Irp1* expression. Collectively, the results suggest that while changes observed on the gene levels in the heart seem to be related to changes in iron load, changes in the liver seem to be more related to oxidative stress and/or NO, which may be induced by altered hepatic iron content. Indeed, superoxide production was elevated in the liver of ION-treated WKY as well as in both SHR groups compared to control WKY, which was not found in the heart. Thus, our data showed considerable differences in the expression of genes involved in iron metabolism in the heart and the liver of rats. In agreement, a recent study by Kasztura et al. [63] has shown that the mechanisms of iron uptake, storage and clearance differ between the liver and heart in the porcine model of heart failure progression.

5. Conclusions

Our results showed that a single administration of IONs intravenously at a relatively low dose was found in the liver and the heart of both rat genotypes 100 min after their infusion. Lower content of ION-derived iron was found in the tissues of SHR compared to WKY as well as in the hearts compared to livers, confirming the hypothesis that high blood pressure significantly alters the biodistribution of IONs with less incorporation into the heart than into the liver. In addition, our results showed differences in the regulation of iron metabolism on gene levels in the heart and liver. In the heart, expressions of various genes involved in iron metabolism, including *Sod* and *Nos*, seem to be mediated predominantly by iron content and regulated by IRP1-mediated mechanisms. In the liver, the expression of genes correlated with *Nfe2l2*, suggesting a predominant effect NRF2–mediated mechanisms in the regulation of iron metabolism due to an altered redox balance and NO bioavailability.

Supplementary Materials: The following supporting information can be downloaded at https://www.mdpi.com/article/10.3390/pharmaceutics15051475/s1. Table S1: Correlations of the gene expressions in the livers and left heart ventricles of rats.

Author Contributions: Conceptualization, I.B.; data curation, I.B.; formal analysis, M.K., A.M., M.S. and I.B.; funding acquisition, J.M. and I.B.; investigation, M.K., A.M., M.S., P.B., M.O. and I.B.; methodology, M.K., M.S., P.B., M.O., J.M. and I.B.; project administration, I.B.; resources, J.M.; software, I.B.; validation, M.K., A.M. and I.B.; visualization, M.K. and I.B.; writing—original draft, A.M.; writing—review and editing, M.K., M.O., J.M. and I.B. All authors have read and agreed to the published version of the manuscript.

Funding: This research was funded by the Slovak Research and Development Agency (grant No. APVV-16-0263), by the Scientific Grant Agency of the Ministry of Education, Science, Research and Sport of the Slovak Republic (grants Nos. 2/0157/21 and 2/0141/21) and by the European Regional Development Fund "Vývoj biomodelov pre zlepšenie hodnotenia účinnosti liekov a látok, ktoré majú potenciál pri liečbe COVID-19 (BIOVID-19)"—ITMS2014+: 313011AVG3.

Institutional Review Board Statement: All of the procedures used in this study were approved by the Ethics Committee of the Centre of Experimental Medicine, Slovak Academy of Sciences; by the State Veterinary and Food Administration of the Slovak Republic, protocol code 3619/16-221 (from 28 October 2016); and were in accordance with the European Union Directive 2010/63/EU.

Informed Consent Statement: Not applicable.

Data Availability Statement: The data presented in this study are available on request from the corresponding author.

Acknowledgments: The authors thank J. Petova and B. Bolgacova for their excellent technical assistance.

Conflicts of Interest: The authors declare no conflict of interest.

References

1. Merle, U.; Fein, E.; Gehrke, S.G.; Stremmel, W.; Kulaksiz, H. The iron regulatory peptide hepcidin is expressed in the heart and regulated by hypoxia and inflammation. *Endocrinology* **2007**, *148*, 2663–2668. [CrossRef] [PubMed]
2. Chifman, J.; Laubenbacher, R.; Torti, S.V. A systems biology approach to iron metabolism. *A Syst. Biol. Approach Blood* **2014**, *844*, 201–225. [CrossRef]
3. Reichert, C.O.; da Cunha, J.; Levy, D.; Maselli, L.M.F.; Bydlowski, S.P.; Spada, C. Hepcidin: Homeostasis and diseases related to iron metabolism. *Acta Haematol.* **2017**, *137*, 220–236. [CrossRef] [PubMed]

4. Yanatori, I.; Kishi, F. DMT1 and iron transport. *Free Radic. Biol. Med.* **2019**, *133*, 55–63. [CrossRef]
5. Eisenstein, R.S.; Blemings, K.P. Iron regulatory proteins, iron responsive elements and iron homeostasis. *J. Nutr.* **1998**, *128*, 2295–2298. [CrossRef] [PubMed]
6. Worwood, M. Ferritin. *Blood Rev.* **1990**, *4*, 259–269. [CrossRef]
7. Basuli, D.; Stevens, R.G.; Torti, F.M.; Torti, S.V. Epidemiological associations between iron and cardiovascular disease and diabetes. *Front. Pharmacol.* **2014**, *5*, 117. [CrossRef]
8. Klip, I.T.; Comin-Colet, J.; Voors, A.A.; Ponikowski, P.; Enjuanes, C.; Banasiak, W.; Lok, D.J.; Rosentryt, P.; Torrens, A.; Polonski, L. Iron deficiency in chronic heart failure: An international pooled analysis. *Am. Heart J.* **2013**, *165*, 575–582.e3. [CrossRef]
9. Seravalle, G.; Dell'Oro, R.; Quarti-Trevano, F.; Spaziani, D.; Bertoli, S.; Airoldi, F.; Mancia, G.; Grassi, G. Sympathetic overactivation in patients with essential hypertension and hepatic iron overload. *Hypertension* **2020**, *76*, 1444–1450. [CrossRef]
10. El Hadi, H.; Di Vincenzo, A.; Vettor, R.; Rossato, M. Relationship between heart disease and liver disease: A two-way street. *Cells* **2020**, *9*, 567. [CrossRef]
11. Liu, X.; Wang, N.; Liu, X.; Deng, R.; Kang, R.; Xie, L. Vascular Repair by Grafting Based on Magnetic Nanoparticles. *Pharmaceutics* **2022**, *14*, 1433. [CrossRef] [PubMed]
12. Lin, Z.; Monteiro-Riviere, N.A.; Riviere, J.E. Pharmacokinetics of metallic nanoparticles. *WIREs Nanomed. Nanobiotechnol.* **2014**, *7*, 189–217. [CrossRef] [PubMed]
13. Micurova, A.; Kluknavsky, M.; Liskova, S.; Balis, P.; Skratek, M.; Okruhlicova, L.; Manka, J.; Bernatova, I. Differences in Distribution and Biological Effects of F_3O_4@ PEG Nanoparticles in Normotensive and Hypertensive Rats—Focus on Vascular Function and Liver. *Biomedicines* **2021**, *9*, 1855. [CrossRef] [PubMed]
14. Nowak-Jary, J.; Machnicka, B. Pharmacokinetics of magnetic iron oxide nanoparticles for medical applications. *J. Nanobiotechnol.* **2022**, *20*, 305. [CrossRef] [PubMed]
15. Oh, N.; Park, J.-H. Endocytosis and exocytosis of nanoparticles in mammalian cells. *Int. J. Nanomed.* **2014**, *9*, 51–63. [CrossRef]
16. Drakesmith, H.; Nemeth, E.; Ganz, T. Ironing out ferroportin. *Cell Metab.* **2015**, *22*, 777–787. [CrossRef]
17. Wang, J.; Pantopoulos, K. Regulation of cellular iron metabolism. *Biochem. J.* **2011**, *434*, 365–381. [CrossRef]
18. Kerins, M.J.; Ooi, A. The roles of NRF2 in modulating cellular iron homeostasis. *Antioxid. Redox Signal.* **2018**, *29*, 1756–1773. [CrossRef]
19. Kobayashi, A.; Kang, M.I.; Okawa, H.; Ohtsuji, M.; Zenke, Y.; Chiba, T.; Yamamoto, M. Oxidative stress sensor Keap1 functions as an adaptor for Cul3-based E3 ligase to regulate proteasomal degradation of Nrf2. *Mol. Cell. Biol.* **2004**, *24*, 7130–7139. [CrossRef]
20. Chen, B.; Lu, Y.; Chen, Y.; Cheng, J. The role of Nrf2 in oxidative stress-induced endothelial injuries. *J. Endocrinol.* **2015**, *225*, R83–R99. [CrossRef]
21. Buckley, B.J.; Marshall, Z.M.; Whorton, A.R. Nitric oxide stimulates Nrf2 nuclear translocation in vascular endothelium. *Biochem. Biophys. Res. Commun.* **2003**, *307*, 973–979. [CrossRef] [PubMed]
22. Ishii, T.; Itoh, K.; Yamamoto, M. Roles of Nrf2 in activation of antioxidant enzyme genes via antioxidant responsive elements. In *Methods in Enzymology*; Academic Press: Cambridge, MA, USA, 2002; Volume 348, pp. 182–190.
23. Duarte, T.L.; Talbot, N.P.; Drakesmith, H. NRF2 and hypoxia-inducible factors: Key players in the redox control of systemic iron homeostasis. *Antioxid. Redox Signal.* **2021**, *35*, 433–452. [CrossRef] [PubMed]
24. Lim, P.J.; Duarte, T.L.; Arezes, J.; Garcia-Santos, D.; Hamdi, A.; Pasricha, S.R.; Drakesmith, H. Nrf2 controls iron homoeostasis in haemochromatosis and thalassaemia via Bmp6 and hepcidin. *Nat. Metab.* **2019**, *1*, 519–531. [CrossRef] [PubMed]
25. Yi, J.-H.; Park, S.-W.; Brooks, N.; Lang, B.T.; Vemuganti, R. PPARγ agonist rosiglitazone is neuroprotective after traumatic brain injury via anti-inflammatory and anti-oxidative mechanisms. *Brain Res.* **2008**, *1244*, 164–172. [CrossRef]
26. Kleinhenz, J.M.; Kleinhenz, D.J.; You, S.; Ritzenthaler, J.D.; Hansen, J.M.; Archer, D.R.; Sutliff, R.L.; Hart, C.M. Disruption of endothelial peroxisome proliferator-activated receptor-γ reduces vascular nitric oxide production. *Am. J. Physiol.—Heart Circ. Physiol.* **2009**, *297*, H1647–H1654. [CrossRef]
27. Vandewalle, B.; Moerman, E.; Lefebvre, B.; Defrance, F.; Gmyr, V.; Lukowiak, B.; Conte, J.K.; Pattou, F. PPARγ-dependent and -independent effects of rosiglitazone on lipotoxic human pancreatic islets. *Biochem. Biophys. Res. Commun.* **2008**, *366*, 1096–1101. [CrossRef]
28. Zhu, M.; Chen, H.; Zhou, S.; Zheng, L.; Li, X.; Chu, R.; Chen, W.; Wang, B.; Wang, M.; Chai, Z. Iron oxide nanoparticles aggravate hepatic steatosis and liver injury in nonalcoholic fatty liver disease through BMP-SMAD-mediated hepatic iron overload. *Nanotoxicology* **2021**, *15*, 761–778. [CrossRef]
29. Al_Hussain, R.S.; Al-Qayim, M.A. In Vivo study the effectiveness of novel biogenic Pr-IONPs in rehomeostasis iron mechanisms in Iron deficiency anemia. *J. Pharm. Sci. Res.* **2018**, *10*, 2007–2013.
30. Yang, L.; Kuang, H.; Zhang, W.; Aguilar, Z.P.; Xiong, Y.; Lai, W.; Xu, H.; Wei, H. Size dependent biodistribution and toxicokinetics of iron oxide magnetic nanoparticles in mice. *Nanoscale* **2015**, *7*, 625–636. [CrossRef]
31. Sharifi, S.; Daghighi, S.; Motazacker, M.M.; Badlou, B.; Sanjabi, B.; Akbarkhanzadeh, A.; Rezaee, F. Superparamagnetic iron oxide nanoparticles alter expression of obesity and T2D-associated risk genes in human adipocytes. *Sci. Rep.* **2013**, *3*, 2173. [CrossRef]
32. Líšková, S.; Bališ, P.; Mičurová, A.; Kluknavský, M.; Okuliarová, M.; Puzserová, A.; Škrátek, M.; Sekaj, I.; Maňka, J.; Valovič, P. Effect of iron oxide nanoparticles on vascular function and nitric oxide production in acute stress-exposed rats. *Physiol. Res.* **2020**, *69*, 1067–1083. [CrossRef] [PubMed]

33. Bernátová, I.; Bališ, P.; Goga, R.; Behuliak, M.; Zicha, J.; Sekaj, I. Lack of reactive oxygen species deteriorates blood pressure regulation in acute stress. *Physiol. Res.* **2016**, *65*, S381–S390. [CrossRef] [PubMed]
34. Andrade, R.G.D.; Veloso, S.R.S.; Castanheira, E.M.S. Shape anisotropic iron oxide-based magnetic nanoparticles: Synthesis and biomedical applications. *Int. J. Mol. Sci.* **2020**, *21*, 2455. [CrossRef] [PubMed]
35. Dalzon, B.; Torres, A.; Reymond, S.; Gallet, B.; Saint-Antonin, F.; Collin-Faure, V.; Rabilloud, T. Influences of nanoparticles characteristics on the cellular responses: The example of iron oxide and macrophages. *Nanomaterials* **2020**, *10*, 266. [CrossRef] [PubMed]
36. Lee, G.K.; Maheshri, N.; Kaspar, B.; Schaffer, D.V. PEG conjugation moderately protects adeno-associated viral vectors against antibody neutralization. *Biotechnol. Bioeng.* **2005**, *92*, 24–34. [CrossRef]
37. Suk, J.; Xu, Q.; Kim, N.; Hanes, J.; Ensign, L.; Sciences, H.; Sciences, M. PEGylation as a strategy for improving nanoparticle-based drug and gene delivery. *Adv. Drug Deliv. Rev.* **2016**, *99*, 28–51. [CrossRef]
38. Yoffe, S.; Leshuk, T.; Everett, P.; Gu, F. Superparamagnetic iron oxide nanoparticles (SPIONs): Synthesis and surface modification techniques for use with MRI and other biomedical applications. *Curr. Pharm. Des.* **2013**, *19*, 493–509. [CrossRef]
39. Škrátek, M.; Dvurečenskij, A.; Kluknavský, M.; Barta, A.; Bališ, P.; Mičurová, A.; Cigáň, A.; Eckstein-Andicsová, A.; Maňka, J.; Bernátová, I. Sensitive SQUID bio-magnetometry for determination and differentiation of biogenic iron and iron oxide nanoparticles in the biological samples. *Nanomaterials* **2020**, *10*, 1993. [CrossRef]
40. Radosinska, J.; Jasenovec, T.; Radosinska, D.; Balis, P.; Puzserova, A.; Skratek, M.; Manka, J.; Bernatova, I. Ultra-small superparamagnetic iron-oxide nanoparticles exert different effects on erythrocytes in normotensive and hypertensive rats. *Biomedicines* **2021**, *9*, 377. [CrossRef]
41. Lowry, O.H.; Rosebrough, N.J.; Farr, A.L.; Randall, R.J. Protein measurement with the Folin phenol reagent. *J. Biol. Chem.* **1951**, *193*, 265–275. [CrossRef]
42. Guzik, T.J.; Channon, K.M. Measurement of vascular reactive oxygen species production by chemiluminescence. In *Hypertension*; Springer: Berlin/Heidelberg, Germany, 2005; pp. 73–89. [CrossRef]
43. Slezak, P.; Puzserova, A.; Balis, P.; Sestakova, N.; Majzunova, M.; Dovinova, I.; Kluknavsky, M.; Bernatova, I. Genotype-related effect of crowding stress on blood pressure and vascular function in young female rats. *BioMed Res. Int.* **2014**, *2014*, 413629. [CrossRef] [PubMed]
44. Kumar, P.; Bulk, M.; Webb, A.; van der Weerd, L.; Oosterkamp, T.H.; Huber, M.; Bossoni, L. A novel approach to quantify different iron forms in ex-vivo human brain tissue. *Sci. Rep.* **2016**, *6*, 38916. [CrossRef] [PubMed]
45. Zysler, R.D.; Lima, E., Jr.; Mansilla, M.V.; Troiani, H.E.; Pisciotti, M.; Gurman, P.; Lamagna, A.; Colombo, L. A new quantitative method to determine the uptake of SPIONs in animal tissue and its application to determine the quantity of nanoparticles in the liver and lung of Balb-c mice exposed to the SPIONs. *J. Biomed. Nanotechnol.* **2013**, *9*, 142–145. [CrossRef] [PubMed]
46. Hashimoto, S.; Oda, T.; Yamada, K.; Takagi, M.; Enomoto, T.; Ohkohchi, N.; Takagi, T.; Kanamori, T.; Ikeda, H.; Yanagihara, H. The measurement of small magnetic signals from magnetic nanoparticles attached to the cell surface and surrounding living cells using a general-purpose SQUID magnetometer. *Phys. Med. Biol.* **2009**, *54*, 2571. [CrossRef]
47. Hautot, D.; Pankhurst, Q.A.; Dobson, J. Superconducting quantum interference device measurements of dilute magnetic materials in biological samples. *Rev. Sci. Instrum.* **2005**, *76*, 045101. [CrossRef]
48. Gunn, A.J.; Seethamraju, R.T.; Hedgire, S.; Elmi, A.; Daniels, G.H.; Harisinghani, M.G. Imaging behavior of the normal adrenal on ferumoxytol-enhanced MRI: Preliminary findings. *Am. J. Roentgenol.* **2013**, *201*, 117–121. [CrossRef]
49. Ravingerová, T.; Kindernay, L.; Barteková, M.; Ferko, M.; Adameová, A.; Zohdi, V.; Bernátová, I.; Ferenczyová, K.; Lazou, A. The molecular mechanisms of iron metabolism and its role in cardiac dysfunction and cardioprotection. *Int. J. Mol. Sci.* **2020**, *21*, 7889. [CrossRef]
50. Rishi, G.; Wallace, D.F.; Subramaniam, V.N. Hepcidin: Regulation of the master iron regulator. *Biosci. Rep.* **2015**, *35*, e00192. [CrossRef]
51. Lakhal-Littleton, S.; Wolna, M.; Chung, Y.J.; Christian, H.C.; Heather, L.C.; Brescia, M.; Ball, V.; Diaz, R.; Santos, A.; Biggs, D. An essential cell-autonomous role for hepcidin in cardiac iron homeostasis. *eLife* **2016**, *5*, e19804. [CrossRef]
52. Vela, D. Balance of cardiac and systemic hepcidin and its role in heart physiology and pathology. *Lab. Investig.* **2018**, *98*, 315–326. [CrossRef]
53. Lakhal-Littleton, S.; Wolna, M.; Carr, C.A.; Miller, J.J.; Christian, H.C.; Ball, V.; Santos, A.; Diaz, R.; Biggs, D.; Stillion, R. Cardiac ferroportin regulates cellular iron homeostasis and is important for cardiac function. *Proc. Natl. Acad. Sci. USA* **2015**, *112*, 3164–3169. [CrossRef] [PubMed]
54. Pongrac, I.M.; Pavičić, I.; Milić, M.; Ahmed, L.B.; Babič, M.; Horák, D.; Vrček, I.V.; Gajović, S. Oxidative stress response in neural stem cells exposed to different superparamagnetic iron oxide nanoparticles. *Int. J. Nanomed.* **2016**, *11*, 1701. [CrossRef]
55. Galaris, D.; Barbouti, A.; Pantopoulos, K. Iron homeostasis and oxidative stress: An intimate relationship. *Biochim. Biophys. Acta (BBA)—Mol. Cell Res.* **2019**, *1866*, 118535. [CrossRef] [PubMed]
56. Bresgen, N.; Eckl, P.M. Oxidative stress and the homeodynamics of iron metabolism. *Biomolecules* **2015**, *5*, 808–847. [CrossRef] [PubMed]
57. Pantopoulos, K.; Weiss, G.; Hentze, M.W. Nitric oxide and oxidative stress (H_2O_2) control mammalian iron metabolism by different pathways. *Mol. Cell. Biol.* **1996**, *16*, 3781–3788. [CrossRef]

58. Smiljić, S.; Nestorović, V.; Savić, S. Modulatory role of nitric oxide in cardiac performance. *Med. Pregl.* **2014**, *67*, 345–352. [CrossRef]
59. Bernatova, I. Endothelial dysfunction in experimental models of arterial hypertension: Cause or consequence? *BioMed Res. Int.* **2014**, *2014*, 598271. [CrossRef]
60. Wilkinson, N.; Pantopoulos, K. The IRP/IRE system in vivo: Insights from mouse models. *Front. Pharmacol.* **2014**, *5*, 176. [CrossRef]
61. Lushchak, O.V.; Piroddi, M.; Galli, F.; Lushchak, V.I. Aconitase post-translational modification as a key in linkage between Krebs cycle, iron homeostasis, redox signaling, and metabolism of reactive oxygen species. *Redox Rep.* **2014**, *19*, 8–15. [CrossRef]
62. Zhang, D.-L.; Ghosh, M.C.; Rouault, T.A. The physiological functions of iron regulatory proteins in iron homeostasis-an update. *Front. Pharmacol.* **2014**, *5*, 124. [CrossRef]
63. Kasztura, M.; Kiczak, L.; Pasławska, U.; Bania, J.; Janiszewski, A.; Tomaszek, A.; Zacharski, M.; Noszczyk-Nowak, A.; Pasławski, R.; Tabiś, A. Hemosiderin Accumulation in Liver Decreases Iron Availability in Tachycardia-Induced Porcine Congestive Heart Failure Model. *Int. J. Mol. Sci.* **2022**, *23*, 1026. [CrossRef] [PubMed]

MDPI AG
Grosspeteranlage 5
4052 Basel
Switzerland
Tel.: +41 61 683 77 34

Pharmaceutics Editorial Office
E-mail: pharmaceutics@mdpi.com
www.mdpi.com/journal/pharmaceutics